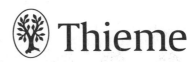

Atlas of Anatomy

Fourth Edition

Edited by

Anne M. Gilroy, MA
Professor Emeritus
Department of Radiology
University of Massachusetts Medical School
Worcester, Massachusetts

Brian R. MacPherson, PhD
Professor and Vice Chair
Department of Neuroscience
University of Kentucky College of Medicine
Lexington, Kentucky

Jamie C. Wikenheiser, PhD
Associate Professor
Department of Anatomy and Neurobiology
UC Irvine School of Medicine
Irvine, California

Based on the work of

Michael Schuenke, MD, PhD
Institute of Anatomy
Christian Albrechts University Kiel
Kiel, Germany

Erik Schulte, MD
Department of Functional and Clinical Anatomy
University Medicine
Johannes Gutenberg University
Mainz, Germany

Udo Schumacher, MD, FRCPath, CBiol, FSB, DSc
Institute of Anatomy and Experimental Morphology
Center for Experimental Medicine
University Cancer Center
University Medical Center Hamburg-Eppendorf
Hamburg, Germany

Illustrations by
Markus Voll
Karl Wesker

2113 illustrations

Thieme

New York · Stuttgart · Delhi · Rio de Janeiro

Table of Contents

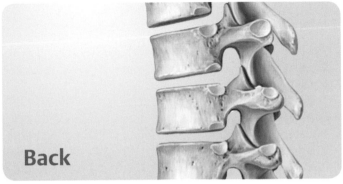

Back

1 Surface Anatomy

2 Bones, Ligaments & Joints

3 Muscles

4 Neurovasculature

5 Sectional & Radiographic Anatomy

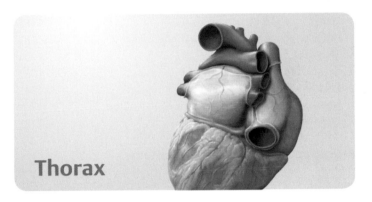

Thorax

6 Surface Anatomy

7 Thoracic Wall

8 Thoracic Cavity

Abdomen

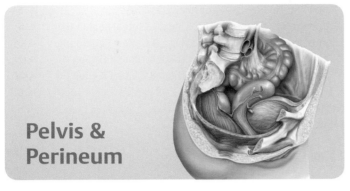

Pelvis & Perineum

Upper Limb

28 Neurovasculature

29 Sectional & Radiographic Anatomy

Lower Limb

30 Surface Anatomy

31 Hip & Thigh

32 Knee & Leg

33 Ankle & Foot

34 Neurovasculature

35 Sectional & Radiographic Anatomy

Head & Neck

36 Surface Anatomy

37 Neck

38 Bones of the Head

39 Muscles of the Skull & Face

40 Cranial Nerves

41 Neurovasculature of the Skull & Face

42 Orbit & Eye

43 Nasal Cavity & Nose

44 Temporal Bone & Ear

45 Oral Cavity & Pharynx

Foreword

This *Atlas of Anatomy*, in my opinion, is the finest single-volume atlas of human anatomy that has ever been created. Two factors make it so: the images and the way they have been organized.

The artists, Markus Voll and Karl Wesker, have created a new standard of excellence in anatomical art. Their graceful use of transparency and their sensitive representation of light and shadow give the reader an accurate three-dimensional understanding of every structure.

The authors have organized the images so that they give just the flow of information a student needs to build up a clear mental image of the human body. Each two-page spread is a self-contained lesson that unobtrusively shows the hand of an experienced and thoughtful teacher. I wish I could have held this book in my hands when I was a student; I envy any student who does so now.

Robert D. Acland, 1941–2016
Louisville, Kentucky   December 2015

Preface

In this new fourth edition of the *Atlas of Anatomy,* we are proud to offer what we believe is our best effort at presenting a clear and accurate story of human anatomy. A significant part of this effort is the addition of our newest co-author, Dr. Jamie C. Wikenheiser from the University of California, Irvine. Jamie's love of anatomy, attention to detail, and proud background in teaching excellence in anatomy at all student levels makes him a highly qualified addition to the editorship of the *Atlas* that will ensure its continued development.

As with previous editions, we have made every attempt to respond to the requests, comments, and critiques of our world-wide users. As always, we recognize that anatomy is a changing science. As concepts and terminology evolve, we feel a responsibility to pass this on and keep these aspects of the *Atlas* updated. Thus, our initial task for this edition was to update and further clarify the material already present in the *Atlas.* Among these modifications was a major revision of the many autonomic innervation wiring schematics. These are now uniformly designed to clearly differentiate between sympathetic and parasympathetic components and pre-and post-ganglionic fibers. We improved many tables by reorganizing and rewording the content and enlarging labels. Sectional and radiographic chapters in each unit, established in the third edition, have been expanded with more than forty additional MR and CT images, now accompanied, as are all sectional images throughout the *Atlas,* by new simplified navigators.

Another focus of this edition was to provide more written and schematic-based information that addresses complex anatomic concepts. This includes new schematics that complement other images, expanded legends that accompany images, and most notably, the addition of almost thirty new clinical boxes (most with illustrations) in every unit. These focus on function, pathology, anatomic variations, clinical procedures, diagnostic techniques, embryological development, and aging.

We continue to try to make difficult areas of anatomy more easily understood through better organization of chapter content and new diagrammatic approaches. The two-page spread that has been so popular in previous editions has been maintained in this edition, but an effort was made to improve their layouts by tabulating some content and adding more than 120 new illustrations and images. In this edition, the reader will notice major changes in two regions. In the abdomen and pelvic units, a greater focus is placed on the peritoneum, mesenteries, and peritoneal spaces. The inguinal region, a difficult area for students, is also expanded with new images and tables, as well as new and revised images of perineal structures. The head and neck unit is the second area of major revisions. In an effort to bring this material into alignment with the way it is usually encountered in the dissection lab, the chapter on the neck now precedes those on the head and includes new artwork that promotes the dissection views. Students will appreciate the reorganization and additional clarifying images of areas such as the cavernous sinus, pterygopalatine and infratemporal fossae, and oral and nasal cavities. Finally, a new expanded overview introduces the brain and nervous system chapter.

As always, we are extremely grateful for the contributions of the many colleagues and reviewers who provide important feedback on earlier editions, alert us to inaccuracies and ambiguities, and share suggestions for new material.

We recognize that our efforts, though important, are just one part of the process that brings this textbook to its final production. The entire Thieme Publishers team has encouraged and supported our efforts throughout this process. Our deep appreciation is extended to the most important contributors: Judith Tomat, Developmental Editor; Delia DeTurris, Acquisitions Editor, and Barbara Chernow, PhD, Production Manager, for their dedication and expertise in their respective fields and their confidence in our ability to produce a quality manuscript.

Anne M. Gilroy
Worcester, Massachusetts

Brian R. MacPherson
Lexington, Kentucky

Jamie C. Wikenheiser
Irvine, California

December 2019

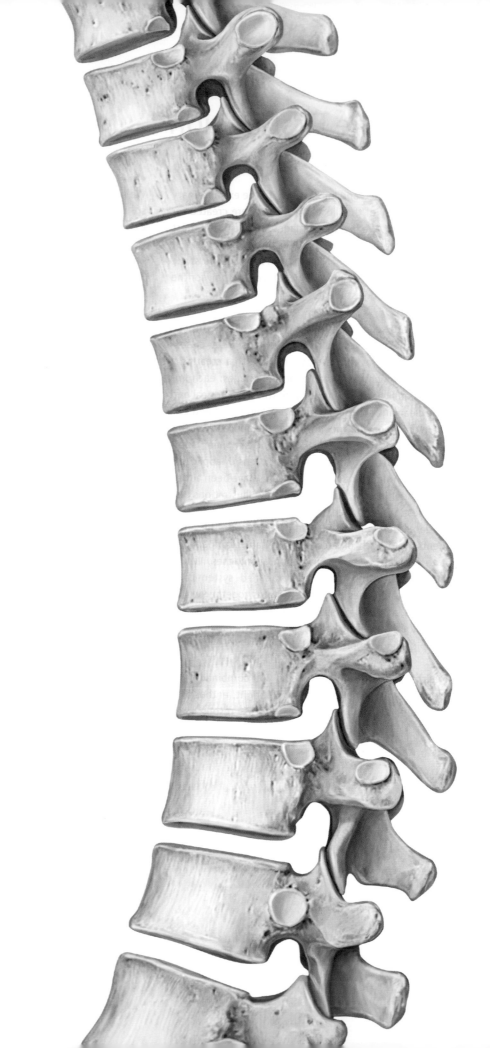

Back

1 Surface Anatomy

2 Bones, Ligaments & Joints

3 Muscles

4 Neurovasculature

5 Sectional & Radiographic Anatomy

2 Bones, Ligaments & Joints
Vertebral Column: Overview

The vertebral column (spine) is divided into four regions: the cervical, thoracic, lumbar, and sacral spines. Both the cervical and lumbar spines demonstrate lordosis (inward curvature); the thoracic and sacral spines demonstrate kyphosis (outward curvature).

Fig. 2.1 **Vertebral column**
Left lateral view.

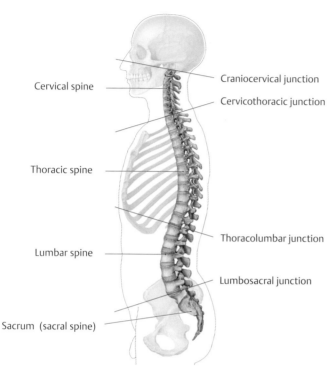

A Regions of the spine.

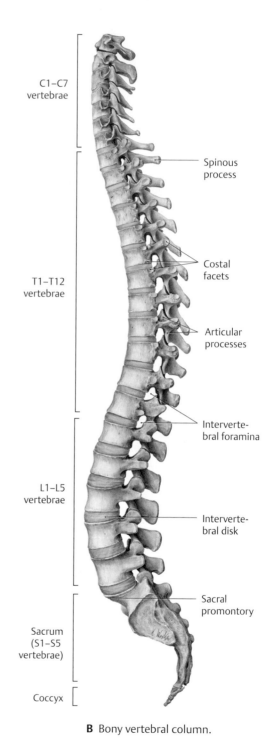

B Bony vertebral column.

Clinical box 2.1

Spinal development
The characteristic curvatures of the adult spine appear over the course of postnatal development, being only partially present in a newborn. The newborn has a "kyphotic" spinal curvature (**A**); lumbar lordosis develops later and becomes stable at puberty (**C**).

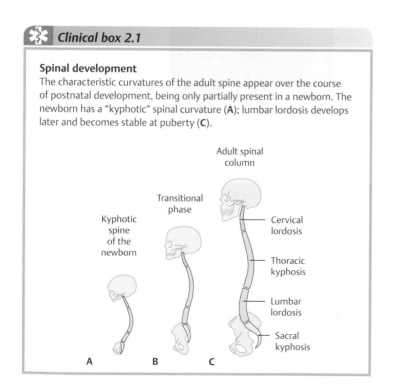

Fig. 2.2 **Normal anatomical position of the spine**
Left lateral view.

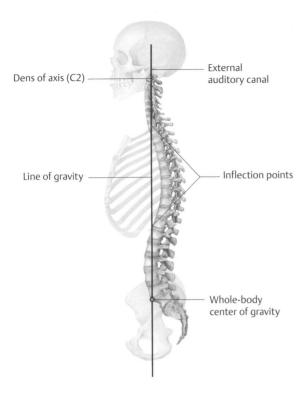

A Line of gravity. The line of gravity passes through certain anatomical landmarks, including the inflection points at the cervicothoracic and thoracolumbar junctions. It continues through the center of gravity (anterior to the sacral promontory) before passing through the hip joint, knee, and ankle.

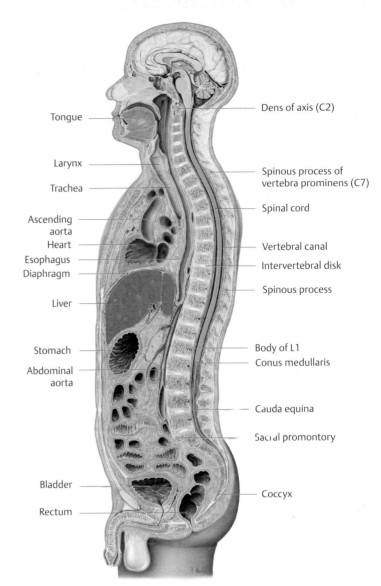

B Midsagittal section through an adult male.

Abnormal Vertebral Column Curvatures

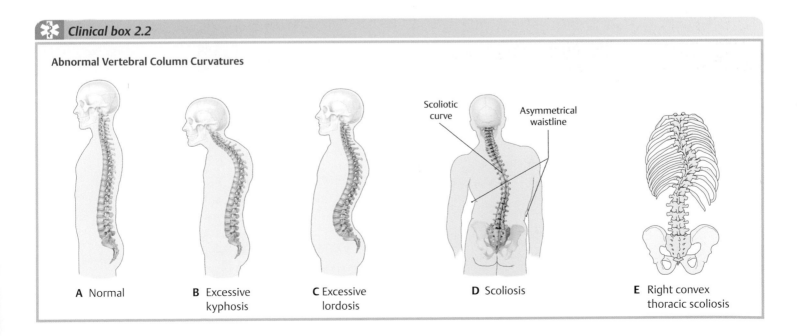

A Normal **B** Excessive kyphosis **C** Excessive lordosis **D** Scoliosis **E** Right convex thoracic scoliosis

Vertebral Column: Elements

Fig. 2.3 **Bones of the vertebral column**

The transverse processes of the lumbar vertebrae are originally rib rudiments and so are named costal processes.

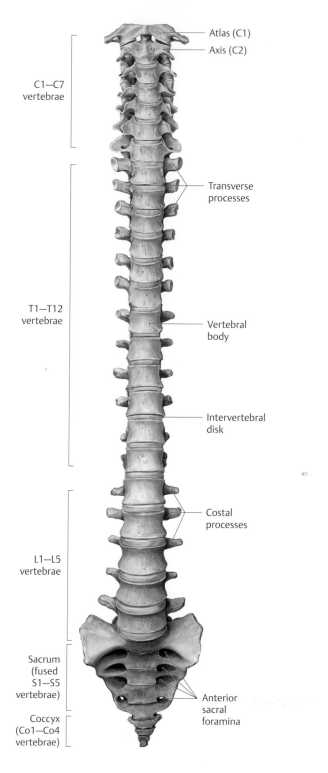

A Anterior view.

B Posterior view.

Fig. 2.4 Structural elements of a vertebra

Left posterosuperior view. With the exception of the atlas (C1) and axis (C2), all vertebrae consist of the same structural elements.

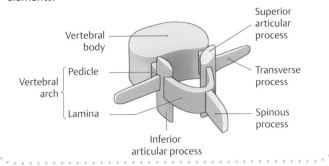

Fig. 2.5 Typical vertebrae

Superior view.

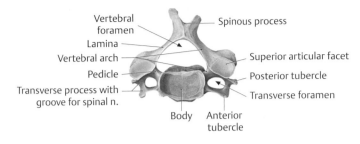

A Cervical vertebra (C4).

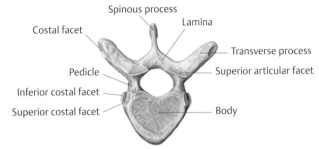

B Thoracic vertebra (T6).

C Lumbar vertebra (L4).

D Sacrum.

Table 2.1		Structural elements of vertebrae			
Vertebrae	**Body**	**Vertebral foramen**	**Transverse processes**	**Articular processes**	**Spinous process**
Cervical vertebrae C3*–C7	Small (kidney-shaped)	Large (triangular)	Small (may be absent on C7); anterior and posterior tubercles enclose transverse foramen	Superoposteriorly and inferoanteriorly; oblique facets: most nearly horizontal	Short (C3–C5); bifid (C3–C6); long (C7)
Thoracic vertebrae T1–T12	Medium (heart-shaped); includes costal facets	Small (circular)	Large and strong; length decreases T1–T12; costal facets (T1–T10)	Posteriorly (slightly laterally) and anteriorly (slightly medially); facets in coronal plane	Long, sloping postero-inferiorly; tip extends to level of vertebral body below
Lumbar vertebrae L1–L5	Large (kidney-shaped)	Medium (triangular)	Called costal processes, long and slender; accessory process on posterior surface	Posteromedially (or medially) and anterolaterally (or laterally); facets nearly in sagittal plane; mammillary process on posterior surface of each superior articular process	Short and broad
Sacral vertebrae (sacrum) S1–S5 (fused)	Decreases from base to apex	Sacral canal	Fused to rudimentary rib (ribs, see **pp. 56–59**)	Superoposteriorly (SI) superior surface of lateral sacrum-auricular surface	Median sacral crest

*C1 (atlas) and C2 (axis) are considered atypical (see **pp. 8–9**).

Cervical Vertebrae

The seven vertebrae of the cervical spine differ most conspicuously from the common vertebral morphology. They are specialized to bear the weight of the head and allow the neck to move in all directions.

C1 and C2 are known as the atlas and axis, respectively. C7 is called the vertebra prominens for its long, palpable spinous process.

Fig. 2.6 Cervical spine
Left lateral view.

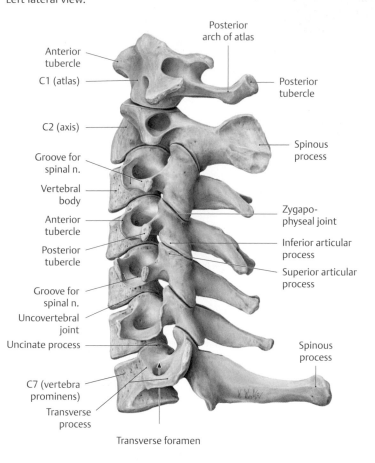

A Bones of the cervical spine, left lateral view.

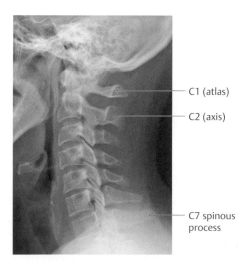

B Radiograph of the cervical spine, left lateral view.

Fig. 2.7 Atlas (C1)

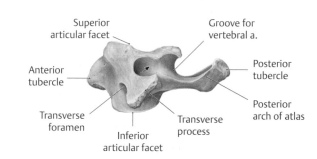

A Left lateral view.

Fig. 2.8 Axis (C2)

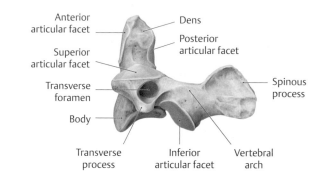

A Left lateral view.

Fig. 2.9 Typical cervical vertebra (C4)

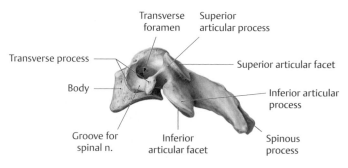

A Left lateral view.

Clinical box 2.3

Injuries in the cervical spine
The cervical spine is prone to hyperextension injuries, such as "whiplash," which can occur when the head extends back much farther than it normally would. The most common injuries of the cervical spine are fractures of the dens of the axis, traumatic spondylolisthesis (anterior slippage of a vertebral body), and atlas fractures. Patient prognosis is largely dependent on the spinal level of the injuries (see p. 42).

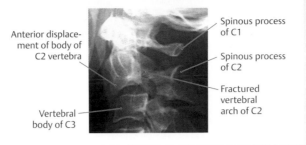

Anterior displacement of body of C2 vertebra

Spinous process of C1

Spinous process of C2

Fractured vertebral arch of C2

Vertebral body of C3

This patient hit the dashboard of his car while not wearing a seat belt. The resulting hyperextension caused the traumatic spondylolisthesis of C2 (axis) with fracture of the vertebral arch of C2, as well as tearing of the ligaments between C2 and C3. This injury is often referred to as "hangman's fracture."

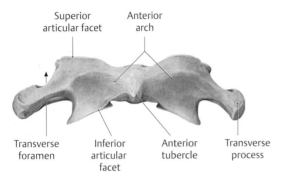

Superior articular facet

Anterior arch

Transverse foramen

Inferior articular facet

Anterior tubercle

Transverse process

B Anterior view.

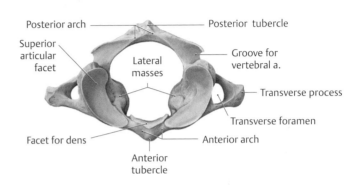

Posterior arch

Posterior tubercle

Superior articular facet

Lateral masses

Groove for vertebral a.

Transverse process

Transverse foramen

Facet for dens

Anterior arch

Anterior tubercle

C Superior view.

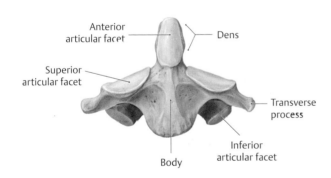

Anterior articular facet

Dens

Superior articular facet

Transverse process

Inferior articular facet

Body

B Anterior view.

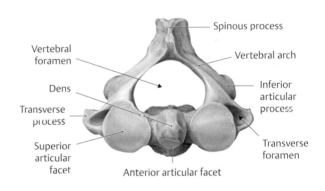

Vertebral foramen

Spinous process

Vertebral arch

Dens

Inferior articular process

Transverse process

Superior articular facet

Anterior articular facet

Transverse foramen

C Superior view.

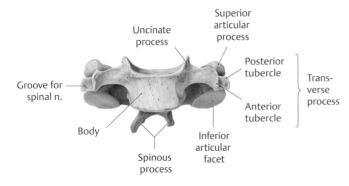

Uncinate process

Superior articular process

Posterior tubercle

Groove for spinal n.

Transverse process

Anterior tubercle

Body

Inferior articular facet

Spinous process

B Anterior view.

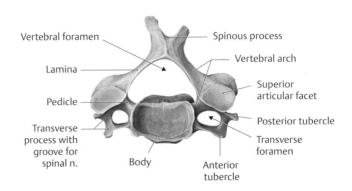

Vertebral foramen

Spinous process

Lamina

Vertebral arch

Pedicle

Superior articular facet

Transverse process with groove for spinal n.

Posterior tubercle

Transverse foramen

Body

Anterior tubercle

C Superior view.

Thoracic & Lumbar Vertebrae

Fig. 2.10 **Thoracic spine**
Left lateral view.

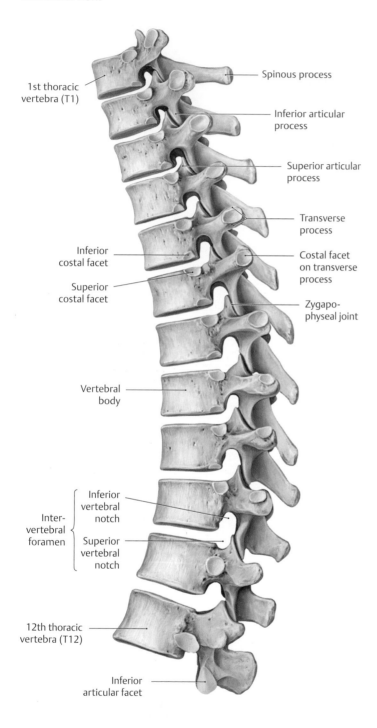

1st thoracic vertebra (T1)

Spinous process

Inferior articular process

Superior articular process

Transverse process

Inferior costal facet

Costal facet on transverse process

Superior costal facet

Zygapophyseal joint

Vertebral body

Inferior vertebral notch

Inter-vertebral foramen

Superior vertebral notch

12th thoracic vertebra (T12)

Inferior articular facet

Fig. 2.11 **Typical thoracic vertebra (T6)**

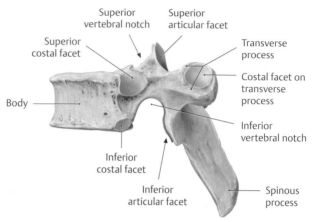

Superior vertebral notch

Superior articular facet

Superior costal facet

Transverse process

Costal facet on transverse process

Body

Inferior vertebral notch

Inferior costal facet

Inferior articular facet

Spinous process

A Left lateral view.

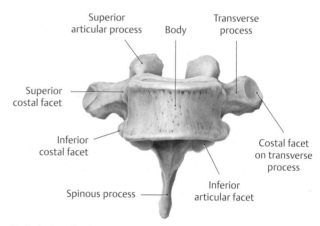

Superior articular process

Body

Transverse process

Superior costal facet

Inferior costal facet

Costal facet on transverse process

Spinous process

Inferior articular facet

B Anterior view.

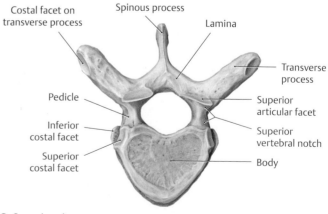

Costal facet on transverse process

Spinous process

Lamina

Transverse process

Pedicle

Superior articular facet

Inferior costal facet

Superior vertebral notch

Superior costal facet

Body

C Superior view.

Fig. 2.12 Lumbar spine

Left lateral view.

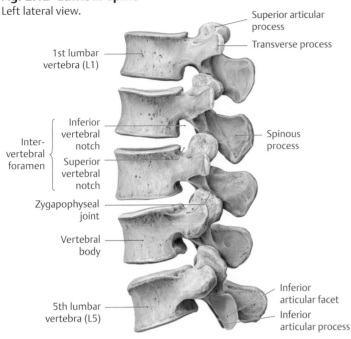

- 1st lumbar vertebra (L1)
- Inter-vertebral foramen
  - Inferior vertebral notch
  - Superior vertebral notch
- Zygapophyseal joint
- Vertebral body
- 5th lumbar vertebra (L5)
- Superior articular process
- Transverse process
- Spinous process
- Inferior articular facet
- Inferior articular process

Fig. 2.13 Typical lumbar vertebra (L4)

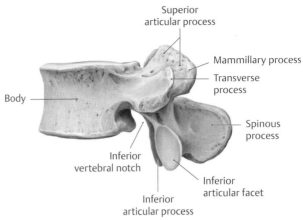

- Body
- Superior articular process
- Mammillary process
- Transverse process
- Spinous process
- Inferior vertebral notch
- Inferior articular facet
- Inferior articular process

A Left lateral view.

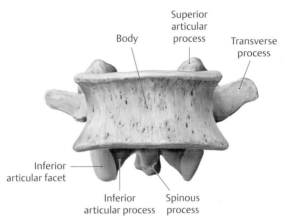

- Body
- Superior articular process
- Transverse process
- Inferior articular facet
- Inferior articular process
- Spinous process

B Anterior view.

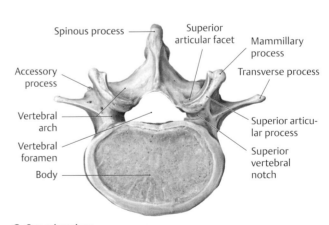

- Spinous process
- Superior articular facet
- Mammillary process
- Accessory process
- Transverse process
- Vertebral arch
- Superior articular process
- Vertebral foramen
- Superior vertebral notch
- Body

C Superior view.

Clinical box 2.4

Osteoporosis

The spine is the structure most affected by degenerative diseases of the skeleton, such as arthrosis and osteoporosis. In osteoporosis, more bone material gets reabsorbed than built up, resulting in a loss of bone mass. Symptoms include compression fractures and resulting back pain.

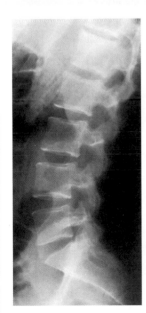

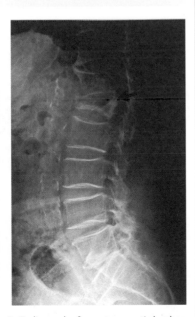

A Radiograph of a normal lumbar spine, left lateral view. (Reproduced from Moeller TB, Reif E. Pocket Atlas of Radiographic Anatomy, 3rd ed. New York, NY: Thieme; 2010.)

B Radiograph of an osteoporotic lumbar spine with a compression fracture at L1 (*arrow*). Note that the vertebral bodies are decreased in density, and the internal trabecular structure is coarse. (Reproduced from Jallo J, Vaccaro AR. Neurotrauma and Critical Care of the Spine, 1st ed. New York, NY: Thieme; 2009.)

Sacrum & Coccyx

The sacrum is formed from five postnatally fused sacral vertebrae. The base of the sacrum articulates with the 5th lumbar vertebra, and the apex articulates with the coccyx, a series of three or four rudimentary vertebrae. See **Fig. 19.1, p. 230.**

Fig. 2.14 **Sacrum and coccyx**

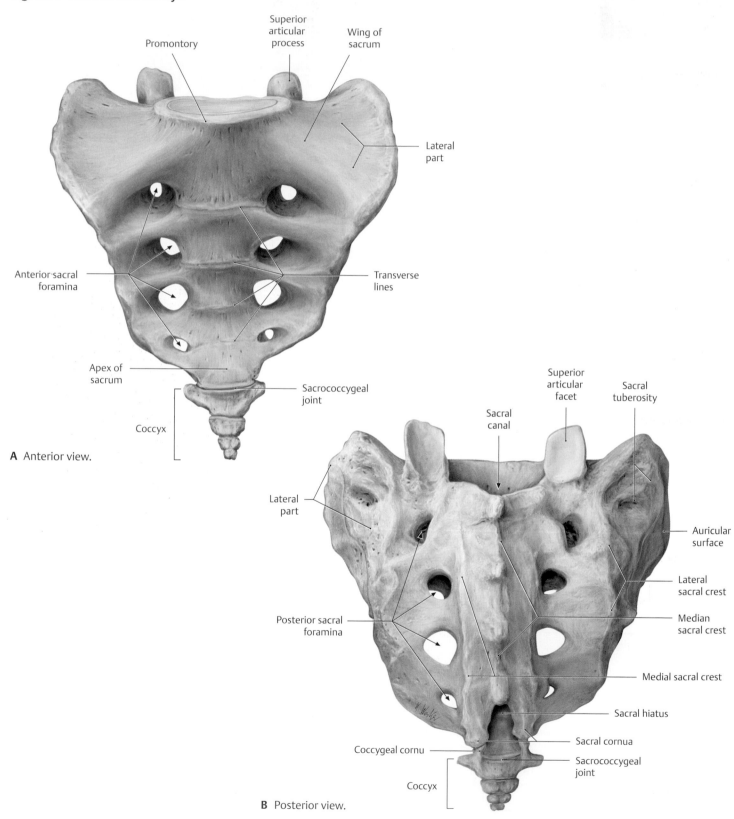

A Anterior view.

B Posterior view.

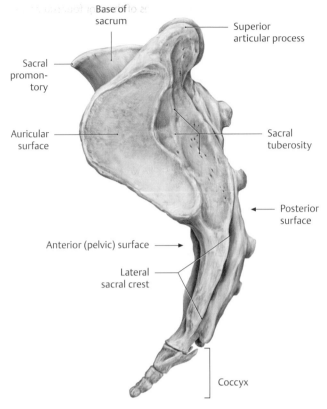

C Left lateral view.

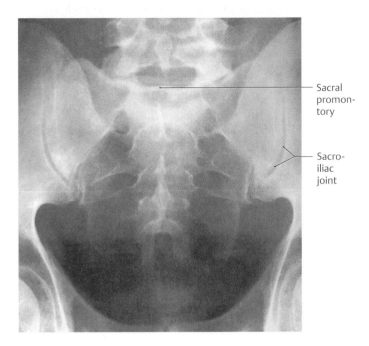

D Radiograph of sacrum, anteroposterior view. (Reproduced from Moeller TB, Reif E. Pocket Atlas of Radiographic Anatomy, 3rd ed. New York, NY: Thieme; 2010.)

Fig. 2.15 Sacrum
Superior view.

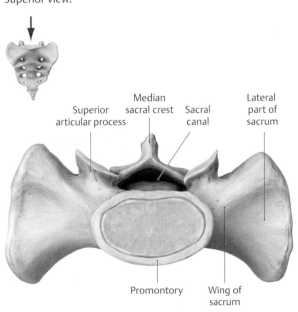

A Base of sacrum, superior view.

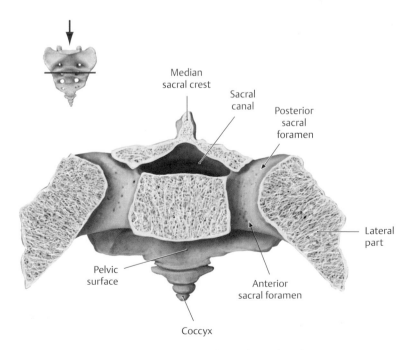

B Transverse section through second sacral vertebra demonstrating anterior and posterior sacral foramina, superior view.

Intervertebral Disks

Midsagittal section of T11–T12, left lateral view. The intervertebral disks occupy the spaces between vertebrae (intervertebral joints, see **p. 16**).

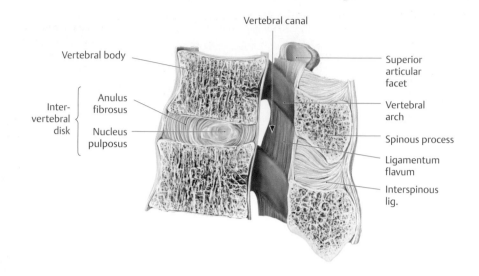

Fig. 2.17 Structure of intervertebral disk
Anterosuperior view with the anterior half of the disk and the right half of the end plate removed. The intervertebral disk consists of an external fibrous ring (anulus fibrosus) and a gelatinous core (nucleus pulposus).

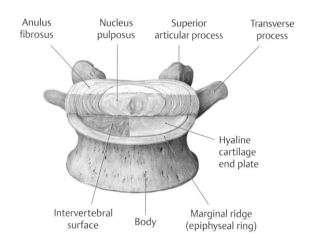

Fig. 2.18 Relation of intervertebral disk to vertebral canal
Fourth lumbar vertebra, superior view.

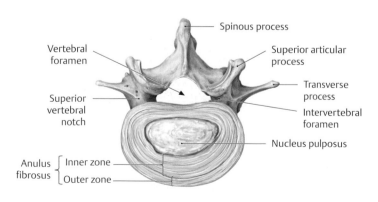

Fig. 2.19 Outer zone of the annulus fibrosus
Anterior view of L3–L4 with intervertebral disk.

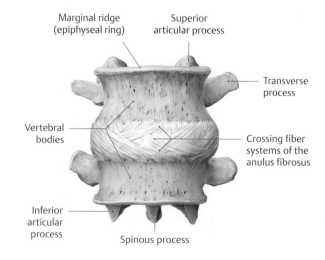

Disk herniation in the lumbar spine

As the stress resistance of the anulus fibrosus declines with age, the tissue of the nucleus pulposus may protrude through weak spots under loading. If the fibrous ring of the anulus ruptures completely, the herniated material may compress the contents of the intervertebral foramen (nerve roots and blood vessels—see posterolateral herniation below). These patients often suffer from severe local back pain. Pain is also felt in the associated dermatome (see **p. 42**). When the motor part of the spinal nerve is affected, the muscles served by that spinal nerve will show weakening. It is an important diagnostic step to test the muscles innervated by a nerve from a certain spinal segment, as well as the sensitivity in the specific dermatome. Example: The first sacral nerve root innervates the gastrocnemius and soleus muscles; thus, standing or walking on toes can be affected (see **p. 446**).

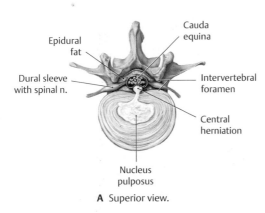

A Superior view.

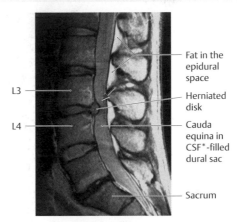

B Midsagittal T2-weighted MRI (magnetic resonance image).

Posterior herniation (A, B) In the MRI, a conspicuously herniated disk at the level of L3–L4 protrudes posteriorly (transligamentous herniation). The dural sac is deeply indented at that level. *CSF (cerebrospinal fluid).

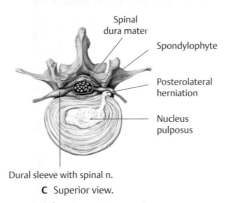

C Superior view.

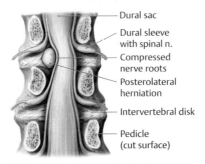

D Posterior view, vertebral arches removed.

Posterolateral herniation (C, D) A posterolateral herniation may compress the spinal nerve as it passes through the intervertebral foramen. If more medially positioned, the herniation may spare the nerve at that level but impact nerves at inferior levels.

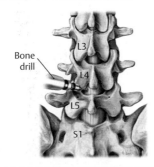

E

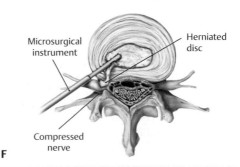

F

Microdiscectomy surgery (**E, F**) is performed in order to remove a portion of a herniated disc that is irritating the nerve root. Through a small incision, the erector spinae muscles are reflected laterally to expose the ligamentum flavum, which is then removed in order to access the nerve roots in the spinal canal. A small portion of the facet joint may be removed to both facilitate access and relieve pressure on the nerve roots. Only the herniated portion of the disk is removed with the remaining tissue left intact.

Joints of the Vertebral Column: Overview

Table 2.2	Joints of the vertebral column	
Craniovertebral joints		
①	Atlanto-occipital joints	Occiput–C1
②	Atlantoaxial joints	C1–C2
Joints of the vertebral bodies		
③	Uncovertebral joints	C3–C7
④	Intervertebral joints	C2–S1
Joints of the vertebral arch		
⑤	Zygapophyseal joints	C2–S1

Fig. 2.20 Zygapophyseal (intervertebral facet) joints

The orientation of the zygapophyseal joints differs between the spinal regions, influencing the degree and direction of movement.

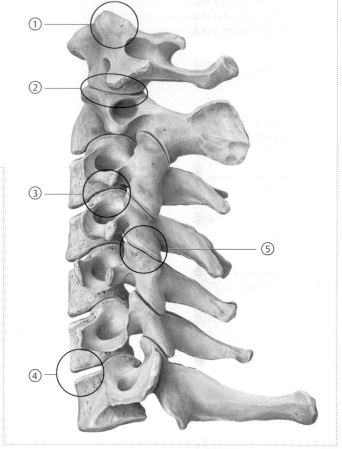

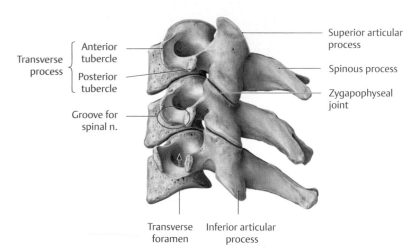

A Cervical region, left lateral view. The zygapophyseal joints lie 45 degrees from the horizontal.

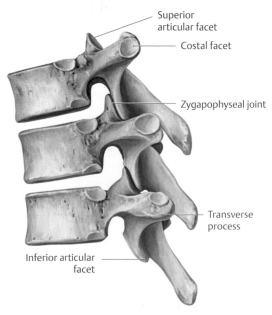

B Thoracic region, left lateral view. The joints lie in the coronal plane.

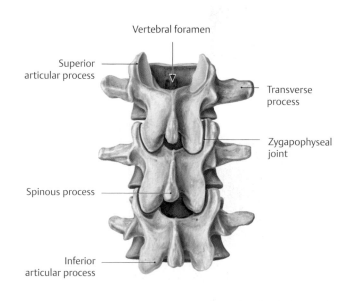

C Lumbar region, posterior view. The joints lie in the sagittal plane.

Fig. 2.21 Uncovertebral joints

Anterior view. Uncovertebral joints form during childhood between the uncinate processes of C3–C7 and the vertebral bodies immediately superior. The joints may result from fissures in the cartilage of the disks that assume an articular character. If the fissures become complete tears, the risk of nucleus pulposus herniation is increased (see **p. 15**).

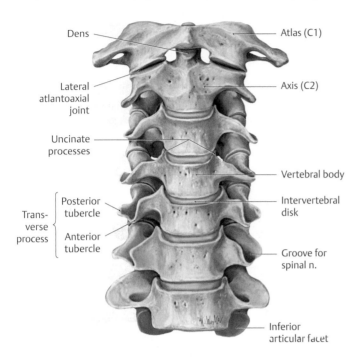

A Uncovertebral joints in the cervical spine of an 18-year-old man, anterior view.

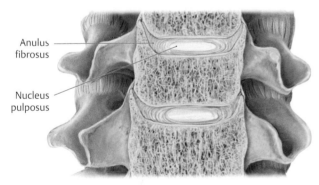

B Uncovertebral joint (enlarged), anterior view of coronal section.

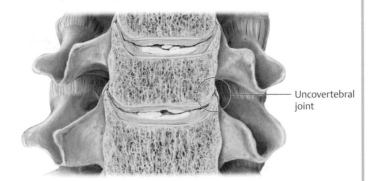

C Uncovertebral joints, split intervertebral disks, anterior view of coronal section.

Clinical box 2.6

Proximity of the spinal nerve and vertebral artery to the uncinate process

The spinal nerve and vertebral artery pass through the intervertebral and transverse foramina, respectively (**A** and **B**). Bony outgrowths (osteophytes) on the uncinate process (**C**) resulting from uncovertebral arthrosis (degeneration) may compress both the nerve and the artery and can lead to chronic pain in the cervical region.

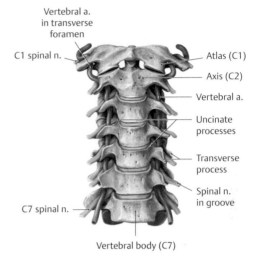

A Cervical spine, anterior view.

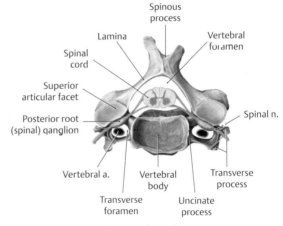

B Fourth cervical vertebra, superior view.

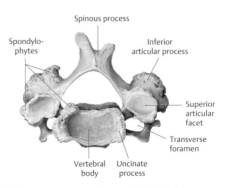

C Advanced uncovertebral arthrosis of the fourth cervical vertebra, superior view.

Joints of the Vertebral Column: Craniovertebral Region

Fig. 2.22 **Craniovertebral joints**

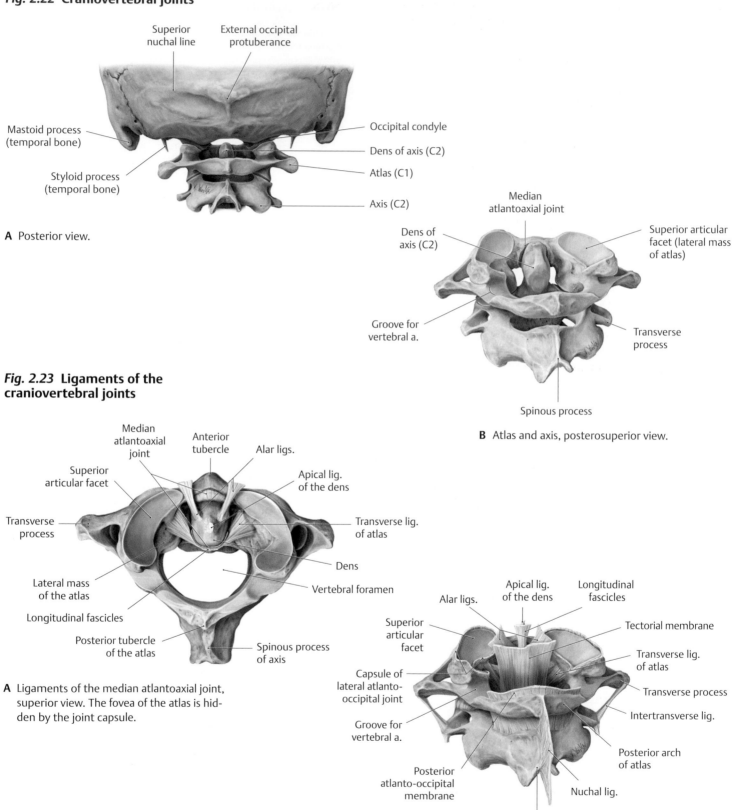

A Posterior view.

B Atlas and axis, posterosuperior view.

Fig. 2.23 **Ligaments of the craniovertebral joints**

A Ligaments of the median atlantoaxial joint, superior view. The fovea of the atlas is hidden by the joint capsule.

B Ligaments of the craniovertebral joints, posterosuperior view. The dens of the axis is hidden by the tectorial membrane.

The atlanto-occipital joints are the two articulations between the convex occipital condyles of the occipital bone and the slightly concave superior articular facets of the atlas (C1). The atlantoaxial joints are the two lateral and one medial articulations between the atlas (C1) and axis (C2).

Fig. 2.24 Dissection of the craniovertebral joint ligaments

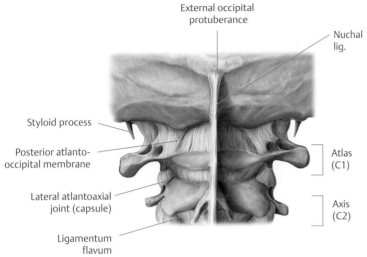

A Nuchal ligament and posterior atlanto-occipital membrane.

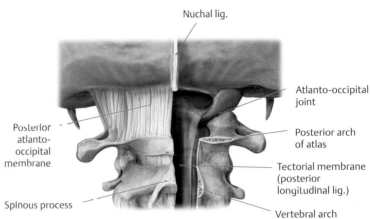

B Posterior longitudinal ligament. *Removed:* Spinal cord; vertebral canal windowed.

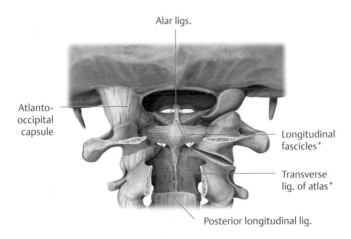

C Cruciform ligament of atlas (*). *Removed:* Tectorial membrane, posterior atlanto-occipital membrane, and vertebral arches.

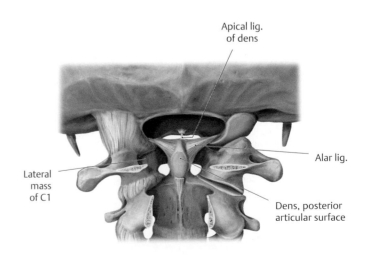

D Alar and apical ligaments. *Removed:* Transverse ligament of atlas.

Vertebral Ligaments: Overview & Cervical Spine

The ligaments of the spinal column bind the vertebrae and enable the spine to withstand high mechanical loads and shearing stresses and limit the range of motion. The ligaments are subdivided into vertebral body ligaments and vertebral arch ligaments.

Fig. 2.25 Vertebral ligaments
Viewed obliquely from the left posterior view.

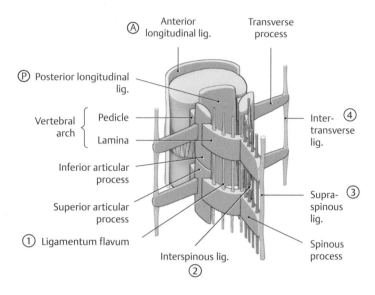

Table 2.3	Vertebral ligaments	
Ligament		**Location**
Vertebral body ligaments		
Ⓐ	Anterior longitudinal lig.	Along anterior surface of vertebral body
Ⓟ	Posterior longitudinal lig.	Along posterior surface of vertebral body
Vertebral arch ligaments		
①	Ligamentum flavum	Between laminae
②	Interspinous lig.	Between spinous process
③	Supraspinous lig.	Along posterior ridge of spinous processes
④	Intertransverse lig.	Between transverse processes
	Nuchal lig.*	Between external occipital protuberance and spinous process of C7

*Corresponds to a supraspinous ligament that is broadened superiorly.

Fig. 2.26 Anterior longitudinal ligament
Anterior view with base of skull removed.

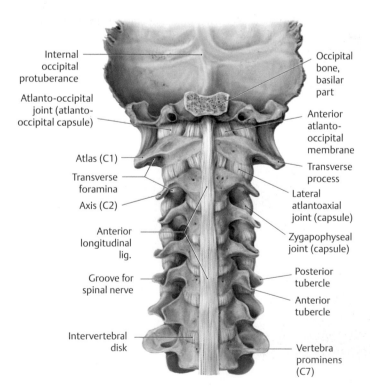

Fig. 2.27 Posterior longitudinal ligament
Posterior view with vertebral canal opened via laminectomy and spinal cord removed. The tectorial membrane is a broadened expansion of the posterior longitudinal ligament.

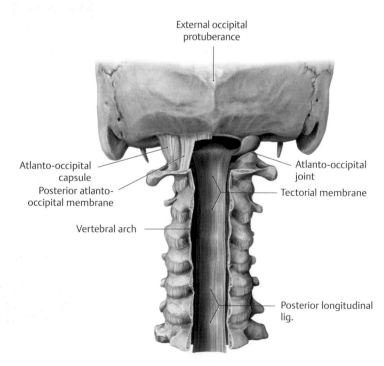

Fig. 2.28 Ligaments of the cervical spine

Mid-sagittal view.

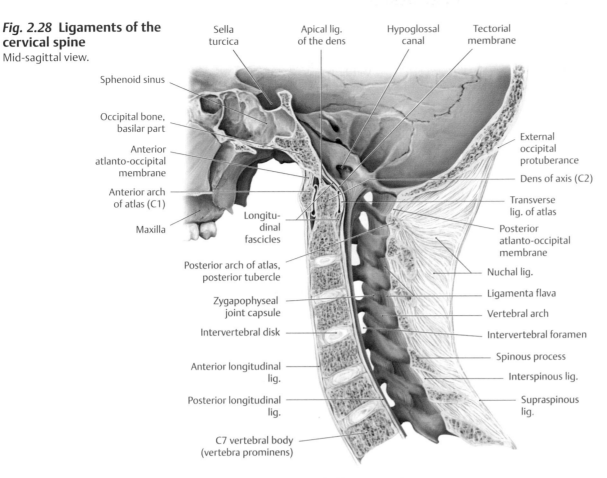

Sella turcica
Apical lig. of the dens
Hypoglossal canal
Tectorial membrane
Sphenoid sinus
Occipital bone, basilar part
Anterior atlanto-occipital membrane
Anterior arch of atlas (C1)
Maxilla
Longitudinal fascicles
Posterior arch of atlas, posterior tubercle
Zygapophyseal joint capsule
Intervertebral disk
Anterior longitudinal lig.
Posterior longitudinal lig.
C7 vertebral body (vertebra prominens)
External occipital protuberance
Dens of axis (C2)
Transverse lig. of atlas
Posterior atlanto-occipital membrane
Nuchal lig.
Ligamenta flava
Vertebral arch
Intervertebral foramen
Spinous process
Interspinous lig.
Supraspinous lig.

A Midsagittal section, left lateral view. The nuchal ligament is the broadened, sagittally oriented part of the supraspinous ligament that extends from the vertebra prominens (C7) to the external occipital protuberance.

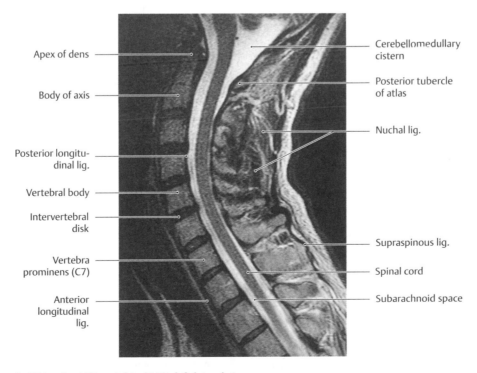

Apex of dens
Body of axis
Posterior longitudinal lig.
Vertebral body
Intervertebral disk
Vertebra prominens (C7)
Anterior longitudinal lig.
Cerebellomedullary cistern
Posterior tubercle of atlas
Nuchal lig.
Supraspinous lig.
Spinal cord
Subarachnoid space

B Midsagittal T2-weighted MRI, left lateral view.

3 Muscles

Muscles of the Back: Overview

The muscles of the back are divided into two groups, the extrinsic and the intrinsic muscles, which are separated by the posterior layer of the thoracolumbar fascia. The superficial extrinsic muscles are considered muscles of the upper limb that have migrated to the back; these muscles are discussed in the Upper Limb, **pp. 312–317.**

Fig. 3.1 **Superficial extrinsic muscles of the back**
Posterior view. *Removed:* Trapezius and latissimus dorsi (right). *Revealed:* Thoracolumbar fascia. *Note:* The posterior layer of the thoracolumbar fascia is reinforced by the aponeurotic origin of the latissimus dorsi.

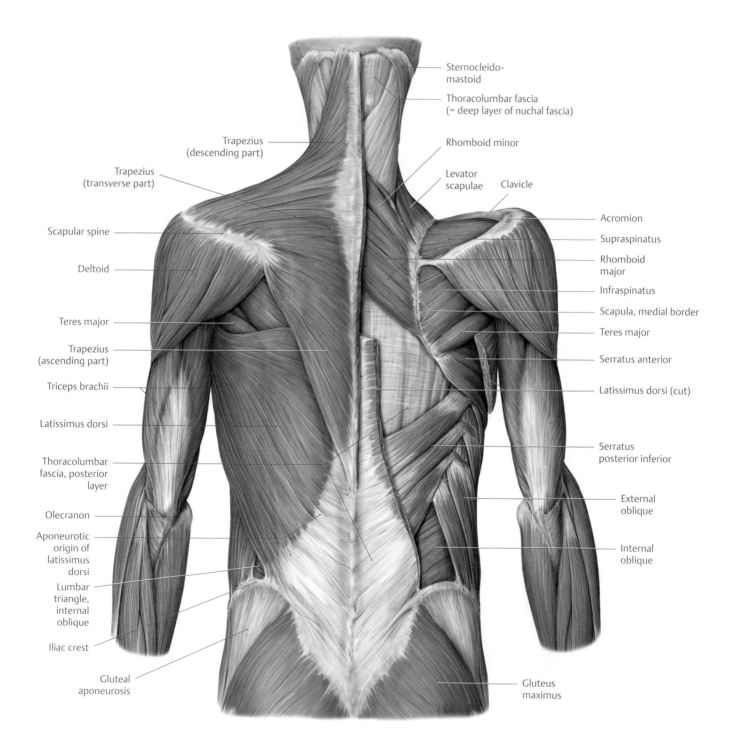

Fig. 3.2 **Thoracolumbar fascia**

Transverse section, superior view. The intrinsic back muscles are sequestered in an osseofibrous canal, formed by the thoracolumbar fascia, the vertebral arches, and the spinous and transverse processes of associated vertebrae. The thoracolumbar fascia consists of a posterior and middle layer that unite at the lateral margin of the intrinsic back muscles. In the neck, the posterior layer blends with the nuchal fascia (deep layer), becoming continuous with the deep cervical fascia (prevertebral layer).

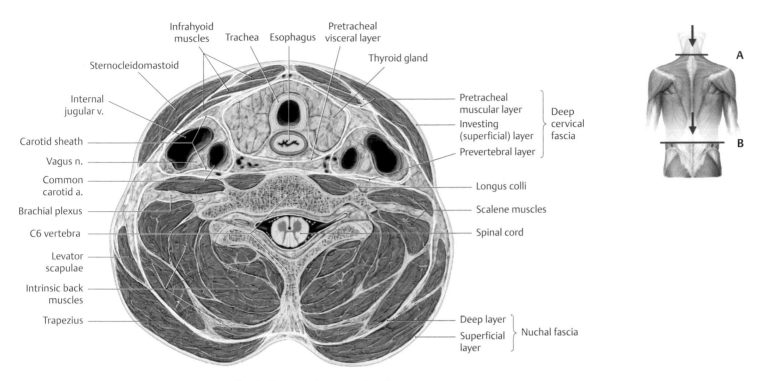

A Transverse section at level of C6 vertebra, superior view.

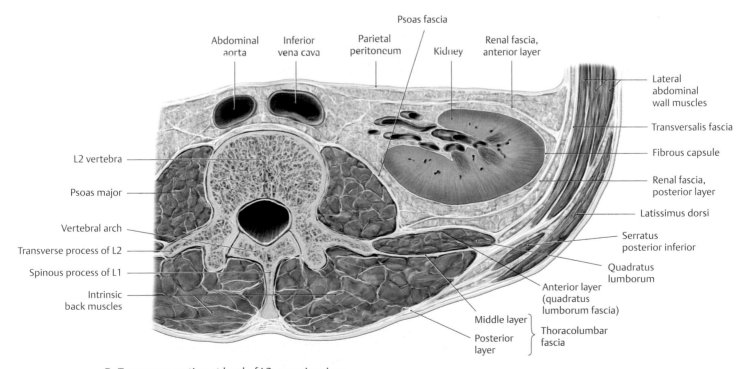

B Transverse section at level of L2, superior view.
Removed: Cauda equina and anterior trunk wall.

25

Intrinsic Muscles of the Back

The extrinsic muscles of the back (trapezius, latissimus dorsi, levator scapulae, and rhomboids) are discussed in the Upper Limb, **pp. 312–313.** The serratus posterior, considered an intermediate extrinsic back muscle, has been included with the superficial intrinsic muscles in this unit.

Fig. 3.5 **Intrinsic muscles of the back**

Posterior view. Sequential dissection of the thoracolumbar fascia, superficial intrinsic muscles, intermediate intrinsic muscles, and deep intrinsic muscles of the back.

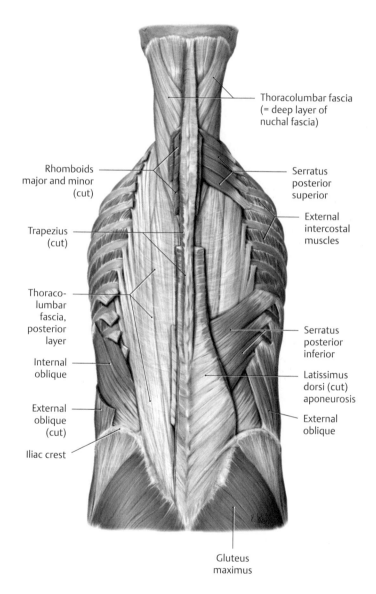

Thoracolumbar fascia (= deep layer of nuchal fascia)

Rhomboids major and minor (cut)

Serratus posterior superior

Trapezius (cut)

External intercostal muscles

Thoraco-lumbar fascia, posterior layer

Serratus posterior inferior

Internal oblique

Latissimus dorsi (cut) aponeurosis

External oblique (cut)

External oblique

Iliac crest

Gluteus maximus

A Thoracolumbar fascia. *Removed:* Shoulder girdles and extrinsic back muscles (except serratus posterior and aponeurotic origin of latissimus dorsi). *Revealed:* Posterior layer of thoracolumbar fascia.

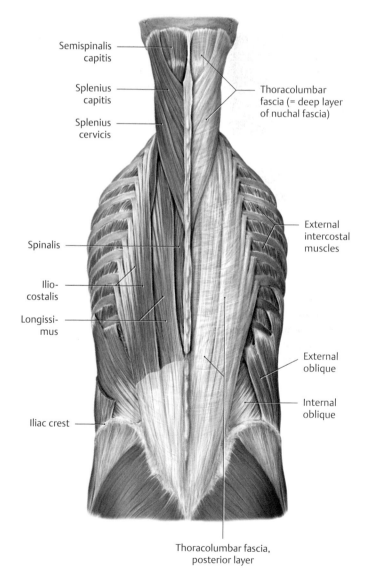

Semispinalis capitis

Splenius capitis

Thoracolumbar fascia (= deep layer of nuchal fascia)

Splenius cervicis

Spinalis

External intercostal muscles

Ilio-costalis

Longissi-mus

External oblique

Internal oblique

Iliac crest

Thoracolumbar fascia, posterior layer

B Superficial and intermediate intrinsic back muscles. *Removed:* Thoracolumbar fascia, posterior layer (left). *Revealed:* Erector spinae and splenius muscles.

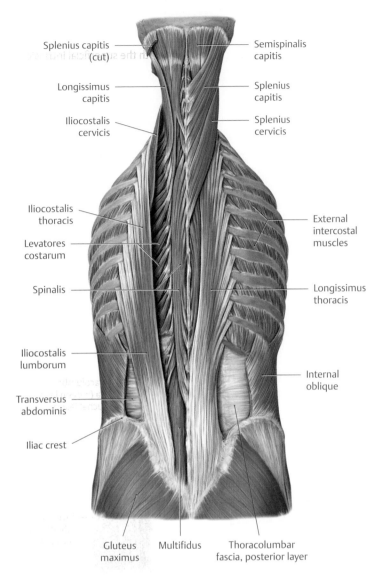

Splenius capitis (cut)

Semispinalis capitis

Longissimus capitis

Splenius capitis

Iliocostalis cervicis

Splenius cervicis

Iliocostalis thoracis

Levatores costarum

External intercostal muscles

Spinalis

Longissimus thoracis

Iliocostalis lumborum

Transversus abdominis

Internal oblique

Iliac crest

Gluteus maximus

Multifidus

Thoracolumbar fascia, posterior layer

C Intermediate and deep intrinsic back muscles. *Removed:* Longissimus thoracis and cervicis, splenius muscles (left); iliocostalis (right). *Note:* The posterior layer of the thoracolumbar fascia gives origin to the internal oblique and transversus abdominis. *Revealed:* Deep muscles of the back.

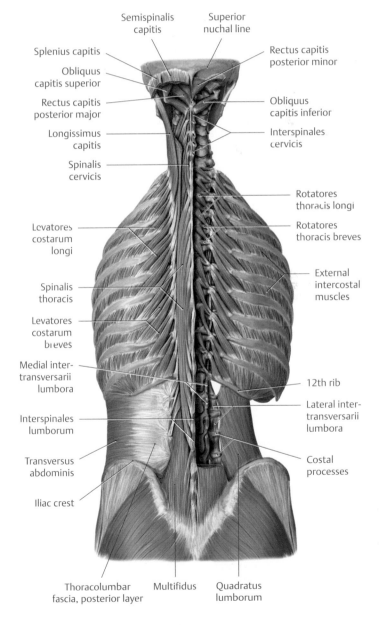

Semispinalis capitis

Superior nuchal line

Splenius capitis

Rectus capitis posterior minor

Obliquus capitis superior

Rectus capitis posterior major

Obliquus capitis inferior

Longissimus capitis

Interspinales cervicis

Spinalis cervicis

Rotatores thoracis longi

Levatores costarum longi

Rotatores thoracis breves

Spinalis thoracis

External intercostal muscles

Levatores costarum breves

Medial inter-transversarii lumbora

12th rib

Interspinales lumborum

Lateral inter-transversarii lumbora

Transversus abdominis

Costal processes

Iliac crest

Thoracolumbar fascia, posterior layer

Multifidus

Quadratus lumborum

D Deep intrinsic back muscles. *Removed:* Superficial and intermediate intrinsic back muscles (all); deep fascial layer and multifidus (right). *Revealed:* Intertransversarii and quadratus lumborum (right).

Muscle Facts (I)

Fig. 3.6 **Short nuchal and craniovertebral joint muscles**

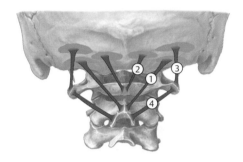

A Posterior view, schematic.

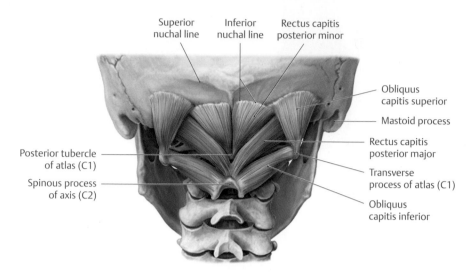

B Suboccipital muscles, posterior view.

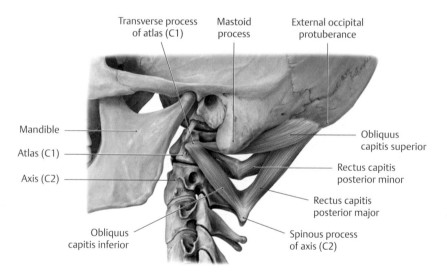

C Suboccipital muscles, left lateral view.

Table 3.1		Short nuchal and craniovertebral joint muscles			
Muscle		**Origin**	**Insertion**	**Innervation**	**Action**
Rectus capitis posterior	① Rectus capitis posterior major	C2 (spinous process)	Occipital bone (inferior nuchal line, middle third)	C1 (posterior ramus = suboccipital n.)	*Bilateral:* Extends head *Unilateral:* Rotates head to same side
	② Rectus capitis posterior minor	C1 (posterior tubercle)	Occipital bone (inferior nuchal line, inner third)		
Obliquus capitis	③ Obliquus capitis superior	C1 (transverse process)	Occipital bone (inferior nuchal line, middle third; above rectus capitis posterior major)		*Bilateral:* Extends head *Unilateral:* Flexes head to same side; rotates to opposite side
	④ Obliquus capitis inferior	C2 (spinous process)	C1 (transverse process)		*Bilateral:* Extends head *Unilateral:* Rotates head to same side

Fig. 3.7 Prevertebral muscles

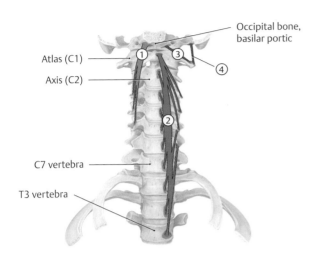

A Anterior view, schematic.

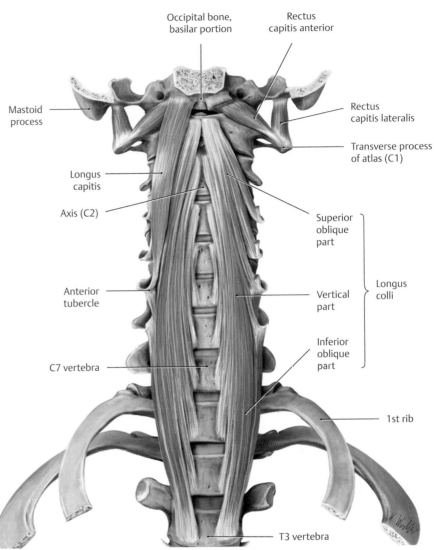

B Prevertebral muscles, anterior view.
Removed: Longus capitis (left); cervical viscera.

Table 3.2	**Prevertebral muscles**				
Muscle		**Origin**	**Insertion**	**Innervation**	**Action**
① Longus capitis		C3–C6 (transverse processes, anterior tubercles)	Occipital bone (basilar part)	Direct branches from cervical plexus (C1–C3)	*Bilateral:* Flexes head *Unilateral:* Flexes and slightly rotates head to same side
② Longus colli (cervicis)	Vertical (medial) part	C5–T3 (anterior sides of vertebral bodies)	C2–C4 (anterior sides of vertebral bodies)	Direct branches from cervical plexus (C2–C6)	*Bilateral:* Flexes cervical spine *Unilateral:* Flexes and rotates cervical spine to same side
	Superior oblique part	C3–C5 (transverse processes, anterior tubercles)	C1 (transverse process, anterior tubercle)		
	Inferior oblique part	T1–T3 (anterior sides of vertebral bodies)	C5–C6 (transverse processes, anterior tubercles)		
③ Rectus capitis anterior		C1 (lateral mass)	Occipital bone (basilar part)	C1 (anterior ramus)	*Bilateral:* Flexion at atlanto-occipital joint *Unilateral:* Lateral flexion at atlanto-occipital joint
④ Rectus capitis lateralis		C1 (transverse process)	Occipital bone (basilar part, lateral to occipital condyles)		

Muscle Facts (II)

The intrinsic back muscles are divided into superficial, intermediate, and deep layers. The serratus posterior muscles are extrinsic back muscles, innervated by the anterior rami of intercostal nerves, not the posterior rami, which innervate the intrinsic back muscles. They are included here as they are encountered in dissection of the back musculature.

Table 3.3		Superficial intrinsic back muscles			
Muscle		**Origin**	**Insertion**	**Innervation**	**Action**
Serratus posterior	① Serratus posterior superior	Nuchal lig.; C7–T3 (spinous processes)	2nd–4th ribs (superior borders)	Spinal nn. T2–T5 (anterior rami)	Elevates ribs
	② Serratus posterior inferior	T11–L2 (spinous processes)	8th–12th ribs (inferior borders, near angles)	Spinal nn. T9–T12 (anterior rami)	Depresses ribs
Splenius	③ Splenius capitis	Nuchal lig.; C7–T3 or T4 (spinous processes)	Lateral 1/3 nuchal line (occipital bone); mastoid process (temporal bone)	Spinal nn. C1–C6 (posterior rami, lateral branches)	*Bilateral:* Extends cervical spine and head *Unilateral:* Laterally flexes and rotates head to the same side
	④ Splenius cervicis	T3–T6 or T7 (spinous processes)	C1–C3/4 (transverse processes)		

Fig. 3.8 Superficial intrinsic back muscles, schematic
Right side, posterior view.

Fig. 3.9 Intermediate intrinsic back muscles, schematic
Right side, posterior view. These muscles are collectively known as the erector spinae.

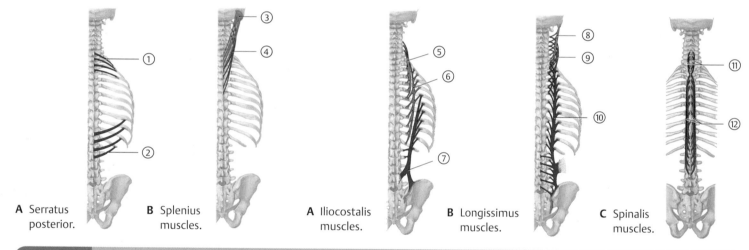

A Serratus posterior. **B** Splenius muscles. **A** Iliocostalis muscles. **B** Longissimus muscles. **C** Spinalis muscles.

Table 3.4		Intermediate intrinsic back muscles (erector spinae)			
Muscle		**Origin**	**Insertion**	**Innervation**	**Action**
Iliocostalis	⑤ Iliocostalis cervicis	3rd–7th ribs	C4–C6 (transverse processes)	Spinal nn. C8–L1 (posterior rami, lateral branches)	*Bilateral:* Extends spine *Unilateral:* Flexes spine laterally to same side
	⑥ Iliocostalis thoracis	7th–12th ribs	1st–6th ribs		
	⑦ Iliocostalis lumborum	Sacrum; iliac crest; thoracolumbar fascia (posterior layer)	6th–12th ribs; thoracolumbar fascia (posterior layer); upper lumbar vertebrae (transverse processes)		
Longissimus	⑧ Longissimus capitis	T1–T3 (transverse processes); C4–C7 (transverse and articular processes)	Temporal bone (mastoid process)	Spinal nn. C1–L5 (posterior rami, lateral branches)	*Bilateral:* Extends head *Unilateral:* Flexes and rotates head to same side
	⑨ Longissimus cervicis	T1–T6 (transverse processes)	C2–C5 (transverse processes)		*Bilateral:* Extends spine *Unilateral:* Flexes spine laterally to same side
	⑩ Longissimus thoracis	Sacrum; iliac crest; lumbar vertebrae (spinous processes); lower thoracic vertebrae (transverse processes)	2nd–12th ribs; thoracic and lumbar vertebrae (transverse processes)		
Spinalis	⑪ Spinalis cervicis	C5–T2 (spinous processes)	C2–C5 (spinous processes)	Spinal nn. (posterior rami)	*Bilateral:* Extends cervical and thoracic spine *Unilateral:* Flexes cervical and thoracic spine to same side
	⑫ Spinalis thoracis	T10–L3 (spinous processes, lateral surfaces)	T2–T8 (spinous processes, lateral surfaces)		

Fig. 3.10 **Superficial and intermediate intrinsic back muscles**
Posterior view.

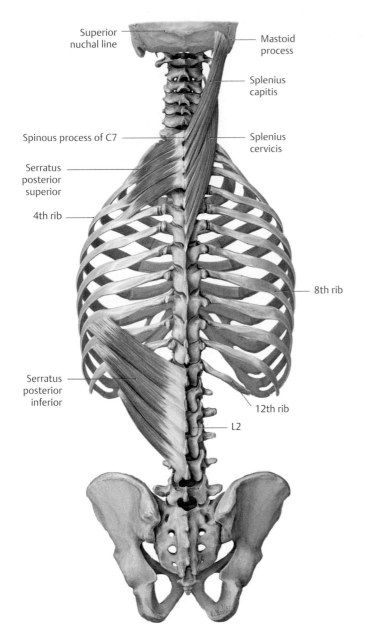

Superior
nuchal line

Mastoid
process

Splenius
capitis

Spinous process of C7

Splenius
cervicis

Serratus
posterior
superior

4th rib

8th rib

Serratus
posterior
inferior

12th rib

L2

A Superficial back muscles:
Splenius and serratus posterior muscles.

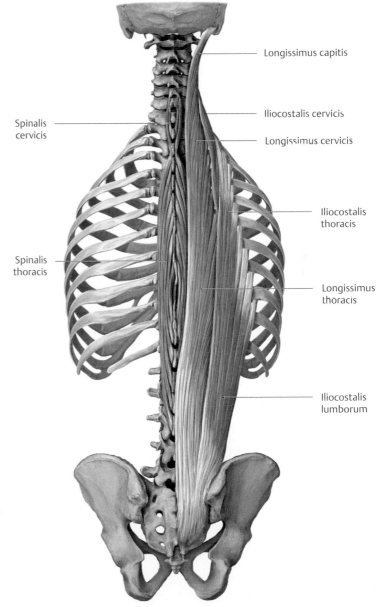

Longissimus capitis

Iliocostalis cervicis

Spinalis
cervicis

Longissimus cervicis

Iliocostalis
thoracis

Spinalis
thoracis

Longissimus
thoracis

Iliocostalis
lumborum

B Intermediate intrinsic back muscles (erector spinae): Iliocostalis,
longissimus, and spinalis muscles.

33

Muscle Facts (III)

The deep intrinsic back muscles are divided into two groups: transversospinalis and deep segmental muscles. The transversospinalis muscles pass between the transverse and spinous processes of the vertebrae.

Table 3.5		Transversospinalis muscles			
Muscle		Origin	Insertion	Innervation	Action
Rotatores	① Rotatores breves	T1–T12 (between transverse and spinous processes of adjacent vertebrae)		Spinal nn. (posterior rami)	*Bilateral:* Extends thoracic spine *Unilateral:* Rotates thoracic spine to opposite side
	② Rotatores longi	T1–T12 (between transverse and spinous processes, skipping one vertebra)			
Multifidus ③		Sacrum, ilium, mamillary processes of L1–L5, transverse and articular processes of T1–T4, C4–C7	Superomedially to spinous processes, skipping two to four vertebrae		*Bilateral:* Extends spine *Unilateral:* Flexes spine to same side, rotates it to opposite side
Semispinalis	④ Semispinalis capitis	C4–T7 (transverse and articular processes)	Occipital bone (between superior and inferior nuchal lines)		*Bilateral:* Extends thoracic and cervical spines and head (stabilizes craniovertebral joints)
	⑤ Semispinalis cervicis	T1–T6 (transverse processes)	C2–C5 (spinous processes)		*Unilateral:* Flexes head, cervical and thoracic spines to same side, rotates to opposite side
	⑥ Semispinalis thoracis	T6–T12 (transverse processes)	C6–T4 (spinous processes)		

Fig. 3.11 Transversospinalis muscles
Posterior view, schematic.

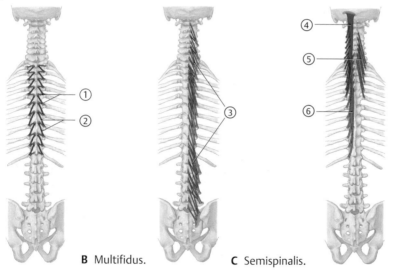

A Rotatores muscles. **B** Multifidus. **C** Semispinalis.

Fig. 3.12 Deep segmental muscles
Posterior view, schematic.

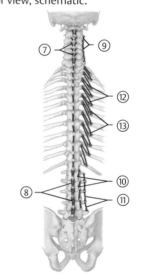

Table 3.6		Deep segmental back muscles			
Muscle		Origin	Insertion	Innervation	Action
Interspinales*	⑦ Interspinales cervicis	C1–C7 (between spinous processes of adjacent vertebrae)		Spinal nn. (posterior rami)	Extends cervical and lumbar spines
	⑧ Interspinales lumbora	L1–L5 (between spinous processes of adjacent vertebrae)			
Inter-transversarii*	Anterior intertransversarii cervices	C2–C7 (between anterior tubercles of adjacent vertebrae)		Spinal nn. (anterior rami)	*Bilateral:* Stabilizes and extends the cervical and lumbar spines
	⑨ Posterior intertransversarii cervices	C2–C7 (between posterior tubercles of adjacent vertebrae)		Spinal nn. (posterior rami)	
	⑩ Medial intertransversarii lumbora	L1–L5 (between mammillary processes of adjacent vertebrae)			*Unilateral:* Flexes the cervical and lumbar spines laterally to same side
	⑪ Lateral intertransversarii lumbora	L1–L5 (between transverse processes of adjacent vertebrae)		Spinal nn. (anterior rami)	
Levatores costarum	⑫ Levatores costarum breves	C7–T11 (transverse processes)	Costal angle of next lower rib	Spinal nn. (posterior rami)	*Bilateral:* Extends thoracic spine *Unilateral:* Flexes thoracic spine to same side, rotates to opposite side
	⑬ Levatores costarum longi		Costal angle of rib two vertebrae below		

*Both the interspinales and intertransversarii muscles traverse the entire spine; only their clinically relevant components have been included.

Fig. 3.13 Deep intrinsic back muscles
Posterior view.

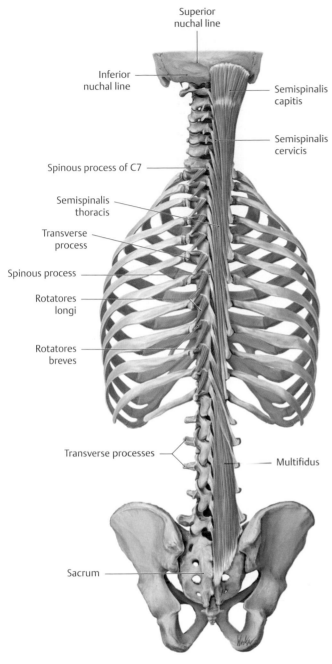

Superior nuchal line

Inferior nuchal line

Semispinalis capitis

Semispinalis cervicis

Spinous process of C7

Semispinalis thoracis

Transverse process

Spinous process

Rotatores longi

Rotatores breves

Transverse processes

Multifidus

Sacrum

A Transversospinalis muscles: Rotatores, multifidus, and semispinalis.

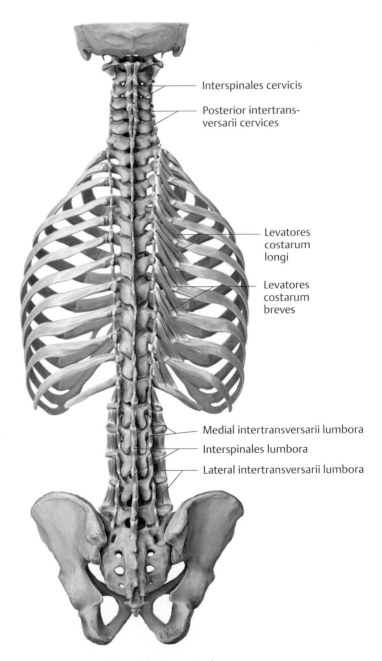

Interspinales cervicis

Posterior intertransversarii cervices

Levatores costarum longi

Levatores costarum breves

Medial intertransversarii lumbora

Interspinales lumbora

Lateral intertransversarii lumbora

B Deep segmental muscles: Interspinales, intertransversarii, and levatores costarum.

4 Neurovasculature
Arteries & Veins of the Back

Fig. 4.1 Arteries of the back

The structures of the back are supplied by branches of the posterior intercostal arteries, which arise from the thoracic aorta or from the subclavian artery.

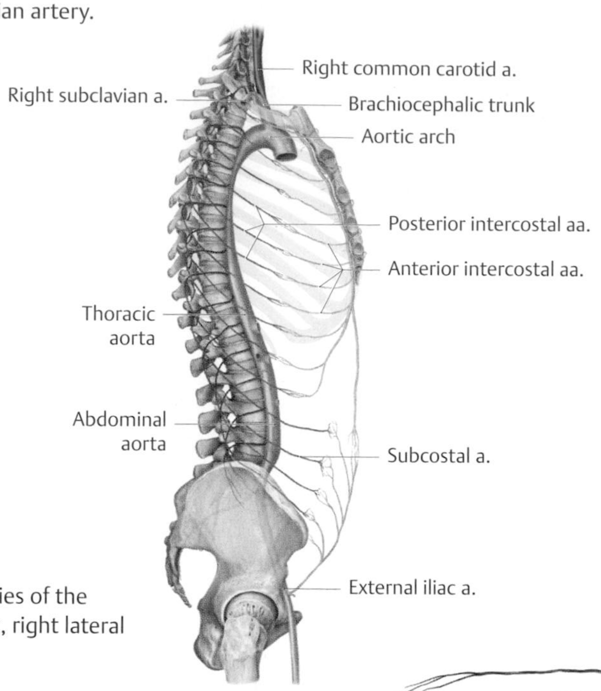

A Arteries of the trunk, right lateral view.

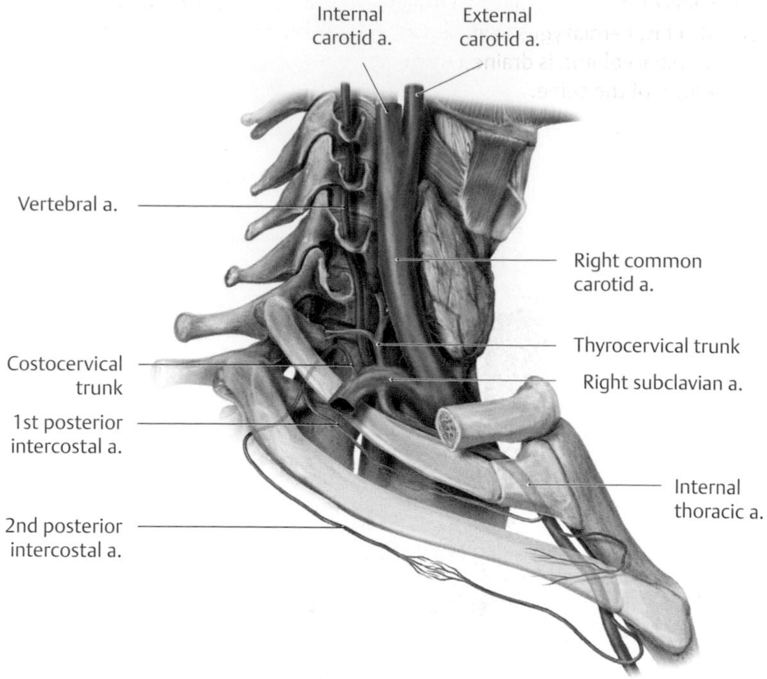

B Vascular supply to the nuchal region, posterolateral view. *Note:* The first and second posterior intercostal arteries arise from the costocervical trunk, a branch of the subclavian artery.

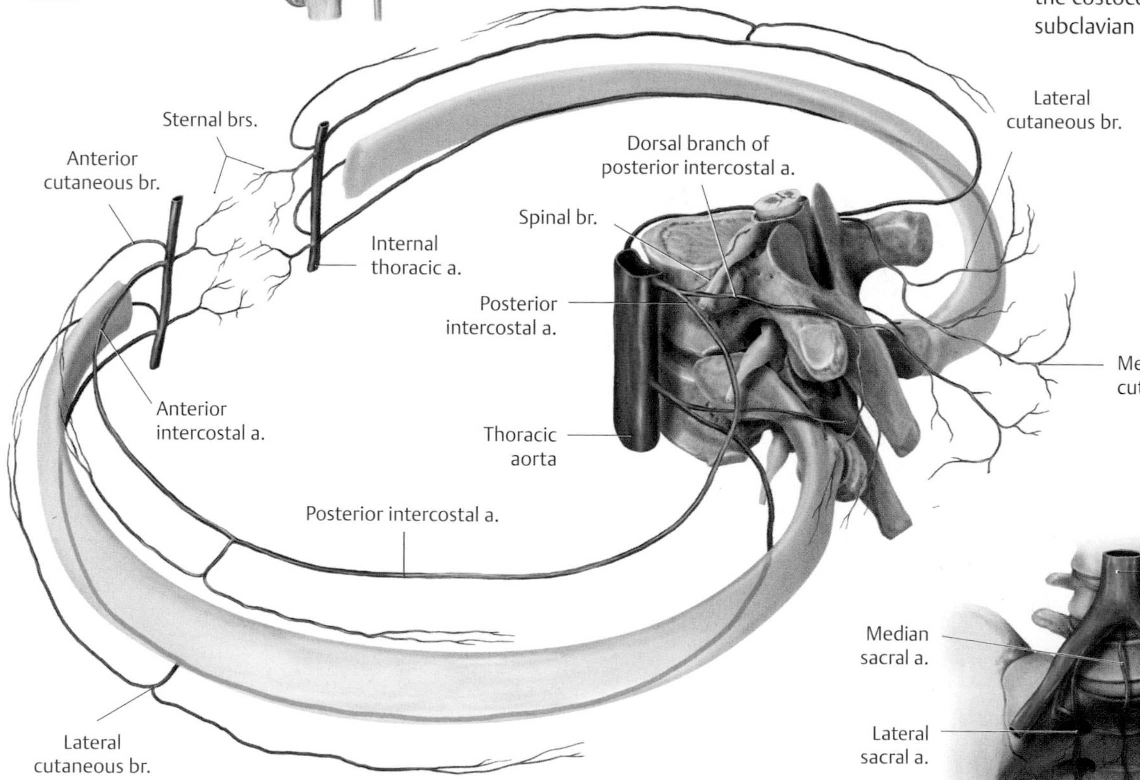

C Posterior intercostal arteries, oblique posterosuperior view. The posterior intercostal arteries give rise to cutaneous and muscular branches, as well as spinal branches that supply the spinal cord.

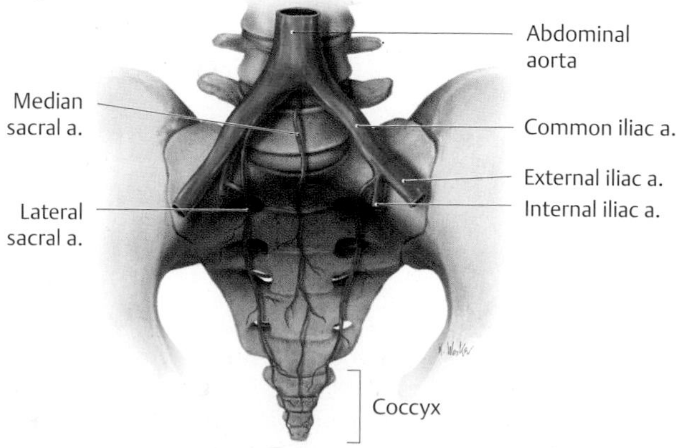

D Vascular supply to the sacrum, anterior view.

Fig. 4.2 Veins of the back

The veins of the back drain into the azygos vein via the posterior intercostal veins, hemiazygos vein, and ascending lumbar veins. The interior of the spinal column is drained by the vertebral venous plexus that runs the length of the spine.

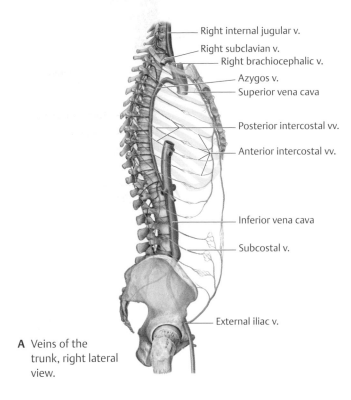

A Veins of the trunk, right lateral view.

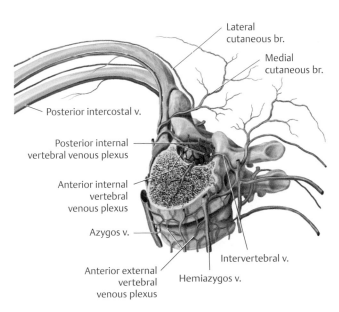

C Intercostal veins and anterior vertebral venous plexus, anterosuperior view. The intercostal veins follow a similar course to the intercostal nerves and arteries (see **pp. 36, 38**). *Note:* The anterior external vertebral venous plexus can be seen communicating with the azygos vein.

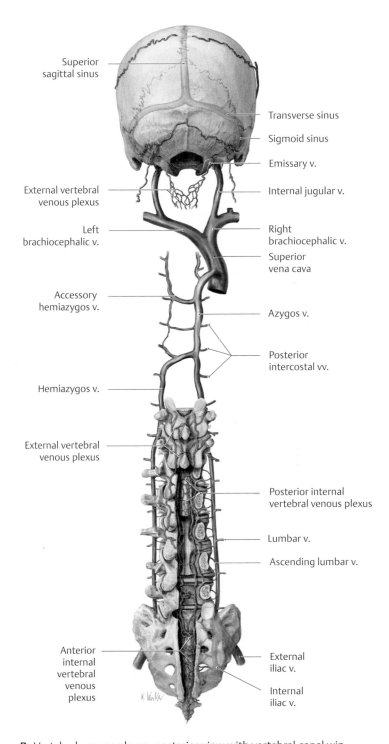

B Vertebral venous plexus, posterior view with vertebral canal windowed in the lumbar and sacral spine. The external vertebral venous plexus communicates with the sigmoid sinus through emissary veins in the skull. The *external* vertebral venous plexus is divided into an anterior and a posterior portion that run along the exterior of the vertebral column. The anterior and posterior *internal* vertebral venous plexus run in the vertebral foramen and drain the spinal cord.

Nerves of the Back

The back receives its innervation from branches of the spinal nerves. The *posterior (dorsal) rami* of the spinal nerves supply most of the intrinsic muscles of the back. The extrinsic muscles of the back are supplied by the *anterior (ventral) rami* of the spinal nerves.

Fig. 4.3 **Nerves of the back**
Cross section of the vertebral column and spinal cord with surrounding musculature, superior view.

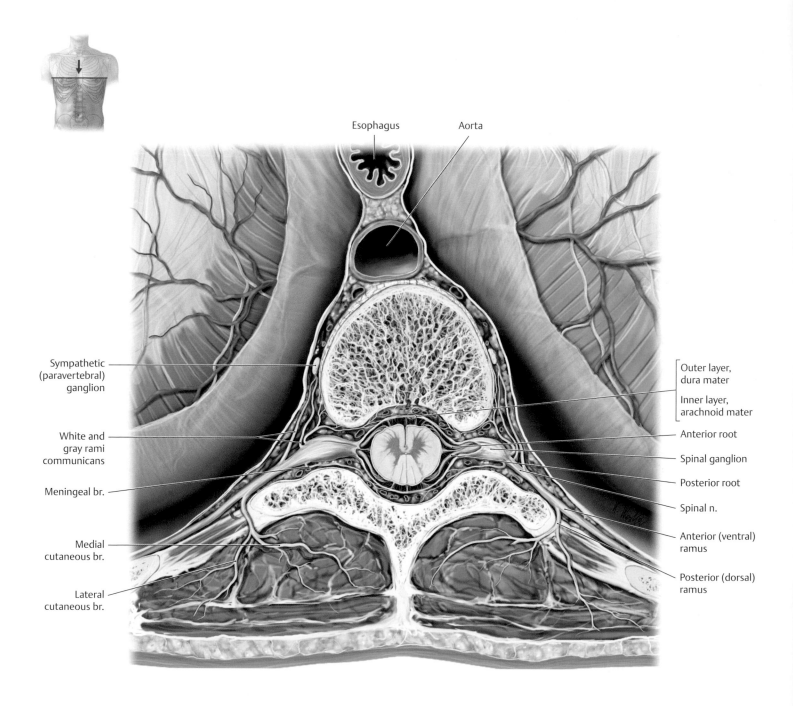

Esophagus

Aorta

Sympathetic (paravertebral) ganglion

Outer layer, dura mater

Inner layer, arachnoid mater

White and gray rami communicans

Anterior root

Spinal ganglion

Meningeal br.

Posterior root

Spinal n.

Medial cutaneous br.

Anterior (ventral) ramus

Lateral cutaneous br.

Posterior (dorsal) ramus

Fig. 4.4 Nerves of the nuchal region

Right side, posterior view.

Table 4.1		Nerves of the nuchal region
Branches		**Function**
Posterior (dorsal) ramus	Suboccipital n. (C1)	Innervates the rectus capitis posterior major and minor; and obliquus capitis superior and inferior
	Greater occipital n. (C2)	Assits in the innervation of the semispinalis capitis muscle and supplies skin behind the auricle and the scalp to the coronal suture
	Third occipital n. (C3)	Assists in the innervation of the semispinalis capitis muscle, the C2-C3 facet joint, and supplies a small area of skin just below the superior nuchal line
Anterior (ventral) ramus	Lesser occipital n. (C2)	Cutaneous only, supplies an area of scalp posterolateral to the auricle, and the skin on the upper third of the medial aspect of the auricle
	Greater auricular n. (C2, C3)	Cutaneous only, supplies an area of skin over the parotid gland, the majority of the pinna, lateral neck, and posterior to the auricle

The anterior rami of C1-C3 also give rise to the ansa cervicalis, which innervates the infrahyoid muscles (see **p. 524).

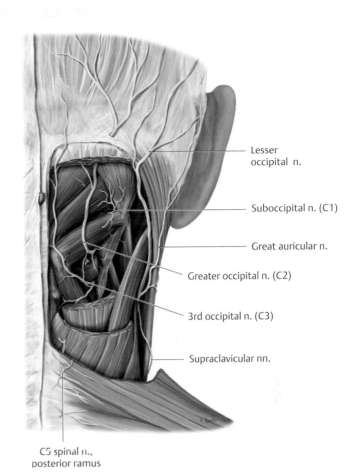

Lesser occipital n.

Suboccipital n. (C1)

Great auricular n.

Greater occipital n. (C2)

3rd occipital n. (C3)

Supraclavicular nn.

C5 spinal n., posterior ramus

Fig. 4.5 Cutaneous innervation of the back

Color denotes the skin areas innervated by (**A**) particular peripheral nerves or (**B**) particular pairs of segmental spinal nerves. Patterns of loss of cutaneous sensation can be helpful in diagnosis of nerve lesions.

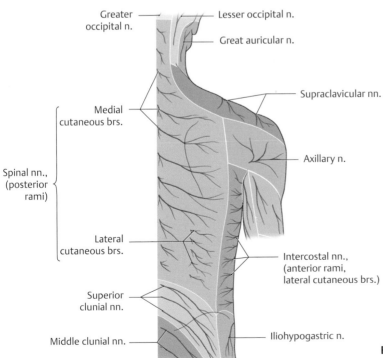

Greater occipital n.

Lesser occipital n.

Great auricular n.

Supraclavicular nn.

Medial cutaneous brs.

Axillary n.

Spinal nn., (posterior rami)

Lateral cutaneous brs.

Intercostal nn., (anterior rami, lateral cutaneous brs.)

Superior clunial nn.

Middle clunial nn.

Iliohypogastric n.

A Cutaneous innervation patterns of specific peripheral nerves.

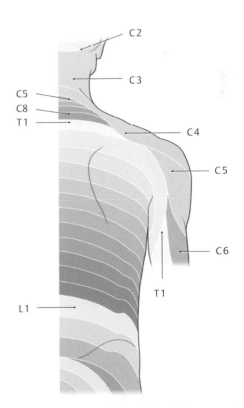

C2

C3

C5

C8

T1

C4

C5

C6

T1

L1

B Dermatomes: Dermatomes are bilateral band-like areas of skin receiving innervation from a single pair of spinal nerves (from a single segment of the spinal cord). *Note:* Spinal nerve C1 is purely motor; consequently there is no C1 dermatome.

Spinal Cord

The dura mater of the cranial cavity is composed of two layers, the periosteal and meningeal. Only the meningeal layer extends into the vertebral canal with the spinal cord. The periosteal layer of dura terminates at the foramen magnum and is replaced in the vertebral canal with the periosteum of the vertebral bone. Due to this structural difference in the two regions, the dural sac is not adherent to the bone of the vertebral canal as it is in the cranial cavity.

Fig. 4.6 **Spinal cord in situ**
Posterior view with vertebral canal windowed.

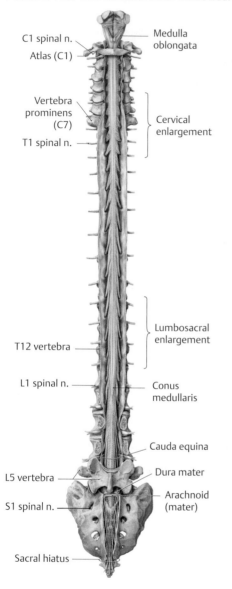

C1 spinal n.
Atlas (C1)
Medulla oblongata
Vertebra prominens (C7)
T1 spinal n.
Cervical enlargement
Lumbosacral enlargement
T12 vertebra
L1 spinal n.
Conus medullaris
Cauda equina
L5 vertebra
Dura mater
S1 spinal n.
Arachnoid (mater)
Sacral hiatus

Fig. 4.7 **Spinal cord and its meningeal layers**
Posterior view. The dura mater is opened and the arachnoid is sectioned. The detailed anatomy of the spinal cord can be found on **pp. 690–691.**

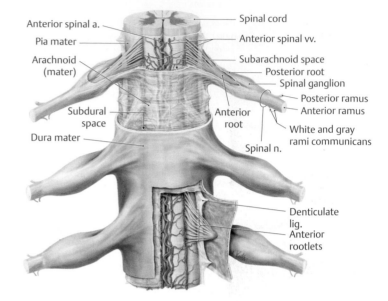

Anterior spinal a.
Pia mater
Arachnoid (mater)
Subdural space
Dura mater
Spinal cord
Anterior spinal vv.
Subarachnoid space
Posterior root
Spinal ganglion
Posterior ramus
Anterior ramus
White and gray rami communicans
Anterior root
Spinal n.
Denticulate lig.
Anterior rootlets

Fig. 4.8 **Cervical spinal cord in situ: Transverse section**
Superior view. Spinal cord at level of C4 vertebra.

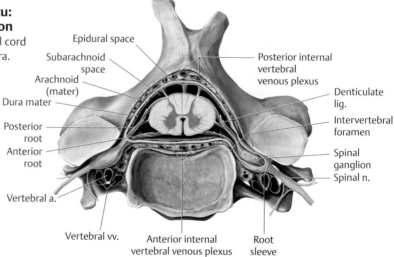

Epidural space
Subarachnoid space
Arachnoid (mater)
Dura mater
Posterior root
Anterior root
Vertebral a.
Vertebral vv.
Anterior internal vertebral venous plexus
Root sleeve
Posterior internal vertebral venous plexus
Denticulate lig.
Intervertebral foramen
Spinal ganglion
Spinal n.

✳ *Clinical box 4.1*

Spina Bifida

Spina bifida is a neural tube defect that occurs when the spine and spinal cord do not form properly. In the United States, it affects about one out of every 1,500 newborns. There are three main types.

- **Spina bifida occulta (A)** is the most common congenital anomaly of the vertebral column in which the laminae of L5 and/or S1 fail to develop. The defect is often hidden and most individuals are unaware they have the condition because there is only a small defect in the vertebrae. There is generally no disturbance of spinal function.
- **Spina bifida (meningocele) (B)** occurs when one or more vertebral arches fail to develop and presents with a herniation or sac of only the meninges. The spinal cord and nerves are normal and not severely affected.

- **Spina bifida (myelomeningocele) (C)** occurs when multiple vertebral arches fail to develop resulting in a herniation of both the meninges and spinal nerves. This is the most severe form exposing the newborn to life threatening infections, bowel and bladder dysfunction, and total paralysis of the lower extremities.

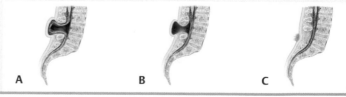

A   B   C

Fig. 4.9 Cauda equina in the vertebral canal

Posterior view. The lamina and posterior surface of the sacrum have been partially removed.

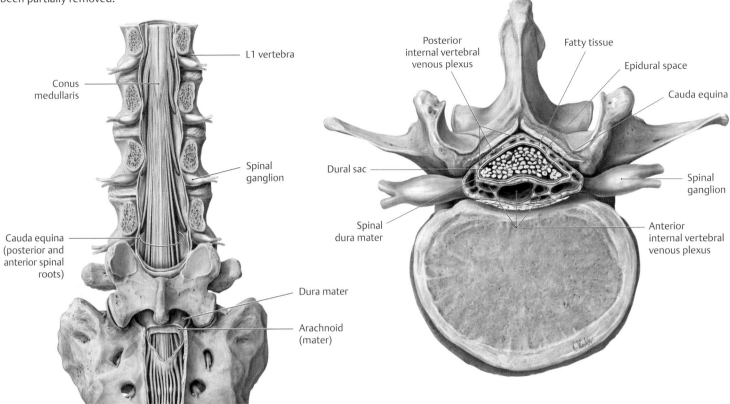

- L1 vertebra
- Conus medullaris
- Spinal ganglion
- Cauda equina (posterior and anterior spinal roots)
- Dura mater
- Arachnoid (mater)
- Sacral hiatus
- Filum terminale

Fig. 4.10 Cauda equina in situ: Transverse section

Superior view. Cauda equina at level of L2 vertebra.

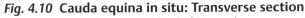

- Posterior internal vertebral venous plexus
- Fatty tissue
- Epidural space
- Cauda equina
- Dural sac
- Spinal ganglion
- Spinal dura mater
- Anterior internal vertebral venous plexus

Fig. 4.11 Spinal cord, dural sac, and vertebral column at different ages.

Anterior view. Longitudinal growth of the spinal cord lags behind that of the vertebral column. At birth, the distal end of the spinal cord, the conus medullaris, is at the level of the L3 vertebral body, but in the average adult it extends to the level of L1/L2. The dural sac always extends into the upper sacrum.

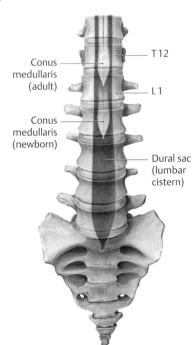

- T 12
- Conus medullaris (adult)
- L 1
- Conus medullaris (newborn)
- Dural sac (lumbar cistern)

Clinical box 4.2

Lumbar puncture

A needle introduced into the dural sac (lumbar cistern) generally slips past the spinal nerve roots without injuring the spinal cord or spinal nerves. Cerebrospinal fluid (CSF) samples are therefore taken between the L3 and L4 vertebrae (2), once the patient has leaned forward to separate the spinous processes of the lumbar spine.

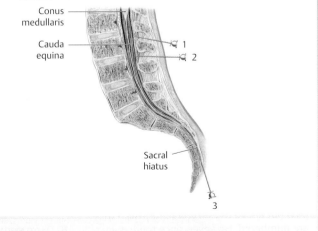

- Conus medullaris
- Cauda equina
- 1
- 2
- Sacral hiatus
- 3

Anesthesia

Lumbar anesthesia may be administered in a similar fashion (2). Epidural anesthesia is administered by placing a catheter in the epidural space without penetrating the dural sac (1). This may also be done by passing a needle through the sacral hiatus (3).

Arteries & Veins of the Spinal Cord

Like the spinal cord itself, the arteries and veins of the spinal cord consist of multiple horizontal systems (blood vessels of the spinal cord segments) that are integrated into a vertical system.

Fig. 4.15 Arteries of the spinal cord

The unpaired anterior and paired posterior spinal arteries typically arise from the vertebral arteries. As they descend within the vertebral canal, the spinal arteries are reinforced by anterior and posterior segmental medullary arteries. Depending on the spinal level, these reinforcing branches may arise from the vertebral, ascending or deep cervical, posterior intercostal, lumbar, or lateral sacral arteries.

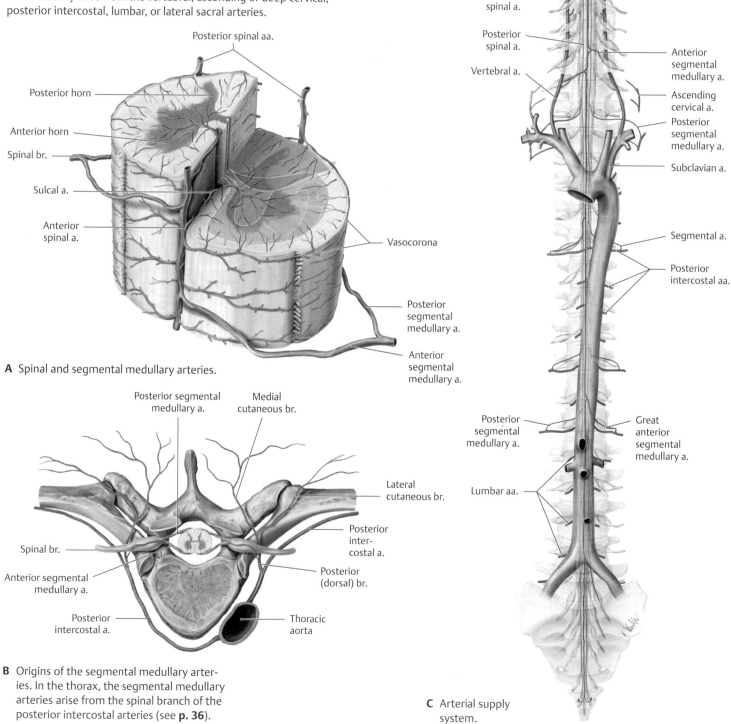

A Spinal and segmental medullary arteries.

B Origins of the segmental medullary arteries. In the thorax, the segmental medullary arteries arise from the spinal branch of the posterior intercostal arteries (see **p. 36**).

C Arterial supply system.

44

Fig. 4.16 Veins of the spinal cord

The interior of the spinal cord drains via venous plexuses into an anterior and a posterior spinal vein. The radicular and spinal veins connect the veins of the spinal cord with the internal vertebral venous plexus. The intervertebral and basivertebral veins connect the internal and external venous plexuses, which drain into the azygos system.

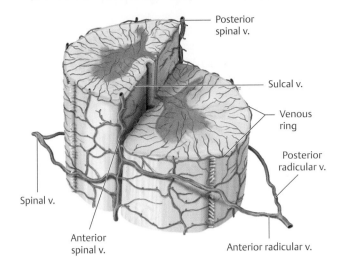

B Spinal and radicular veins.

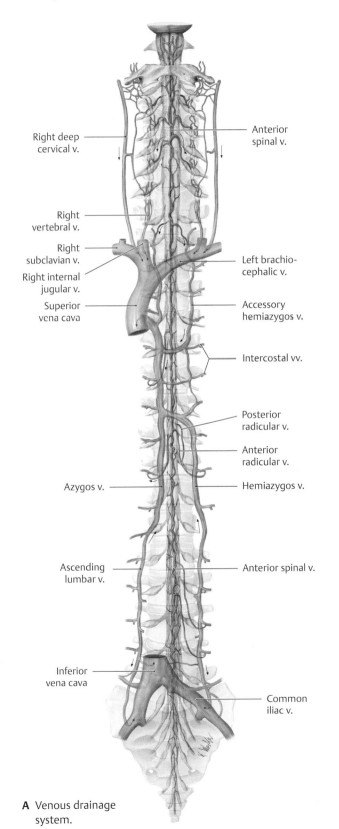

A Venous drainage system.

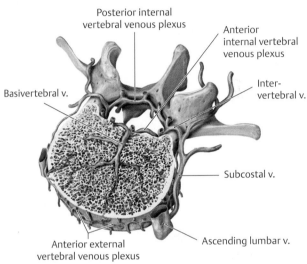

C Vertebral venous plexuses.

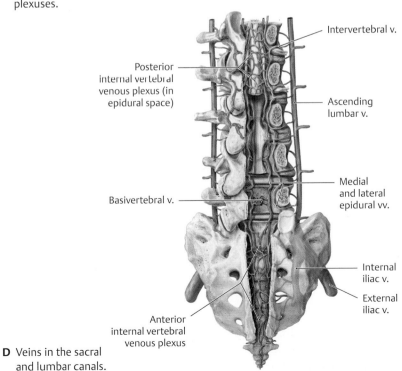

D Veins in the sacral and lumbar canals.

***Fig. 4.17* Neurovasculature of the nuchal region**

Posterior view. *Removed:* Trapezius, sterno-cleidomastoid, and semispinalis capitis.
Revealed: Suboccipital region.

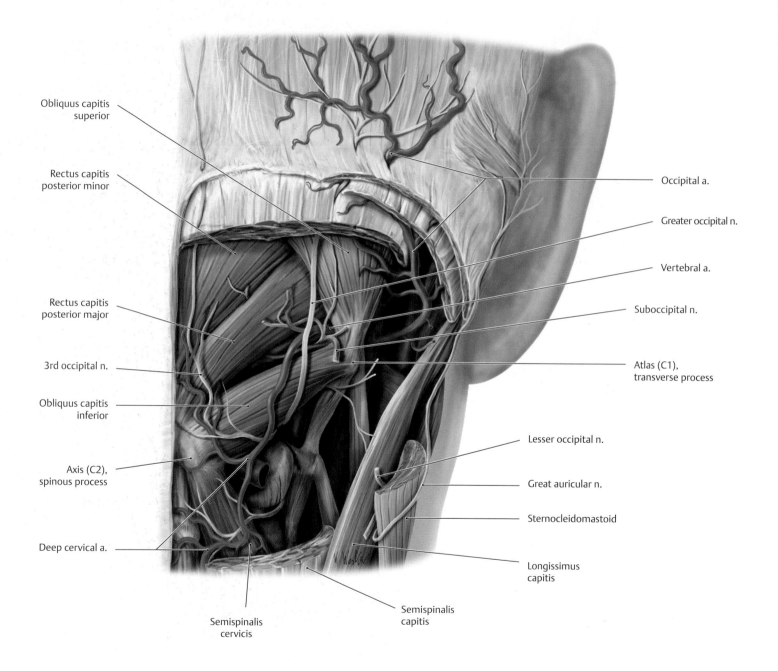

Obliquus capitis superior

Rectus capitis posterior minor

Rectus capitis posterior major

3rd occipital n.

Obliquus capitis inferior

Axis (C2), spinous process

Deep cervical a.

Semispinalis cervicis

Semispinalis capitis

Occipital a.

Greater occipital n.

Vertebral a.

Suboccipital n.

Atlas (C1), transverse process

Lesser occipital n.

Great auricular n.

Sternocleidomastoid

Longissimus capitis

Fig. 4.18 Neurovasculature of the back

Posterior view. *Removed:* Muscle fascia (except posterior layer of thoracolumbar fascia); latissimus dorsi (right). *Reflected:* Trapezius (right). *Revealed:* Transverse cervical artery in the deep scapular region. See **p. 72** for the course of the intercostal vessels.

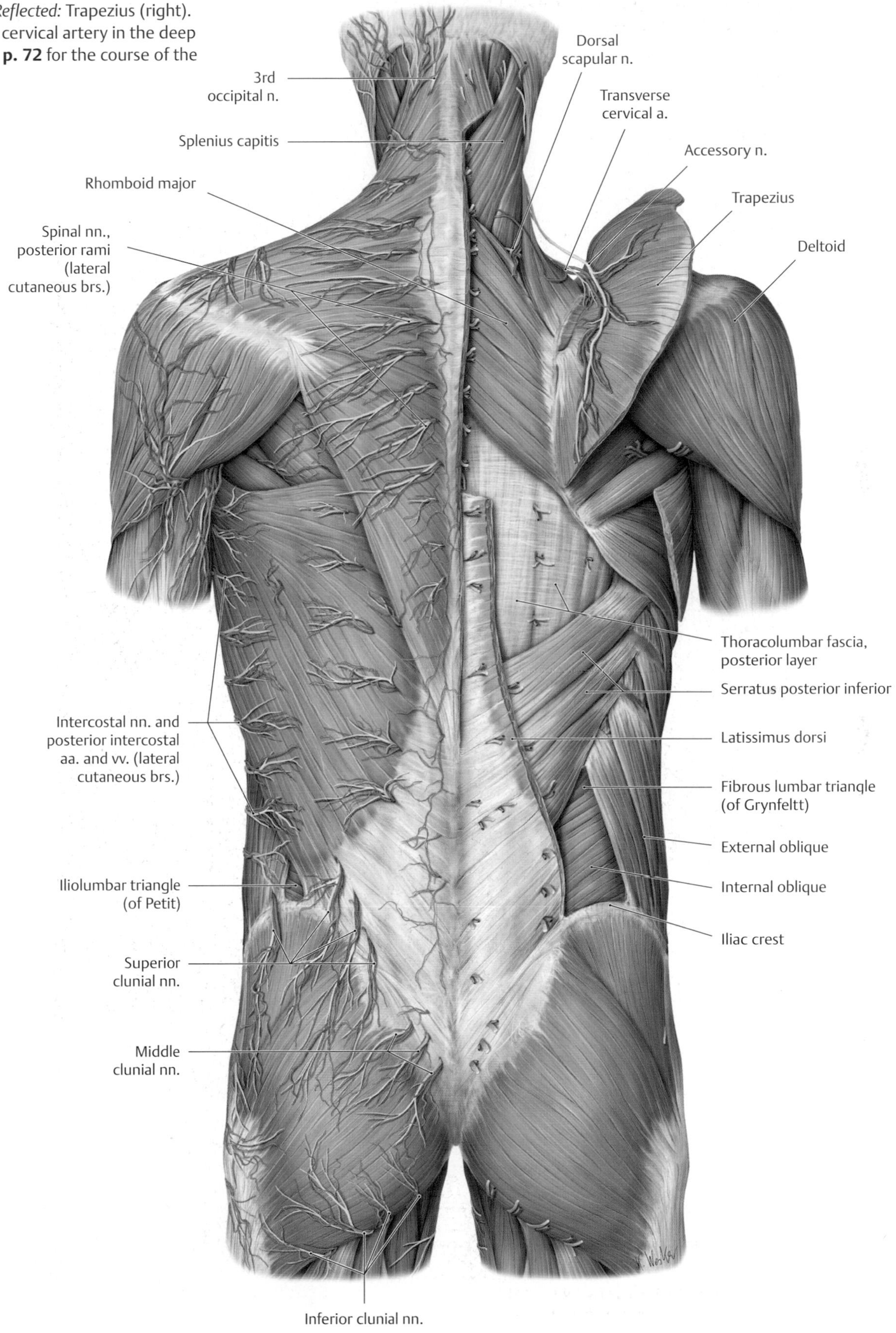

3rd occipital n.

Splenius capitis

Rhomboid major

Spinal nn., posterior rami (lateral cutaneous brs.)

Intercostal nn. and posterior intercostal aa. and vv. (lateral cutaneous brs.)

Iliolumbar triangle (of Petit)

Superior clunial nn.

Middle clunial nn.

Inferior clunial nn.

Dorsal scapular n.

Transverse cervical a.

Accessory n.

Trapezius

Deltoid

Thoracolumbar fascia, posterior layer

Serratus posterior inferior

Latissimus dorsi

Fibrous lumbar triangle (of Grynfeltt)

External oblique

Internal oblique

Iliac crest

5 Sectional & Radiographic Anatomy
Radiographic Anatomy of the Back (I)

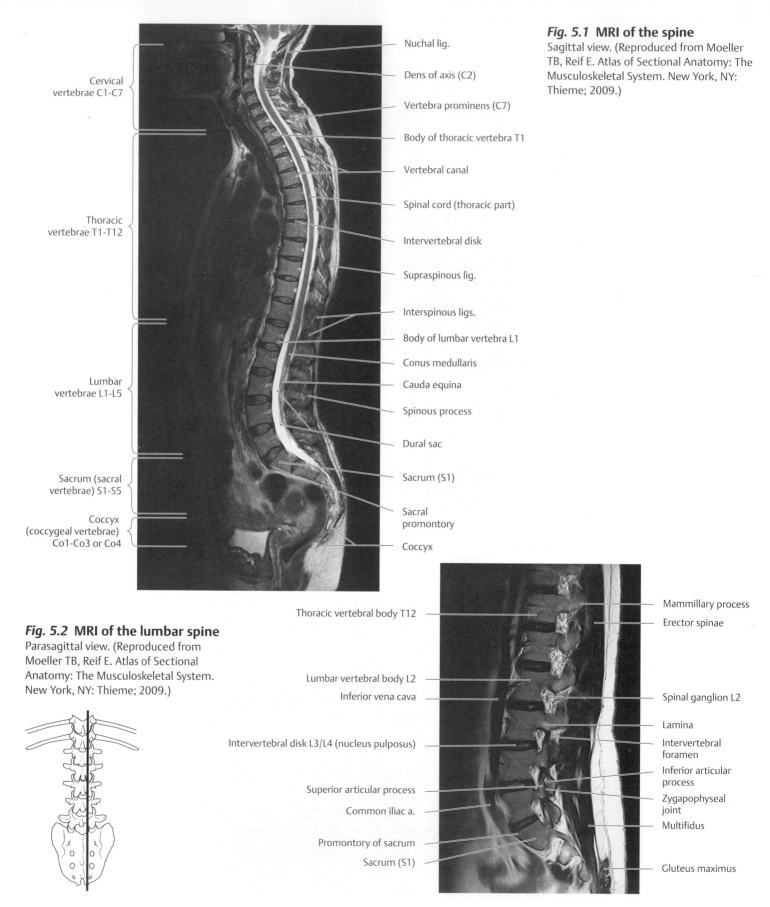

Cervical vertebrae C1–C7

Thoracic vertebrae T1–T12

Lumbar vertebrae L1–L5

Sacrum (sacral vertebrae) S1–S5

Coccyx (coccygeal vertebrae) Co1–Co3 or Co4

Nuchal lig.

Dens of axis (C2)

Vertebra prominens (C7)

Body of thoracic vertebra T1

Vertebral canal

Spinal cord (thoracic part)

Intervertebral disk

Supraspinous lig.

Interspinous ligs.

Body of lumbar vertebra L1

Conus medullaris

Cauda equina

Spinous process

Dural sac

Sacrum (S1)

Sacral promontory

Coccyx

Fig. 5.1 MRI of the spine
Sagittal view. (Reproduced from Moeller TB, Reif E. Atlas of Sectional Anatomy: The Musculoskeletal System. New York, NY: Thieme; 2009.)

Fig. 5.2 MRI of the lumbar spine
Parasagittal view. (Reproduced from Moeller TB, Reif E. Atlas of Sectional Anatomy: The Musculoskeletal System. New York, NY: Thieme; 2009.)

Thoracic vertebral body T12

Lumbar vertebral body L2

Inferior vena cava

Intervertebral disk L3/L4 (nucleus pulposus)

Superior articular process

Common iliac a.

Promontory of sacrum

Sacrum (S1)

Mammillary process

Erector spinae

Spinal ganglion L2

Lamina

Intervertebral foramen

Inferior articular process

Zygapophyseal joint

Multifidus

Gluteus maximus

Fig. 5.3 Radiograph of the cervical spine

Lateral view. (Reproduced from Moeller TB, Reif E. Pocket Atlas of Radiographic Anatomy, 3rd ed. New York, NY: Thieme; 2010.)

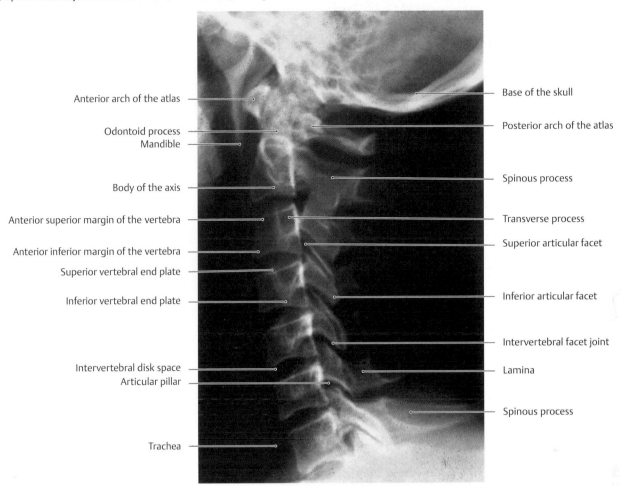

Anterior arch of the atlas

Odontoid process
Mandible

Body of the axis

Anterior superior margin of the vertebra

Anterior inferior margin of the vertebra

Superior vertebral end plate

Inferior vertebral end plate

Intervertebral disk space
Articular pillar

Trachea

Base of the skull

Posterior arch of the atlas

Spinous process

Transverse process

Superior articular facet

Inferior articular facet

Intervertebral facet joint

Lamina

Spinous process

Fig. 5.4 Radiograph of the thoracic spine

Anteroposterior view. Lower thoracic region. (Reproduced from Moeller TB, Reif E. Pocket Atlas of Radiographic Anatomy, 3rd ed. New York, NY: Thieme; 2010.)

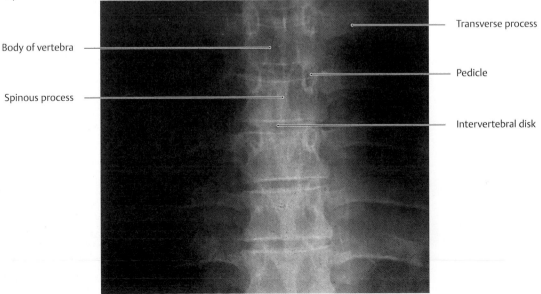

Body of vertebra

Spinous process

Transverse process

Pedicle

Intervertebral disk

Fig. 5.5 Radiograph of the lumbar spine

Lateral view. (Reproduced from Moeller TB, Reif E. Pocket Atlas of Radiographic Anatomy, 3rd ed. New York, NY: Thieme; 2010.)

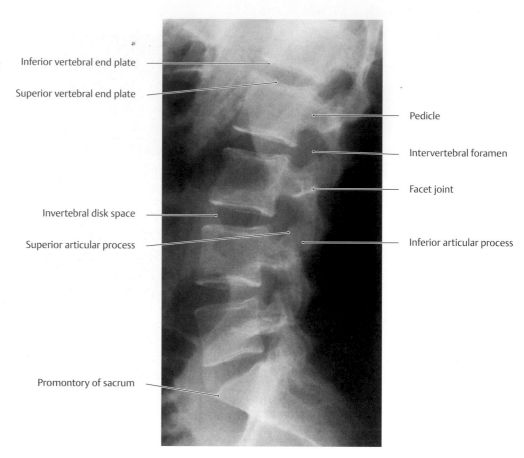

Inferior vertebral end plate

Superior vertebral end plate

Pedicle

Intervertebral foramen

Facet joint

Invertebral disk space

Superior articular process

Inferior articular process

Promontory of sacrum

Fig. 5.6 Radiograph of the lumbar spine

Oblique view. (Reproduced from Moeller TB, Reif E. Pocket Atlas of Radiographic Anatomy, 3rd ed. New York, NY: Thieme; 2010.)

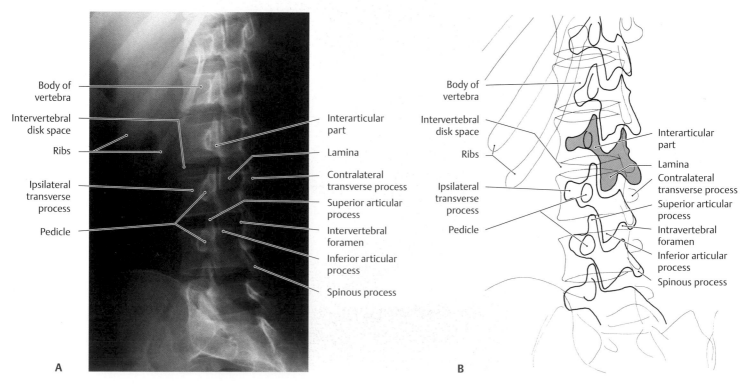

Body of vertebra

Intervertebral disk space

Ribs

Ipsilateral transverse process

Pedicle

Interarticular part

Lamina

Contralateral transverse process

Superior articular process

Intervertebral foramen

Inferior articular process

Spinous process

Body of vertebra

Intervertebral disk space

Ribs

Ipsilateral transverse process

Pedicle

Interarticular part

Lamina

Contralateral transverse process

Superior articular process

Intravertebral foramen

Inferior articular process

Spinous process

A

B

Fig. 5.7 MRI of the sacrum I

Oblique view. (Reproduced from Moeller TB, Reif E. Atlas of Sectional Anatomy: The Musculoskeletal System. New York, NY: Thieme; 2009.)

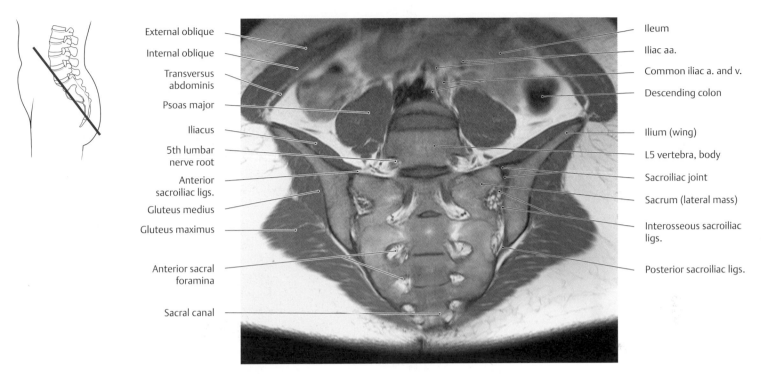

External oblique — Internal oblique — Transversus abdominis — Psoas major — Iliacus — 5th lumbar nerve root — Anterior sacroiliac ligs. — Gluteus medius — Gluteus maximus — Anterior sacral foramina — Sacral canal

Ileum — Iliac aa. — Common iliac a. and v. — Descending colon — Ilium (wing) — L5 vertebra, body — Sacroiliac joint — Sacrum (lateral mass) — Interosseous sacroiliac ligs. — Posterior sacroiliac ligs.

Fig. 5.8 MRI of the sacrum II

Oblique view. (Reproduced from Moeller TB, Reif E. Atlas of Sectional Anatomy: The Musculoskeletal System. New York, NY: Thieme; 2009.)

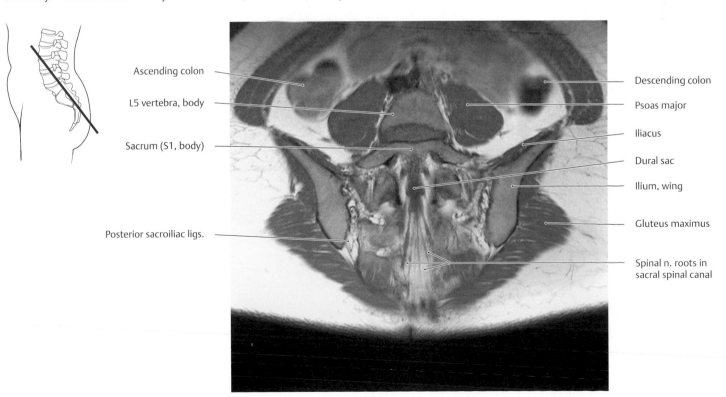

Ascending colon — L5 vertebra, body — Sacrum (S1, body) — Posterior sacroiliac ligs.

Descending colon — Psoas major — Iliacus — Dural sac — Ilium, wing — Gluteus maximus — Spinal n. roots in sacral spinal canal

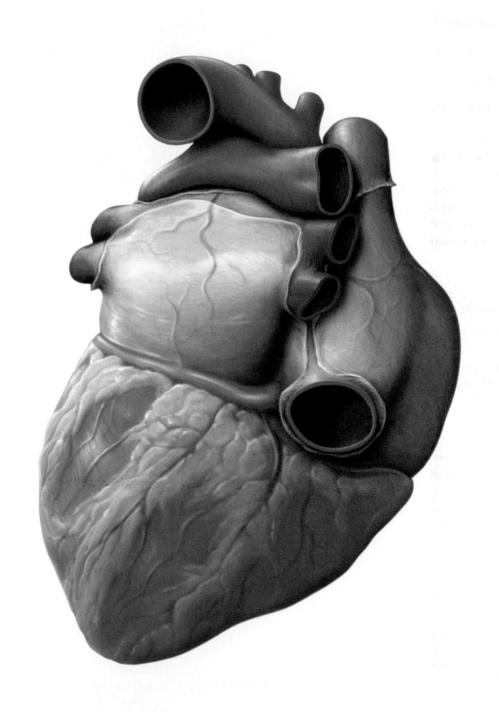

Thorax

6 Surface Anatomy

Surface Anatomy

***Fig. 6.1* Regions of the thorax**
Anterior view.

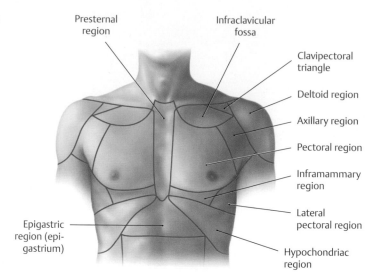

Presternal region

Infraclavicular fossa

Clavipectoral triangle

Deltoid region

Axillary region

Pectoral region

Inframammary region

Lateral pectoral region

Hypochondriac region

Epigastric region (epi-gastrium)

***Fig. 6.2* Palpable structures of the thorax**
Anterior view.

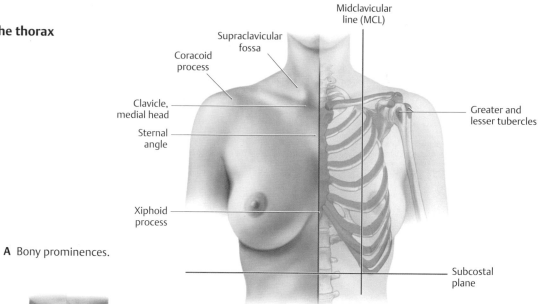

Midclavicular line (MCL)

Supraclavicular fossa

Coracoid process

Clavicle, medial head

Sternal angle

Greater and lesser tubercles

Xiphoid process

Subcostal plane

A Bony prominences.

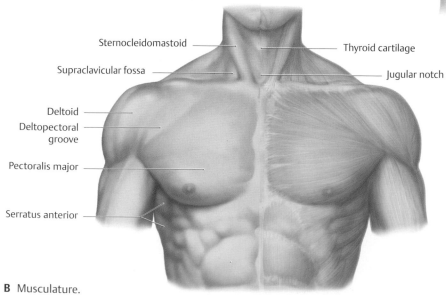

Sternocleidomastoid

Thyroid cartilage

Supraclavicular fossa

Jugular notch

Deltoid

Deltopectoral groove

Pectoralis major

Serratus anterior

B Musculature.

Fig. 6.3 **Vertical reference lines of the thorax**

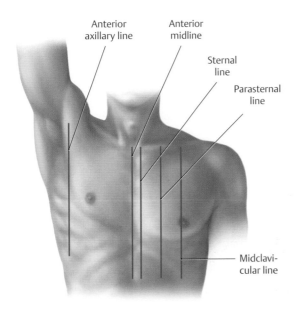

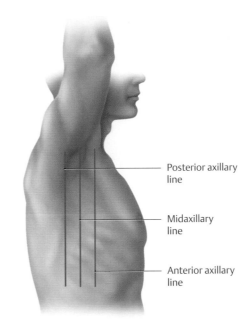

A Anterior view.

B Right lateral view.

Fig. 6.4 **Pleural cavities and lungs projected onto the thoracic skeleton**

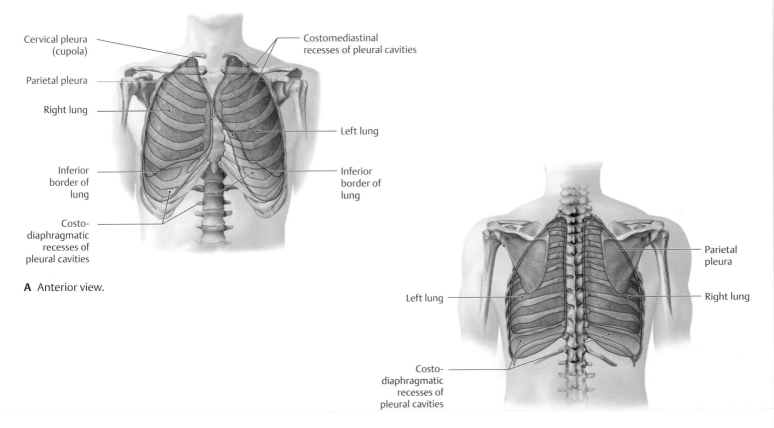

A Anterior view.

B Posterior view.

7 Thoracic Wall
Thoracic Skeleton

The thoracic skeleton consists of 12 thoracic vertebrae (**p. 10**), 12 pairs of ribs with costal cartilages, and the sternum. In addition to participating in respiratory movements, it provides a measure of protection to vital organs. The female thorax is generally narrower and shorter than the male equivalent.

Fig. 7.1 **Thoracic skeleton**

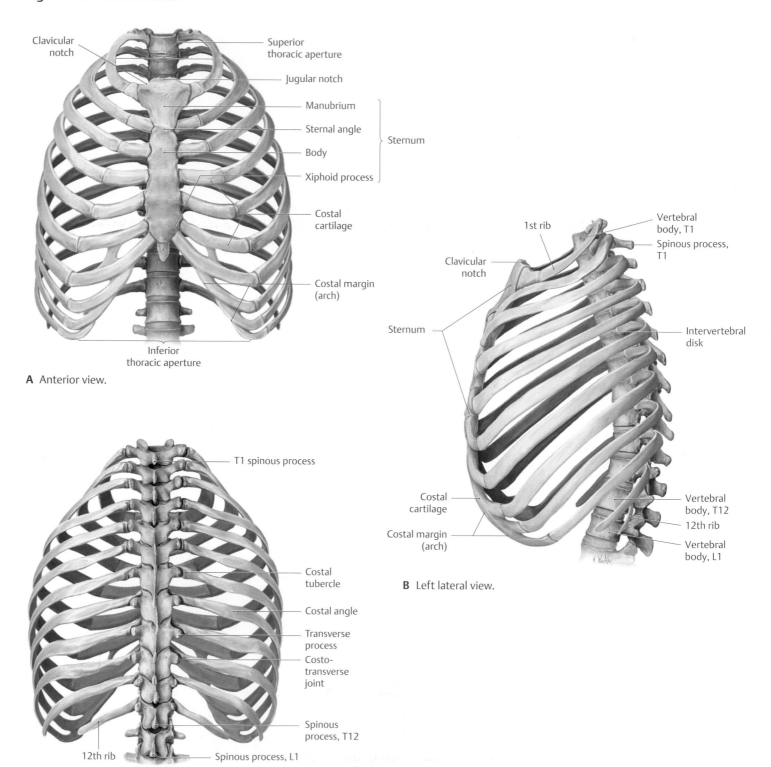

A Anterior view.

B Left lateral view.

C Posterior view.

Fig. 7.2 Structure of a thoracic segment
Superior view of 6th rib pair.

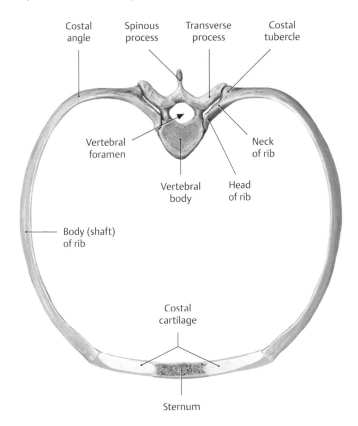

Costal angle · Spinous process · Transverse process · Costal tubercle · Vertebral foramen · Neck of rib · Vertebral body · Head of rib · Body (shaft) of rib · Costal cartilage · Sternum

Table 7.1	Elements of a thoracic segment		
Vertebra			
Rib	Bony part (costal bone)		Head
			Neck
			Costal tubercle
			Body (including costal angle)
	Costal part (costal cartilage)		
Sternum (articulates with costal cartilage of true ribs only; see **Fig. 7.3**)			

Fig. 7.3 Types of ribs
Left lateral view.

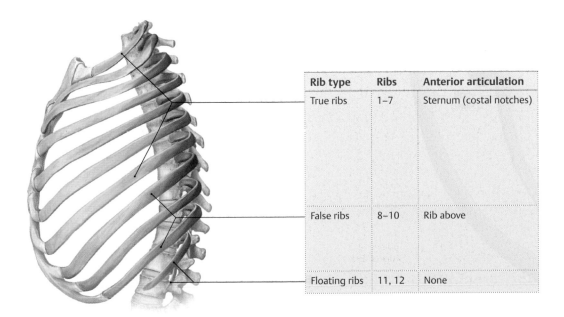

Rib type	Ribs	Anterior articulation
True ribs	1–7	Sternum (costal notches)
False ribs	8–10	Rib above
Floating ribs	11, 12	None

Joints of the Thoracic Cage

The diaphragm is the chief muscle for quiet respiration (see **p. 64**).
The muscles of the thoracic wall (see **p. 62**) contribute to deep (forced) inspiration.

Fig. 7.6 **Rib cage movement**

Full inspiration (red); full expiration (blue). In deep inspiration, there is an increase in transverse and anteroposterior (AP) dimensions, as well as the infrasternal angle. Note the red lines (inspiration dimensions) on the diagrams are longer than the blue ones (expiration dimensions) below. The downward movement of the diaphragm further increases the volume of the thoracic cavity.

Inspiration

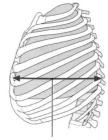

Infrasternal angle

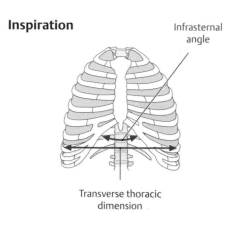

Transverse thoracic dimension

Anteroposterior (AP) dimension

Expiration

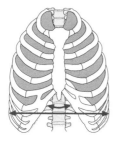

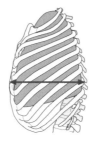

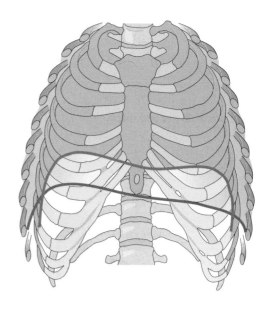

A Anterior view.

B Left lateral view.

C Position of diaphragm during respiration. Blue line = expiration, red line = inspiration.

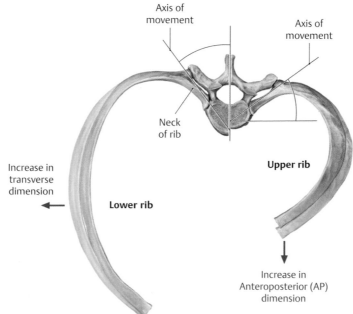

Axis of movement

Axis of movement

Neck of rib

Upper rib

Increase in transverse dimension

Lower rib

Increase in Anteroposterior (AP) dimension

D Axes of rib movement, superior view.

Fig. 7.7 **Sternocostal joints**

Anterior view with right half of sternum sectioned frontally. True joints are generally found only at ribs 2 to 5; ribs 1, 6, and 7 attach to the sternum by synchondroses.

Fig. 7.8 **Costovertebral joints**

Two synovial joints make up the costovertebral articulation of each rib. The costal tubercle of each rib articulates with the costal facet of its accompanying vertebra (**A**). The head of most ribs articulates with the vertebra of its own number and the vertebra immediately superior. Ribs 1, 11, and 12 typically articulate only with their own vertebrae.

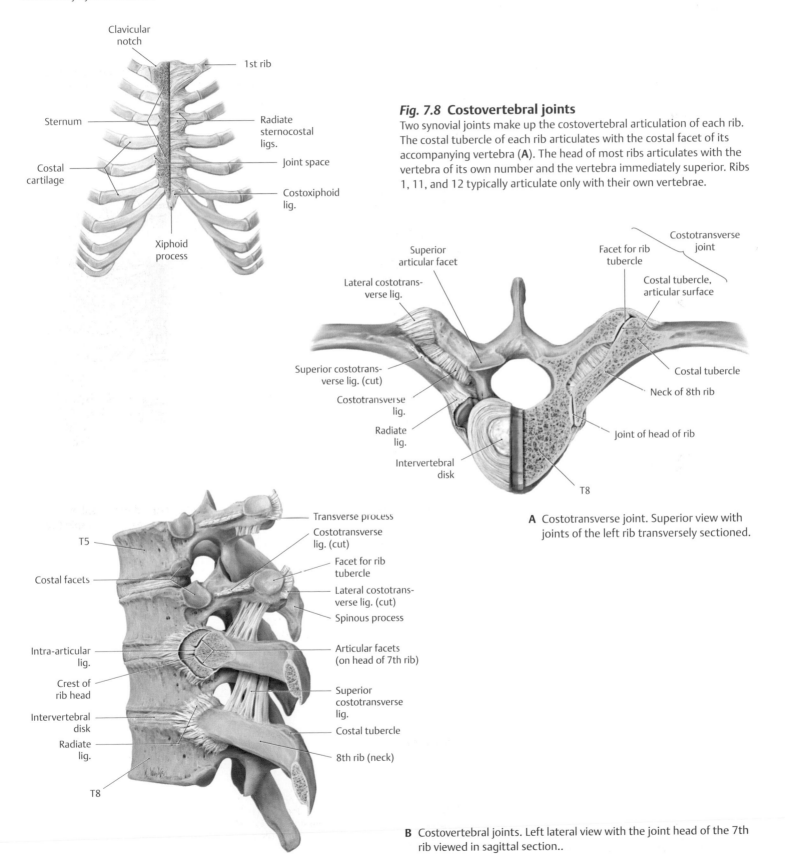

A Costotransverse joint. Superior view with joints of the left rib transversely sectioned.

B Costovertebral joints. Left lateral view with the joint head of the 7th rib viewed in sagittal section..

Thoracic Wall Muscle Facts

The muscles of the thoracic wall are primarily responsible for ribcage movement during respiration, although other muscles aid in *deep* inspiration: the pectoralis major and serratus anterior are discussed with the shoulder (see **pp. 318–319**), and the serratus posterior is discussed with the back (see **p. 32**).

Fig. 7.9 **Muscles of the thoracic wall**

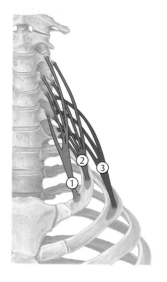

A Scalene muscles, anterior view.

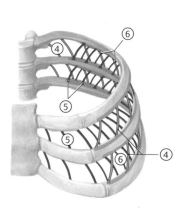

B Intercostal muscles, anterior view.

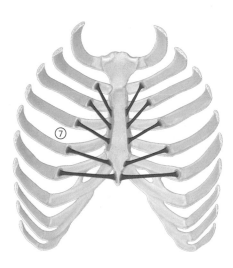

C Transversus thoracis, posterior view.

Table 7.2	**Muscles of the thoracic wall**				
Muscle		**Origin**	**Insertion**	**Innervation**	**Action**
Scalene mm.	① Anterior scalene m.	C3–C6 (transverse processes, anterior tubercles)	1st rib (anterior scalene tubercle)	Anterior rami of C4–C6 spinal nn.	*With ribs mobile*: Elevates upper ribs (inspiration) *With ribs fixed*: Flexes cervical spine to same side (unilateral); flexes neck (bilateral)
	② Middle scalene m.	C1–C2 (transverse processes) C3–C7 (transverse processes, posterior tubercles)	1st rib (posterior to groove for subclavian a.)	Anterior rami of C3–C8 spinal nn.	
	③ Posterior scalene m.	C5–C7 (transverse processes, posterior tubercles)	2nd rib (outer surface)	Anterior rami of C6–C8 spinal nn.	
Intercostal mm.	④ External intercostal mm.	Lower margin of rib to upper margin of next lower rib (courses obliquely forward and downward from costal tubercle to chondro-osseous junction)		1st to 11th intercostal nn.	Elevates ribs (inspiration); supports intercostal spaces; stabilizes chest wall
	⑤ Internal intercostal mm.	Lower margin of rib to upper margin of next lower rib (courses obliquely forward and upward from costal angle to sternum)			Depresses ribs (expiration); supports intercostal spaces, stabilizes chest wall
	⑥ Innermost intercostal mm.				
Subcostal mm.		Lower margin of lower ribs to inner surface of ribs two to three ribs below		Adjacent intercostal nn.	Depresses ribs (expiration)
⑦ Transversus thoracis m.		Sternum and xiphoid process (inner surface)	2nd to 6th ribs (costal cartilage, inner surface)	2nd to 6th intercostal nn.	Weakly depresses ribs (expiration)

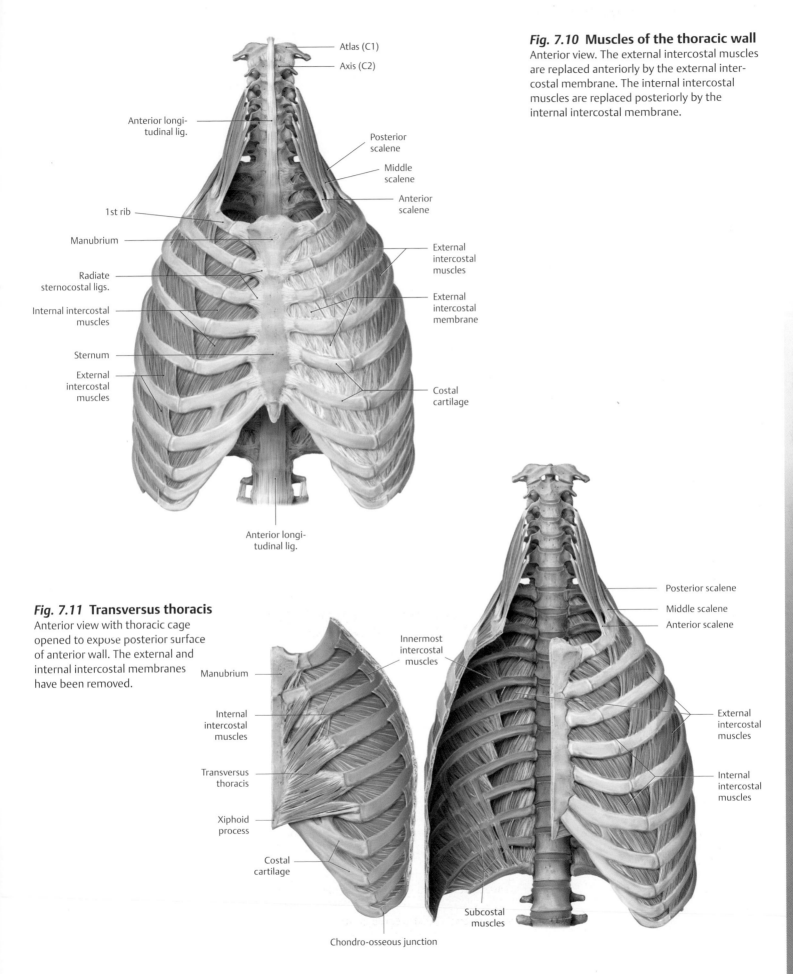

Atlas (C1)

Axis (C2)

Anterior longi-
tudinal lig.

Posterior
scalene

Middle
scalene

Anterior
scalene

1st rib

Manubrium

External
intercostal
muscles

Radiate
sternocostal ligs.

External
intercostal
membrane

Internal intercostal
muscles

Sternum

External
intercostal
muscles

Costal
cartilage

Anterior longi-
tudinal lig.

Fig. 7.10 Muscles of the thoracic wall
Anterior view. The external intercostal muscles
are replaced anteriorly by the external intercostal membrane. The internal intercostal
muscles are replaced posteriorly by the
internal intercostal membrane.

Fig. 7.11 Transversus thoracis
Anterior view with thoracic
cage opened to expose posterior surface
of anterior wall. The external and
internal intercostal membranes
have been removed.

Manubrium

Internal
intercostal
muscles

Transversus
thoracis

Xiphoid
process

Costal
cartilage

Chondro-osseous junction

Innermost
intercostal
muscles

Posterior scalene

Middle scalene

Anterior scalene

External
intercostal
muscles

Internal
intercostal
muscles

Subcostal
muscles

Diaphragm

Fig. 7.12 **Diaphragm**

The diaphragm, which separates the thorax from the abdomen, has two asymmetric domes and three apertures (for the aorta, vena cava, and esophagus; see **Fig. 7.13C**).

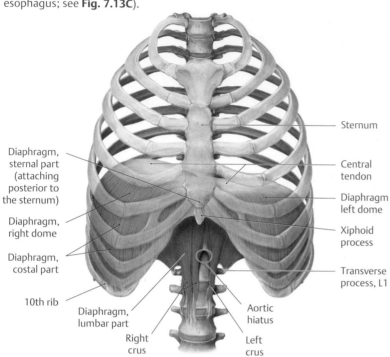

Diaphragm, sternal part (attaching posterior to the sternum)

Diaphragm, right dome

Diaphragm, costal part

10th rib

Diaphragm, lumbar part

Right crus

Sternum

Central tendon

Diaphragm left dome

Xiphoid process

Transverse process, L1

Aortic hiatus

Left crus

A Anterior view.

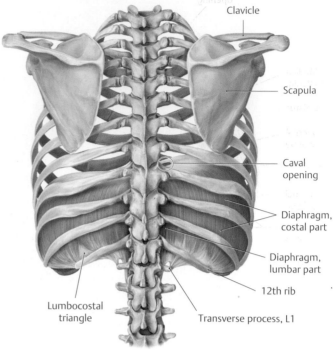

Clavicle

Scapula

Caval opening

Diaphragm, costal part

Diaphragm, lumbar part

12th rib

Transverse process, L1

Lumbocostal triangle

B Posterior view.

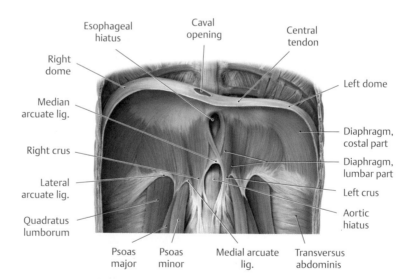

Esophageal hiatus

Caval opening

Central tendon

Right dome

Median arcuate lig.

Right crus

Lateral arcuate lig.

Quadratus lumborum

Left dome

Diaphragm, costal part

Diaphragm, lumbar part

Left crus

Aortic hiatus

Psoas major

Psoas minor

Medial arcuate lig.

Transversus abdominis

C Coronal section with diaphragm in intermediate position.

Table 7.3	**Diaphragm**				
Muscle		**Origin**	**Insertion**	**Innervation**	**Action**
Diaphragm	Costal part	7th to 12th ribs (inner surface; lower margin of costal arch)	Central tendon	Phrenic n. (C3–C5, cervical plexus)	Principal muscle of respiration (diaphragmatic and thoracic breathing); aids in compressing abdominal viscera (abdominal press)
	Lumbar part	Medial part: L1–L3 vertebral bodies, intervertebral disks, and anterior longitudinal lig. as right and left crura			
		Lateral parts: lateral and medial arcuate ligs.			
	Sternal part	Xiphoid process (posterior surface)			

Fig. 7.13 Diaphragm in situ

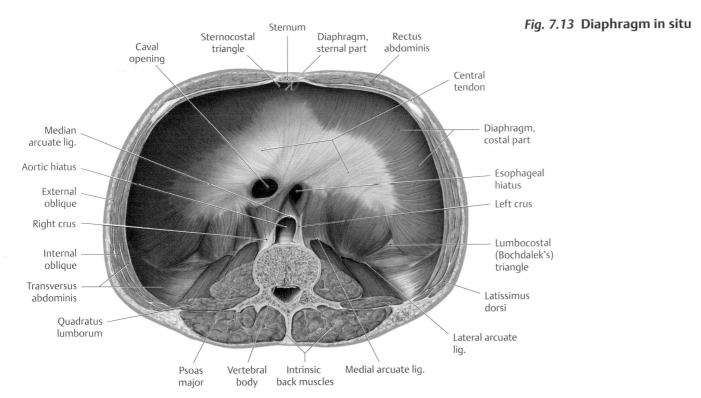

Caval opening
Sternocostal triangle
Sternum
Diaphragm, sternal part
Rectus abdominis
Central tendon
Median arcuate lig.
Diaphragm, costal part
Aortic hiatus
Esophageal hiatus
External oblique
Left crus
Right crus
Internal oblique
Lumbocostal (Bochdalek's) triangle
Transversus abdominis
Latissimus dorsi
Quadratus lumborum
Lateral arcuate lig.
Psoas major
Vertebral body
Intrinsic back muscles
Medial arcuate lig.

A Inferior view.

Sternum
Diaphragm, sternal part
Central tendon
Caval opening
Diaphragm, costal part
Intercostal muscles
Aortic hiatus
Esophageal hiatus
T8
Rib
Intrinsic back muscles
Parietal pleura, costal part

B Superior view.

T8
Inferior vena cava
Esophagus
T10
T12
Aorta

C Diaphragmatic apertures, left lateral view.

Neurovascular Topography of the Thoracic Wall

Fig. 7.26 Anterior structures
Anterior view (see Chapter 4 for neurovasculature of the back).

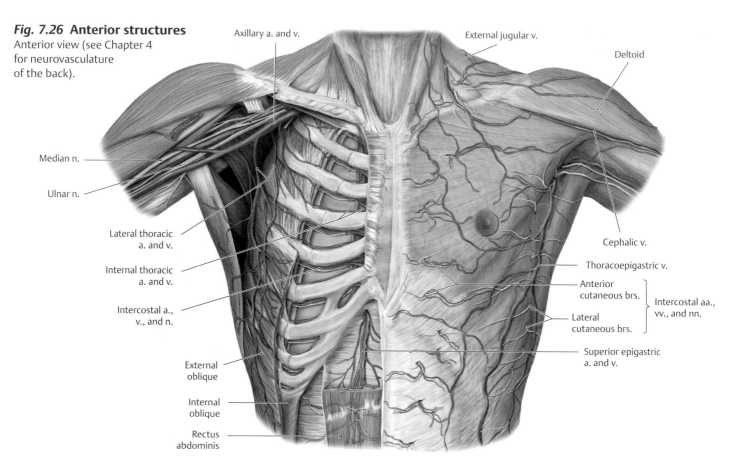

Labels: Axillary a. and v. · External jugular v. · Deltoid · Median n. · Ulnar n. · Lateral thoracic a. and v. · Internal thoracic a. and v. · Intercostal a., v., and n. · External oblique · Internal oblique · Rectus abdominis · Cephalic v. · Thoracoepigastric v. · Anterior cutaneous brs. · Lateral cutaneous brs. · Intercostal aa., vv., and nn. · Superior epigastric a. and v.

⚕ **Clinical box 7.1**

Insertion of a chest tube

Abnormal fluid collection in the pleural space (e.g., pleural effusion due to bronchial carcinoma) may necessitate the insertion of a chest tube. Generally, the optimal puncture site in a sitting patient is at the level of the 4th or 5th intercostal space in the mid to anterior axillary line, immediately behind the lateral edge of the pectoralis major. The drain should always be introduced at the upper margin of a rib to avoid injuring the intercostal vein, artery, and nerve. See **Clinical box 10.5** on **p. 123** for details on collapsed lungs.

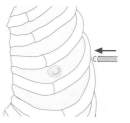

Labels: Pleural effusion · Parietal pleura · Visceral pleura · Rib · Pleural space · Innermost intercostal · Pectoralis major · Costal groove · Intercostal v., a., and n. · Endothoracic fascia · Chest tube · Puncture site · Internal and external intercostal muscles

A Coronal section, anterior view.

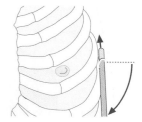

B Drainage tube is inserted perpendicular to chest wall.

C At ribs, the tube is angled and advanced parallel to the chest wall in the subcutaneous plane.

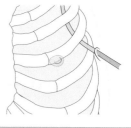

D At the superior margin of the rib, the tube is passed through the intercostal muscles and advanced into the pleural cavity.

Fig. 7.27 Intercostal structures in cross section

Transverse section, anterosuperior view. The relationship of the intercostal vessels in the costal groove, from superior to inferior, is vein, artery, and nerve (see clinical box, **p. 72**).

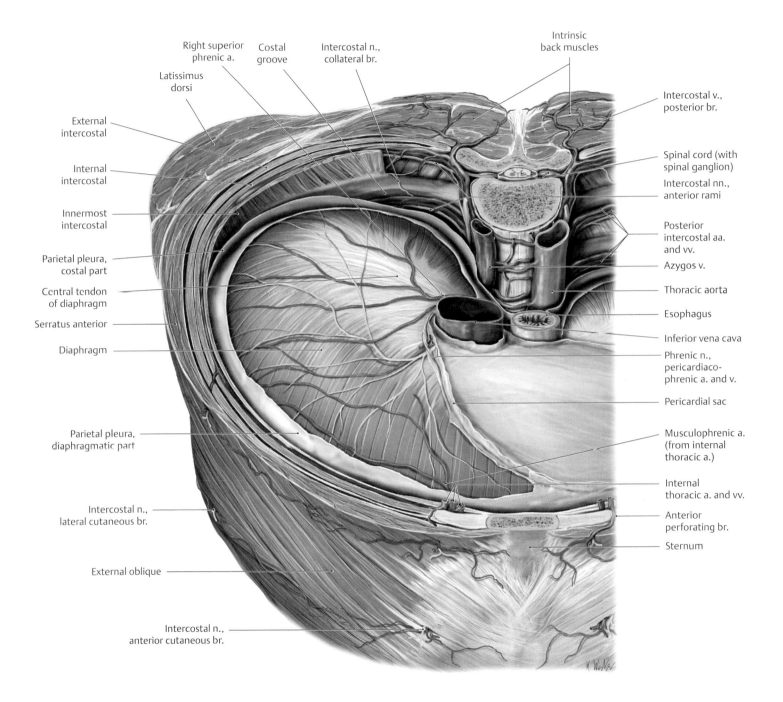

Right superior
phrenic a.

Costal
groove

Intercostal n.,
collateral br.

Latissimus
dorsi

Intrinsic
back muscles

External
intercostal

Intercostal v.,
posterior br.

Internal
intercostal

Spinal cord (with
spinal ganglion)

Intercostal nn.,
anterior rami

Innermost
intercostal

Posterior
intercostal aa.
and vv.

Parietal pleura,
costal part

Azygos v.

Central tendon
of diaphragm

Thoracic aorta

Serratus anterior

Esophagus

Diaphragm

Inferior vena cava

Phrenic n.,
pericardiaco-
phrenic a. and v.

Pericardial sac

Parietal pleura,
diaphragmatic part

Musculophrenic a.
(from internal
thoracic a.)

Internal
thoracic a. and vv.

Intercostal n.,
lateral cutaneous br.

Anterior
perforating br.

Sternum

External oblique

Intercostal n.,
anterior cutaneous br.

8 Thoracic Cavity

Divisions of the Thoracic Cavity

The thoracic cavity is divided into three large spaces: the mediastinum (**p. 90**) and the two pleural (pulmonary) cavities (**p. 112**).

***Fig. 8.1* Thoracic cavity**
Coronal section, anterior view.

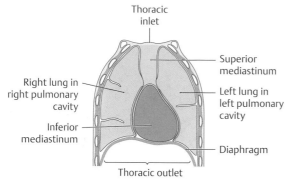

A Divisions of the thoracic cavity.

Table 8.1	Major structures of the thoracic cavity		
Mediastinum	Superior mediastinum		Thymus, great vessels, trachea, esophagus, and thoracic duct
	Inferior mediastinum	Anterior	Thymus (especially in children)
		Middle	Heart, pericardium, and roots of great vessels
		Posterior	Thoracic aorta, thoracic duct, esophagus, and azygos venous system
Pulmonary cavities	Right pulmonary cavity		Right lung
	Left pulmonary cavity		Left lung

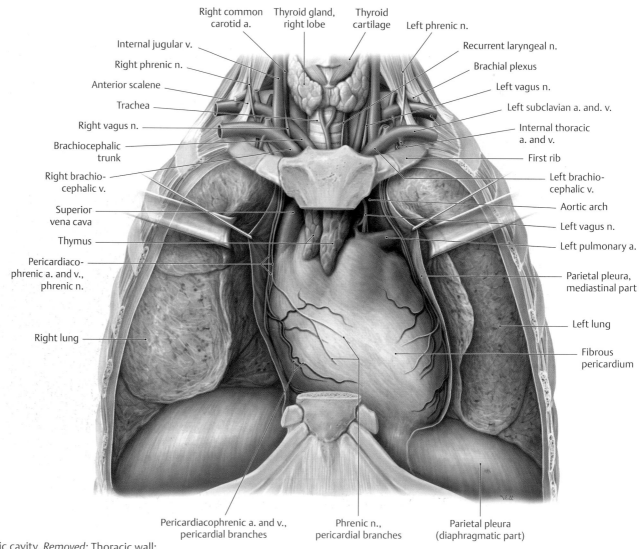

B Opened thoracic cavity. *Removed:* Thoracic wall; connective tissue of anterior mediastinum.

Fig. 8.2 Divisions of the mediastinum

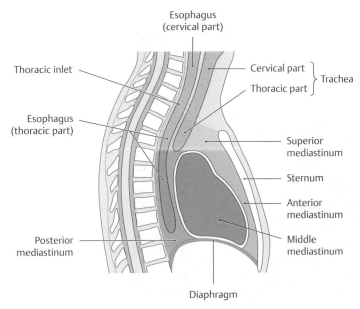

A Midsagittal section, lateral view.

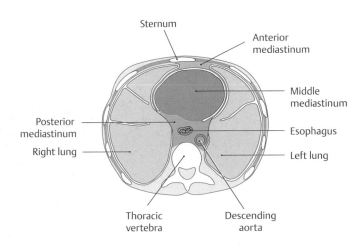

B Transverse section, inferior view.

Fig. 8.3 Transverse sections of the thorax

Computed tomography (CT) scan of thorax, inferior view.

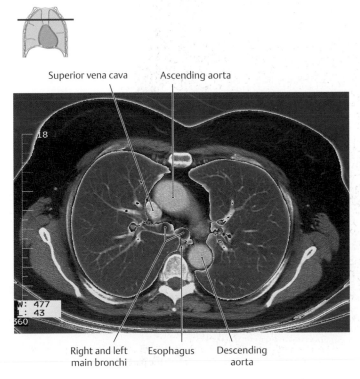

A Superior mediastinum.

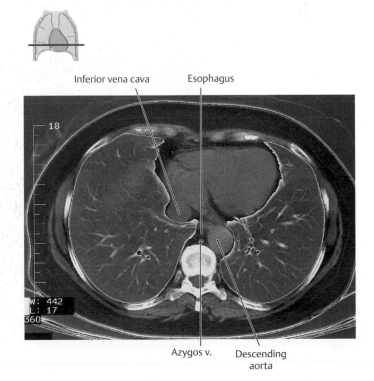

B Inferior mediastinum.

Arteries of the Thoracic Cavity

The arch of the aorta has three major branches: the brachiocephalic trunk, left common carotid artery, and left subclavian artery. After the aortic arch, the aorta begins its descent, becoming the thoracic aorta at the level of the sternal angle and the abdominal aorta once it passes through the aortic hiatus in the diaphragm.

Fig. 8.4 **Thoracic aorta**

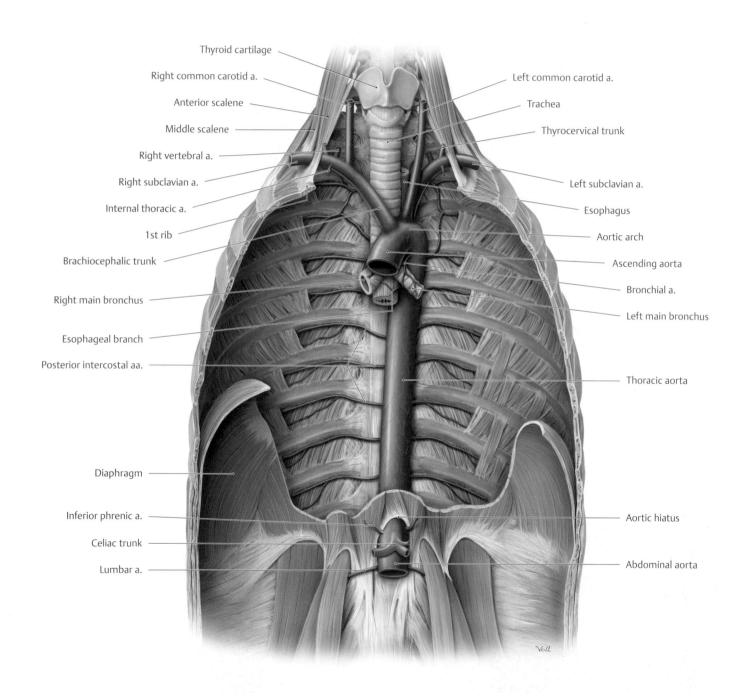

A Thoracic aorta in situ, anterior view. *Removed:* Heart, lungs, portions of diaphragm.

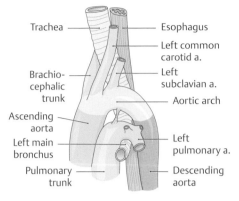

B Parts of the aorta, left lateral view. *Note:* The aortic arch begins and ends at the level of the sternal angle (see **p. 58**).

Table 8.2	**Branches of the thoracic aorta**

The thoracic organs are supplied by direct branches from the thoracic aorta, as well as indirect branches from the subclavian arteries.

Part of aorta	Branches			Region supplied
○ Ascending aorta	Right and left coronary aa.			Heart Bronchi, trachea, esophagus
○ Arch of aorta	Brachiocephalic trunk	Right subclavian a.		See left subclavian a.
		Right common carotid a.		Head and neck
	Left common carotid a.			
	Left subclavian a.	Vertebral a.		
		Internal thoracic a.	Anterior intercostal aa.	Anterior chest wall
			Thymic brs.	Thymus
			Mediastinal brs.	Posterior mediastinum
			Pericardiacophrenic a.	Pericardium, diaphragm
		Thyrocervical trunk	Inferior thyroid a.	Esophagus, trachea, thyroid gland
		Costocervical trunk	Superior intercostal a.	Chest wall
○ Descending aorta	Visceral brs.			Bronchi, trachea, esophagus
	Parietal brs.	Posterior intercostal aa.		Posterior chest wall
		Superior phrenic aa.		Diaphragm

✳ Clinical box 8.1

Aortic dissection

A tear in the inner wall (intima) of the aorta allows blood to separate the layers of the aortic wall, creating a "false lumen" and potentially resulting in life-threatening aortic rupture. Symptoms are dyspnea (shortness of breath) and sudden onset of excruciating pain. Acute aortic dissections occur most often in the ascending aorta and generally require surgery. More distal aortic dissections may be treated conservatively, provided there are no complications (e.g., obstruction of blood supply to the organs, in which case a stent may be inserted to restore perfusion). Aortic dissections occurring at the base of a coronary artery may cause myocardial infarction.

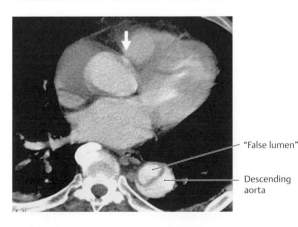

A Aortic dissection. Parts of the intima are still attached to the connective tissue in the wall of the aorta (*arrow*).

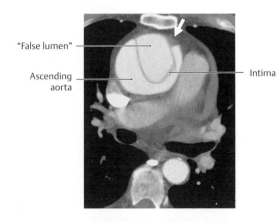

B The flow in the coronary arteries is intact (*arrow*).

Veins of the Thoracic Cavity

The superior vena cava is formed by the union of the two brachio-cephalic veins at the level of the T2–T3 junction. It receives blood drained by the azygos system (the inferior vena cava has no tributaries in the thorax).

***Fig. 8.5* Superior vena cava and azygos system**

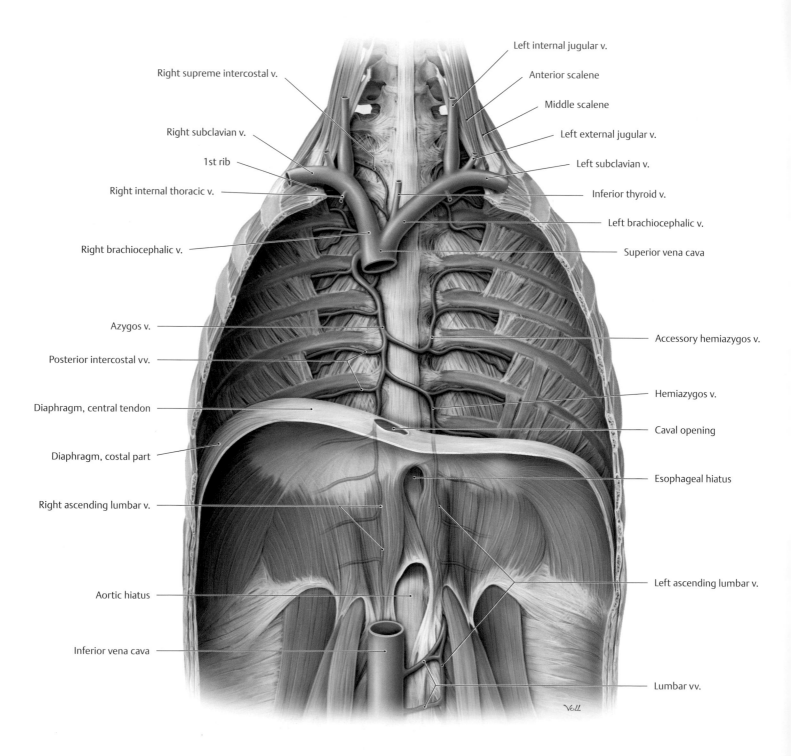

A Veins of the thoracic cavity (viscera removed), anterior view of opened thorax (posterior thoracic wall).

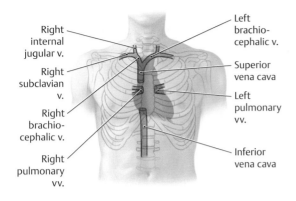

Right internal jugular v.

Left brachio-cephalic v.

Right subclavian v.

Superior vena cava

Right brachio-cephalic v.

Left pulmonary vv.

Right pulmonary vv.

Inferior vena cava

B Projection of venae cavae onto chest, anterior view.

Table 8.3	Thoracic tributaries of the superior vena cava			
Major vein	**Tributaries**			**Region drained**
Brachiocephalic vv.	Inferior thyroid v.			Esophagus, trachea, thyroid gland
	Internal jugular vv.			Head, neck, upper limb
	External jugular vv.			
	Subclavian vv.			
	Supreme intercostal vv.			
	Pericardial vv.			
	Left superior intercostal v.			
Azygos system (left side: accessory hemiazygos v.; right side: azygos v.)	Visceral brs.			Trachea, bronchi, esophagus
	Parietal brs.	Posterior intercostal vv.		Inner chest wall and diaphragm
		Superior phrenic vv.		
		Right superior intercostal v.		
Internal thoracic v.	Thymic vv.			Thymus
	Mediastinal tributaries			Posterior mediastinum
	Anterior intercostal vv.			Anterior chest wall
	Pericardiacophrenic v.			Pericardium
	Musculophrenic v.			Diaphragm

Note: Structures of the superior mediastinum may also drain directly to the brachiocephalic veins via the tracheal, esophageal, and mediastinal veins.

Fig. 8.6 Azygos system
Anterior view.

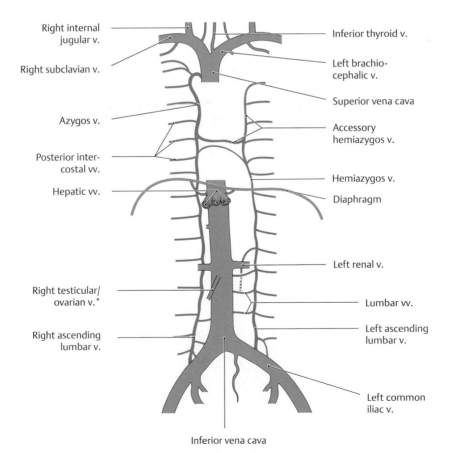

Right internal jugular v.

Inferior thyroid v.

Right subclavian v.

Left brachio-cephalic v.

Superior vena cava

Azygos v.

Accessory hemiazygos v.

Posterior inter-costal vv.

Hemiazygos v.

Hepatic vv.

Diaphragm

Left renal v.

Right testicular/ovarian v.*

Lumbar vv.

Right ascending lumbar v.

Left ascending lumbar v.

Left common iliac v.

Inferior vena cava

*The left testicular/ovarian vein drains to the left renal vein.

Lymphatics of the Thoracic Cavity

The body's chief lymph vessel is the thoracic duct. Beginning in the abdomen at the level of L1 at the *cisterna chyli*, the thoracic duct empties into the junction of the left internal jugular and subclavian veins. The right lymphatic duct drains to the right junction of the internal jugular and subclavian veins.

Fig. 8.7 Lymphatic trunks in the thorax
Anterior view of opened thorax.

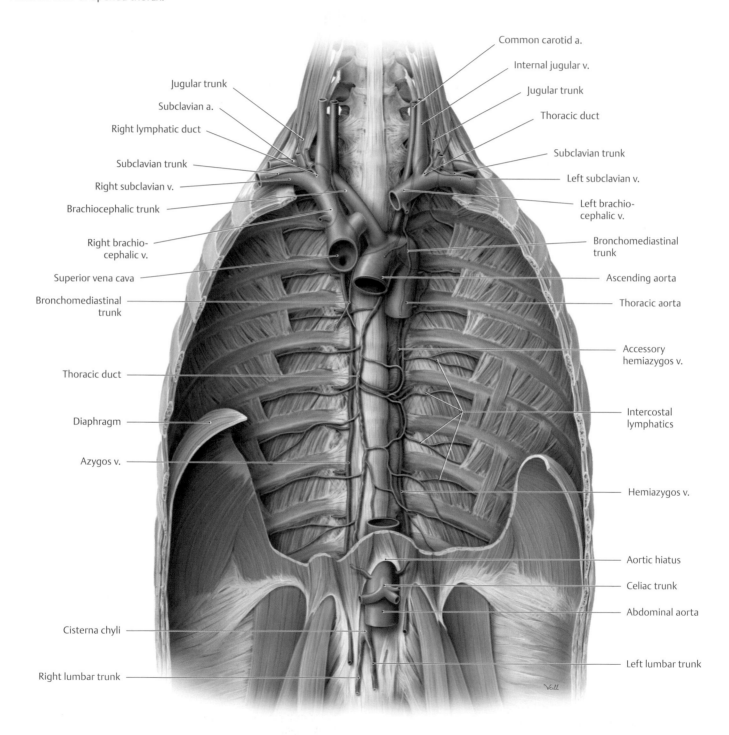

Labels on the figure:
- Jugular trunk
- Subclavian a.
- Right lymphatic duct
- Subclavian trunk
- Right subclavian v.
- Brachiocephalic trunk
- Right brachio-cephalic v.
- Superior vena cava
- Bronchomediastinal trunk
- Thoracic duct
- Diaphragm
- Azygos v.
- Cisterna chyli
- Right lumbar trunk
- Common carotid a.
- Internal jugular v.
- Jugular trunk
- Thoracic duct
- Subclavian trunk
- Left subclavian v.
- Left brachio-cephalic v.
- Bronchomediastinal trunk
- Ascending aorta
- Thoracic aorta
- Accessory hemiazygos v.
- Intercostal lymphatics
- Hemiazygos v.
- Aortic hiatus
- Celiac trunk
- Abdominal aorta
- Left lumbar trunk

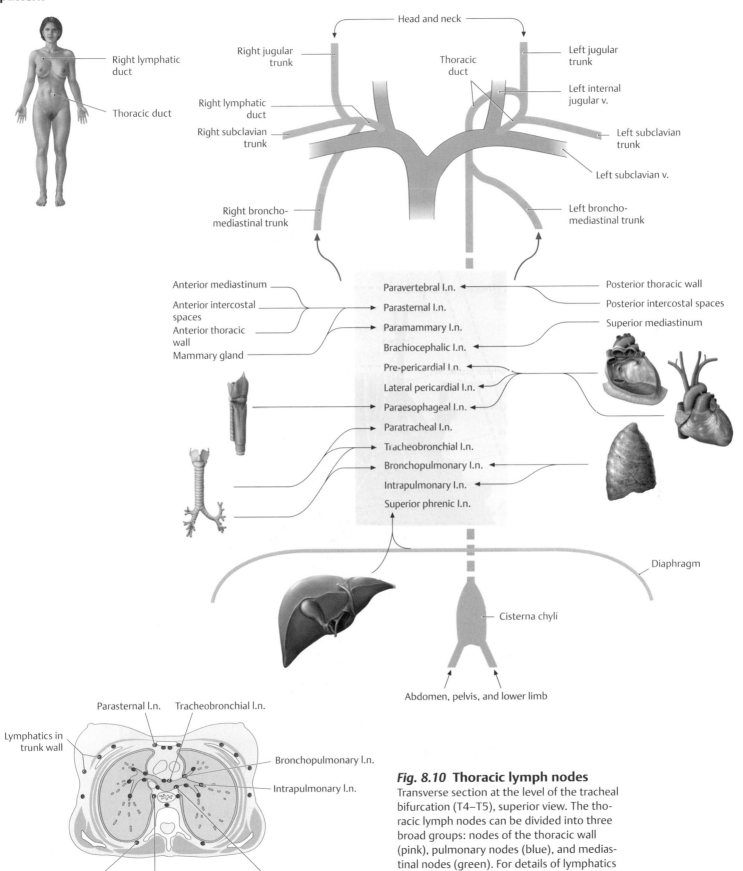

Fig. 8.8 Lymphatic drainage pattern

Right lymphatic duct

Thoracic duct

Fig. 8.9 Lymphatic pathways in the thorax

Head and neck

Right jugular trunk

Thoracic duct

Left jugular trunk

Left internal jugular v.

Right lymphatic duct

Right subclavian trunk

Left subclavian trunk

Left subclavian v.

Right broncho-mediastinal trunk

Left broncho-mediastinal trunk

Anterior mediastinum

Paravertebral l.n.

Posterior thoracic wall

Anterior intercostal spaces

Parasternal l.n.

Posterior intercostal spaces

Anterior thoracic wall

Paramammary l.n.

Superior mediastinum

Mammary gland

Brachiocephalic l.n.

Pre-pericardial l.n.

Lateral pericardial l.n.

Paraesophageal l.n.

Paratracheal l.n.

Tracheobronchial l.n.

Bronchopulmonary l.n.

Intrapulmonary l.n.

Superior phrenic l.n.

Diaphragm

Cisterna chyli

Abdomen, pelvis, and lower limb

Parasternal l.n.   Tracheobronchial l.n.

Lymphatics in trunk wall

Bronchopulmonary l.n.

Intrapulmonary l.n.

Intercostal l.n.   Paraesophageal l.n.   Paratracheal l.n.

Fig. 8.10 Thoracic lymph nodes

Transverse section at the level of the tracheal bifurcation (T4–T5), superior view. The thoracic lymph nodes can be divided into three broad groups: nodes of the thoracic wall (pink), pulmonary nodes (blue), and mediastinal nodes (green). For details of lymphatics of the mediastinum, see **pp. 110–111.**

9 Mediastinum
Mediastinum: Overview

The mediastinum is the space in the thorax between the pleural sacs of the lungs. It is divided into two parts: superior and inferior. The inferior mediastinum is further divided into anterior, middle, and posterior portions.

Fig. 9.1 Divisions of the mediastinum

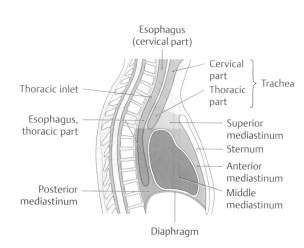

A Schematic.

Table 9.1	Contents of the mediastinum			
	○ **Superior mediastinum**	**Inferior mediastinum**		
		○ *Anterior*	● *Middle*	● *Posterior*
Organs	• Thymus • Trachea • Esophagus	• Thymus, inferior aspects (especially in children)	• Heart • Pericardium	• Esophagus
Arteries	• Aortic arch • Brachiocephalic trunk • Left common carotid a. • Left subclavian a.	• Smaller vessels	• Ascending aorta • Pulmonary trunk and brs. • Pericardiacophrenic aa.	• Thoracic aorta and brs.
Veins and lymph vessels	• Superior vena cava • Brachiocephalic vv. • Thoracic duct and right lymphatic duct	• Smaller vessels, lymphatics, and l.n.	• Superior vena cava • Azygos v. • Pulmonary vv. • Pericardiacophrenic vv.	• Azygos v. • Accessory hemiazygos and hemiazygos vv. • Thoracic duct
Nerves	• Vagus nn. • Left recurrent laryngeal n. • Cardiac nn. • Phrenic nn.	• None	• Phrenic nn.	• Vagus nn.

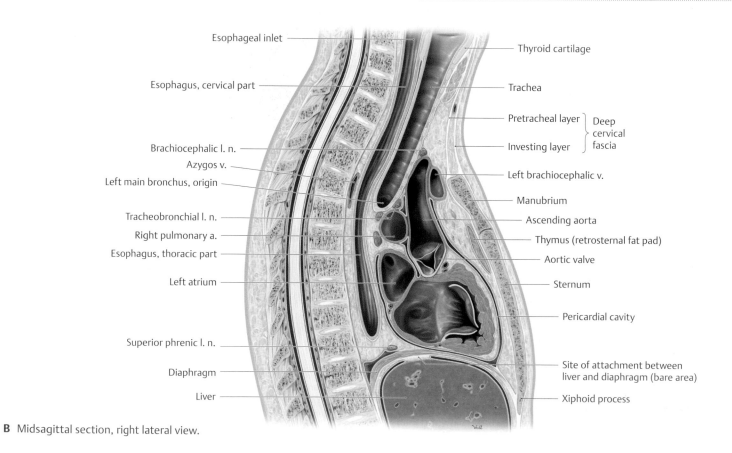

B Midsagittal section, right lateral view.

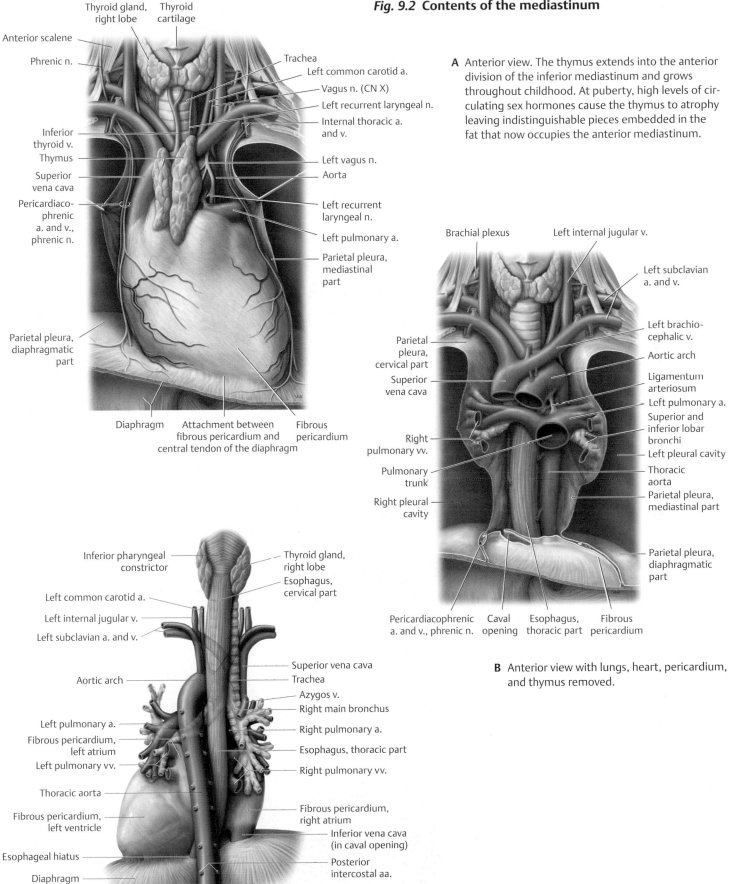

Fig. 9.2 Contents of the mediastinum

Thyroid gland, right lobe
Thyroid cartilage
Anterior scalene
Phrenic n.
Thyroid gland, right lobe
Trachea
Left common carotid a.
Vagus n. (CN X)
Left recurrent laryngeal n.
Internal thoracic a. and v.
Inferior thyroid v.
Thymus
Left vagus n.
Aorta
Superior vena cava
Pericardiaco-phrenic a. and v., phrenic n.
Left recurrent laryngeal n.
Left pulmonary a.
Parietal pleura, mediastinal part
Parietal pleura, diaphragmatic part
Diaphragm
Attachment between fibrous pericardium and central tendon of the diaphragm
Fibrous pericardium

A Anterior view. The thymus extends into the anterior division of the inferior mediastinum and grows throughout childhood. At puberty, high levels of circulating sex hormones cause the thymus to atrophy leaving indistinguishable pieces embedded in the fat that now occupies the anterior mediastinum.

Brachial plexus
Left internal jugular v.
Left subclavian a. and v.
Parietal pleura, cervical part
Superior vena cava
Left brachio-cephalic v.
Aortic arch
Ligamentum arteriosum
Left pulmonary a.
Superior and inferior lobar bronchi
Right pulmonary vv.
Left pleural cavity
Pulmonary trunk
Thoracic aorta
Right pleural cavity
Parietal pleura, mediastinal part
Parietal pleura, diaphragmatic part
Pericardiacophrenic a. and v., phrenic n.
Caval opening
Esophagus, thoracic part
Fibrous pericardium

B Anterior view with lungs, heart, pericardium, and thymus removed.

Inferior pharyngeal constrictor
Thyroid gland, right lobe
Esophagus, cervical part
Left common carotid a.
Left internal jugular v.
Left subclavian a. and v.
Superior vena cava
Trachea
Aortic arch
Azygos v.
Right main bronchus
Left pulmonary a.
Right pulmonary a.
Fibrous pericardium, left atrium
Left pulmonary vv.
Esophagus, thoracic part
Right pulmonary vv.
Thoracic aorta
Fibrous pericardium, left ventricle
Fibrous pericardium, right atrium
Inferior vena cava (in caval opening)
Esophageal hiatus
Posterior intercostal aa.
Diaphragm

C Posterior view.

Mediastinum: Structures

Fig. 9.3 **Mediastinum**

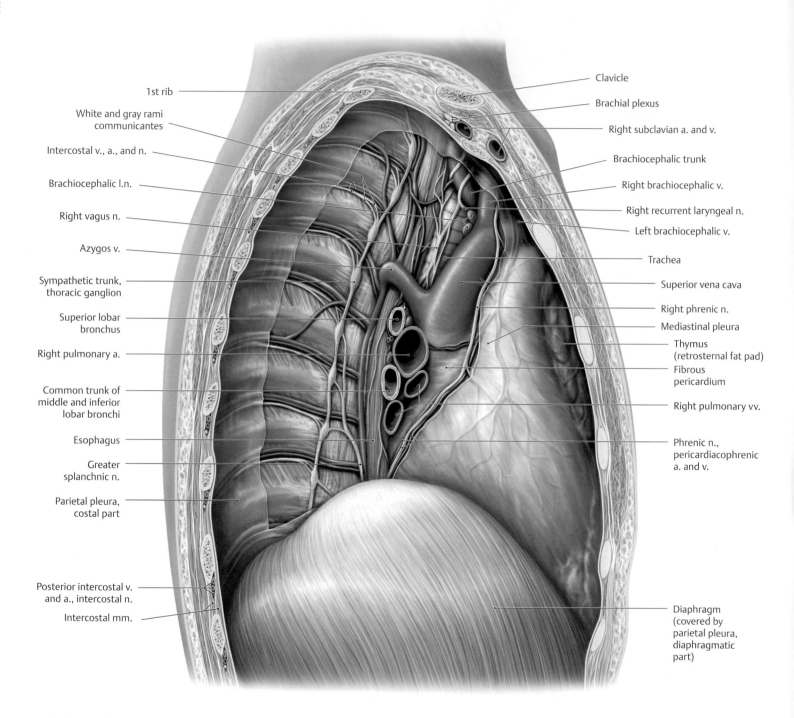

1st rib

White and gray rami communicantes

Intercostal v., a., and n.

Brachiocephalic l.n.

Right vagus n.

Azygos v.

Sympathetic trunk, thoracic ganglion

Superior lobar bronchus

Right pulmonary a.

Common trunk of middle and inferior lobar bronchi

Esophagus

Greater splanchnic n.

Parietal pleura, costal part

Posterior intercostal v. and a., intercostal n.

Intercostal mm.

Clavicle

Brachial plexus

Right subclavian a. and v.

Brachiocephalic trunk

Right brachiocephalic v.

Right recurrent laryngeal n.

Left brachiocephalic v.

Trachea

Superior vena cava

Right phrenic n.

Mediastinal pleura

Thymus (retrosternal fat pad)

Fibrous pericardium

Right pulmonary vv.

Phrenic n., pericardiacophrenic a. and v.

Diaphragm (covered by parietal pleura, diaphragmatic part)

A Right lateral view, parasagittal section. Note the many structures passing between the superior and inferior (middle and posterior) mediastinum.

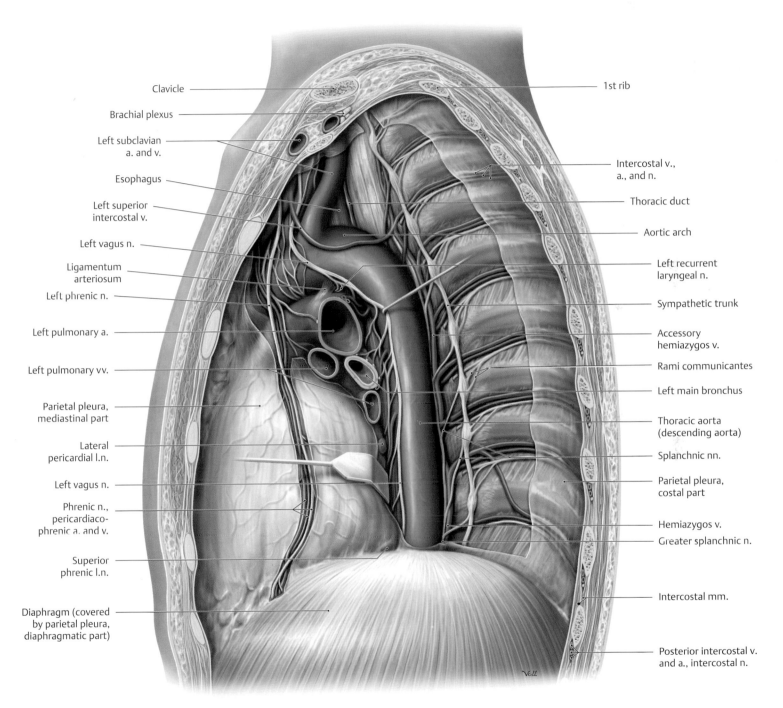

Clavicle

Brachial plexus

Left subclavian
a. and v.

Esophagus

Left superior
intercostal v.

Left vagus n.

Ligamentum
arteriosum

Left phrenic n.

Left pulmonary a.

Left pulmonary vv.

Parietal pleura,
mediastinal part

Lateral
pericardial l.n.

Left vagus n.

Phrenic n.,
pericardiaco-
phrenic a. and v.

Superior
phrenic l.n.

Diaphragm (covered
by parietal pleura,
diaphragmatic part)

1st rib

Intercostal v.,
a., and n.

Thoracic duct

Aortic arch

Left recurrent
laryngeal n.

Sympathetic trunk

Accessory
hemiazygos v.

Rami communicantes

Left main bronchus

Thoracic aorta
(descending aorta)

Splanchnic nn.

Parietal pleura,
costal part

Hemiazygos v.

Greater splanchnic n.

Intercostal mm.

Posterior intercostal v.
and a., intercostal n.

B Left lateral view, parasagittal section. *Removed:* Left lung and parietal
pleura. *Revealed:* Posterior mediastinal structures.

Heart: Functions & Relations

The heart pumps the blood: unoxygenated blood to the lungs and oxygenated blood throughout the body. It is located posterior to the sternum in the middle portion of the mediastinum in the pericardial cavity, located between the right and left pleural cavities containing the lungs. The apex of the cone-shaped heart points anteriorly and to the left in the thoracic cavity.

Fig. 9.4 Circulation

Oxygenated blood is shown in red; deoxygenated blood in blue. See **p. 104** for prenatal circulation.

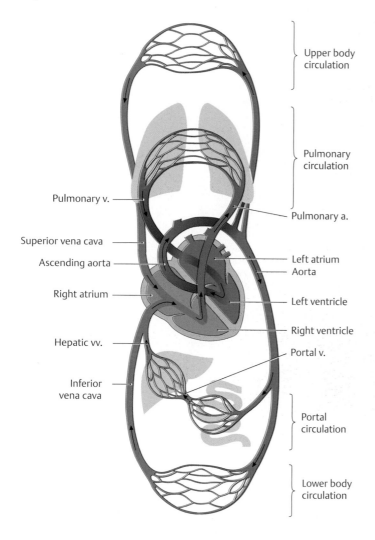

Fig. 9.5 Topographical relations of the heart

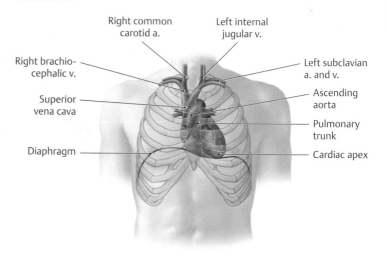

A Projection of the heart and great vessels onto chest, anterior view.

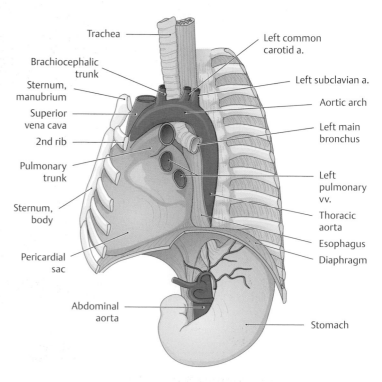

B Left lateral view. *Removed:* Left thoracic wall and left lung.

Fig. 9.6 Heart in situ

A Anterior view of the opened thorax with the thymus removed and flaps of the anterior layer of the pericardial sac reflected to reveal the heart.

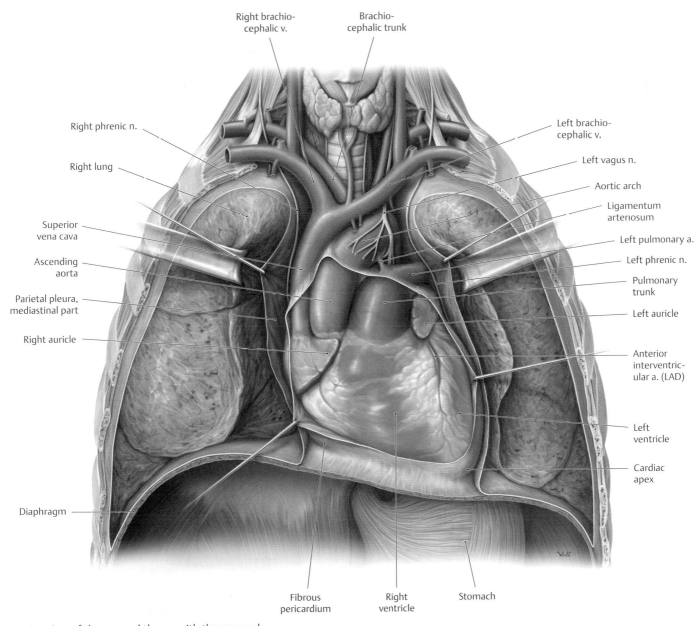

Aortic arch

Superior vena cava

Fibrous pericardium (= external layer)

Serous pericardium, visceral layer (epicardium)

Left lung

Serous pericardium, parietal layer

Parietal pleura, mediastinal part

Cardiac surface

Diaphragm

Right brachio-cephalic v.

Brachio-cephalic trunk

Right phrenic n.

Right lung

Superior vena cava

Ascending aorta

Parietal pleura, mediastinal part

Right auricle

Diaphragm

Left brachio-cephalic v.

Left vagus n.

Aortic arch

Ligamentum arteriosum

Left pulmonary a.

Left phrenic n.

Pulmonary trunk

Left auricle

Anterior interventric-ular a. (LAD)

Left ventricle

Cardiac apex

Fibrous pericardium

Right ventricle

Stomach

B Anterior view of the opened thorax with thymus and anterior pericardium removed to reveal the heart.

Heart: Surfaces & Chambers

Note the reflection of visceral serous pericardium to become parietal serous pericardium.

Fig. 9.11 Surfaces of the heart

The heart has three surfaces: anterior (sternocostal), posterior (base), and inferior (diaphragmatic).

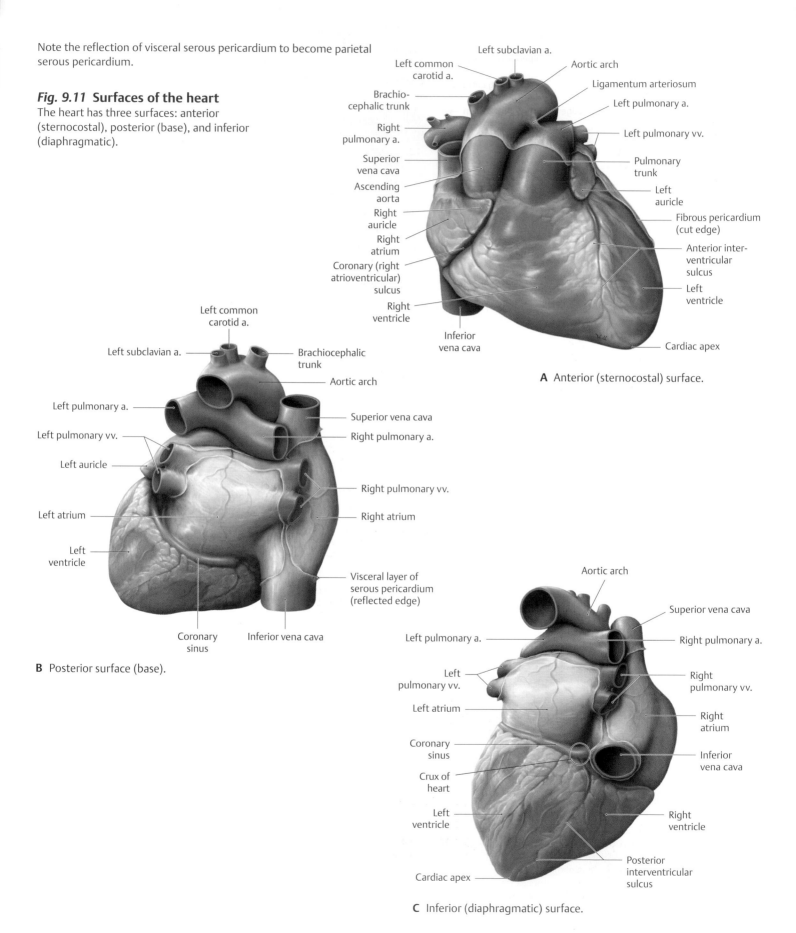

A Anterior (sternocostal) surface.

B Posterior surface (base).

C Inferior (diaphragmatic) surface.

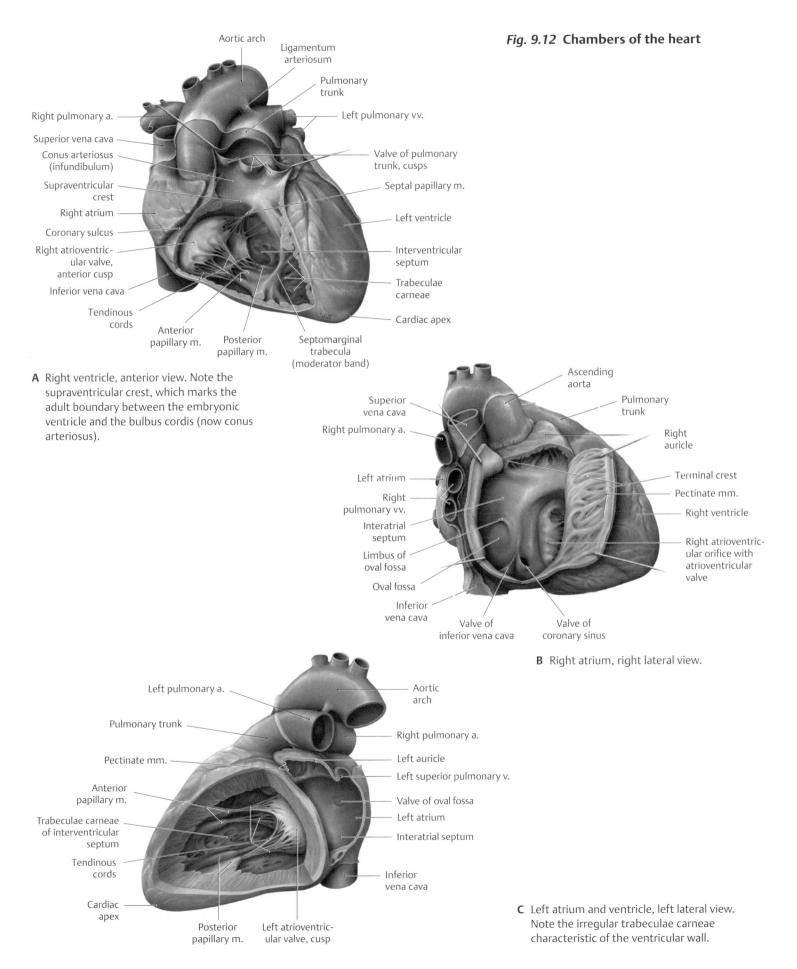

Fig. 9.12 Chambers of the heart

A Right ventricle, anterior view. Note the supraventricular crest, which marks the adult boundary between the embryonic ventricle and the bulbus cordis (now conus arteriosus).

Aortic arch
Ligamentum arteriosum
Pulmonary trunk
Right pulmonary a.
Left pulmonary vv.
Superior vena cava
Conus arteriosus (infundibulum)
Valve of pulmonary trunk, cusps
Supraventricular crest
Septal papillary m.
Right atrium
Left ventricle
Coronary sulcus
Right atrioventricular valve, anterior cusp
Interventricular septum
Inferior vena cava
Trabeculae carneae
Tendinous cords
Cardiac apex
Anterior papillary m.
Posterior papillary m.
Septomarginal trabecula (moderator band)

B Right atrium, right lateral view.

Superior vena cava
Right pulmonary a.
Ascending aorta
Pulmonary trunk
Right auricle
Left atrium
Right pulmonary vv.
Terminal crest
Pectinate mm.
Right ventricle
Interatrial septum
Limbus of oval fossa
Right atrioventricular orifice with atrioventricular valve
Oval fossa
Inferior vena cava
Valve of inferior vena cava
Valve of coronary sinus

C Left atrium and ventricle, left lateral view. Note the irregular trabeculae carneae characteristic of the ventricular wall.

Left pulmonary a.
Aortic arch
Pulmonary trunk
Right pulmonary a.
Pectinate mm.
Left auricle
Left superior pulmonary v.
Anterior papillary m.
Valve of oval fossa
Trabeculae carneae of interventricular septum
Left atrium
Tendinous cords
Interatrial septum
Cardiac apex
Inferior vena cava
Posterior papillary m.
Left atrioventricular valve, cusp

97

Fig. 9.16 Coronary arteries and cardiac veins

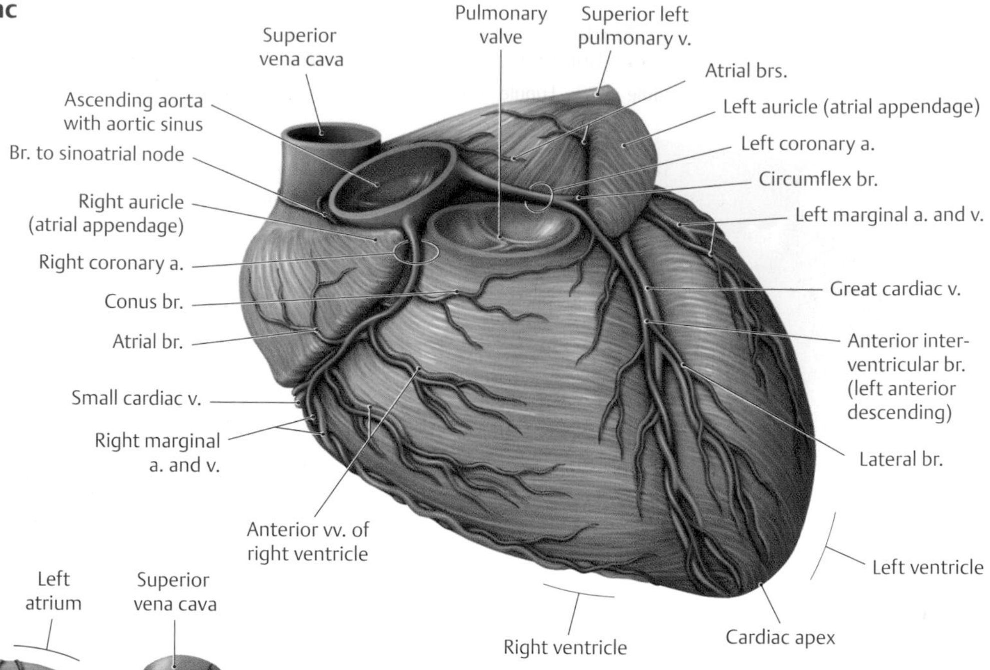

Superior vena cava
Ascending aorta with aortic sinus
Br. to sinoatrial node
Right auricle (atrial appendage)
Right coronary a.
Conus br.
Atrial br.
Small cardiac v.
Right marginal a. and v.
Anterior vv. of right ventricle

Pulmonary valve
Superior left pulmonary v.
Atrial brs.
Left auricle (atrial appendage)
Left coronary a.
Circumflex br.
Left marginal a. and v.
Great cardiac v.
Anterior inter-ventricular br. (left anterior descending)
Lateral br.
Left ventricle
Right ventricle
Cardiac apex

A Anterior view.

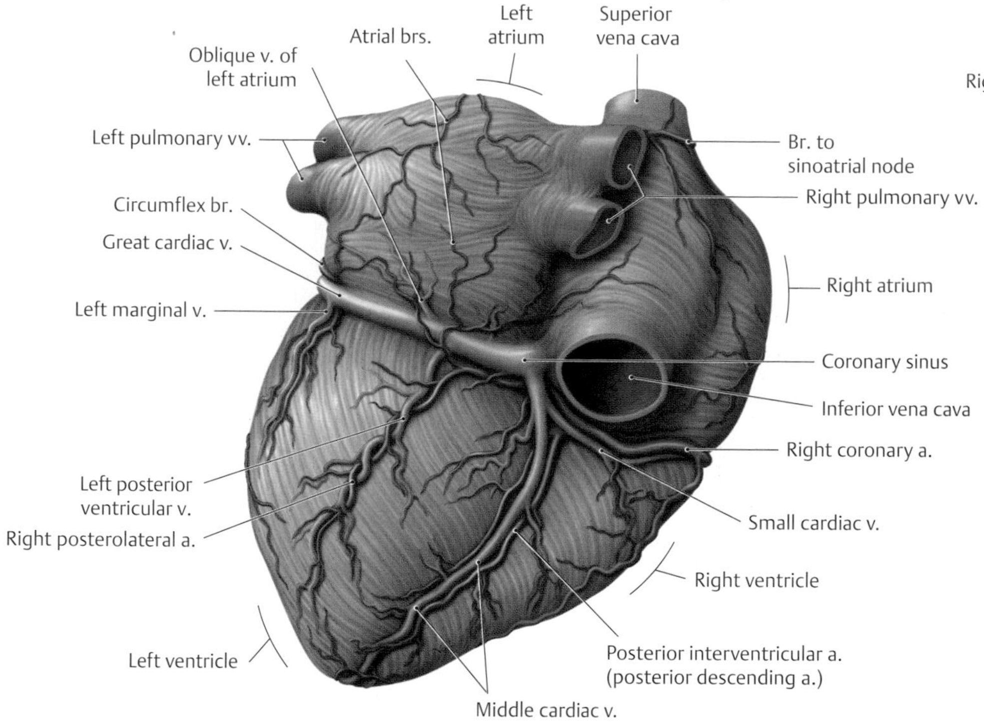

Oblique v. of left atrium
Left pulmonary vv.
Circumflex br.
Great cardiac v.
Left marginal v.
Left posterior ventricular v.
Right posterolateral a.
Left ventricle
Middle cardiac v.

Atrial brs.
Left atrium
Superior vena cava
Br. to sinoatrial node
Right pulmonary vv.
Right atrium
Coronary sinus
Inferior vena cava
Right coronary a.
Small cardiac v.
Right ventricle
Posterior interventricular a. (posterior descending a.)

B Posteroinferior view. *Note:* The right and left coronary arteries typically anastomose posteriorly at the left atrium and ventricle.

Table 9.3	Branches of the coronary arteries
Left coronary artery	**Right coronary artery**
Circumflex br. • Atrial br. • Left marginal a. • Posterior left ventricular br.	Br. to SA node
	Conus br.
	Atrial br.
	Right marginal a.
Anterior interventricular br. (left anterior descending) • Conus br. • Lateral br. • Interventricular septal brs.	Posterior interventricular br. (posterior descending) • Interventricular septal brs.
	Br. to AV node
	Right posterolateral a.
AV, atrioventricular; SA, sinoatrial.	

Table 9.4	Divisions of the cardiac veins	
Vein	**Tributaries**	**Drainage to**
Anterior cardiac vv. (not shown)		Right atrium
Great cardiac v.	Anterior interventricular v.	Coronary sinus
	Left marginal v.	
	Oblique v. of left atrium	
Left posterior ventricular v.		
Middle cardiac v. (posterior interventricular v.)		
Small cardiac v.	Anterior vv. of right ventricle	
	Right marginal v.	

Fig. 9.17 Distribution of the coronary arteries

Anterior and posterior views of the heart, with superior views of transverse sections through the ventricles. The "distribution" of the coronary arteries refers to the area of the myocardium supplied by each artery, as seen in the transverse views, but the term "dominance" refers to the artery that gives rise to the posterior interventricular artery, as seen in the anterior and posterior views. Right coronary artery and branches (green); left coronary artery and branches (red).

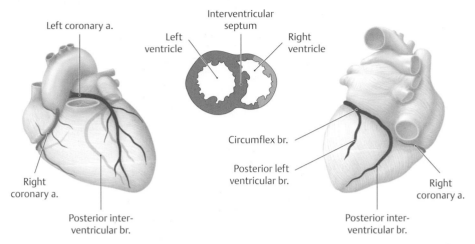

A Left coronary dominance (15–17%).

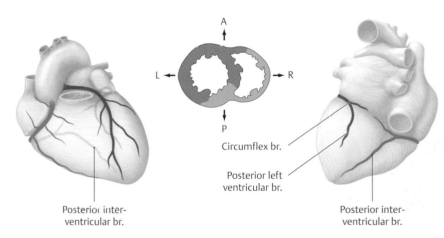

B Balanced distribution, right coronary artery dominance (67–70%).

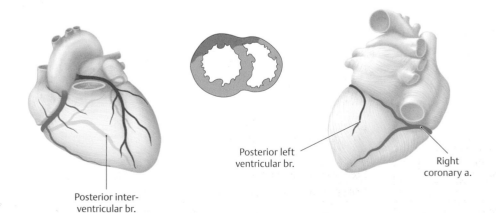

C Right coronary dominance (~15%).

 Clinical box 9.3

Disturbed coronary blood flow

Although the coronary arteries are connected by structural anastomoses, they are end arteries from a functional standpoint. The most frequent cause of deficient blood flow is *atherosclerosis*, a narrowing of the coronary lumen due to plaque-like deposits on the vessel wall. When the decrease in luminal size (stenosis) reaches a critical point, coronary blood flow is restricted, causing chest pain (*angina pectoris*). Initially, this pain is induced by physical effort, but eventually it persists at rest, often radiating to characteristic sites (e.g., medial side of left upper limb, left side of head and neck). A myocardial infarction occurs when deficient blood supply causes myocardial tissue to die (necrosis). The location and extent of the infarction depends on the stenosed vessel (see **A–E**, after Heinecker).

A Supra-apical anterior infarction.

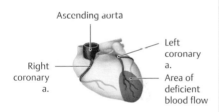

B Apical anterior infarction.

C Anterior lateral infarction.

D Posterior lateral infarction.

E Posterior infarction.

Conduction & Innervation of the Heart

Contraction of cardiac muscle is modulated by the cardiac conduction system. This system of specialized myocardial cells (Purkinje fibers) generates and conducts excitatory impulses in the heart. The conduction system contains two nodes, both located in the right atrium: the sinoatrial (SA) node, known as the pacemaker, and the atrioventricular (AV) node.

Fig. 9.18 Cardiac conduction system

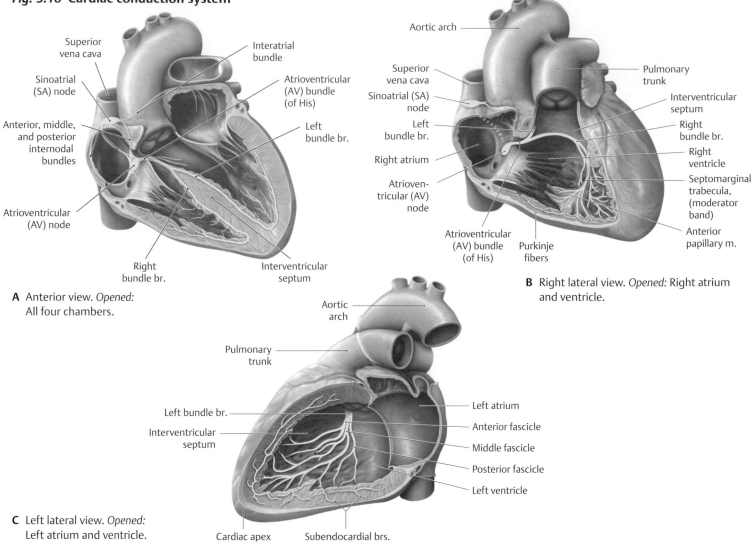

A Anterior view. *Opened:* All four chambers.

B Right lateral view. *Opened:* Right atrium and ventricle.

C Left lateral view. *Opened:* Left atrium and ventricle.

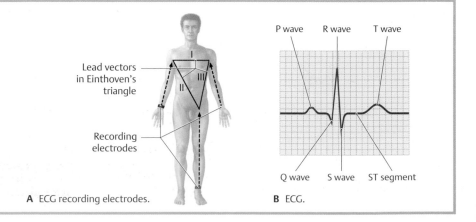

✴ *Clinical box 9.4*

Electrocardiogram (ECG)

The cardiac impulse (a physical dipole) travels across the heart and may be detected with electrodes. The use of three electrodes that separately record electrical activity of the heart along three axes or vectors (Einthoven limb leads) generates an electrocardiogram (ECG). The ECG graphs the cardiac cycle ("heartbeat"), reducing it to a series of waves, segments, and intervals. These ECG components can be used to determine whether cardiac impulses are normal or abnormal (e.g., myocardial infarction, chamber enlargement). *Note:* Although only three leads are required, a standard ECG examination includes at least two others (Goldberger, Wilson leads).

A ECG recording electrodes.

B ECG.

Sympathetic innervation: Preganglionic neurons from T1 to T6 spinal cord segments send fibers to synapse on postganglionic neurons in the cervical and upper thoracic sympathetic ganglia. The three cervical cardiac nerves and thoracic cardiac branches contribute to the cardiac plexus. Parasympathetic innervation: Preganglionic neurons and fibers reach the heart via cardiac branches, some of which also arise in the cervical region. They synapse on postganglionic neurons near the SA node and along the coronary arteries.

Fig. 9.19 Autonomic innervation of the heart

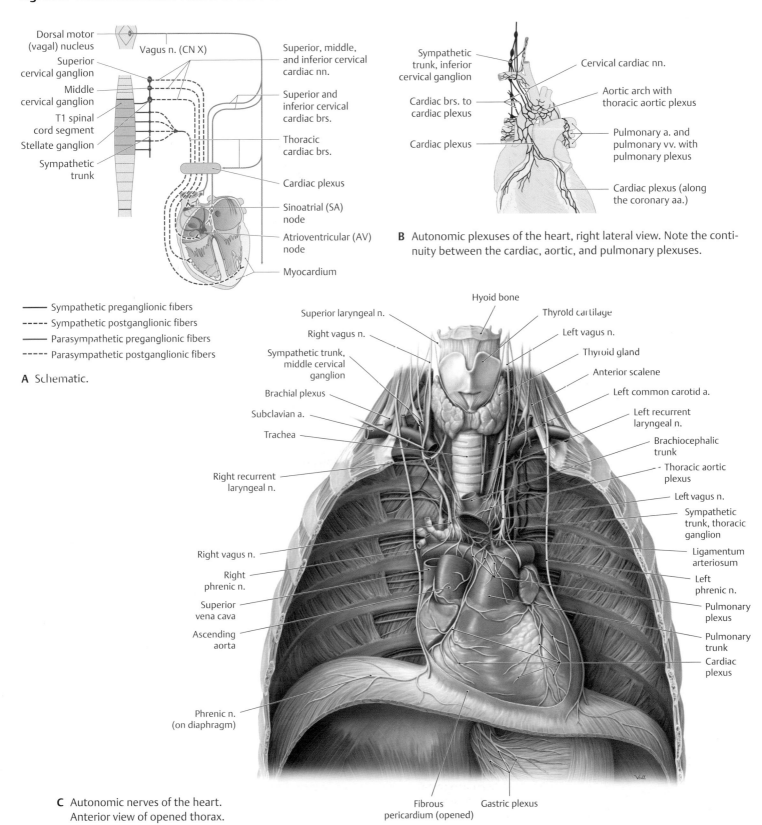

Dorsal motor (vagal) nucleus
Vagus n. (CN X)
Superior cervical ganglion
Middle cervical ganglion
T1 spinal cord segment
Stellate ganglion
Sympathetic trunk

Superior, middle, and inferior cervical cardiac nn.
Superior and inferior cervical cardiac brs.
Thoracic cardiac brs.
Cardiac plexus
Sinoatrial (SA) node
Atrioventricular (AV) node
Myocardium

——— Sympathetic preganglionic fibers
----- Sympathetic postganglionic fibers
——— Parasympathetic preganglionic fibers
----- Parasympathetic postganglionic fibers

A Schematic.

Sympathetic trunk, inferior cervical ganglion
Cardiac brs. to cardiac plexus
Cardiac plexus

Cervical cardiac nn.
Aortic arch with thoracic aortic plexus
Pulmonary a. and pulmonary vv. with pulmonary plexus
Cardiac plexus (along the coronary aa.)

B Autonomic plexuses of the heart, right lateral view. Note the continuity between the cardiac, aortic, and pulmonary plexuses.

Hyoid bone
Superior laryngeal n.
Right vagus n.
Sympathetic trunk, middle cervical ganglion
Brachial plexus
Subclavian a.
Trachea
Right recurrent laryngeal n.
Right vagus n.
Right phrenic n.
Superior vena cava
Ascending aorta
Phrenic n. (on diaphragm)

Thyroid cartilage
Left vagus n.
Thyroid gland
Anterior scalene
Left common carotid a.
Left recurrent laryngeal n.
Brachiocephalic trunk
Thoracic aortic plexus
Left vagus n.
Sympathetic trunk, thoracic ganglion
Ligamentum arteriosum
Left phrenic n.
Pulmonary plexus
Pulmonary trunk
Cardiac plexus

Fibrous pericardium (opened)
Gastric plexus

C Autonomic nerves of the heart. Anterior view of opened thorax.

Pre- & Postnatal Circulation

Fig. 9.20 **Prenatal circulation**
After Fritsch and Kühnel.

① Oxygenated and nutrient-rich fetal blood from the placenta passes to the fetus via the umbilical *vein*.

② Approximately half of this blood bypasses the liver (via the ductus venosus) and enters the inferior vena cava. The remainder enters the portal vein to supply the liver with nutrients and oxygen.

③ Blood entering the right atrium from the inferior vena cava bypasses the right ventricle (as the lungs are not yet functioning) to enter the left atrium via the oval foramen, a right-to-left shunt.

④ Blood from the superior vena cava enters the right atrium, passes to the right ventricle, and moves into the pulmonary trunk. Most of this blood enters the aorta via the ductus arteriosus, a right-to-left shunt.

⑤ The partially oxygenated blood in the aorta returns to the placenta via the paired umbilical arteries that arise from the internal iliac arteries.

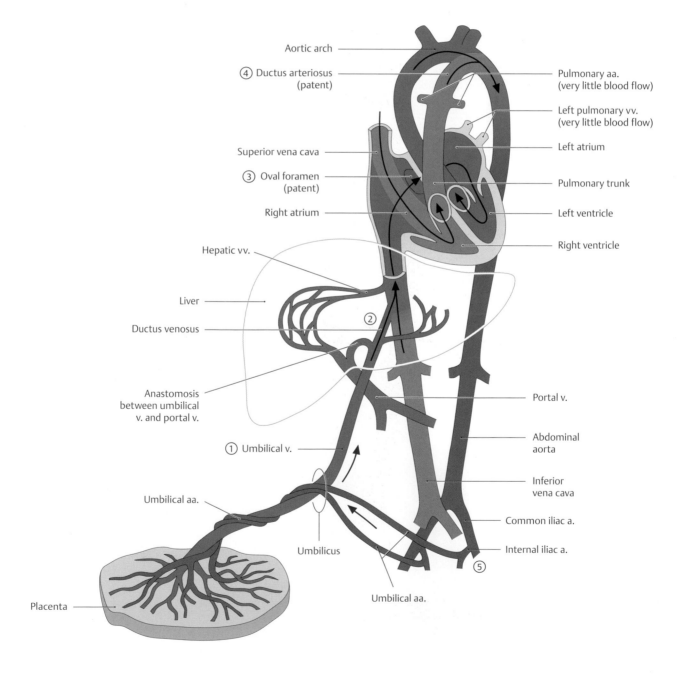

Fig. 9.21 Postnatal circulation

After Fritsch and Kühnel.

① As pulmonary respiration begins at birth, pulmonary blood pressure falls, causing blood from the right pulmonary trunk to enter the pulmonary arteries.

② The foramen ovale and ductus arteriosus close, eliminating the fetal right-to-left shunts. The pulmonary and systemic circulations in the heart are now separate.

③ As the infant is separated from the placenta, the umbilical arteries occlude (except for the proximal portions), along with the umbilical vein and ductus venosus.

④ Blood to be metabolized now passes through the liver.

Table 9.5	Derivatives of fetal circulatory structures
Fetal structure	**Adult remnant**
Ductus arteriosus	Ligamentum arteriosum
Foramen ovale	Oval fossa (fossa ovalis)
Ductus venosus	Ligamentum venosum
Umbilical v.	Round lig. of the liver (ligamentum teres)
Umbilical a.	Medial umbilical lig.

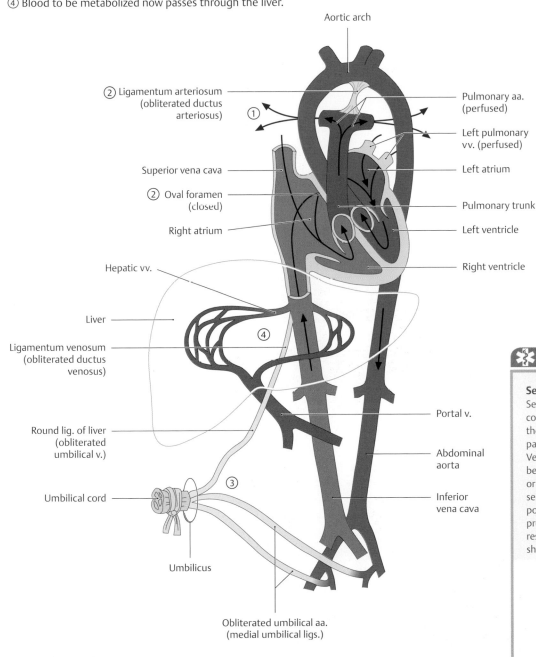

Clinical box 9.5

Septal defects

Septal defects, the most common type of congenital heart defect, allow blood from the left chambers of the heart to improperly pass into the right chambers during systole. Ventricular septal defect (VSD, shown below) is a defect in either the membranous or muscular portion of the ventricular septum—most commonly the membranous portion. Patent foramen ovale, the most prevalent form of *atrial* septal defect (ASD), results from improper closure of the fetal shunt. LV, left ventricle; RV, right ventricle.

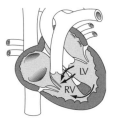

Esophagus

The esophagus is divided into three parts: cervical (C6–T1), thoracic (T1 to the esophageal hiatus of the diaphragm), and abdominal (the diaphragm to the cardiac orifice of the stomach). It descends slightly to the right of the thoracic aorta and pierces the diaphragm slightly to the left, just below the xiphoid process of the sternum.

Fig. 9.22 Esophagus: Location and constrictions

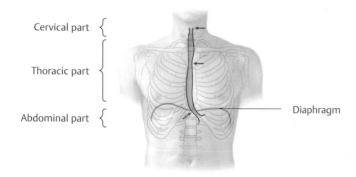

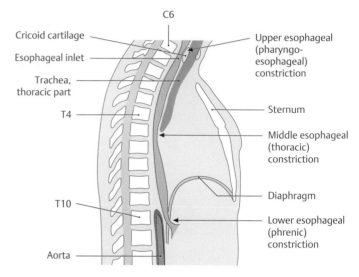

A Projection of esophagus onto chest wall. Esophageal constrictions are indicated with arrows.

B Esophageal constrictions, right lateral view.

Fig. 9.23 Esophagus in situ
Anterior view.

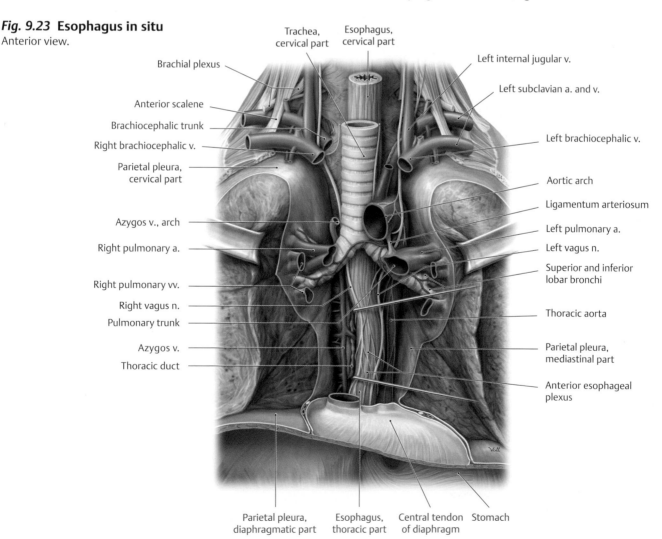

Fig. 9.24 Structure of the esophagus

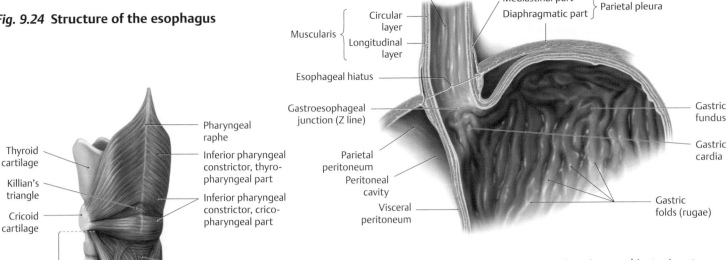

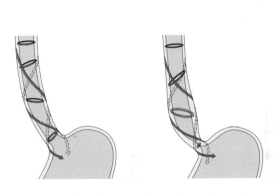

B Esophagogastric junction, anterior view. A true sphincter is not identifiable at this junction; instead, the diaphragmatic muscle of the esophageal hiatus functions as a sphincter. It is often referred to as the "Z line" because of its zigzag form.

A Esophageal wall, oblique left posterior view. Pharynx (**p. 650**); trachea (**p. 120**).

C Functional architecture of esophageal muscle.

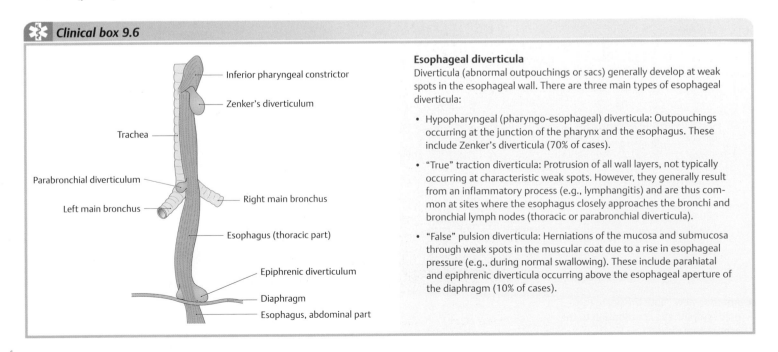

Clinical box 9.6

Esophageal diverticula

Diverticula (abnormal outpouchings or sacs) generally develop at weak spots in the esophageal wall. There are three main types of esophageal diverticula:

- Hypopharyngeal (pharyngo-esophageal) diverticula: Outpouchings occurring at the junction of the pharynx and the esophagus. These include Zenker's diverticula (70% of cases).

- "True" traction diverticula: Protrusion of all wall layers, not typically occurring at characteristic weak spots. However, they generally result from an inflammatory process (e.g., lymphangitis) and are thus common at sites where the esophagus closely approaches the bronchi and bronchial lymph nodes (thoracic or parabronchial diverticula).

- "False" pulsion diverticula: Herniations of the mucosa and submucosa through weak spots in the muscular coat due to a rise in esophageal pressure (e.g., during normal swallowing). These include parahiatal and epiphrenic diverticula occurring above the esophageal aperture of the diaphragm (10% of cases).

Neurovasculature of the Esophagus

Sympathetic innervation: Preganglionic fibers arise from the T2–T6 spinal cord segments. Postganglionic fibers arise from the sympathetic trunk to join the esophageal plexus. Parasympathetic innervation: Preganglionic fibers arise from the dorsal vagal nucleus and travel in the vagus nerves to form the extensive esophageal plexus. *Note:* The postganglionic neurons are in the wall of the esophagus. Fibers to the cervical portion of the esophagus travel in the recurrent laryngeal nerves.

Fig. 9.25 Autonomic innervation of the esophagus

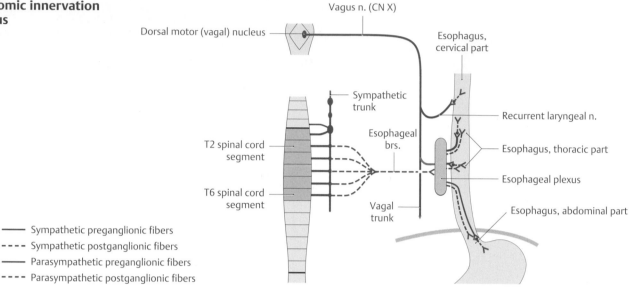

—— Sympathetic preganglionic fibers
---- Sympathetic postganglionic fibers
—— Parasympathetic preganglionic fibers
---- Parasympathetic postganglionic fibers

Fig. 9.26 Esophageal plexus

The left and right vagus nerves initially descend on the left and right sides of the esophagus. As they begin to contribute to the esophageal plexus, they shift to anterior and posterior positions, respectively. As the vagus nerves continue into the abdomen, they are named the anterior and posterior vagal trunks.

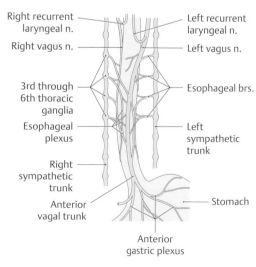

A Anterior view. Note the postganglionic sympathetic contribution to the esophageal plexus.

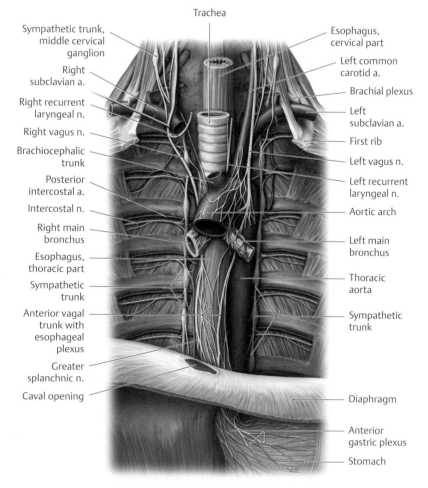

B Esophageal plexus in situ. Anterior view.

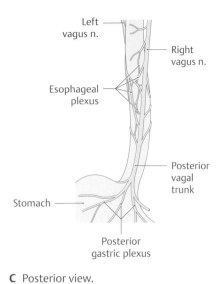

C Posterior view.

Fig. 9.28 Esophageal veins
Anterior view.

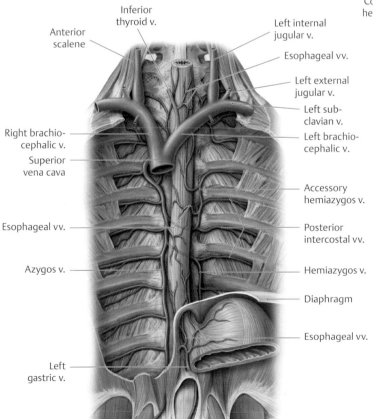

Fig. 9.27 Esophageal arteries
Anterior view.

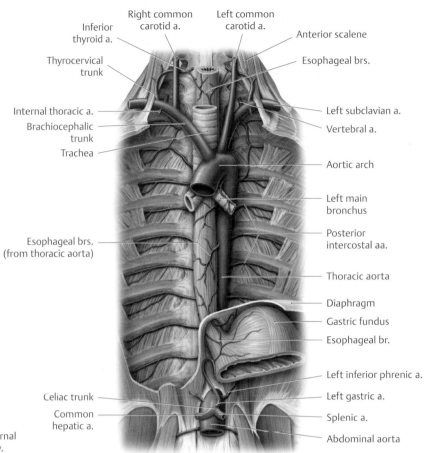

Table 9.6	Blood vessels of the esophagus	
Part	**Origin of esophageal arteries**	**Drainage of esophageal veins**
Cervical	Inferior thyroid a.	Inferior thyroid v.
	Rarely direct brs. from thyrocervical trunk or common carotid a.	Left brachiocephalic v.
Thoracic	Aorta (four or five esophageal aa.)	Upper left: Accessory hemiazygos v. or left brachiocephalic v.
		Lower left: Hemiazygos v.
		Right side: Azygos v.
Abdominal	Left gastric a.	Left gastric v.

Lymphatics of the Mediastinum

The superior phrenic lymph nodes drain lymph from the diaphragm, pericardium, lower esophagus, lung, and liver into the broncho-mediastinal trunk. The inferior phrenic lymph nodes, found in the abdomen, collect lymph from the diaphragm and lower lobes of the lung and convey it to the lumbar trunk. *Note:* The pericardium may also drain superiorly to the brachiocephalic lymph nodes.

***Fig. 9.29* Lymph nodes of the mediastinum and thoracic cavity**
Left anterior oblique view.

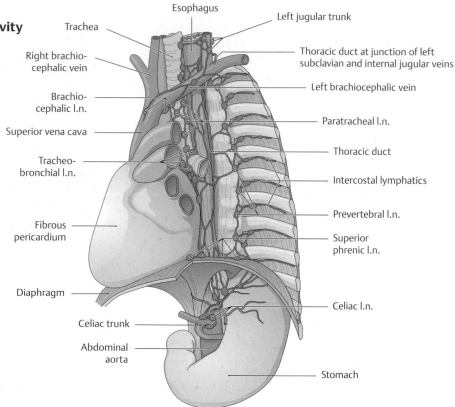

***Fig. 9.30* Lymphatic drainage of the heart**
A unique "crossed" drainage pattern exists in the heart: lymph from the left atrium and ventricle drains to the right venous junction, whereas lymph from the right atrium and ventricle drains to the left venous junction.

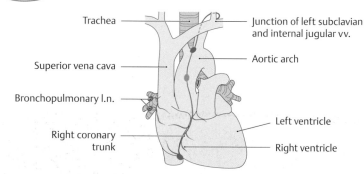

B Lymphatic drainage of the right chambers, anterior view.

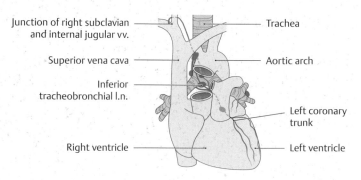

A Lymphatic drainage of the left chambers, anterior view.

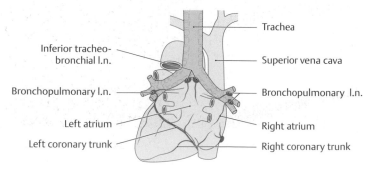

C Posterior view.

The paraesophageal nodes drain the esophagus. Lymphatic drainage of the cervical part of the esophagus is primarily cranial, to the deep cervical lymph nodes and then to the jugular trunk. The thoracic part of the esophagus drains to the bronchomediastinal trunks in two parts: the upper half drains cranially, and the lower half drains inferiorly via the superior phrenic lymph nodes. The bronchopulmonary and paratracheal nodes drain lymph from the lungs, bronchi, and trachea into the bronchomediastinal trunk (see **p. 128**).

***Fig. 9.31* Mediastinal lymph nodes**

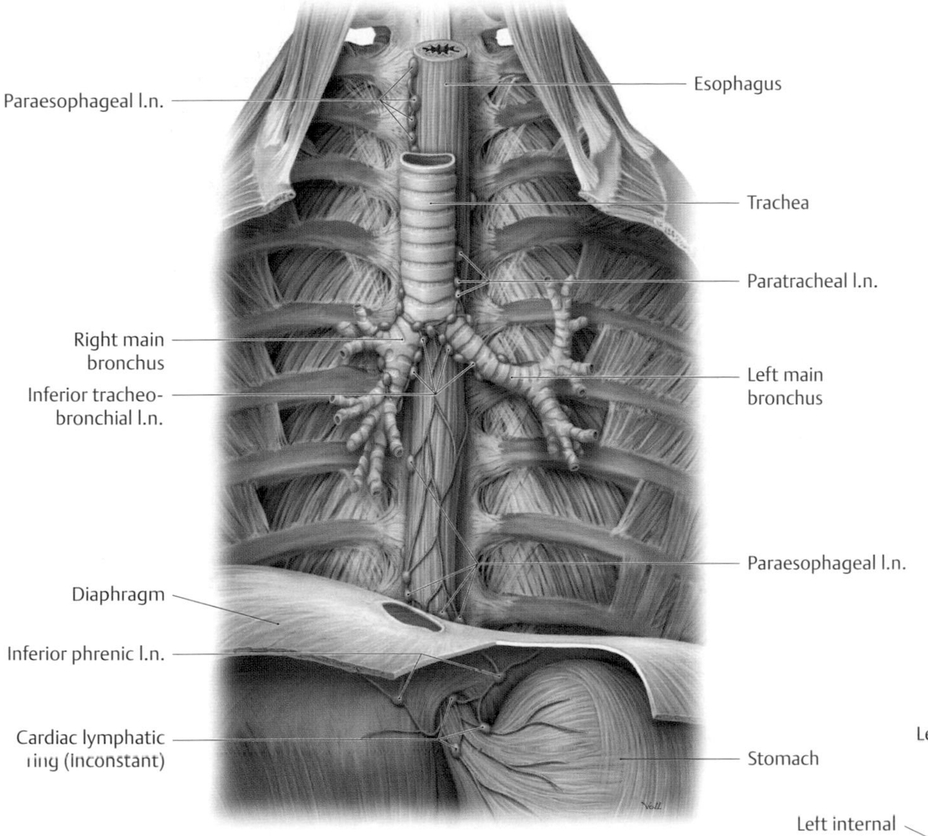

A Anterior view of opened thorax.

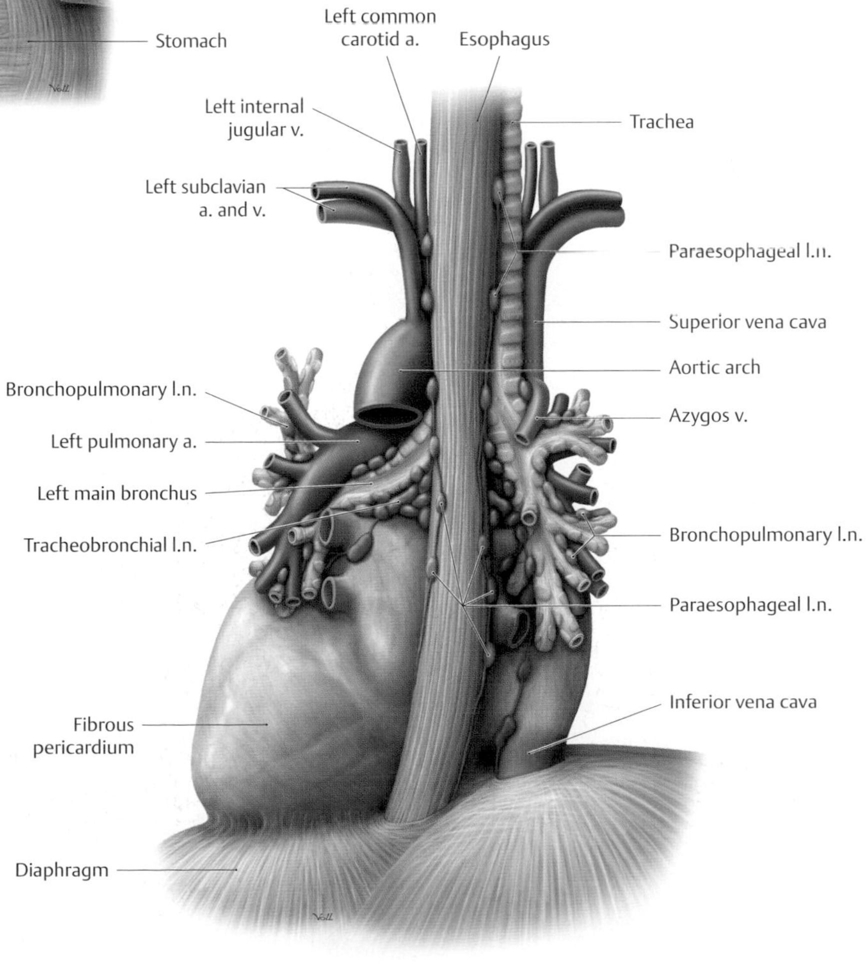

B Posterior view of mediastinal lymph nodes.

10 Pulmonary Cavities

Pulmonary Cavities

The paired pulmonary cavities contain the left and right lungs. They are completely separated from each other by the mediastinum and are under negative atmospheric pressure (see respiratory mechanics, **pp. 122–123**). The left pulmonary cavity is slightly smaller than the right, especially anteriorly, due to the asymmetrical position of the heart in the mediastinum, with the greater mass on the left. This causes a shift of some of the boundaries of the parietal pleura and lung on the left side at the level of the heart, as reflected in the difference in thoracic landmarks found at the intersection of the anterior border of the pulmonary cavities with certain reference lines on the left and right.

Fig. 10.1 Boundaries of the lungs and pulmonary cavities

The upper red dot on each reference line is the inferior boundary of the lung and the lower blue dot is the inferior boundary of the pulmonary cavity.

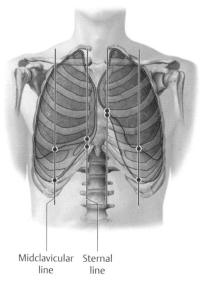

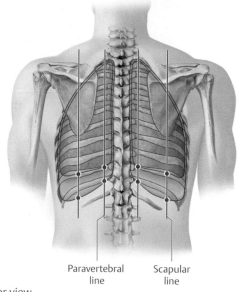

Midclavicular line Sternal line

A Anterior view.

Paravertebral line Scapular line

B Posterior view.

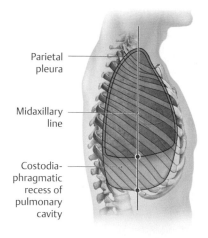

Parietal pleura

Midaxillary line

Costodiaphragmatic recess of pulmonary cavity

C Right lateral view.

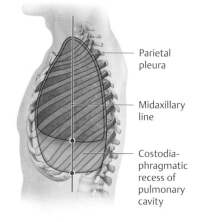

Parietal pleura

Midaxillary line

Costodiaphragmatic recess of pulmonary cavity

D Left lateral view.

Table 10.1	Pulmonary cavity boundaries and reference points			
Reference line	Right lung	Right parietal pleura	Left lung	Left parietal pleura
Sternal line (STL)	6th rib	7th rib	4th rib	4th rib
Midclavicular line (MCL)	6th rib	8th costal cartilage	6th rib	8th rib
Midaxillary line (MAL)	8th rib	10th rib	8th rib	10th rib
Scapular line (SL)	10th rib	11th rib	10th rib	11th rib
Paravertebral line (PV)	10th rib	T12 vertebra	10th rib	T12 vertebra

Fig. 10.2 **Parietal pleura**

The pulmonary cavity is bounded by two serous layers. The visceral pleura covering the lungs, and parietal pleura lining the inner surfaces of the thoracic cavity. The four divisions of the parietal pleura (costal, diaphragmatic, mediastinal, and cervical) are continuous.

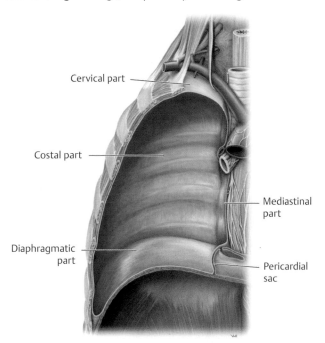

A Parts of the parietal pleura. *Opened:* Right pleural cavity, anterior view.

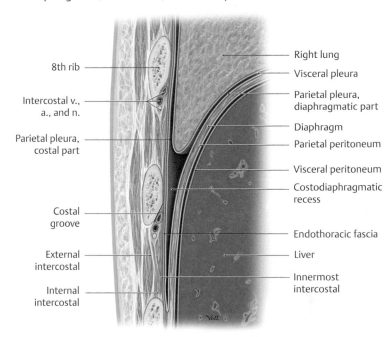

B Costodiaphragmatic recess, coronal section, anterior view. Reflection of the diaphragmatic pleura onto the inner thoracic wall (becoming the costal pleura) forms the costodiaphraqmatic recess.

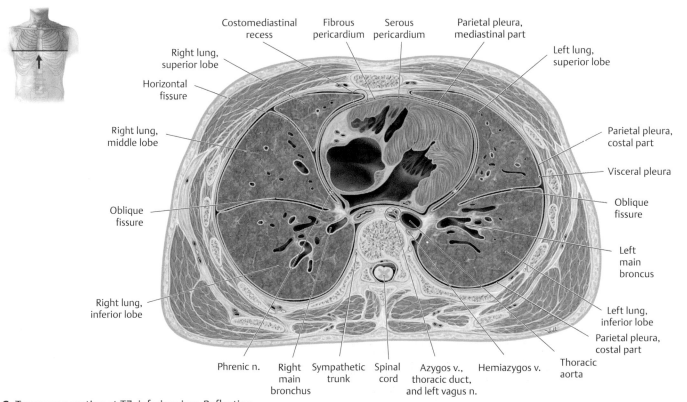

C Transverse section at T7, inferior view. Reflection of the costal pleura onto the pericardium forms the costomediastinal recess.

Pleura: Subdivisions, Recesses & Innervation

Fig. 10.3 Pleura and its divisions

The anterior thoracic wall and costal portion of the parietal pleura have been removed to show the lungs in situ.

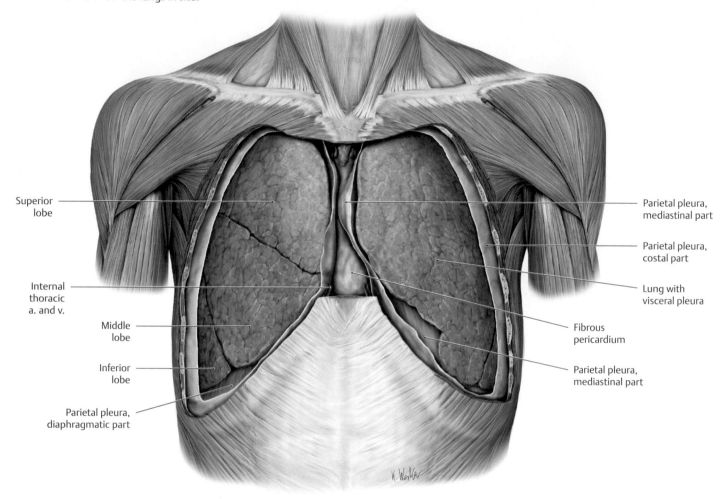

Superior lobe

Internal thoracic a. and v.

Middle lobe

Inferior lobe

Parietal pleura, diaphragmatic part

Parietal pleura, mediastinal part

Parietal pleura, costal part

Lung with visceral pleura

Fibrous pericardium

Parietal pleura, mediastinal part

Fig. 10.4 Innervation of the pleura

The costal and cervical portions and the periphery of the diaphragmatic portion of the parietal pleura are innervated by the intercostal nerves. The mediastinal and central portions of the diaphragmatic pleura are innervated by the phrenic nerves. The visceral pleura covering the lung itself receives its innervation from the autonomic nervous system.

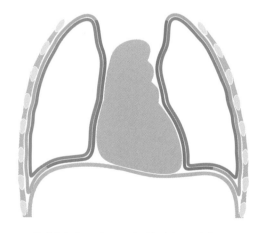

Parietal pleura innervated by intercostal nn.

Parietal pleura innervated by phrenic n.

Visceral pleura innervated by autonomic nn.

Fig. 10.5 Costomediastinal and costodiaphragmatic recesses

On the left side of the thorax, an examiner's fingertips are placed in the costomediastinal and costodiaphragmatic recesses. These recesses are formed by the acute reflection of the costal part of the parietal pleura onto the fibrous pericardium as mediastinal pleura (costomediastinal) or on to the diaphragm as diaphragmatic pleura (costodiaphragmatic).

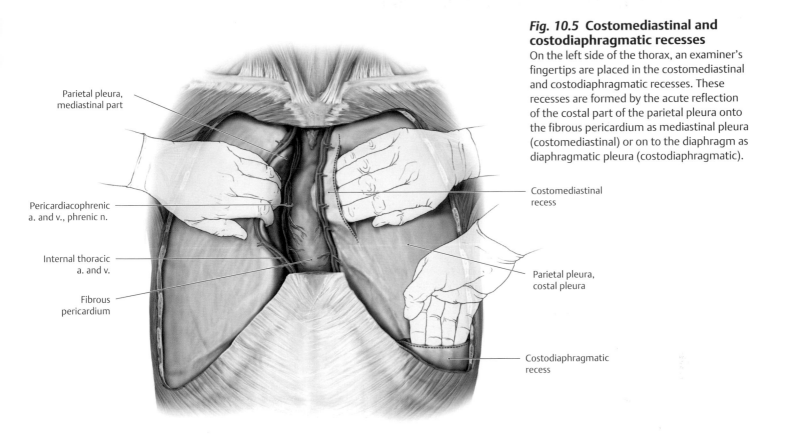

Parietal pleura, mediastinal part

Pericardiacophrenic a. and v., phrenic n.

Internal thoracic a. and v.

Fibrous pericardium

Costomediastinal recess

Parietal pleura, costal pleura

Costodiaphragmatic recess

Fig. 10.6 Pleural recesses

Transverse section at T8, superior view.

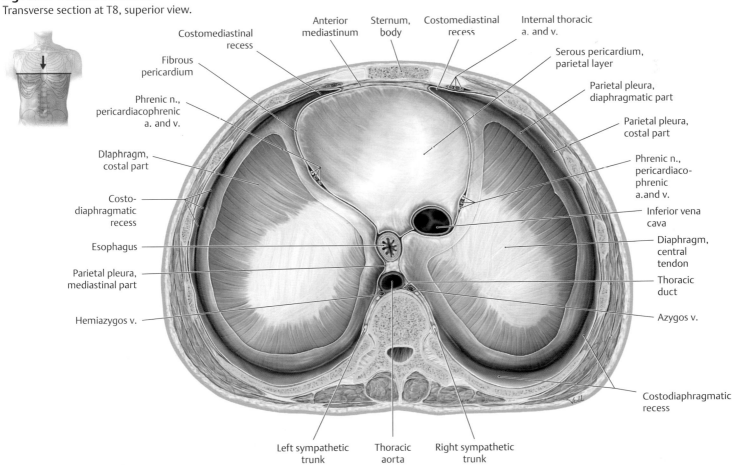
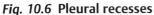

Costomediastinal recess

Fibrous pericardium

Phrenic n., pericardiacophrenic a. and v.

Diaphragm, costal part

Costo-diaphragmatic recess

Esophagus

Parietal pleura, mediastinal part

Hemiazygos v.

Anterior mediastinum

Sternum, body

Costomediastinal recess

Internal thoracic a. and v.

Serous pericardium, parietal layer

Parietal pleura, diaphragmatic part

Parietal pleura, costal part

Phrenic n., pericardiaco-phrenic a. and v.

Inferior vena cava

Diaphragm, central tendon

Thoracic duct

Azygos v.

Costodiaphragmatic recess

Left sympathetic trunk

Thoracic aorta

Right sympathetic trunk

Lungs

Fig. 10.7 Lungs in situ

The left and right lungs occupy the full volume of the pleural cavity. Note that the left lung is slightly smaller than the right due to the asymmetrical position of the heart.

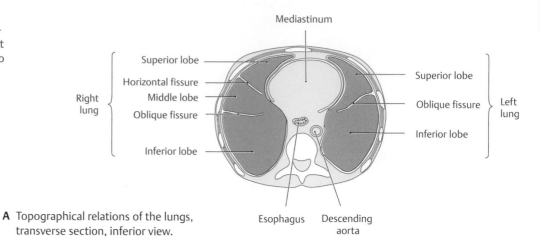

A Topographical relations of the lungs, transverse section, inferior view.

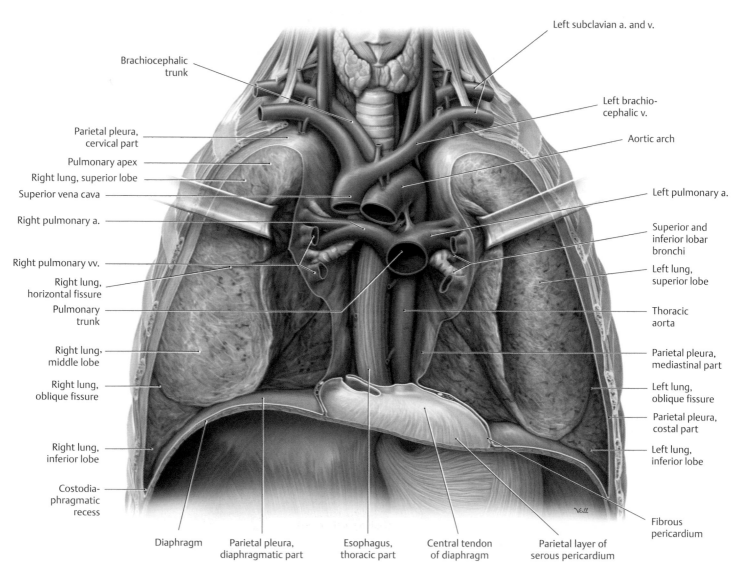

B Anterior view with lungs retracted.

Fig. 10.8 Gross anatomy of the lungs

The oblique and horizontal fissures divide the right lung into three lobes: superior, middle, and inferior. The oblique fissure divides the left lung into two lobes: superior and inferior. The apex of each lung extends into the root of the neck. The hilum is the location at which the bronchi and neurovascular structures connect to the lung.

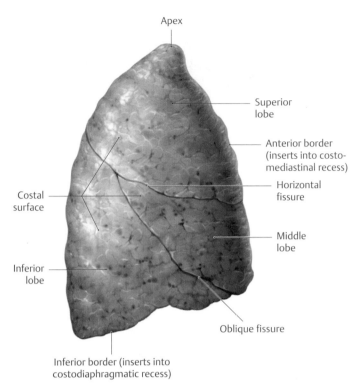

Apex
Superior lobe
Anterior border (inserts into costo-mediastinal recess)
Horizontal fissure
Costal surface
Middle lobe
Inferior lobe
Oblique fissure
Inferior border (inserts into costodiaphragmatic recess)

A Right lung, lateral view.

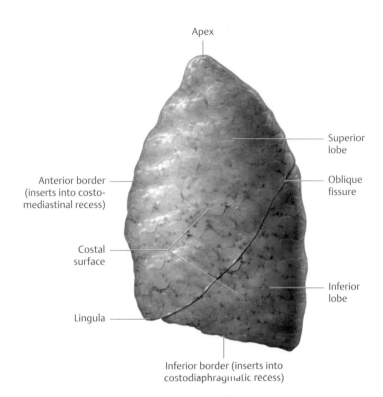

Apex
Superior lobe
Oblique fissure
Anterior border (inserts into costo-mediastinal recess)
Costal surface
Inferior lobe
Lingula
Inferior border (inserts into costodiaphragmatic recess)

B Left lung, lateral view.

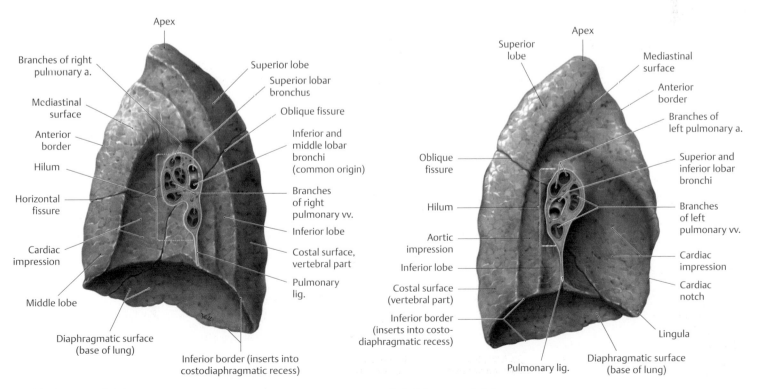

Apex
Branches of right pulmonary a.
Superior lobe
Superior lobar bronchus
Mediastinal surface
Oblique fissure
Anterior border
Inferior and middle lobar bronchi (common origin)
Hilum
Branches of right pulmonary vv.
Horizontal fissure
Inferior lobe
Cardiac impression
Costal surface, vertebral part
Pulmonary lig.
Middle lobe
Diaphragmatic surface (base of lung)
Inferior border (inserts into costodiaphragmatic recess)

C Right lung, medial view.

Apex
Superior lobe
Mediastinal surface
Anterior border
Branches of left pulmonary a.
Oblique fissure
Superior and inferior lobar bronchi
Hilum
Branches of left pulmonary vv.
Aortic impression
Inferior lobe
Cardiac impression
Costal surface (vertebral part)
Cardiac notch
Inferior border (inserts into costo-diaphragmatic recess)
Lingula
Pulmonary lig.
Diaphragmatic surface (base of lung)

D Left lung, medial view.

117

Bronchopulmonary Segments of the Lungs

The lung lobes are subdivided into bronchopulmonary segments, the smallest resectable portion of a lung, each supplied by a tertiary (segmental) bronchus. *Note*: These subdivisions are not defined by surface boundaries but by origin.

Fig. 10.9 Segmentation of the lung

Anterior view. See **pp. 120–121** for details of the trachea and bronchial tree.

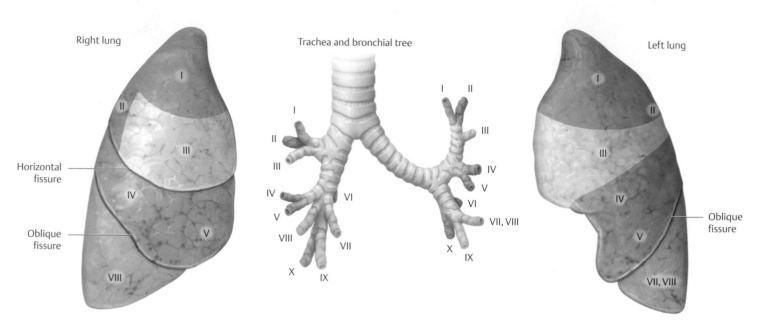

Fig. 10.10 Anteroposterior bronchogram

Anterior view of right lung.

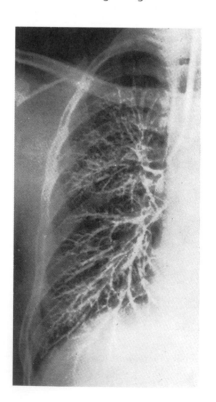

Table 10.2	Segmental architecture of the lungs		
Each segment is supplied by a segmental bronchus of the same name (e.g., the apical segmental bronchus supplies the apical segment). See **pp. 120–121** for details of the trachea and bronchial tree.			
Right lung		**Left lung**	
Superior lobe			
I	Apical segment	Apicoposterior segment	I
II	Posterior segment		II
III	Anterior segment		III
Middle lobe		**Lingula**	
IV	Lateral segment	Superior lingular segment	IV
V	Medial segment	Inferior lingular segment	V
Inferior lobe			
VI	Superior segment		VI
VII	Medial basal segment		VII
VIII	Anterior basal segment		VIII
IX	Lateral basal segment		IX
X	Posterior basal segment		X

Fig. 10.11 Right lung: Bronchopulmonary segments

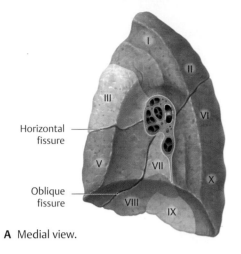

A Medial view.

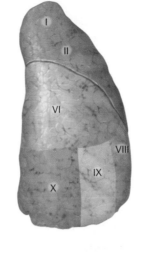

B Posterior view.

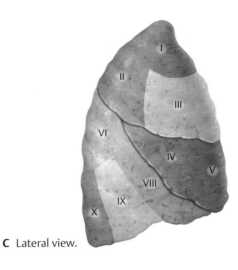

C Lateral view.

Fig. 10.12 Left lung: Bronchopulmonary segments

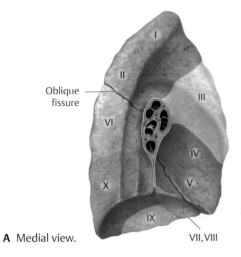

A Medial view.

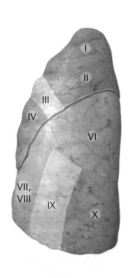

B Posterior view.

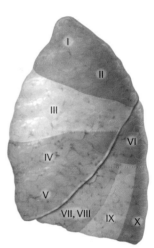

C Lateral view.

✳ *Clinical box 10.1*

Lung resections

Lung cancer, emphysema, or tuberculosis may necessitate the surgical removal of damaged portions of the lung. Surgeons exploit the anatomical subdivision of the lungs into lobes and segments when excising damaged tissue.

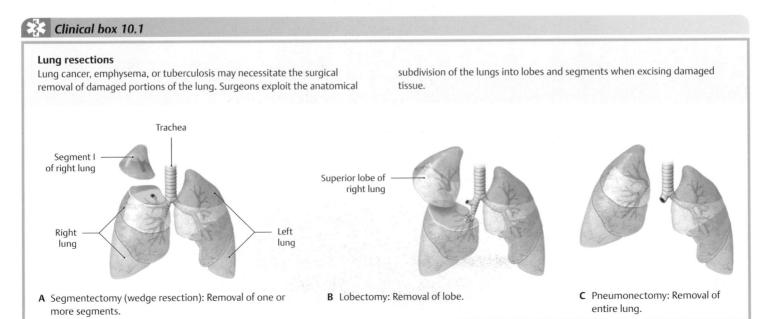

A Segmentectomy (wedge resection): Removal of one or more segments.

B Lobectomy: Removal of lobe.

C Pneumonectomy: Removal of entire lung.

Trachea & Bronchial Tree

At or near the level of the sternal angle (T4/T5), the lowest tracheal cartilage extends anteroposteriorly, forming the carina. The trachea bifurcates at the carina into the right and left main bronchi. Each bronchus gives off lobar branches to the corresponding lung.

Fig. 10.13 **Trachea**
See **p. 530** for the structures of the thyroid.

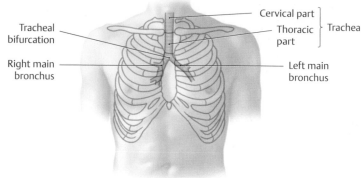

A Projection of trachea onto chest.

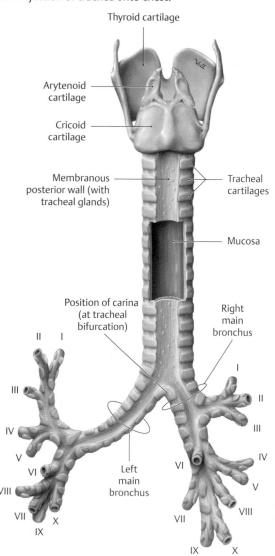

C Posterior view with opened posterior wall.

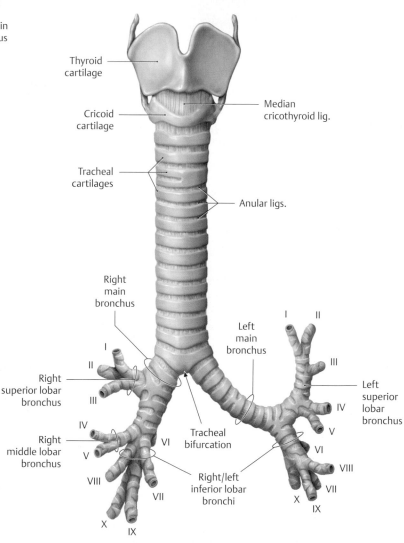

B Anterior view.

✚ **Clinical box 10.2**

Foreign body aspiration

Toddlers are at particularly high risk of potentially fatal aspiration of foreign bodies. In general, foreign bodies are more likely to become lodged in the right main bronchus than the left: the left bronchus diverges more sharply at the tracheal bifurcation to pass more horizontally over the heart, whereas the right bronchus is relatively straight and more in line with the trachea.

The conducting portion of the bronchial tree extends from the tracheal bifurcation to the terminal bronchiole, inclusive. The respiratory portion consists of the respiratory bronchiole, alveolar ducts, alveolar sacs, and alveoli.

Fig. 10.14 Bronchial tree

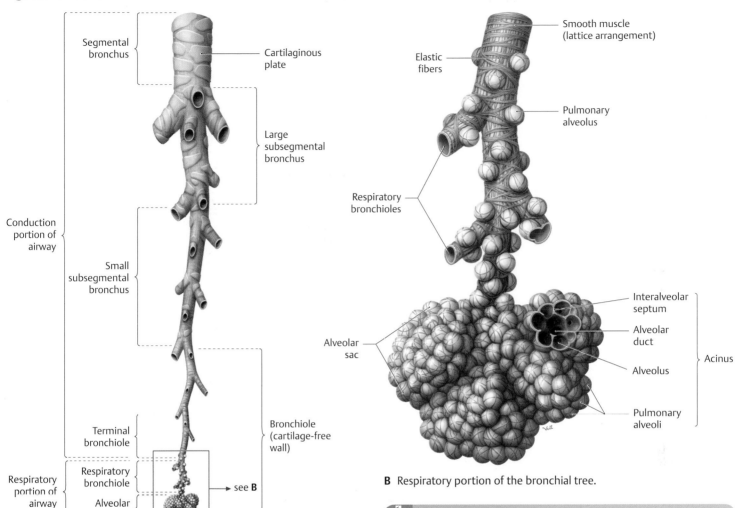

A Divisions of the bronchial tree.

B Respiratory portion of the bronchial tree.

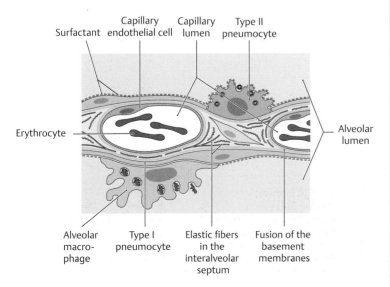

C Epithelial lining of the alveoli.

Respiratory Mechanics

The mechanics of respiration are based on a rhythmic increase and decrease in thoracic volume, with an associated expansion and contraction of the lungs. *Inspiration* (red): Contraction of the diaphragm leaflets lowers the diaphragm into the inspiratory position, increasing the volume of the pleural cavity along the vertical axis. Contraction of the thoracic muscles (external intercostals with the scalene, intercartilaginous, and posterior serratus muscles) elevates the ribs, expanding the pleural cavity along the sagittal and transverse axes (**Fig. 10.16A,B**). Surface tension in the pleural space causes the visceral and parietal pleura to adhere; thus, changes in thoracic volume alter the volume of the lungs. This is particularly evident in the pleural recesses: at functional residual capacity

(resting position between inspiration and expiration), the lung does not fully occupy the pleural cavity. As the pleural cavity expands, a negative intrapleural pressure is generated. The air pressure differential results in an influx of air (inspiration). *Expiration* (blue): During passive expiration, the muscles of the thoracic cage relax and the diaphragm returns to its expiratory position. Contraction of the lungs increases the pulmonary pressure and expels air from the lungs. For forcible expiration, the internal intercostal muscles (with the transverse thoracic and subcostal mucosa) can actively lower the rib cage more rapidly and to a greater extent than through passive elastic recoil.

Fig. 10.15 Respiratory changes in thoracic volume
Inspiratory position (red); expiratory position (blue).

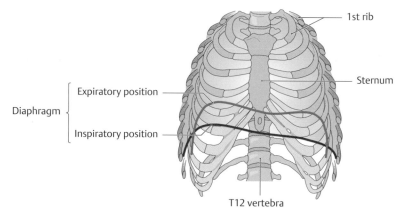

Fig. 10.16 Inspiration: Pleural cavity expansion

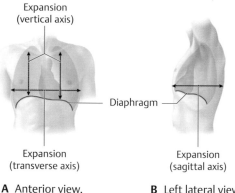

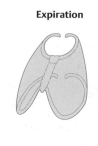

Inspiration

A Anterior view.　　**B** Left lateral view.　　**C** Anterolateral view.

Fig. 10.18 Respiratory changes in lung volume

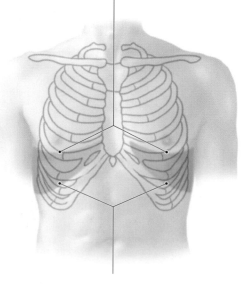

Inferior border of lung (full expiration)

Inferior border of lung (full inspiration)

Fig. 10.17 Expiration: Pleural cavity contraction

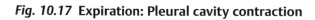

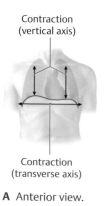

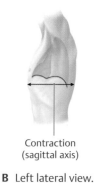

Expiration

A Anterior view.　　**B** Left lateral view.　　**C** Anterolateral view.

Fig. 10.19 Inspiration: Lung expansion

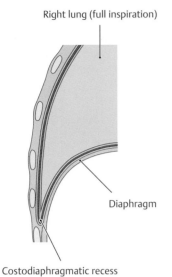

Right lung (full inspiration)

Diaphragm

Costodiaphragmatic recess

Fig. 10.20 Expiration: Lung contraction

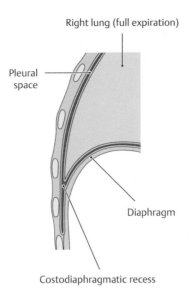

Right lung (full expiration)

Pleural space

Diaphragm

Costodiaphragmatic recess

Fig. 10.21 Movements of the lung and bronchial tree

As the volume of the lung changes with the volume of the thoracic cavity, the entire bronchial tree moves within the lung. These structural movements are more pronounced in portions of the bronchial tree distant from the pulmonary hilum.

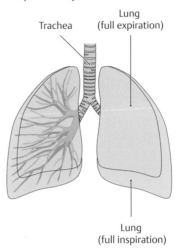

Trachea

Lung (full expiration)

Lung (full inspiration)

Clinical box 10.4

Pneumothorax

The pleural space is normally sealed from the outside environment. Injury to the parietal pleura, visceral pleura, or lung allows air to enter the pleural cavity (pneumothorax). The lung collapses due to its inherent elasticity, and the patient's ability to breathe is compromised. The uninjured lung continues to function under normal pressure variations, resulting in "mediastinal flutter": the mediastinum shifts toward the normal side during inspiration and returns to the midline during expiration. Tension (valve) pneumothorax occurs when traumatically detached and displaced tissue covers the defect in the thoracic wall from the inside. This mobile flap allows air to enter, but not escape, the pleural cavity, causing a pressure buildup. The mediastinum shifts to the normal side, which may cause kinking of the great vessels and prevent the return of venous blood to the heart. Without treatment, tension pneumothorax is invariably fatal.

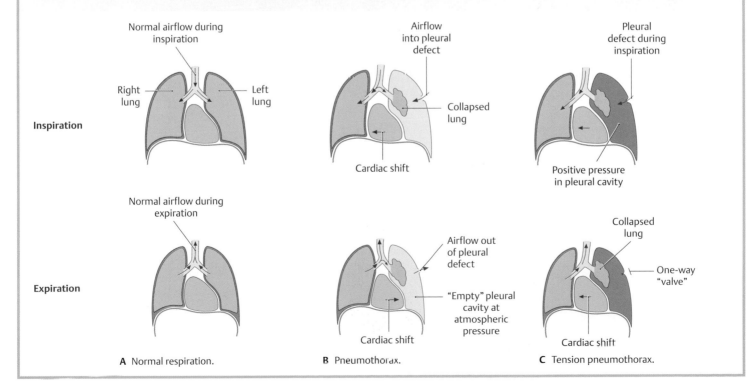

Inspiration

Normal airflow during inspiration

Right lung

Left lung

Airflow into pleural defect

Collapsed lung

Cardiac shift

Pleural defect during inspiration

Positive pressure in pleural cavity

Expiration

Normal airflow during expiration

Airflow out of pleural defect

"Empty" pleural cavity at atmospheric pressure

Cardiac shift

Collapsed lung

One-way "valve"

Cardiac shift

A Normal respiration.   **B** Pneumothorax.   **C** Tension pneumothorax.

Pulmonary Arteries & Veins

The pulmonary trunk arises from the right ventricle and divides into a left and right pulmonary artery for each lung. The paired pulmonary veins open into the left atrium on each side. The pulmonary arteries accompany and follow the branching of the bronchial tree, whereas the pulmonary veins do not, being located at the margins of the pulmonary lobules.

***Fig. 10.22* Pulmonary arteries and veins**
Anterior view.

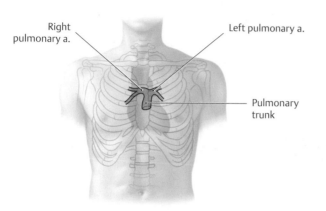

A Projection of pulmonary arteries on chest wall.

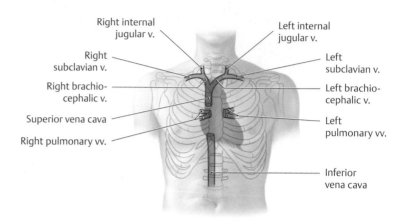

B Projection of pulmonary veins on chest wall.

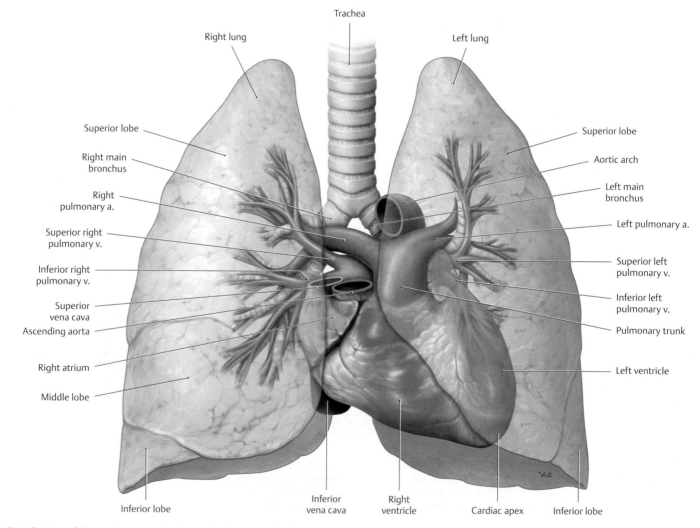

C Distribution of the pulmonary arteries and veins, anterior view.

Fig. 10.23 Pulmonary arteries

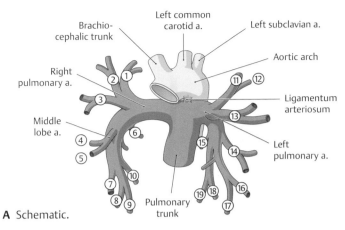

A Schematic.

Table 10.3	Pulmonary arteries and their branches	
Right pulmonary artery	**Left pulmonary artery**	
Superior lobe arteries		
①	Apical segmental a.	⑪
②	Posterior segmental a.	⑫
③	Anterior segmental a.	⑬
Middle lobe arteries		
④	Lateral segmental a.	Lingular a.	⑭
⑤	Medial segmental a.		
Inferior lobe arteries		
⑥	Superior segmental a.	⑮
⑦	Anterior basal segmental a.	⑯
⑧	Lateral basal segmental a.	⑰
⑨	Posterior basal segmental a.	⑱
⑩	Medial basal segmental a.	⑲

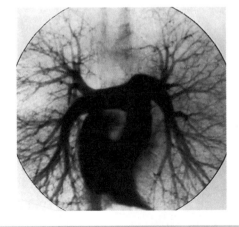

B Pulmonary arteriogram, arterial phase, anterior view. (Reproduced from Moeller TB, Reif E. Pocket Atlas of Radiographic Anatomy, 3rd ed. New York, NY: Thieme; 2010.)

Fig. 10.24 Pulmonary veins

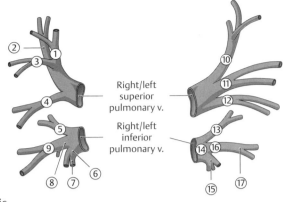

A Schematic.

Table 10.4	Pulmonary veins and their tributaries	
Right pulmonary vein	**Left pulmonary vein**	
Superior pulmonary veins		
①	Apical v.	Apicoposterior v.	⑩
②	Posterior v.		
③	Anterior v.	Anterior v.	⑪
④	Middle lobe v.	Lingular v.	⑫
Inferior pulmonary veins		
⑤	Superior v.	⑬
⑥	Common basal v.	⑭
⑦	Inferior basal v.	⑮
⑧	Superior basal v.	⑯
⑨	Anterior basal v.	⑰

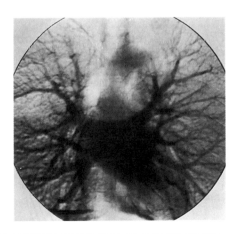

B Pulmonary arteriogram, venous phase, anterior view. (Reproduced from Moeller TB, Reif E. Pocket Atlas of Radiographic Anatomy, 3rd ed. New York, NY: Thieme; 2010.)

Clinical box 10.5

Pulmonary embolism
Potentially life-threatening pulmonary embolism occurs when blood clots migrate through the venous system and become lodged in one of the arteries supplying the lungs. Symptoms include dyspnea (difficulty breathing) and tachycardia (increased heart rate). Most pulmonary emboli originate from stagnant blood in the veins of the lower limb and pelvis (venous thromboemboli). Causes include immobilization, disordered blood coagulation, and trauma. *Note*: A thromboembolus is a thrombus (blood clot) that has migrated (embolized).

Lymphatics of the Pleural Cavity

The lungs and bronchi are drained by two lymphatic drainage systems. The peribronchial network follows the bronchial tree, draining lymph from the bronchi and most of the lungs. The subpleural network collects lymph from the peripheral lung and visceral pleura.

Fig. 10.29 Lymphatic drainage of the pleural cavity and thoracic wall

A Peribronchial network, coronal section, anterior view. (Intra)pulmonary nodes along the bronchial tree drain lymph from the lungs into the bronchopulmonary (hilar) nodes. Lymph then passes sequentially through the inferior and superior tracheobronchial nodes, paratracheal nodes, bronchomediastinal trunk, and finally to the right lymphatic or thoracic duct. *Note*: Significant amounts of lymph from the left lower lobe drain to the right superior tracheobronchial nodes.

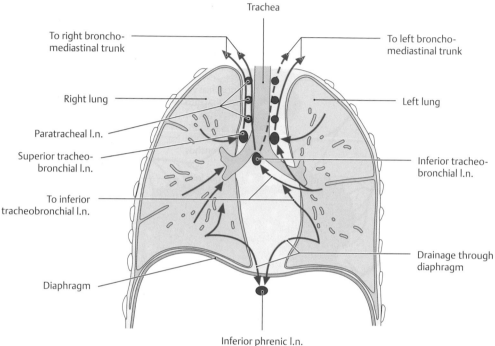

B Subpleural and thoracic wall networks, transverse section, superior view.

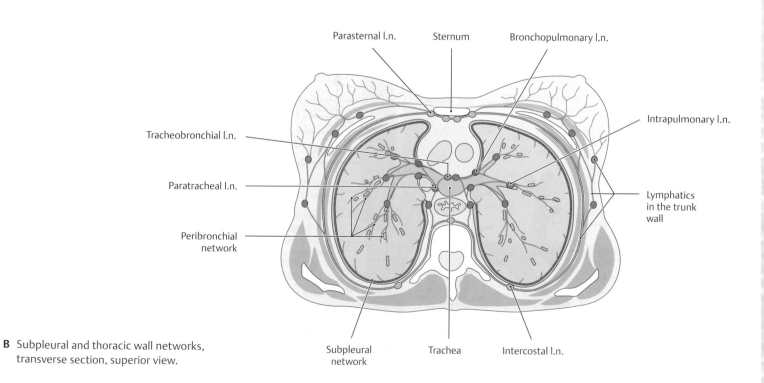

Fig. 10.30 **Lymph nodes of the pleural cavity**
Anterior view of pulmonary nodes.

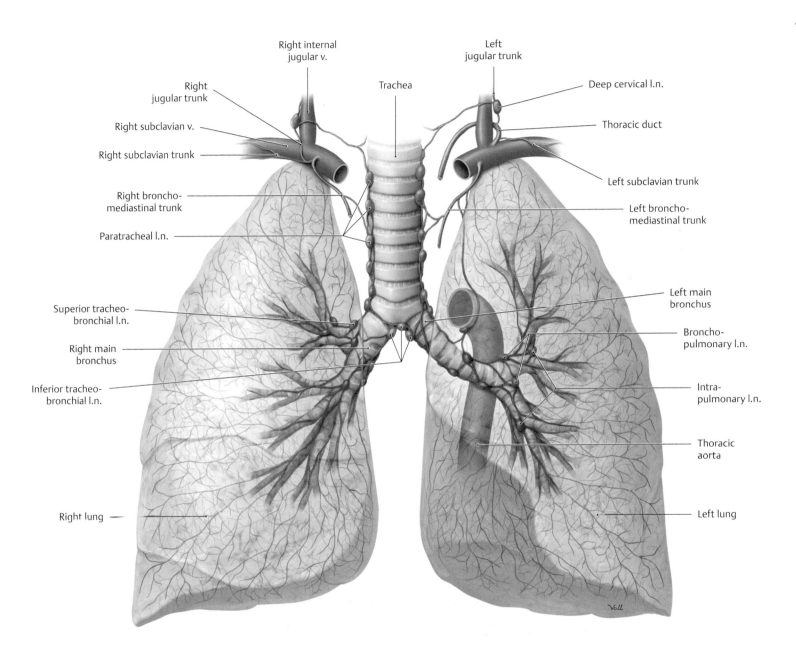

✦ Clinical box 10.6

Carcinoma of the Lung

Carcinoma of the lung accounts for ≈ 20% of all cancers and is mainly caused by cigarette smoking. It arises first in the lining of the bronchi and metastasizes quickly to bronchopulmonary lymph nodes and subsequently to other node groups, including supraclavicular nodes. It can also spread via the blood to the lungs, brain, bone, and suprarenal glands. Lung cancer can invade adjacent structures such as the phrenic nerve, resulting in paralysis of a hemidiaphragm, or the recurrent laryngeal nerve, resulting in hoarseness due to paralysis of the vocal cord.

Radiographic Anatomy of the Thorax (I)

Fig. 11.6
(Reproduced from Lange S. Radiologische Diagnostik der Thoraxerkrankungen, 4th ed. Stuttgart: Thieme; 2010.)

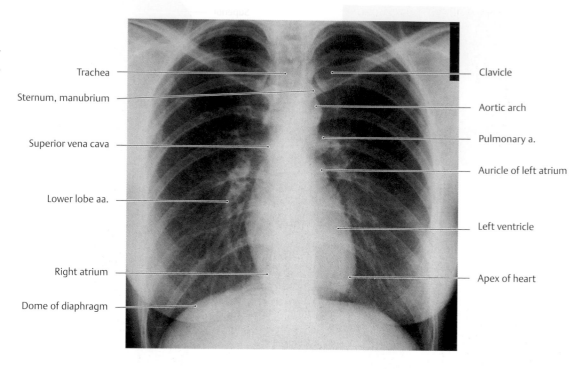

Trachea

Sternum, manubrium

Superior vena cava

Lower lobe aa.

Right atrium

Dome of diaphragm

Clavicle

Aortic arch

Pulmonary a.

Auricle of left atrium

Left ventricle

Apex of heart

A Posterior-anterior (PA) chest radiograph. Anterior view.

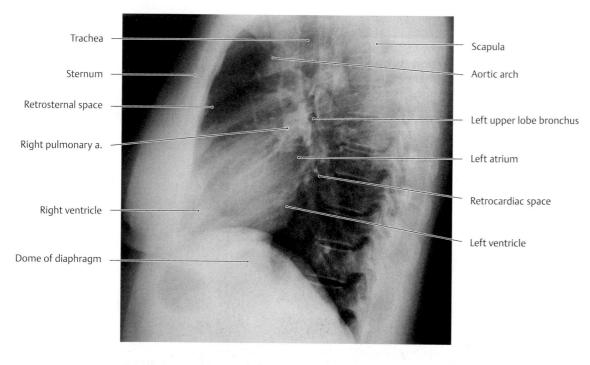

Trachea

Sternum

Retrosternal space

Right pulmonary a.

Right ventricle

Dome of diaphragm

Scapula

Aortic arch

Left upper lobe bronchus

Left atrium

Retrocardiac space

Left ventricle

B Left lateral chest radiograph.

Fig. 11.7 Left bronchogram

Anteroposterior view. (Reproduced from Moeller TB, Reif E. Pocket Atlas of Radiographic Anatomy, 3rd ed. New York, NY: Thieme; 2010.)

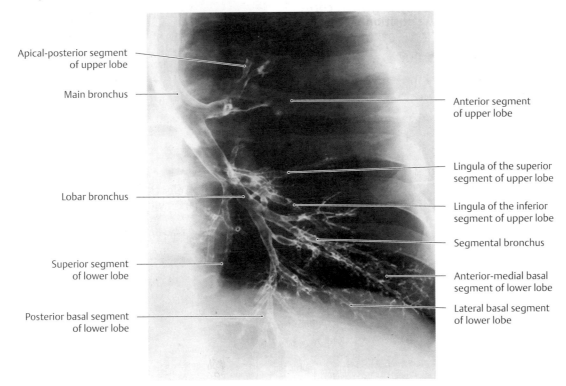

Apical-posterior segment of upper lobe

Main bronchus

Lobar bronchus

Superior segment of lower lobe

Posterior basal segment of lower lobe

Anterior segment of upper lobe

Lingula of the superior segment of upper lobe

Lingula of the inferior segment of upper lobe

Segmental bronchus

Anterior-medial basal segment of lower lobe

Lateral basal segment of lower lobe

Fig. 11.8 MRI of the thorax

Coronal view. (Reproduced from Moeller TB, Reif E. Pocket Atlas of Sectional Anatomy, Vol 2, 3rd ed. New York, NY: Thieme; 2007.)

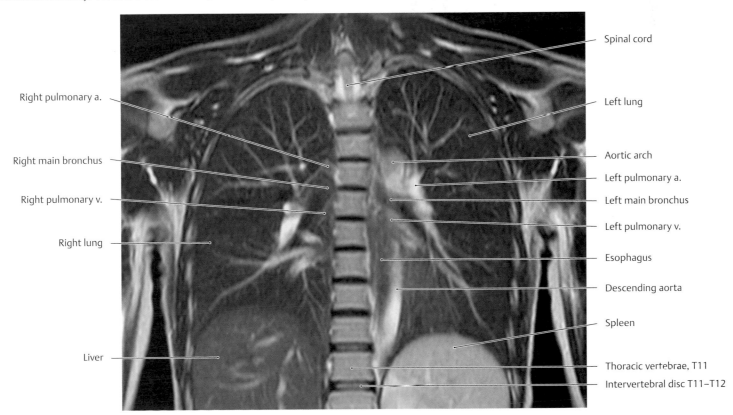

Right pulmonary a.

Right main bronchus

Right pulmonary v.

Right lung

Liver

Spinal cord

Left lung

Aortic arch

Left pulmonary a.

Left main bronchus

Left pulmonary v.

Esophagus

Descending aorta

Spleen

Thoracic vertebrae, T11

Intervertebral disc T11–T12

Radiographic Anatomy of the Thorax (III)

***Fig. 11.14* CT of the thorax**
(Reproduced from Moeller TB, Reif E.
Pocket Atlas of Sectional Anatomy, Vol 2,
4th ed. New York, NY: Thieme; 2014.)

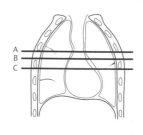

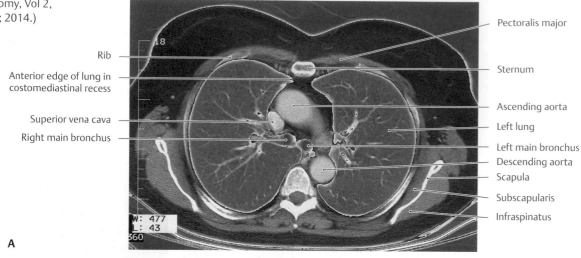

Rib

Anterior edge of lung in
costomediastinal recess

Superior vena cava

Right main bronchus

Pectoralis major

Sternum

Ascending aorta

Left lung

Left main bronchus

Descending aorta

Scapula

Subscapularis

Infraspinatus

A

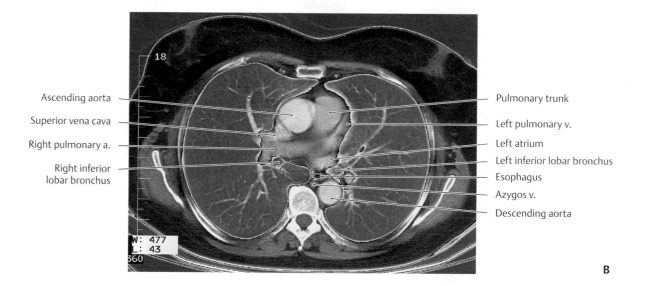

Ascending aorta

Superior vena cava

Right pulmonary a.

Right inferior
lobar bronchus

Pulmonary trunk

Left pulmonary v.

Left atrium

Left inferior lobar bronchus

Esophagus

Azygos v.

Descending aorta

B

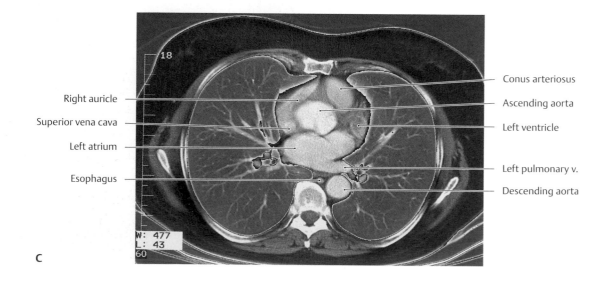

Right auricle

Superior vena cava

Left atrium

Esophagus

Conus arteriosus

Ascending aorta

Left ventricle

Left pulmonary v.

Descending aorta

C

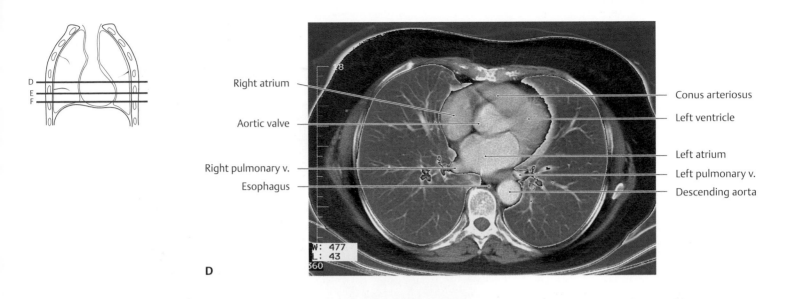

Right atrium — Conus arteriosus

Aortic valve — Left ventricle

Right pulmonary v. — Left atrium
Esophagus — Left pulmonary v.
— Descending aorta

D

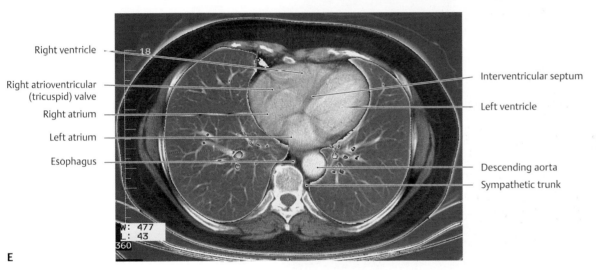

Right ventricle — Interventricular septum

Right atrioventricular
(tricuspid) valve — Left ventricle

Right atrium

Left atrium

Esophagus — Descending aorta
— Sympathetic trunk

E

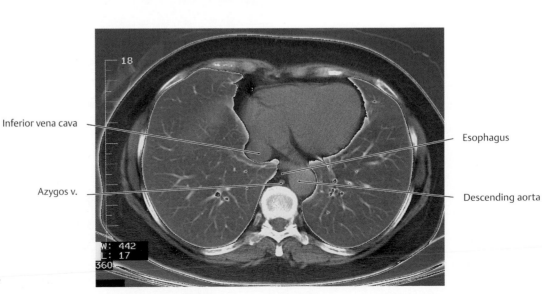

Inferior vena cava — Esophagus

Azygos v. — Descending aorta

F

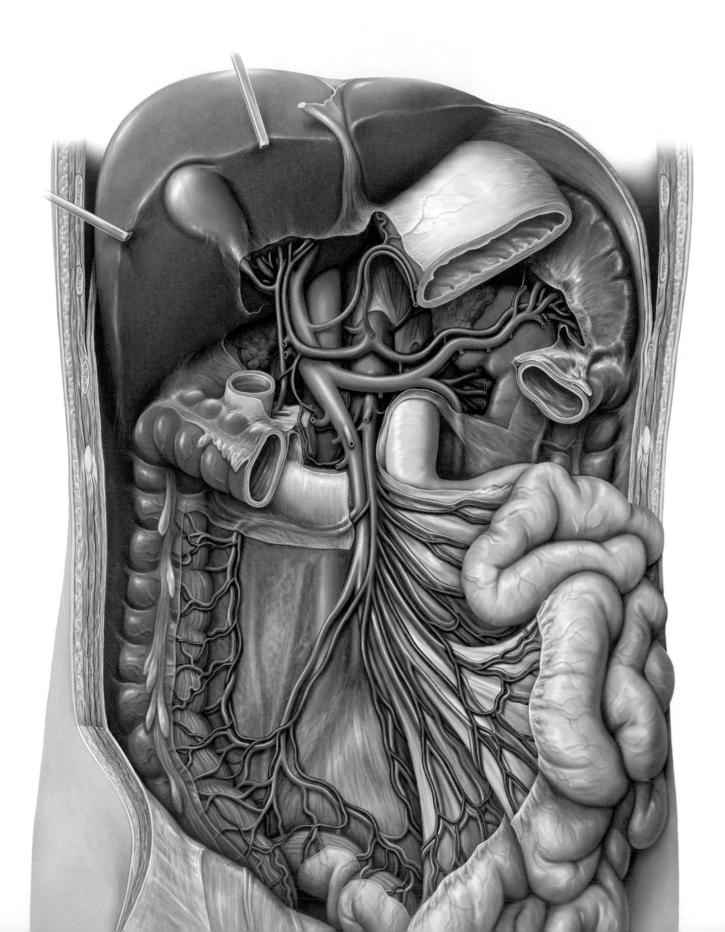

Abdomen

13 Abdominal Wall

Bony Framework for the Abdominal Wall

Fig. 13.1 Bony framework of the abdomen

Anterior view. These bones are the site of attachment for the muscles and ligaments of the anterolateral abdominal wall and form a bony cage that protects certain abdominal organs.

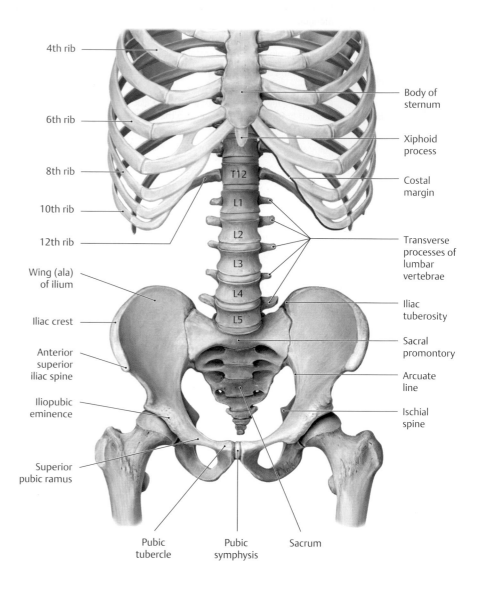

4th rib

6th rib

8th rib

10th rib

12th rib

Wing (ala) of ilium

Iliac crest

Anterior superior iliac spine

Iliopubic eminence

Superior pubic ramus

T12
L1
L2
L3
L4
L5

Body of sternum

Xiphoid process

Costal margin

Transverse processes of lumbar vertebrae

Iliac tuberosity

Sacral promontory

Arcuate line

Ischial spine

Pubic tubercle   Pubic symphysis   Sacrum

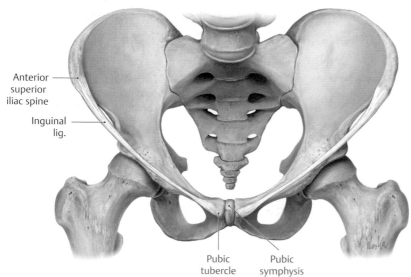

Anterior superior iliac spine

Inguinal lig.

Pubic tubercle   Pubic symphysis

Fig 13.2 The inguinal ligament

Male pelvis, anterosuperior view.
The inguinal ligament is a palpable landmark that forms the demarcation between the abdominal wall and thigh. It is formed by the inferior edge of the external oblique apo-neurosis, the most superficial of the anterior abdominal wall muscles. The inguinal ligament attaches laterally to the anterior superior iliac spine and medially to the pubic tubercle. It is important clinically as it forms the floor of the inguinal canal (see **Table 13.2**) and the roof of the retro-inguinal space (see **Fig. 34.31**).

Fig. 13.3 Abdominal wall muscle attachment sites

Left hip bone. Muscle origins are in red, insertions in blue.

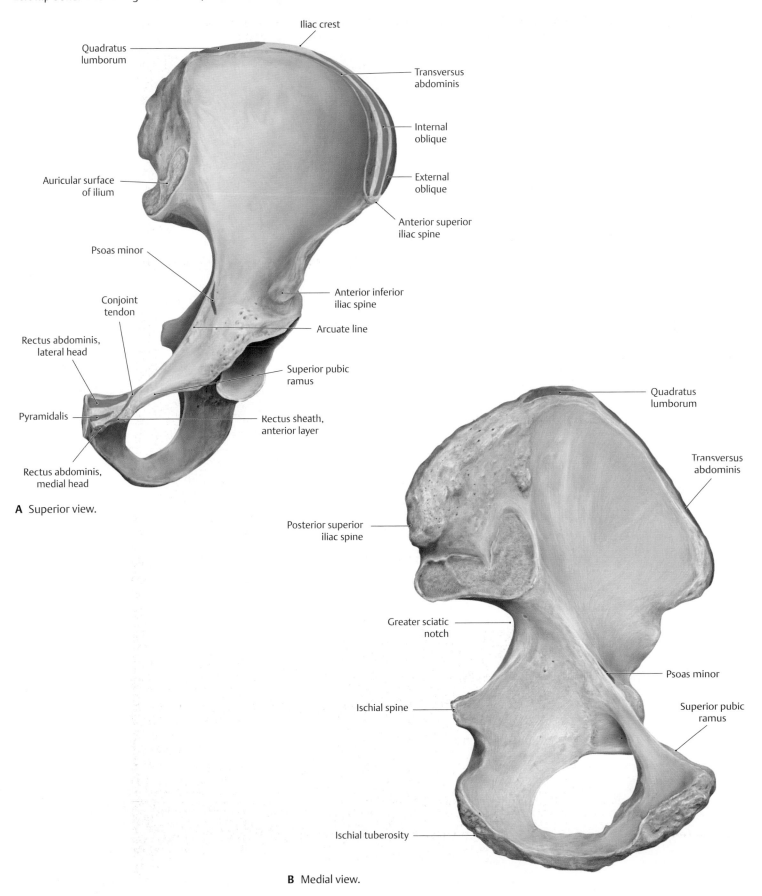

Quadratus lumborum

Iliac crest

Transversus abdominis

Internal oblique

External oblique

Auricular surface of ilium

Anterior superior iliac spine

Psoas minor

Anterior inferior iliac spine

Conjoint tendon

Arcuate line

Rectus abdominis, lateral head

Superior pubic ramus

Pyramidalis

Rectus sheath, anterior layer

Rectus abdominis, medial head

A Superior view.

Quadratus lumborum

Transversus abdominis

Posterior superior iliac spine

Greater sciatic notch

Psoas minor

Ischial spine

Superior pubic ramus

Ischial tuberosity

B Medial view.

Muscles of the Anterolateral Abdominal Wall

The muscles of the anterolateral abdominal wall consist of the external and internal obliques and the transversus abdominis. The posterior or deep abdominal wall muscles (notably the psoas major) are functionally hip muscles (see **p. 148**).

Fig. 13.4 **Muscles of the abdominal wall**
Right side, anterior view.

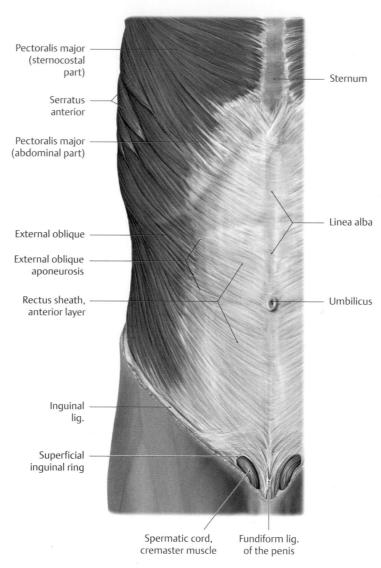

Pectoralis major (sternocostal part)

Serratus anterior

Pectoralis major (abdominal part)

External oblique

External oblique aponeurosis

Rectus sheath, anterior layer

Inguinal lig.

Superficial inguinal ring

Sternum

Linea alba

Umbilicus

Spermatic cord, cremaster muscle

Fundiform lig. of the penis

A Superficial abdominal wall muscles.

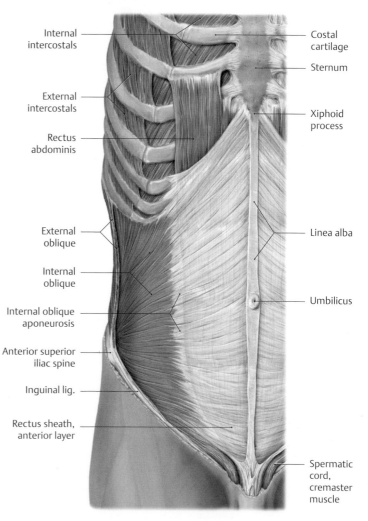

Internal intercostals

External intercostals

Rectus abdominis

External oblique

Internal oblique

Internal oblique aponeurosis

Anterior superior iliac spine

Inguinal lig.

Rectus sheath, anterior layer

Costal cartilage

Sternum

Xiphoid process

Linea alba

Umbilicus

Spermatic cord, cremaster muscle

B *Removed:* External oblique, pectoralis major, and serratus anterior.

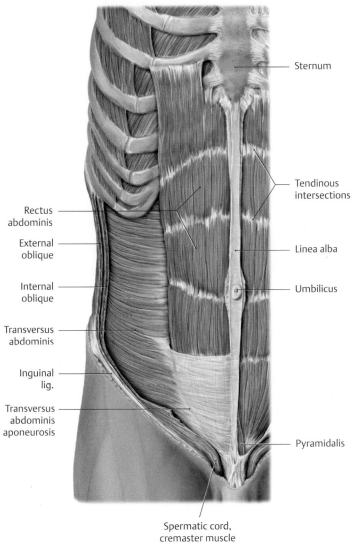

Rectus
abdominis

External
oblique

Internal
oblique

Transversus
abdominis

Inguinal
lig.

Transversus
abdominis
aponeurosis

Sternum

Tendinous
intersections

Linea alba

Umbilicus

Pyramidalis

Spermatic cord,
cremaster muscle

C *Removed:* External and internal obliques.

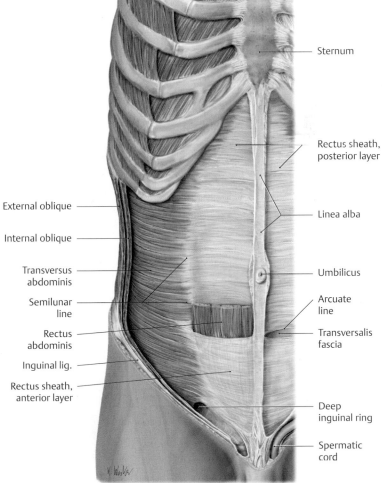

External oblique

Internal oblique

Transversus
abdominis

Semilunar
line

Rectus
abdominis

Inguinal lig.

Rectus sheath,
anterior layer

Sternum

Rectus sheath,
posterior layer

Linea alba

Umbilicus

Arcuate
line

Transversalis
fascia

Deep
inguinal ring

Spermatic
cord

D *Removed:* Rectus abdominis.

145

Rectus Sheath & Posterior Abdominal Wall

Fig. 13.5 **The rectus sheath**

The rectus sheath encloses the rectus abdominis and pyramidalis muscles on either side of the midline. Its anterior and posterior layers are formed by the aponeuroses of the anterolateral muscles as they split to pass around the rectus muscles. An arcuate line marks the inferior extent of the posterior layer, the point at which all of the aponeuroses pass anterior to the rectus muscles.

A Posterior (interior) view of the anterior abdominal wall. Peritoneum and transversalis fascia have been removed on the left side to reveal the rectus sheath.

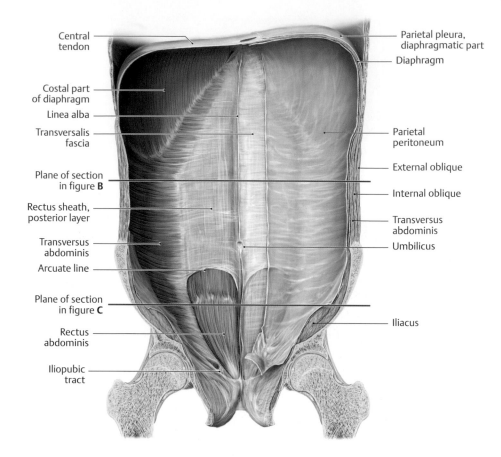

Central tendon

Costal part of diaphragm

Linea alba

Transversalis fascia

Plane of section in figure **B**

Rectus sheath, posterior layer

Transversus abdominis

Arcuate line

Plane of section in figure **C**

Rectus abdominis

Iliopubic tract

Parietal pleura, diaphragmatic part

Diaphragm

Parietal peritoneum

External oblique

Internal oblique

Transversus abdominis

Umbilicus

Iliacus

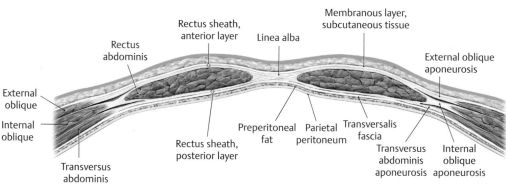

Rectus sheath, anterior layer

Rectus abdominis

Linea alba

Membranous layer, subcutaneous tissue

External oblique aponeurosis

External oblique

Internal oblique

Transversus abdominis

Rectus sheath, posterior layer

Preperitoneal fat

Parietal peritoneum

Transversalis fascia

Transversus abdominis aponeurosis

Internal oblique aponeurosis

B Section through the abdominal wall superior to the arcuate line.

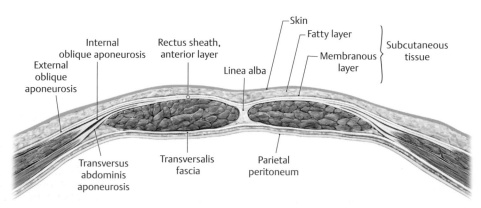

Internal oblique aponeurosis

External oblique aponeurosis

Rectus sheath, anterior layer

Linea alba

Skin

Fatty layer

Membranous layer

Subcutaneous tissue

Transversus abdominis aponeurosis

Transversalis fascia

Parietal peritoneum

C Section through the abdominal wall inferior to the arcuate line.

Fig. 13.6 Muscles of the posterior abdominal wall

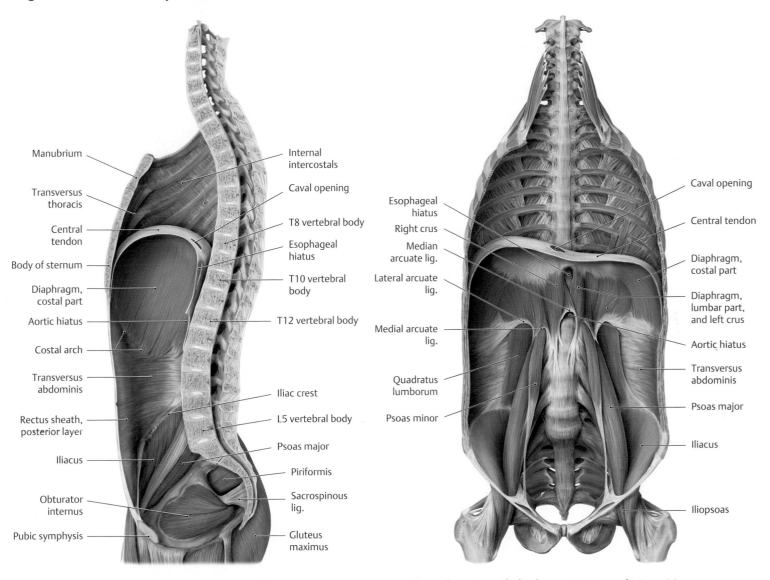

Manubrium

Transversus thoracis

Central tendon

Body of sternum

Diaphragm, costal part

Aortic hiatus

Costal arch

Transversus abdominis

Rectus sheath, posterior layer

Iliacus

Obturator internus

Pubic symphysis

Internal intercostals

Caval opening

T8 vertebral body

Esophageal hiatus

T10 vertebral body

T12 vertebral body

Iliac crest

L5 vertebral body

Psoas major

Piriformis

Sacrospinous lig.

Gluteus maximus

A Midsagittal section with diagraphm in intermediate position.

Esophageal hiatus

Right crus

Median arcuate lig.

Lateral arcuate lig.

Medial arcuate lig.

Quadratus lumborum

Psoas minor

Caval opening

Central tendon

Diaphragm, costal part

Diaphragm, lumbar part, and left crus

Aortic hiatus

Transversus abdominis

Psoas major

Iliacus

Iliopsoas

B Coronal section with diaphragm in intermediate position.

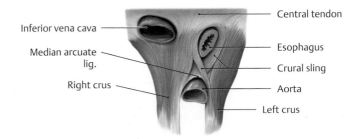

Inferior vena cava

Median arcuate lig.

Right crus

Central tendon

Esophagus

Crural sling

Aorta

Left crus

C Apertures of the diaphragm with vessels transected. Anterior view.
The caval opening is located to the right of the midline, those for the esophagus and aorta are to the left. Note that the crura of the diaphragm typically extend inferiorly as far as the L3 vertebra on the right and L2 vertebra on the left.

 Clinical box 13.1

Diaphragmatic hernias
In diaphragmatic hernias, abdominal viscera prolapse into the thorax through a congenital or acquired opening in the diaphragm. By far the most common herniation site is the esophageal hiatus, accounting for 90% of cases. "Sliding" hernias, which account for 85% of these hiatal hernias, occur when the distal end of the esophagus and the cardia of the stomach slide upward into the thorax through the esophageal hiatus.

Abdominal Wall Muscle Facts

Fig. 13.7 Anterior abdominal wall muscles
Anterior view.

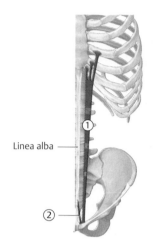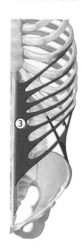

Linea alba

Fig. 13.8 Anterolateral abdominal wall muscles
Anterior view.

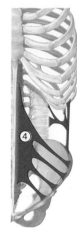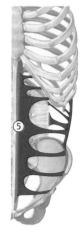

A External oblique.　**B** Internal oblique.　**C** Transversus abdominis.

Fig. 13.9 Posterior abdominal wall muscles
Anterior view. The psoas major and iliacus are together known as the iliopsoas inferiorly.

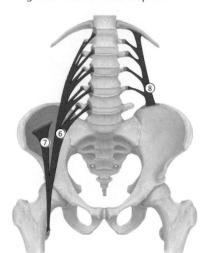

Table 13.1	Abdominal wall muscles				
Muscle	**Origin**	**Insertion**	**Innervation**	**Action**	
Anterior abdominal wall muscles					
① Rectus abdominis	*Lateral head:* Crest of pubis to pubic tubercle *Medial head:* Anterior region of pubic symphysis	Cartilages of 5th to 7th ribs, xiphoid process of sternum	Intercostal nn. (T5–T11) , subcostal n. (T12)	Flexes trunk, compresses abdomen, stabilizes pelvis	
② Pyramidalis	Pubis (anterior to rectus abdominis)	Linea alba (runs within the rectus sheath)	Subcostal n. (T12)	Tenses linea alba	
Anterolateral abdominal wall muscles					
③ External oblique	5th to 12th ribs (outer surface)	Linea alba, pubic tubercle, anterior iliac crest	Intercostal nn. (T7–T11) , subcostal n. (T12)	*Unilateral:* Flexes trunk to same side, rotates trunk to opposite side (external oblique) or same side (internal oblique)	
④ Internal oblique	Thoracolumbar fascia (deep layer), iliac crest (intermediate line), anterior superior iliac spine, iliopsoas fascia	10th to 12th ribs (lower borders), linea alba (anterior and posterior layers)	Intercostal nn. (T7–T11) , subcostal n. (T12) iliohypogastric n., ilioinguinal n.	*Bilateral:* Flexes trunk, compresses abdomen, stabilizes pelvis	
⑤ Transversus abdominis	7th to 12th costal cartilages (inner surfaces), thoracolumbar fascia (deep layer), iliac crest, anterior superior iliac spine (inner lip), iliopsoas fascia	Linea alba, pubic crest		*Unilateral:* Rotates trunk to same side *Bilateral:* Compresses abdomen	
Posterior abdominal wall muscles					
Psoas minor* (see **Fig. 31.19**)	T12, L1 vertebrae and intervertebral disk (lateral surfaces)	Pectineal line, iliopubic ramus, iliac fascia; lowermost fibers may reach inguinal lig.		Weak flexor of the trunk	
⑥ Psoas major	Superficial layer	T12–L4 vertebral bodies and associated intervertebral disks (lateral surfaces)	Femur (lesser trochanter), joint insertion as iliopsoas muscle	L1–L2 (L3) spinal nn.	Hip joint: Flexion and external rotation Lumbar spine (with femur fixed): *Unilateral:* Contraction flexes trunk laterally *Bilateral:* Contraction raises trunk from supine position
	Deep layer	L1–L5 (costal processes)			
⑦ Iliacus	Iliac fossa		Femoral n. (L2–L4)		
⑧ Quadratus lumborum	Iliac crest and iliolumbar lig. (not shown)	12th rib, L1–L4 vertebrae (costal processes)	Subcostal n. (T12), L1–L4 spinal nn.	*Unilateral:* Flexes trunk to same side *Bilateral:* Bearing down and expiration, stabilizes 12th rib	

* Approximately 50% of the population has this muscle. For the diaphragm see **pp. 64–65**.

Fig. 13.10 Anterior, anterolateral, and posterior abdominal wall muscles

Anterior view.

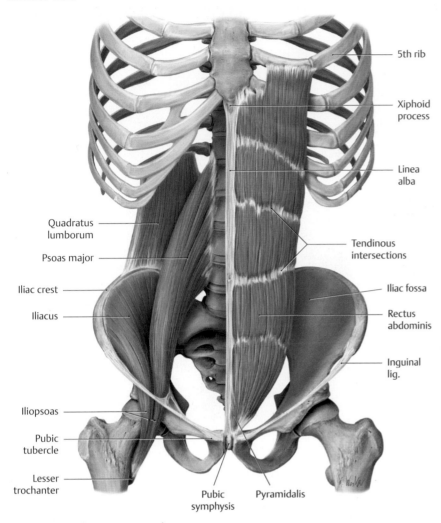

Quadratus lumborum

Psoas major

Iliac crest

Iliacus

Iliopsoas

Pubic tubercle

Lesser trochanter

5th rib

Xiphoid process

Linea alba

Tendinous intersections

Iliac fossa

Rectus abdominis

Inguinal lig.

Pubic symphysis

Pyramidalis

A Anterior and posterior muscles.

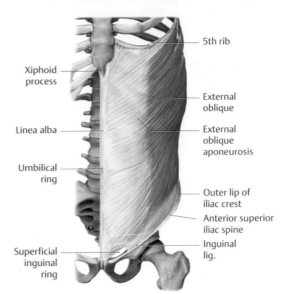

Xiphoid process

Linea alba

Umbilical ring

Superficial inguinal ring

5th rib

External oblique

External oblique aponeurosis

Outer lip of iliac crest

Anterior superior iliac spine

Inguinal lig.

B External oblique.

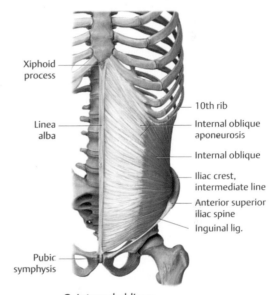

Xiphoid process

Linea alba

Pubic symphysis

10th rib

Internal oblique aponeurosis

Internal oblique

Iliac crest, intermediate line

Anterior superior iliac spine

Inguinal lig.

C Internal oblique.

Fig. 13.11 Anterior and lateral abdominal wall muscles as a functional unit

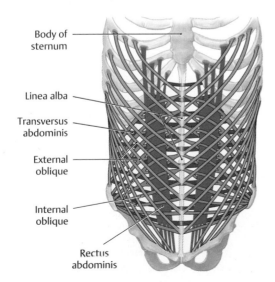

Body of sternum

Linea alba

Transversus abdominis

External oblique

Internal oblique

Rectus abdominis

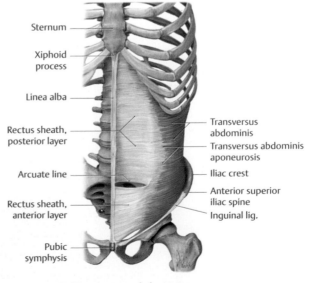

Sternum

Xiphoid process

Linea alba

Rectus sheath, posterior layer

Arcuate line

Rectus sheath, anterior layer

Pubic symphysis

Transversus abdominis

Transversus abdominis aponeurosis

Iliac crest

Anterior superior iliac spine

Inguinal lig.

D Transversus abdominis.

Inguinal Region & Canal

The inguinal region is the junction of the anterior abdominal wall and the anterior thigh. The inguinal canal in the male is an important site for the passage of structures into and out of the abdominal cavity (e.g., components of the spermatic cord).

Fig. 13.12 Inguinal region
Right side, anterior view.

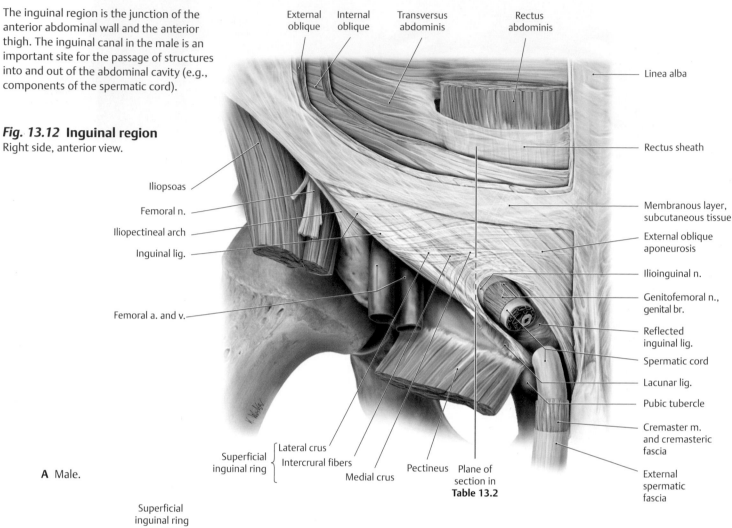

A Male.

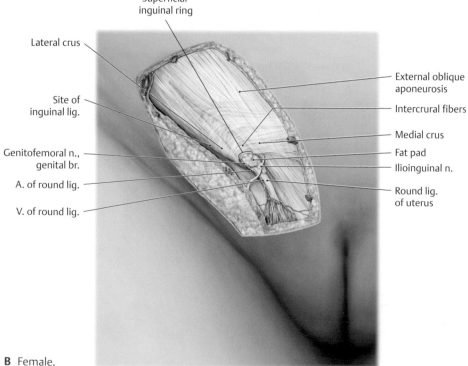

B Female.

Table 13.2	Structures of the inguinal canal		
Structures			**Formed by**
Wall	Anterior wall	①	External oblique aponeurosis
	Roof	②	Internal oblique m.
		③	Transversus abdominis m.
	Posterior wall	④	Transversalis fascia
		⑤	Parietal peritoneum
	Floor	⑥	Inguinal lig. (densely interwoven fibers of the lower external oblique aponeurosis and adjacent fascia lata of the thigh)
Openings	Superficial inguinal ring		Opening in external oblique aponeurosis; bounded by medial and lateral crus, intercrural fibers, and reflected inguinal lig.
	Deep inguinal ring		Outpouching of the transversalis fascia lateral to the lateral umbilical fold (inferior epigastric vessels)

Sagittal section through plane in **Fig. 13.12A.**

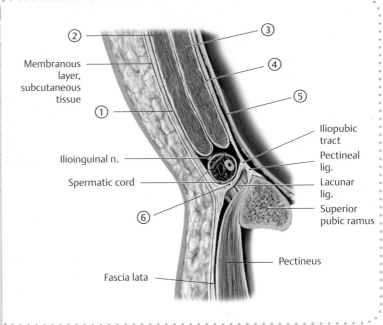

Fig. 13.13 Dissection of the male inguinal region
Right side, anterior view.

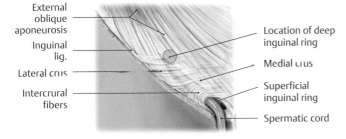

A Superficial layer.

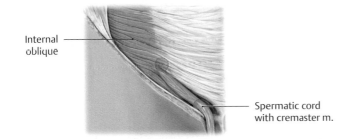

B *Removed:* External oblique aponeurosis.

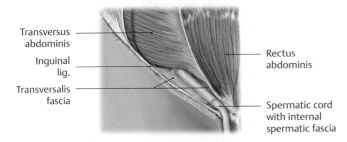

C *Removed:* Internal oblique m.

Fig. 13.14 Opening of the inguinal canal
Right side, anterior view.

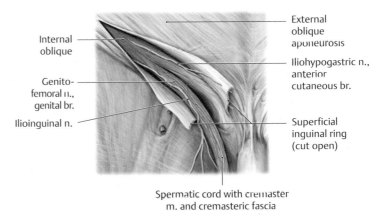

A *Divided:* External oblique aponeurosis.

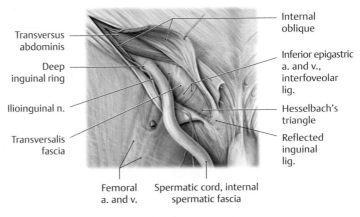

B *Divided:* Internal oblique and cremaster mm.

Inguinal Region & Inguinal Hernias

Fig. 13.15 Sites of herniation through the anterior abdominal wall

Coronal section, male, posterior (internal) view.

A The three fossae of the anterior abdominal wall (circled) are sites of potential herniation through the wall.

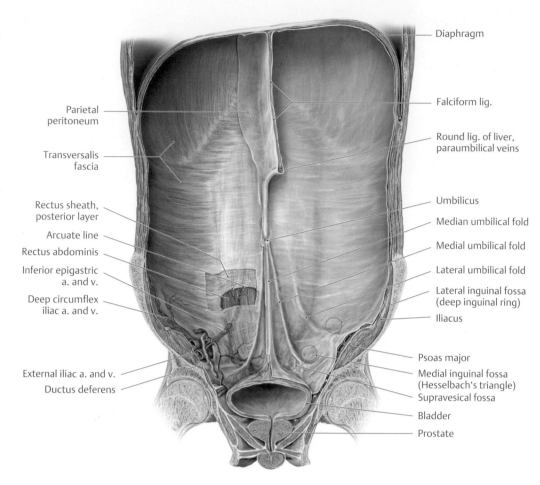

Diaphragm

Falciform lig.

Round lig. of liver, paraumbilical veins

Parietal peritoneum

Transversalis fascia

Umbilicus

Median umbilical fold

Medial umbilical fold

Rectus sheath, posterior layer

Arcuate line

Rectus abdominis

Lateral umbilical fold

Inferior epigastric a. and v.

Lateral inguinal fossa (deep inguinal ring)

Deep circumflex iliac a. and v.

Iliacus

External iliac a. and v.

Ductus deferens

Psoas major

Medial inguinal fossa (Hesselbach's triangle)

Supravesical fossa

Bladder

Prostate

B Internal hernial openings in the male inguinal region. Detail from **A.** Peritoneum and transversalis fascia have been removed to reveal the hernia openings. Color shading indicates openings for supravesical (*green*), indirect (*teal*) and direct (*purple*) hernias (see **Table 13.3**).

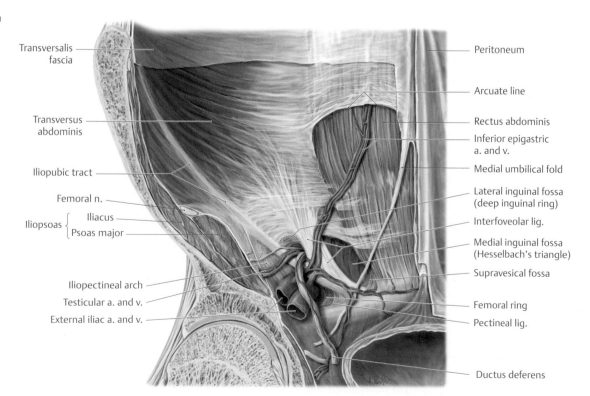

Transversalis fascia

Peritoneum

Arcuate line

Transversus abdominis

Rectus abdominis

Inferior epigastric a. and v.

Iliopubic tract

Medial umbilical fold

Femoral n.

Lateral inguinal fossa (deep inguinal ring)

Iliopsoas { Iliacus

Psoas major }

Interfoveolar lig.

Medial inguinal fossa (Hesselbach's triangle)

Supravesical fossa

Iliopectineal arch

Testicular a. and v.

External iliac a. and v.

Femoral ring

Pectineal lig.

Ductus deferens

Fig. 13.16 Schematic of the male inguinal canal and its relation to structures of the abdominal wall
Right side, anterior view.

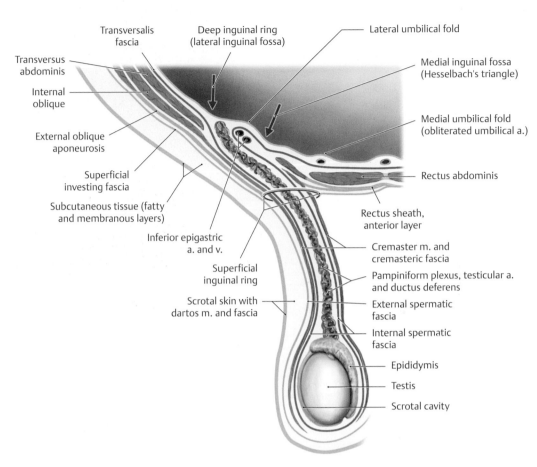

Transversalis fascia

Deep inguinal ring (lateral inguinal fossa)

Lateral umbilical fold

Transversus abdominis

Internal oblique

External oblique aponeurosis

Superficial investing fascia

Subcutaneous tissue (fatty and membranous layers)

Inferior epigastric a. and v.

Superficial inguinal ring

Scrotal skin with dartos m. and fascia

Medial inguinal fossa (Hesselbach's triangle)

Medial umbilical fold (obliterated umbilical a.)

Rectus abdominis

Rectus sheath, anterior layer

Cremaster m. and cremasteric fascia

Pampiniform plexus, testicular a. and ductus deferens

External spermatic fascia

Internal spermatic fascia

Epididymis

Testis

Scrotal cavity

Table 13.3	**Hernias of the inguinal region**

Most inguinal hernias occur in males. All are located above the inguinal ligament and, if large enough, protrude externally through the superficial ring. However, the internal site of origin, and therefore structure of the hernia sac (covering), differ among types. Femoral hernias, more common in women, originate at the femoral ring below the inguinal ligament and emerge at the saphenous opening in the thigh.

Hernia type	Site of origin	Hernia sac
Indirect inguinal (congenital or acquired)	Lateral inguinal fossa (deep inguinal ring) lateral to inferior epigastric vessels	Peritoneum, transversalis fascia, cremaster m.
Direct inguinal (acquired)	Medial inguinal fossa (Hesselbach's triangle), medial to inferior epigastric vessels	Peritoneum, transversalis fascia
Femoral	Femoral ring, inferior to inguinal lig.	Cribiform fascia of saphenous opening

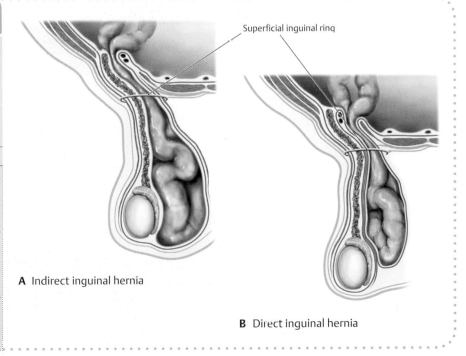

Superficial inguinal ring

A Indirect inguinal hernia

B Direct inguinal hernia

153

Scrotum & Spermatic Cord

The coverings of the scrotum, testis, and spermatic cord are continuations of muscular and fascial layers of the anterior abdominal wall, as are those of the inguinal canal.

***Fig. 13.17* Scrotum and spermatic cord**
Anterior view.

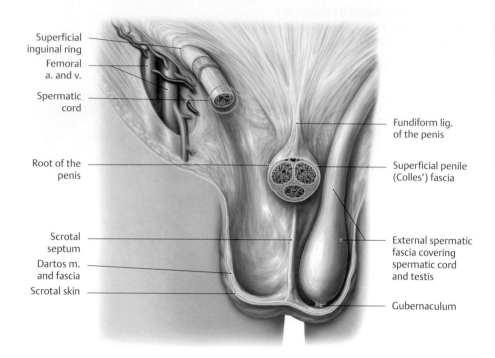

- Superficial inguinal ring
- Femoral a. and v.
- Spermatic cord
- Root of the penis
- Scrotal septum
- Dartos m. and fascia
- Scrotal skin
- Fundiform lig. of the penis
- Superficial penile (Colles') fascia
- External spermatic fascia covering spermatic cord and testis
- Gubernaculum

A Structure and contents of the scrotum.

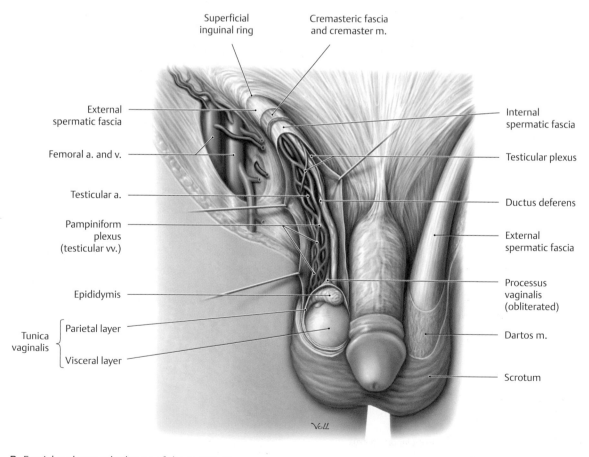

- Superficial inguinal ring
- Cremasteric fascia and cremaster m.
- External spermatic fascia
- Femoral a. and v.
- Testicular a.
- Pampiniform plexus (testicular vv.)
- Epididymis
- Tunica vaginalis { Parietal layer / Visceral layer }
- Internal spermatic fascia
- Testicular plexus
- Ductus deferens
- External spermatic fascia
- Processus vaginalis (obliterated)
- Dartos m.
- Scrotum

Voll

B Fascial and muscular layers of the spermatic cord have been opened to reveal its contents.

Table 13.4	Contents of the spermatic cord
Surrounding layer	**Contents**
External spermatic fascia	① Ilioinguinal n.
Cremasteric muscle	② Cremasteric a. and v.
	③ Genitofemoral n., genital br.
Internal spermatic fascia	④ A. and v. of ductus deferens
	⑤ Ductus deferens
	⑥ Testicular a.
	⑦ Processus vaginalis (obliterated)
	⑧ Testicular (nerve) plexus
	⑨ Pampiniform (venous) plexus

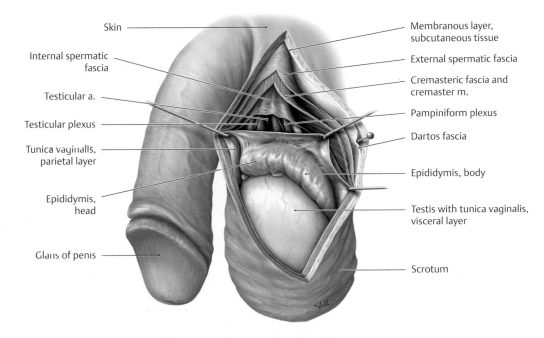

Fig. 13.18 Testis and epididymis

Left lateral view.

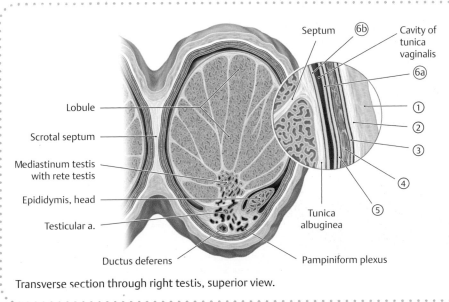

Transverse section through right testis, superior view.

Table 13.5	Coverings of the testis	
Covering layer		**Derived from**
①	Scrotal skin	Abdominal skin
②	Dartos m. and fascia	Membranous layer, subcutaneous tissue
③	External spermatic fascia	External oblique aponeurosis and superficial investing fascia
④	Cremaster m. and cremasteric fascia	Internal oblique m.
⑤	Internal spermatic fascia	Transversalis fascia
⑥a	Tunica vaginalis, parietal layer	Peritoneum
⑥b	Tunica vaginalis, visceral layer	

* The transversus abdominis has no contribution to the spermatic cord or covering of the testis.

14 Abdominal Cavity & Spaces

Divisions of the Abdominopelvic Cavity

***Fig. 14.1* Organs of the abdominopelvic cavity**

Midsagittal section, male, viewed from the left.

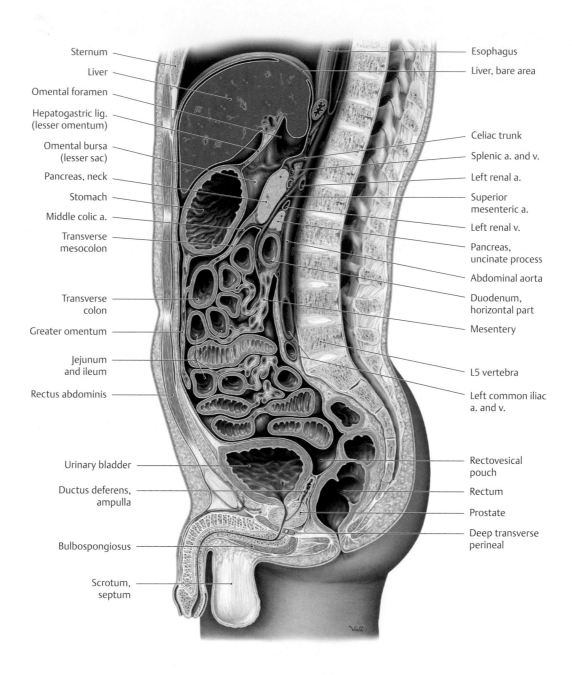

Sternum

Liver

Omental foramen

Hepatogastric lig. (lesser omentum)

Omental bursa (lesser sac)

Pancreas, neck

Stomach

Middle colic a.

Transverse mesocolon

Transverse colon

Greater omentum

Jejunum and ileum

Rectus abdominis

Urinary bladder

Ductus deferens, ampulla

Bulbospongiosus

Scrotum, septum

Esophagus

Liver, bare area

Celiac trunk

Splenic a. and v.

Left renal a.

Superior mesenteric a.

Left renal v.

Pancreas, uncinate process

Abdominal aorta

Duodenum, horizontal part

Mesentery

L5 vertebra

Left common iliac a. and v.

Rectovesical pouch

Rectum

Prostate

Deep transverse perineal

✳ Clinical box 14.1

Acute abdominal pain

Acute abdominal pain ("acute abdomen") may be so severe that the abdominal wall becomes extremely sensitive to touch ("guarding") and the intestines stop functioning. Causes include organ inflammation such as appendicitis, perforation due to a gastric ulcer (see **p. 167**), or organ blockage by a stone, tumor, etc. In women, gynecological processes or ectopic pregnancies may produce severe abdominal pain.

Fig. 14.2 Divisions of the pelvic and abdominal cavities

Each column of diagrams shows a midsagittal section viewed from the left side, as well as two axial sections, one at the L1 level and the other at the lower part of the sacrum, both viewed from below.

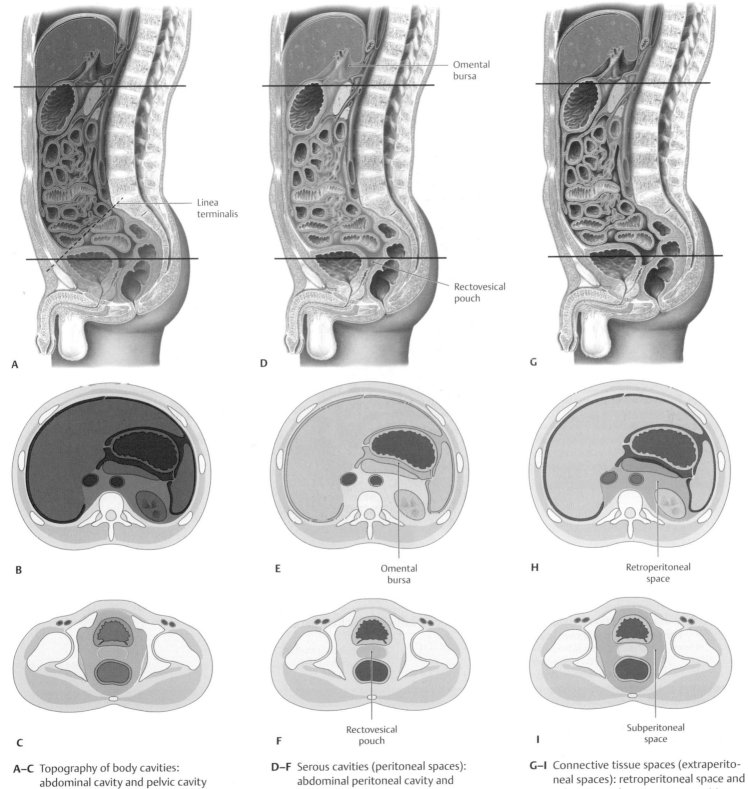

A–C Topography of body cavities: abdominal cavity and pelvic cavity (imaginary line separating the two cavities is the linea terminalis).

D–F Serous cavities (peritoneal spaces): abdominal peritoneal cavity and pelvic peritoneal cavity.

G–I Connective tissue spaces (extraperitoneal spaces): retroperitoneal space and subperitoneal space; serous cavities and extraperitoneal spaces are separated by peritoneum.

Mesenteries & Peritoneal Recesses

The peritoneal cavity is divided into the large greater sac and small omental bursa (lesser sac). The greater omentum is an apron-like fold of peritoneum suspended from the greater curvature of the stomach and covering the anterior surface of the transverse colon. The attach-ment of the transverse mesocolon on the anterior surface of the descending part of the duodenum and the pancreas divides the peritoneal cavity into a supracolic compartment (liver, gallbladder, and stomach) and an infracolic compartment (intestines).

Fig. 14.7 **Dissection of the peritoneal cavity**
Anterior view.

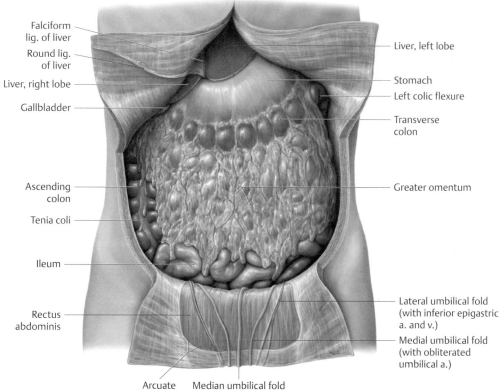

Falciform lig. of liver
Round lig. of liver
Liver, right lobe
Gallbladder
Ascending colon
Tenia coli
Ileum
Rectus abdominis
Arcuate line
Median umbilical fold (with obliterated urachus)
Liver, left lobe
Stomach
Left colic flexure
Transverse colon
Greater omentum
Lateral umbilical fold (with inferior epigastric a. and v.)
Medial umbilical fold (with obliterated umbilical a.)

A Greater sac. *Retracted:* Abdominal wall.

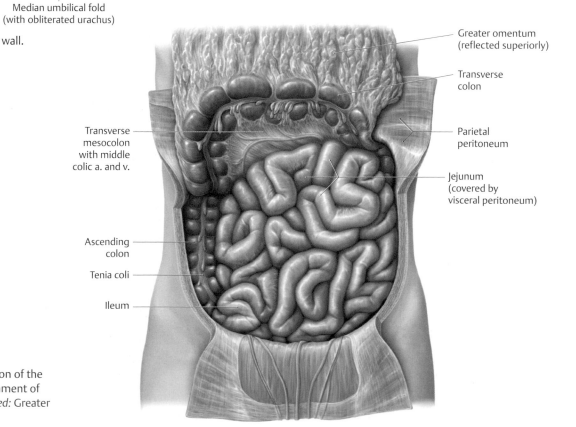

Transverse mesocolon with middle colic a. and v.
Ascending colon
Tenia coli
Ileum
Greater omentum (reflected superiorly)
Transverse colon
Parietal peritoneum
Jejunum (covered by visceral peritoneum)

B Infracolic compartment, the portion of the peritoneal cavity below the attachment of the transverse mesocolon. *Reflected:* Greater omentum and transverse colon.

C Mesentery (of the small intestine). *Reflected:* Greater omentum, transverse colon, small intestine.

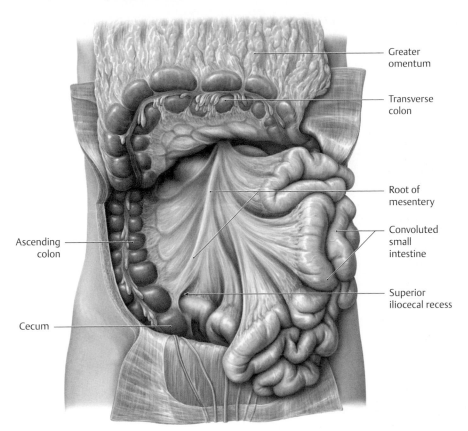

Greater omentum

Transverse colon

Root of mesentery

Convoluted small intestine

Superior iliocecal recess

Ascending colon

Cecum

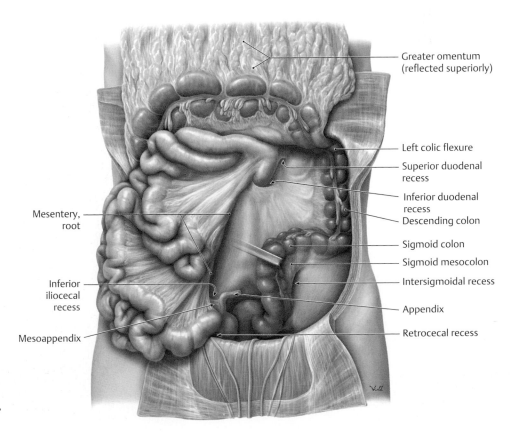

Greater omentum (reflected superiorly)

Left colic flexure

Superior duodenal recess

Inferior duodenal recess

Descending colon

Sigmoid colon

Sigmoid mesocolon

Intersigmoidal recess

Appendix

Retrocecal recess

Mesentery, root

Inferior iliocecal recess

Mesoappendix

D Mesenteries and mesenteric recesses in the infracolic compartment. *Reflected:* Greater omentum, transverse colon, small intestines, and sigmoid colon.

Lesser Omentum & Omental Bursa

The omental bursa, or lesser sac, is the portion of the peritoneal cavity behind the stomach and the lesser omentum (a double-layered peritoneal structure connecting the lesser curvature of the stomach and the proximal part of the duodenum to the liver). The omental bursa communicates with the greater sac via the omental (epiploic) foramen, located posterior to the free edge of the lesser omentum.

Fig. 14.8 The lesser omentum
Anterior view with liver retracted superiorly.
The arrow points to the omental foramen, the opening into the omental bursa, posterior to the lesser omentum.

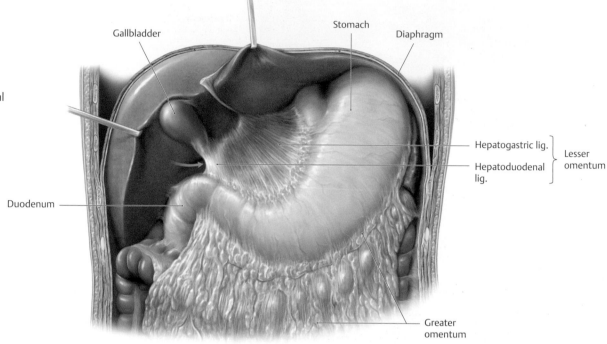

Gallbladder — Stomach — Diaphragm — Hepatogastric lig. — Hepatoduodenal lig. } Lesser omentum — Duodenum — Greater omentum

Fig. 14.9 Omental bursa in situ
Anterior view. *Divided:* Gastrocolic ligament.
Retracted: Liver. *Reflected:* Stomach.

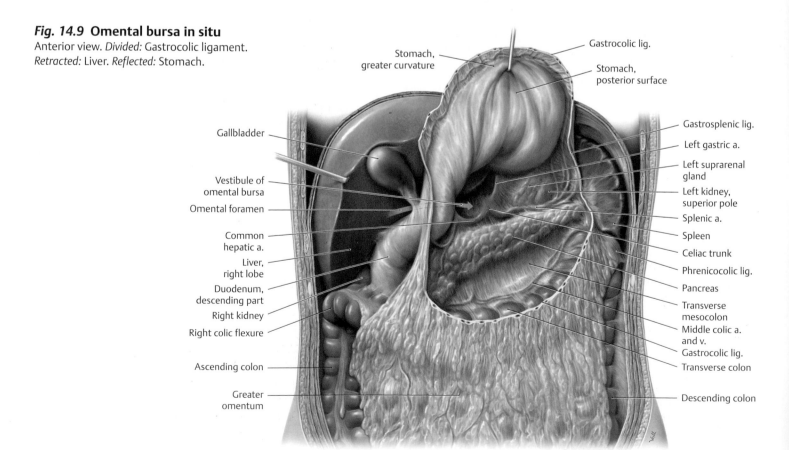

Stomach, greater curvature — Gastrocolic lig. — Stomach, posterior surface — Gastrosplenic lig. — Left gastric a. — Left suprarenal gland — Left kidney, superior pole — Splenic a. — Spleen — Celiac trunk — Phrenicocolic lig. — Pancreas — Transverse mesocolon — Middle colic a. and v. — Gastrocolic lig. — Transverse colon — Descending colon
Gallbladder — Vestibule of omental bursa — Omental foramen — Common hepatic a. — Liver, right lobe — Duodenum, descending part — Right kidney — Right colic flexure — Ascending colon — Greater omentum

Fig. 14.10 Location of the omental bursa

Transverse section, inferior view.

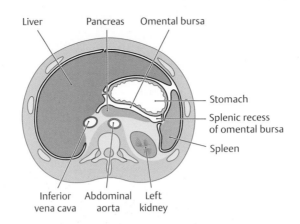

Fig. 14.11 Boundaries and walls of the omental bursa (lesser sac)

Anterior view.

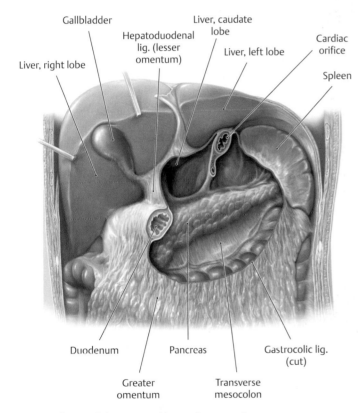

A Boundaries of the omental bursa (lesser sac).

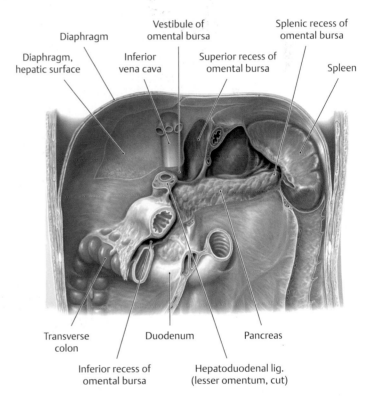

B Posterior wall of the omental bursa (lesser sac).

Table 14.3	Boundaries of the omental bursa	
Direction	**Boundary**	**Recess**
Anterior	Lesser omentum, gastrocolic lig.	—
Inferior	Transverse mesocolon	Inferior recess
Superior	Liver (with caudate lobe)	Superior recess
Posterior	Pancreas, aorta (abdominal part), celiac trunk, splenic a. and v., gastrosplenic fold, left suprarenal gland, left kidney (superior pole)	—
Right	Liver, duodenal bulb	—
Left	Spleen, gastrosplenic lig.	Splenic recess

Table 14.4	Boundaries of the omental foramen
The communication between the greater sac and lesser sac (omental bursa) is the omental (epiploic) foramen (see arrow in **Fig. 14.9**).	
Direction	**Boundary**
Anterior	Hepatoduodenal lig. with the portal v., proper hepatic a., and bile duct
Inferior	Duodenum (superior part)
Posterior	Inferior vena cava, diaphragm (right crus)
Superior	Liver (caudate lobe)

Mesenteries & Posterior Abdominal Wall

Fig. 14.12 Mesenteric attachments of intraperitoneal organs

Anterior view. *Removed:* Stomach, jejunum and ileum, and transverse and sigmoid colons. *Retracted:* Liver.

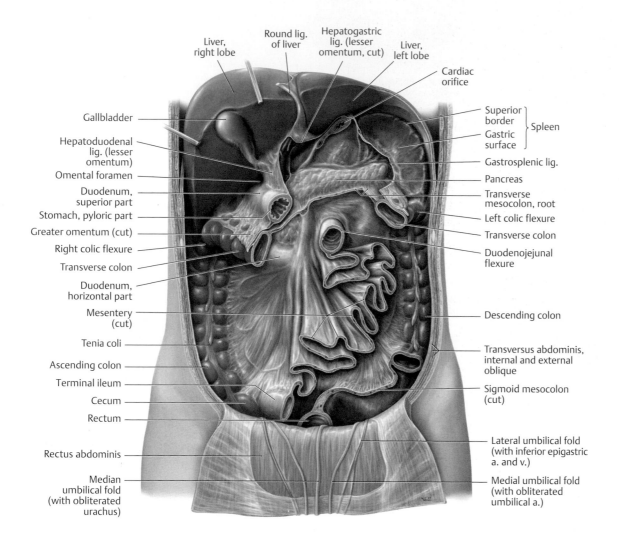

Liver, right lobe — Round lig. of liver — Hepatogastric lig. (lesser omentum, cut) — Liver, left lobe — Cardiac orifice

Superior border — Spleen
Gastric surface

Gallblader
Gastrosplenic lig.

Hepatoduodenal lig. (lesser omentum)
Pancreas

Omental foramen
Transverse mesocolon, root

Duodenum, superior part
Left colic flexure

Stomach, pyloric part
Transverse colon

Greater omentum (cut)
Duodenojejunal flexure

Right colic flexure

Transverse colon

Duodenum, horizontal part

Mesentery (cut)
Descending colon

Tenia coli

Ascending colon
Transversus abdominis, internal and external oblique

Terminal ileum
Sigmoid mesocolon (cut)

Cecum

Rectum

Rectus abdominis
Lateral umbilical fold (with inferior epigastric a. and v.)

Median umbilical fold (with obliterated urachus)
Medial umbilical fold (with obliterated umbilical a.)

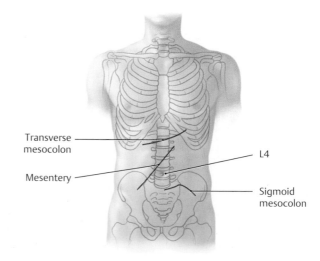

Transverse mesocolon

Mesentery

L4

Sigmoid mesocolon

Fig. 14.13 Location of mesenteric sites of connection to the abdominal wall

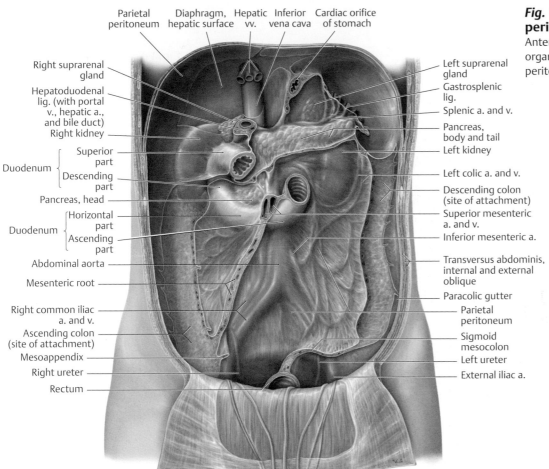

Fig. 14.14 Posterior wall of the peritoneal cavity

Anterior view. *Removed:* All intraperitoneal organs. *Revealed:* Structures of the retroperitoneum (see **Table 14.2** and **p. 250**).

Parietal peritoneum · Diaphragm, hepatic surface · Hepatic vv. · Inferior vena cava · Cardiac orifice of stomach

Right suprarenal gland
Hepatoduodenal lig. (with portal v., hepatic a., and bile duct)
Right kidney
Duodenum { Superior part / Descending part
Pancreas, head
Duodenum { Horizontal part / Ascending part
Abdominal aorta
Mesenteric root
Right common iliac a. and v.
Ascending colon (site of attachment)
Mesoappendix
Right ureter
Rectum

Left suprarenal gland
Gastrosplenic lig.
Splenic a. and v.
Pancreas, body and tail
Left kidney
Left colic a. and v.
Descending colon (site of attachment)
Superior mesenteric a. and v.
Inferior mesenteric a.
Transversus abdominis, internal and external oblique
Paracolic gutter
Parietal peritoneum
Sigmoid mesocolon
Left ureter
External iliac a.

Fig. 14.15 Drainage spaces and recesses within the peritoneal cavity

Anterior view.

Subhepatic recess · Subphrenic recess · Left paracolic gutter
Hepato-renal recess
Right paracolic gutter
Right infracolic space · Left infracolic space

A Anterior view with the greater omentum and small intestine removed; preferred metastatic sites (see blue stars).

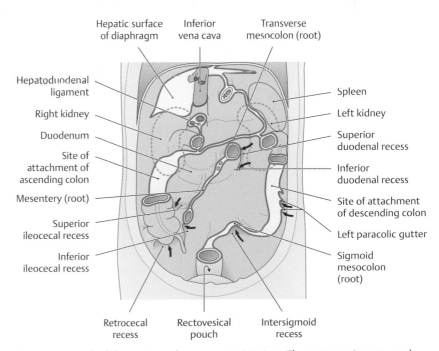

Hepatic surface of diaphragm · Inferior vena cava · Transverse mesocolon (root)
Hepatoduodenal ligament
Right kidney
Duodenum
Site of attachment of ascending colon
Mesentery (root)
Superior ileocecal recess
Inferior ileocecal recess
Spleen
Left kidney
Superior duodenal recess
Inferior duodenal recess
Site of attachment of descending colon
Left paracolic gutter
Sigmoid mesocolon (root)
Retrocecal recess · Rectovesical pouch · Intersigmoid recess

B Posterior wall of the peritoneal cavity, anterior view. The mesenteric roots and sites of organ attachment create partially bounded spaces (recesses or sulci) where peritoneal fluid can flow freely.

15 Internal Organs
Stomach

Fig. 15.1 Stomach: Location

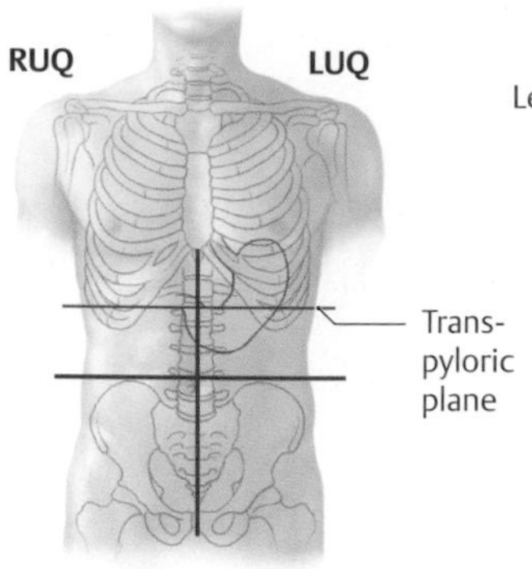

RUQ   LUQ

Trans-
pyloric
plane

A Anterior view.

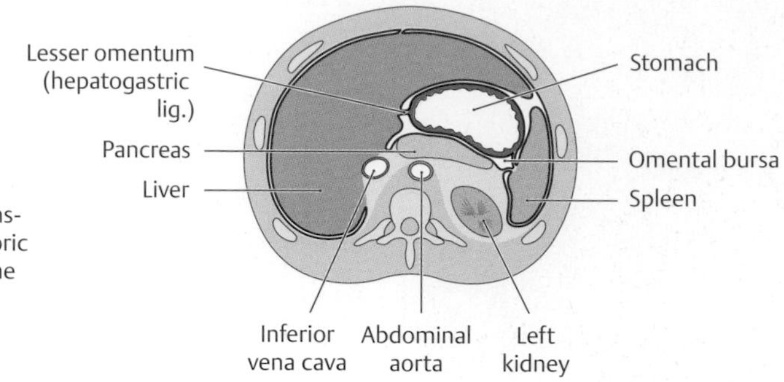

Lesser omentum
(hepatogastric
lig.)

Pancreas

Liver

Inferior
vena cava   Abdominal
aorta   Left
kidney

Stomach

Omental bursa

Spleen

B Transverse section, inferior view.

Fig. 15.2 Relations of the stomach

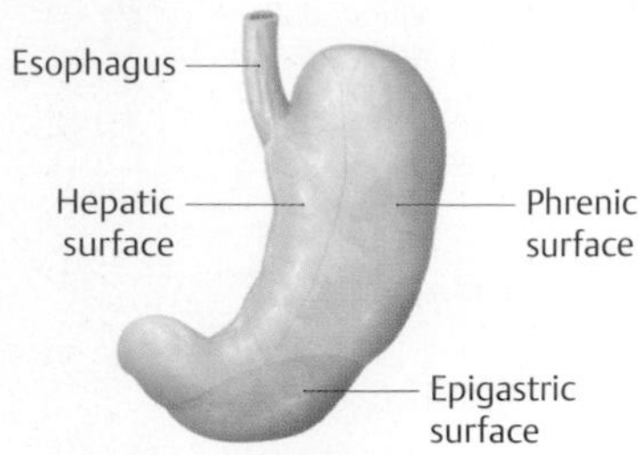

Esophagus

Hepatic
surface

Phrenic
surface

Epigastric
surface

A Anterior view.

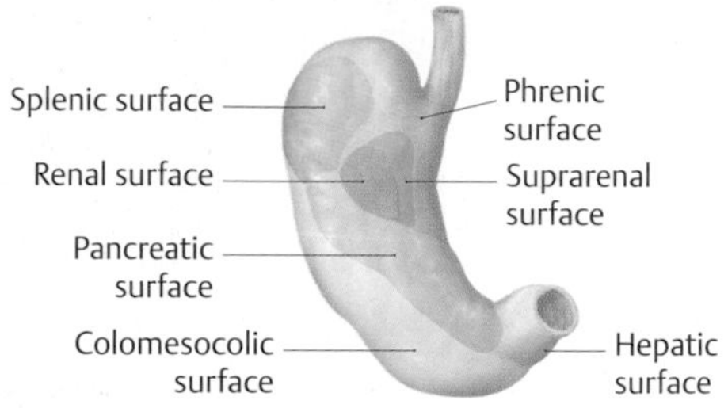

Splenic surface

Renal surface

Pancreatic
surface

Colomesocolic
surface

Phrenic
surface

Suprarenal
surface

Hepatic
surface

B Posterior view.

Fig. 15.3 Stomach
Anterior view.

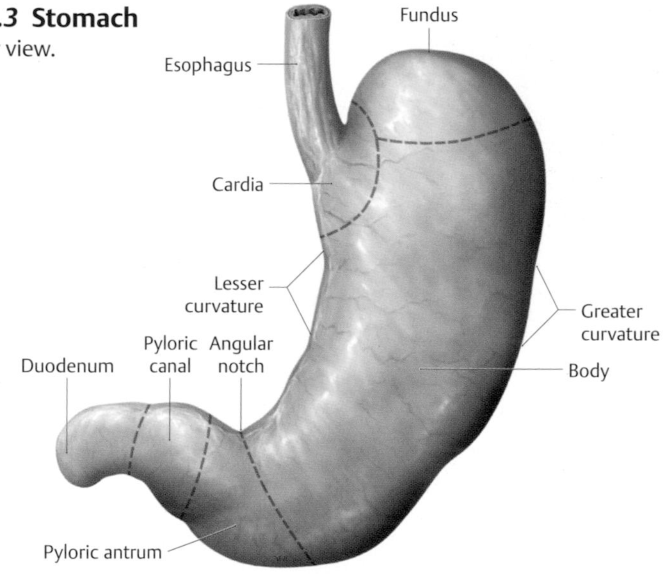

Esophagus

Cardia

Lesser
curvature

Pyloric   Angular
canal   notch

Duodenum

Fundus

Greater
curvature

Body

Pyloric antrum

A Anterior wall.

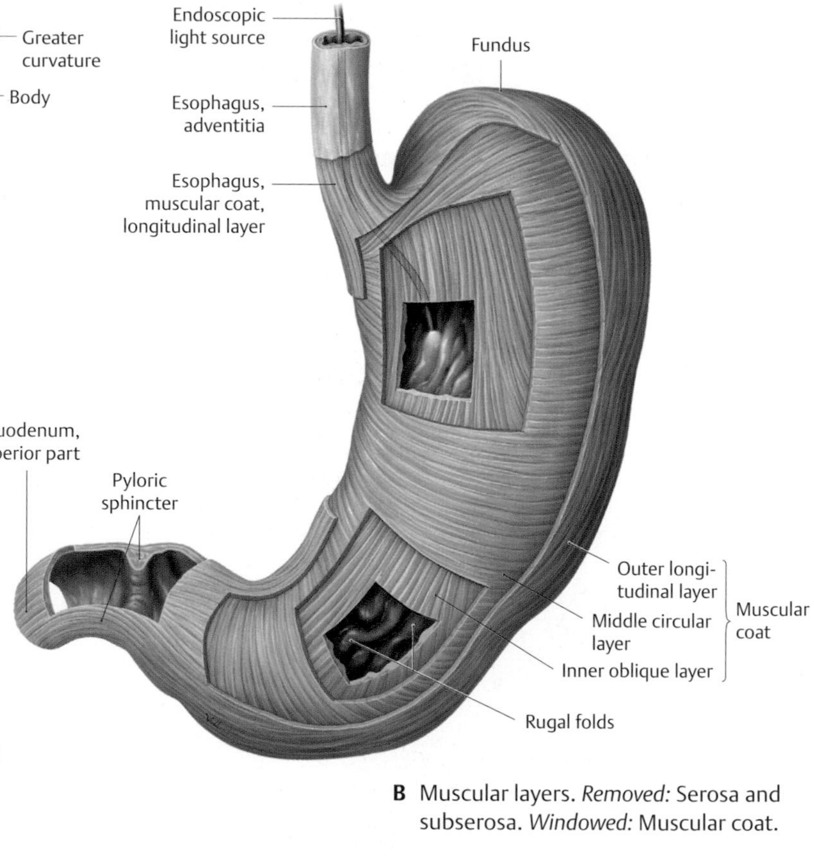

Esophagus

Cardia

Duodenum

Pyloric
sphincter   Angular
notch

Pyloric
orifice

Body with
longitudinal
rugal folds

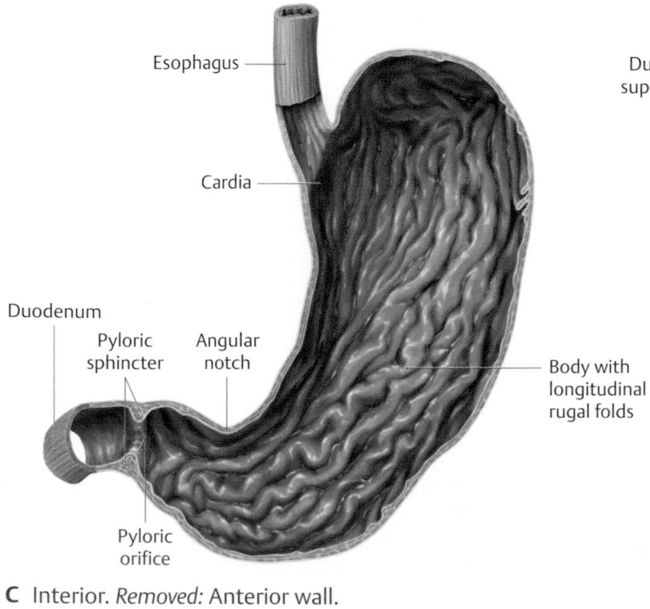

C Interior. *Removed:* Anterior wall.

Endoscopic
light source

Esophagus,
adventitia

Esophagus,
muscular coat,
longitudinal layer

Duodenum,
superior part

Pyloric
sphincter

Fundus

Outer longi-
tudinal layer

Middle circular
layer

Inner oblique layer

Muscular
coat

Rugal folds

B Muscular layers. *Removed:* Serosa and
subserosa. *Windowed:* Muscular coat.

The stomach, an intraperitoneal organ, resides primarily in the left upper quadrant. Double layers of peritoneum extend superiorly from its lesser curvature as the lesser omentum and inferiorly from its greater curvature as the greater omentum.

Fig. 15.4 Stomach in situ

Anterior view of the opened upper abdomen. Arrow indicates the omental foramen.

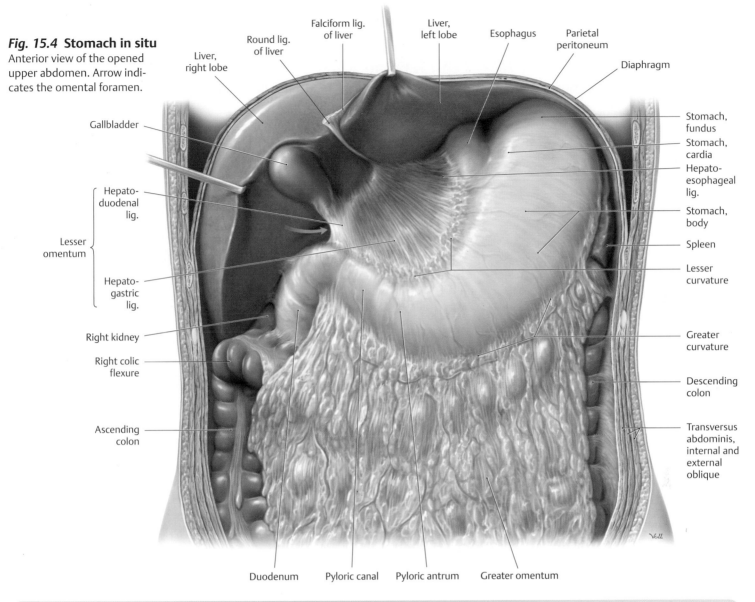

Clinical box 15.1

Gastritis and gastric ulcers

Gastritis and gastric ulcers, the two most common diseases of the stomach, are associated with increased acid production and are caused by alcohol, drugs such as aspirin, and the bacterium *Helicobacter pylori*. Symptoms include lessened appetite, pain, and even bleeding, which manifests as black stool or dark brown material, often described as resembling "coffee grounds," in vomit. Gastritis is limited to the inner surface of the stomach, whereas gastric ulcers extend into the stomach wall. In these endoscopic images, the gastric ulcer in **C** is covered with fibrin and shows hematin spots.

A Body of normal stomach.

B Normal pyloric antrum.

C Gastric ulcer.

Duodenum

The small intestine consists of the duodenum, jejunum, and ileum. The duodenum is primarily retroperitoneal and is divided into four parts: superior, descending, horizontal, and ascending.

Fig. 15.5 **Duodenum: Location**
Anterior view.

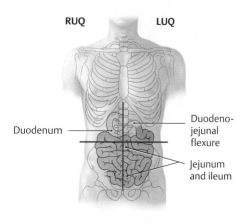

RUQ   LUQ

Duodenum

Duodeno-
jejunal
flexure

Jejunum
and ileum

Fig. 15.6 **Parts of the duodenum**
Anterior view.

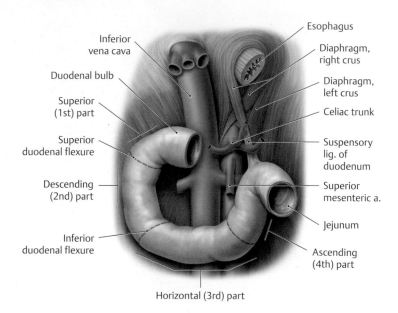

Inferior
vena cava

Duodenal bulb

Superior
(1st) part

Superior
duodenal flexure

Descending
(2nd) part

Inferior
duodenal flexure

Esophagus

Diaphragm,
right crus

Diaphragm,
left crus

Celiac trunk

Suspensory
lig. of
duodenum

Superior
mesenteric a.

Jejunum

Ascending
(4th) part

Horizontal (3rd) part

Fig. 15.7 **Duodenum**
Anterior view with the anterior wall opened.

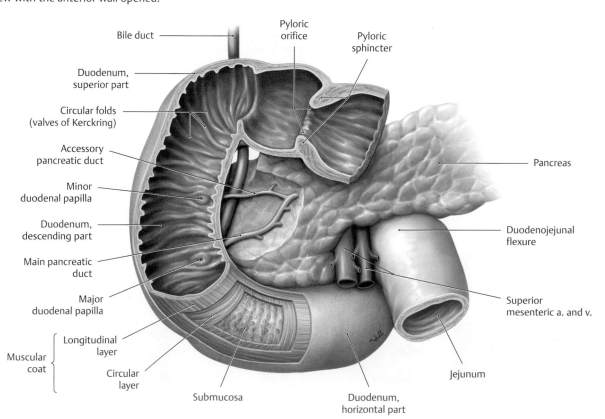

Bile duct

Duodenum,
superior part

Circular folds
(valves of Kerckring)

Accessory
pancreatic duct

Minor
duodenal papilla

Duodenum,
descending part

Main pancreatic
duct

Major
duodenal papilla

Muscular
coat {
Longitudinal
layer

Circular
layer

Submucosa

Pyloric
orifice

Pyloric
sphincter

Pancreas

Duodenojejunal
flexure

Superior
mesenteric a. and v.

Jejunum

Duodenum,
horizontal part

Fig. 15.8 **Duodenum in situ**

Anterior view. *Removed:* Stomach, liver, small intestine, and large portions of the transverse colon. *Thinned:* Retroperitoneal fat and connective tissue.

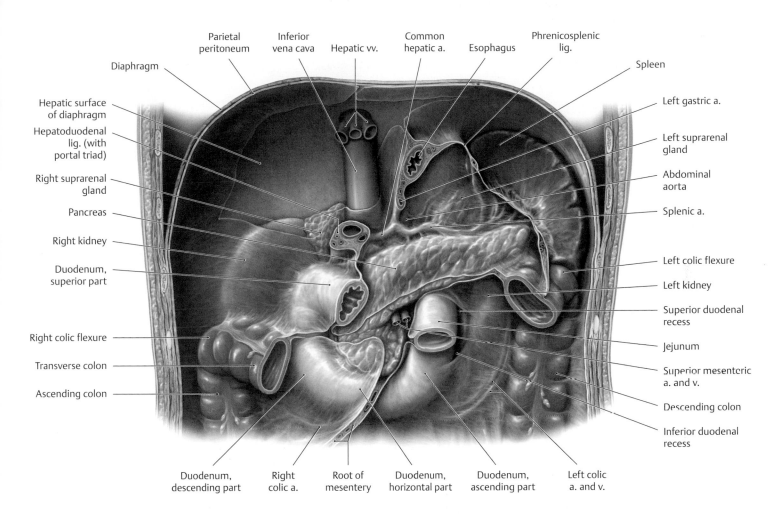

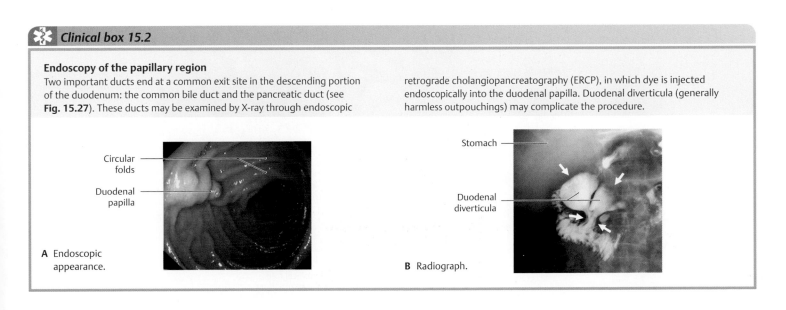

Endoscopy of the papillary region

Two important ducts end at a common exit site in the descending portion of the duodenum: the common bile duct and the pancreatic duct (see **Fig. 15.27**). These ducts may be examined by X-ray through endoscopic retrograde cholangiopancreatography (ERCP), in which dye is injected endoscopically into the duodenal papilla. Duodenal diverticula (generally harmless outpouchings) may complicate the procedure.

A Endoscopic appearance.

B Radiograph.

Jejunum & Ileum

Fig. 15.9 Jejunum and ileum: Location
Anterior view. The intraperitoneal jejunum and ileum are enclosed by the mesentery proper.

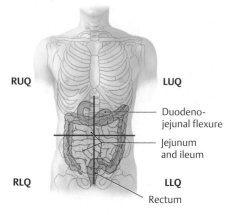

RUQ

LUQ

Duodeno-jejunal flexure

Jejunum and ileum

RLQ

LLQ

Rectum

Fig. 15.10 Mucosal appearance of the jejunum and ileum
Macroscopic views of the longitudinally opened small intestine.

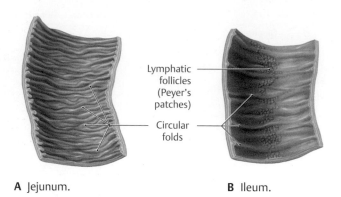

Lymphatic follicles (Peyer's patches)

Circular folds

A Jejunum.

B Ileum.

Fig. 15.11 Jejunum and ileum in situ
Anterior view. *Reflected:* Transverse colon.

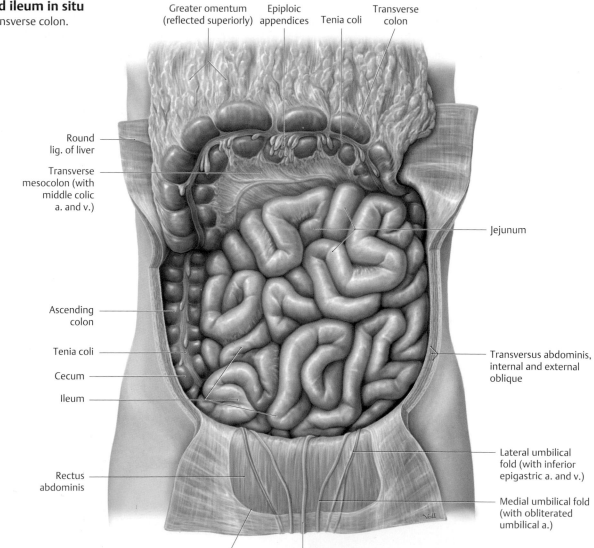

Greater omentum (reflected superiorly)

Epiploic appendices

Tenia coli

Transverse colon

Round lig. of liver

Transverse mesocolon (with middle colic a. and v.)

Jejunum

Ascending colon

Tenia coli

Cecum

Ileum

Transversus abdominis, internal and external oblique

Lateral umbilical fold (with inferior epigastric a. and v.)

Rectus abdominis

Medial umbilical fold (with obliterated umbilical a.)

Arcuate line

Median umbilical fold (with obliterated urachus)

Clinical box 15.3

Crohn's disease

Crohn's disease, a chronic inflammation of the digestive tract, occurs most often in the terminal ileum (30% of cases). Patients are generally young and suffer from abdominal pain, nausea, elevated body temperature, and diarrhea. Initially, these symptoms can be confused with appendicitis. Complications of the chronic inflammation in Crohn's disease often lead to fistula formation (seen here in figure **B** as an abnormal passage between two gastrointestinal regions).

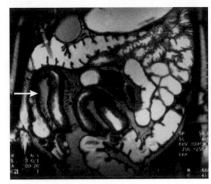

A MRI showing thickened wall of terminal ileum. (arrow).

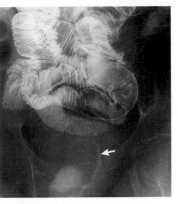

B Double-contrast radiograph, showing ileorectal fistula (arrow).

Fig. 15.12 Mesentery of the small intestine

Anterior view. *Removed:* Stomach, jejunum, and ileum. *Reflected:* Liver.

Liver, right lobe
Round lig. of liver
Hepatogastric lig.
Liver, left lobe
Esophagus
Gallbladder
Lesser omentum, hepatoduodenal lig.
Omental foramen
Duodenum, superior part
Stomach, pyloric part
Greater omentum
Right colic flexure
Transverse colon
Duodenum, horizontal part
Mesentery (cut edge)
Tenia coli
Ascending colon
Terminal ileum
Cecum
Rectum
Spleen
Gastrosplenic lig.
Pancreas
Transverse mesocolon, root
Left colic flexure
Transverse colon
Duodenojejunal flexure
Descending colon
Sigmoid mesocolon (cut edge)

Cecum, Appendix & Colon

The ascending and descending colon are normally secondarily retro-peritoneal, but are sometimes suspended by a short mesentery from the posterior abdominal wall. *Note*: In the clinical setting, the left colic flexure is often referred to as the splenic flexure and the right colic flexure, as the hepatic flexure.

Fig. 15.13 Large intestine: Location
Anterior view.

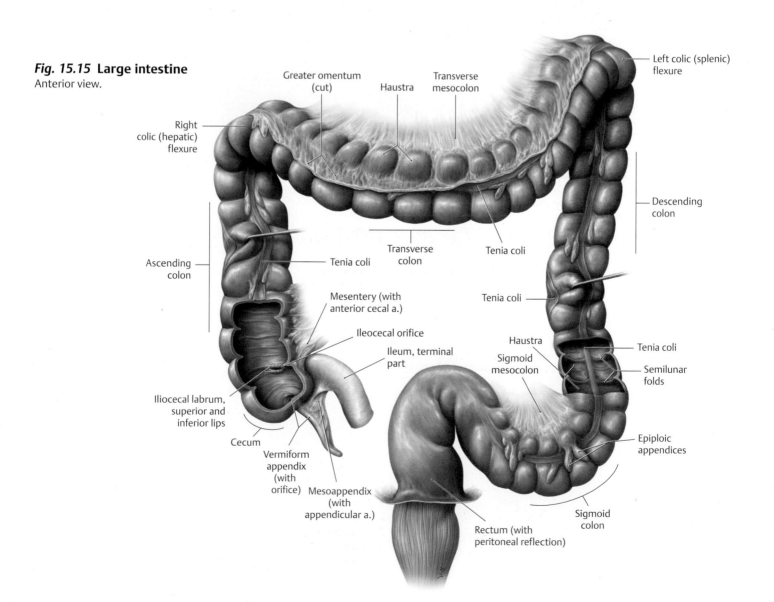

RUQ

LUQ

Right colic flexure

Left colic flexure

Ascending colon

Transverse colon

Descending colon

Cecum

Sigmoid colon

RLQ

LLQ

Rectum

Fig. 15.14 Ileocecal orifice
Anterior view of longitudinal coronal section.

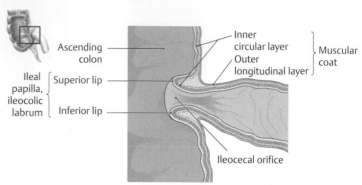

Ascending colon

Inner circular layer

Outer longitudinal layer

Muscular coat

Ileal papilla, ileocolic labrum

Superior lip

Inferior lip

Ileocecal orifice

Fig. 15.15 Large intestine
Anterior view.

Greater omentum (cut)

Haustra

Transverse mesocolon

Left colic (splenic) flexure

Right colic (hepatic) flexure

Descending colon

Ascending colon

Tenia coli

Transverse colon

Tenia coli

Tenia coli

Mesentery (with anterior cecal a.)

Ileocecal orifice

Ileum, terminal part

Haustra

Tenia coli

Sigmoid mesocolon

Semilunar folds

Iliocecal labrum, superior and inferior lips

Cecum

Vermiform appendix (with orifice)

Mesoappendix (with appendicular a.)

Epiploic appendices

Sigmoid colon

Rectum (with peritoneal reflection)

Fig. 15.16 Large intestine in situ

Anterior view. *Reflected:* Transverse colon and greater omentum. *Removed:* Intraperitoneal small intestine.

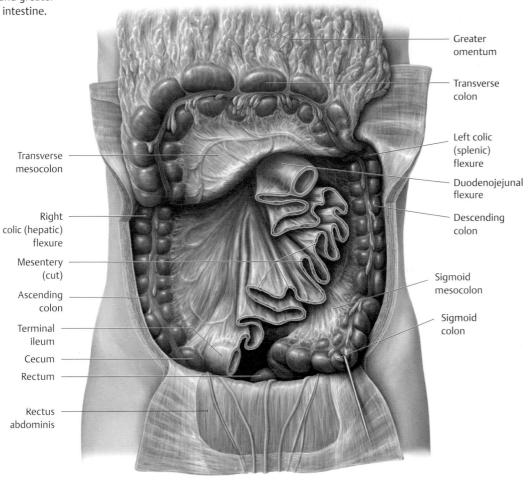

Greater omentum

Transverse colon

Left colic (splenic) flexure

Duodenojejunal flexure

Descending colon

Transverse mesocolon

Right colic (hepatic) flexure

Mesentery (cut)

Ascending colon

Terminal ileum

Cecum

Rectum

Rectus abdominis

Sigmoid mesocolon

Sigmoid colon

 Clinical box 15.4

Colitis

Ulcerative colitis is a chronic inflammation of the large intestine, often starting in the rectum. Typical symptoms include diarrhea (sometimes with blood), pain, weight loss, and inflammation of other organs. Patients are also at higher risk for colorectal carcinomas.

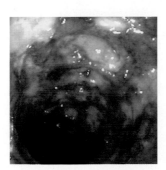

A Colonoscopy of ulcerative colitis.

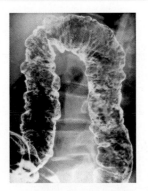

B Early-phase colitis. Double-contrast radiograph, anterior view.

Clinical box 15.5

Colon carcinoma

Malignant tumors of the colon and rectum are among the most frequent solid tumors. More than 90% occur in patients over the age of 50. In early stages, the tumor may be asymptomatic; later symptoms include loss of appetite, changes in bowel movements, and weight loss. Blood in the stools is particularly incriminating, necessitating a thorough examination. Hemorrhoids are not a sufficient explanation for blood in stools unless all other tests (including a colonoscopy) are negative.

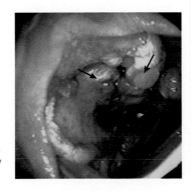

Colonoscopy of colon carcinoma. The tumor (*black arrows*) partially blocks the lumen of the colon.

Liver: Overview

Fig. 15.17 Liver: Location

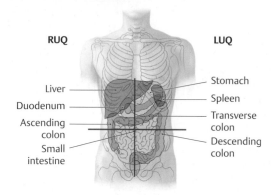

A Anterior view.

RUQ

LUQ

Liver
Duodenum
Ascending colon
Small intestine

Stomach
Spleen
Transverse colon
Descending colon

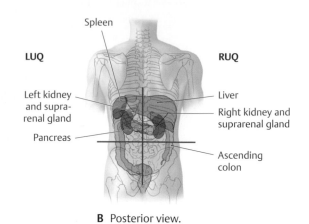

B Posterior view.

Spleen

LUQ

RUQ

Left kidney and supra-renal gland
Pancreas

Liver
Right kidney and suprarenal gland
Ascending colon

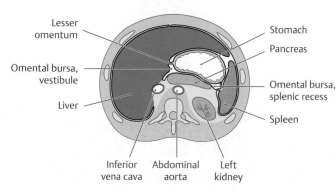

C Transverse section, inferior view.

Lesser omentum
Omental bursa, vestibule
Liver

Stomach
Pancreas
Omental bursa, splenic recess
Spleen

Inferior vena cava
Abdominal aorta
Left kidney

Fig. 15.18 Relations of the liver

Visceral (inferior) surface, inferior view.

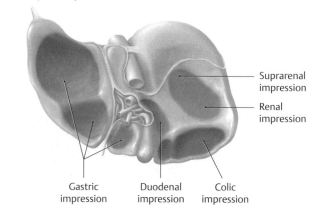

Suprarenal impression
Renal impression

Gastric impression
Duodenal impression
Colic impression

Fig. 15.19 Liver in situ

Anterior view. The liver is intraperitoneal except for its "bare area" (see **Fig. 15.21**); its mesenteries include the falciform, coronary, and triangular ligaments (see **Fig. 15.22**).

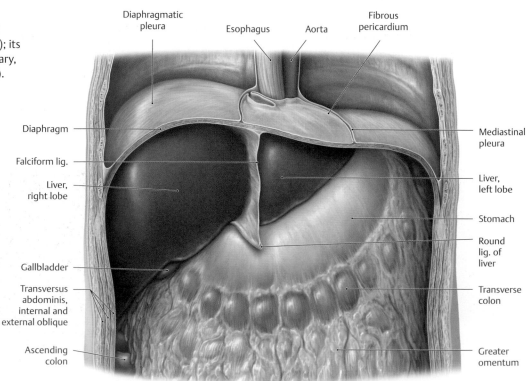

Diaphragmatic pleura
Esophagus
Aorta
Fibrous pericardium

Diaphragm
Falciform lig.
Liver, right lobe

Gallbladder
Transversus abdominis, internal and external oblique
Ascending colon

Mediastinal pleura
Liver, left lobe
Stomach
Round lig. of liver
Transverse colon
Greater omentum

Fig. 15.20 Liver in situ: Inferior surface

The liver is retracted to show the gallbladder on its inferior surface.

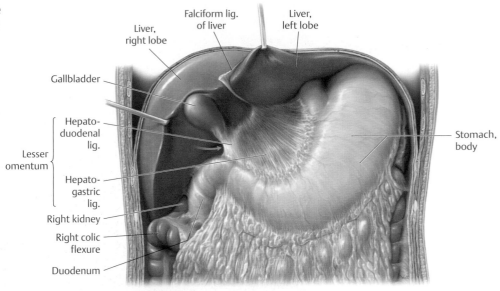

- Falciform lig. of liver
- Liver, left lobe
- Liver, right lobe
- Gallbladder
- Hepato-duodenal lig.
- Lesser omentum
- Hepato-gastric lig.
- Right kidney
- Right colic flexure
- Duodenum
- Stomach, body

Fig. 15.21 Attachment of liver to diaphragm

- Left triangular lig.
- Bare area
- Coronary lig.
- Right triangular lig.

A Diaphragmatic surface of the liver, posterior view.

- Parietal peritoneum
- Inferior vena cava
- Abdominal aorta
- Hepatic surface of diaphragm (no parietal peritoneum)
- Right suprarenal gland
- Right kidney
- Duodenum
- Stomach
- Spleen
- Hepato-duodenal lig.
- Pancreas

B Hepatic surface of the diaphragm, anterior view.

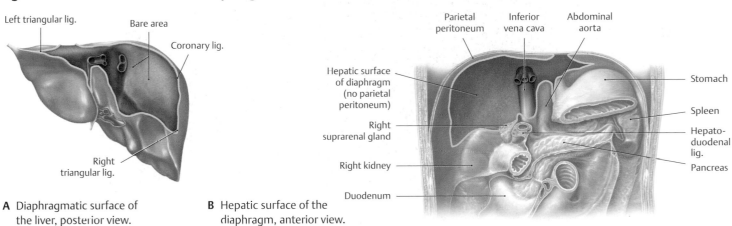

Clinical box 15.6

Hepatic cirrhosis

Hepatic cirrhosis is a condition leading to irreversible fibrosis of the liver parenchyma. Alcohol abuse is the leading cause (70% of cases) followed by hepatitis B. Portal hypertension with the development of collateral vessels is a common result arising in approximately 30% of cases.

Changes associated with advanced hepatic cirrhosis. All three sequences show multiple regenerating nodules in the liver, creating a nodular surface contour. Only the caudate lobe (**B**, *arrow*) is less affected by the changes and still shows a relatively normal signal.

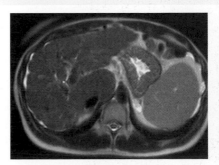

A T2W sequence. (Reproduced from Krombach GA, Mahnken AH. Body Imaging: Thorax and Abdomen. New York, NY: Thieme; 2018.)

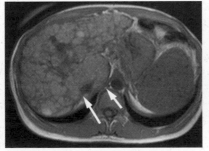

B T1W sequence. (Reproduced from Krombach GA, Mahnken AH. Body Imaging: Thorax and Abdomen. New York, NY: Thieme; 2018.)

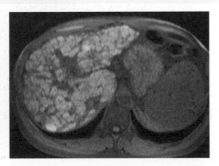

C Fat-suppressed T1W sequence. (Reproduced from Krombach GA, Mahnken AH. Body Imaging: Thorax and Abdomen. New York, NY: Thieme; 2018.)

Liver: Lobes & Segments

Fig. 15.22 Surfaces of the liver

The liver is divided into four lobes by its ligaments: right, left, caudate, and quadrate. The falciform ligament, a double layer of parietal peritoneum that reflects off the anterior abdominal wall and extends to the liver, spreading out over its surface as visceral peritoneum, divides the liver into right and left anatomical lobes. The round ligament of the liver is found in the free edge of the falciform ligament and is the obliterated umbilical vein, which once extended from the umbilicus to the liver.

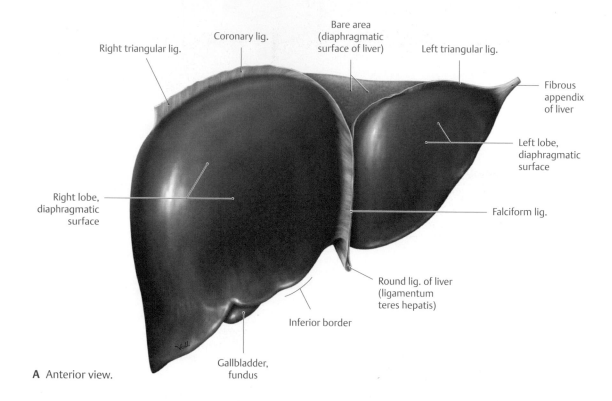

A Anterior view.

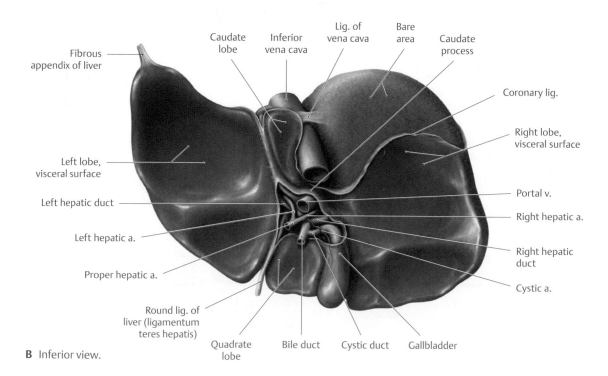

B Inferior view.

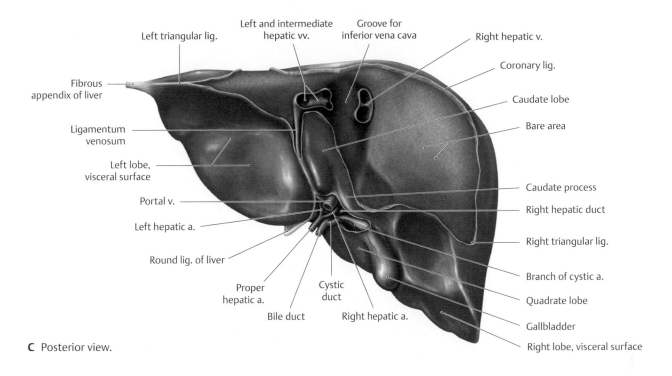

C Posterior view.

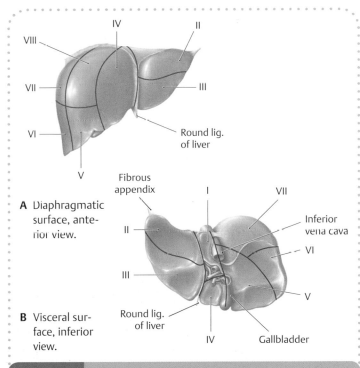

A Diaphragmatic surface, anterior view.

B Visceral surface, inferior view.

Fig. 15.23 Segmentation of the liver

The liver is divided into functional divisions, which are further divided into segments (see **Table 15.1**). Each segment is served by tertiary branches of the hepatic artery, the portal vein, and the common hepatic duct, which together make up the portal triad.

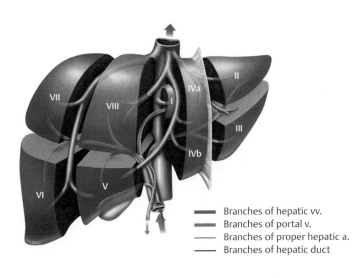

— Branches of hepatic vv.
— Branches of portal v.
— Branches of proper hepatic a.
— Branches of hepatic duct

Table 15.1	Hepatic segments		
Part	**Division**	**Segment**	
Left part	Posterior part	I	Caudate lobe
	Left lateral division	II	Left posterolateral
		III	Left anterolateral
	Left medial division	IV	Left medial
Right part	Right medial division	V	Right anteromedial
		VI	Right anterolateral
	Right lateral division	VII	Right posterolateral
		VIII	Right posteromedial

Gallbladder & Bile Ducts

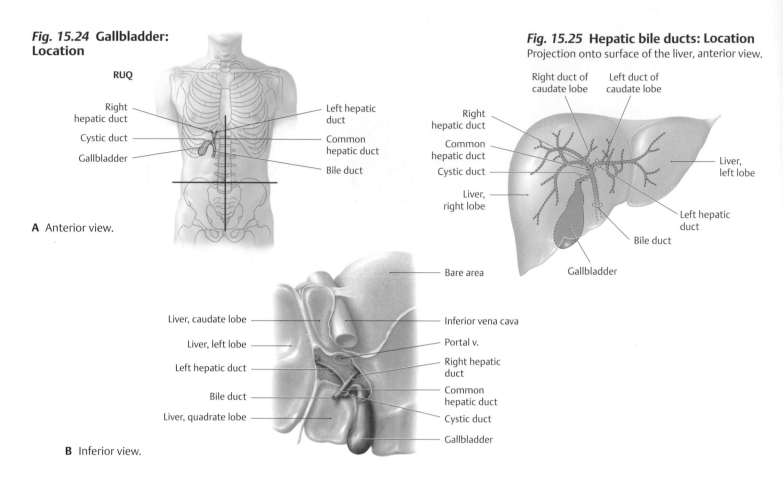

Fig. 15.24 Gallbladder: Location

RUQ

Right hepatic duct
Cystic duct
Gallbladder
Left hepatic duct
Common hepatic duct
Bile duct

A Anterior view.

Fig. 15.25 Hepatic bile ducts: Location
Projection onto surface of the liver, anterior view.

Right duct of caudate lobe
Left duct of caudate lobe
Right hepatic duct
Common hepatic duct
Cystic duct
Liver, right lobe
Liver, left lobe
Left hepatic duct
Bile duct
Gallbladder

Bare area
Liver, caudate lobe
Liver, left lobe
Left hepatic duct
Bile duct
Liver, quadrate lobe
Inferior vena cava
Portal v.
Right hepatic duct
Common hepatic duct
Cystic duct
Gallbladder

B Inferior view.

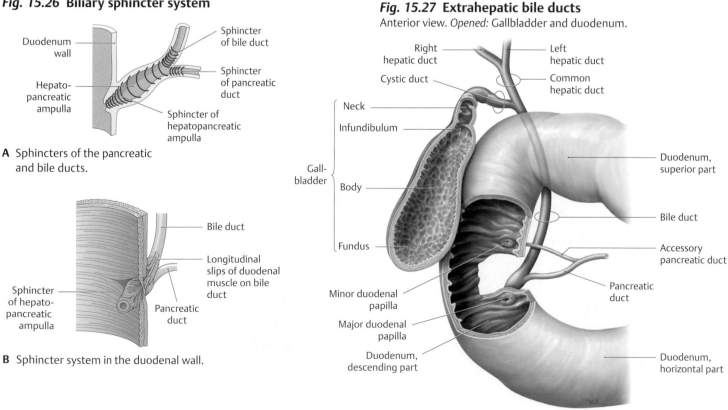

Fig. 15.26 Biliary sphincter system

Duodenum wall
Hepato-pancreatic ampulla
Sphincter of bile duct
Sphincter of pancreatic duct
Sphincter of hepatopancreatic ampulla

A Sphincters of the pancreatic and bile ducts.

Bile duct
Sphincter of hepato-pancreatic ampulla
Pancreatic duct
Longitudinal slips of duodenal muscle on bile duct

B Sphincter system in the duodenal wall.

Fig. 15.27 Extrahepatic bile ducts
Anterior view. *Opened:* Gallbladder and duodenum.

Right hepatic duct
Cystic duct
Neck
Infundibulum
Gall-bladder
Body
Fundus
Minor duodenal papilla
Major duodenal papilla
Duodenum, descending part
Left hepatic duct
Common hepatic duct
Duodenum, superior part
Bile duct
Accessory pancreatic duct
Pancreatic duct
Duodenum, horizontal part

Fig. 15.28 Biliary tract in situ

Anterior view. *Removed:* Stomach, small intestine, transverse colon, and large portions of the liver. The gallbladder is intraperitoneal, covered by visceral peritoneum where it is not attached to the liver.

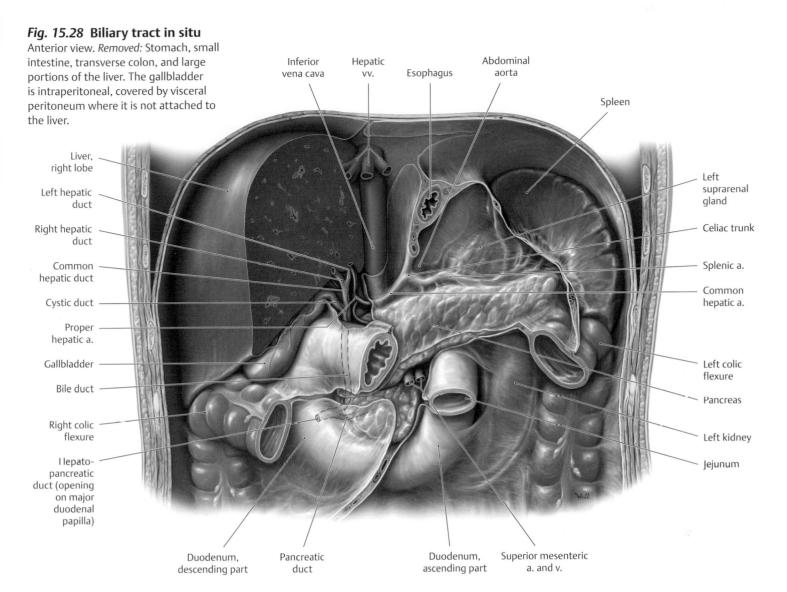

Inferior vena cava — Hepatic vv. — Esophagus — Abdominal aorta — Spleen — Left suprarenal gland — Celiac trunk — Splenic a. — Common hepatic a. — Left colic flexure — Pancreas — Left kidney — Jejunum

Liver, right lobe — Left hepatic duct — Right hepatic duct — Common hepatic duct — Cystic duct — Proper hepatic a. — Gallbladder — Bile duct — Right colic flexure — Hepato-pancreatic duct (opening on major duodenal papilla)

Duodenum, descending part — Pancreatic duct — Duodenum, ascending part — Superior mesenteric a. and v.

Fig. 15.29 MR Cholangiopancreatography

(Reproduced from Moeller TB, Reif E. Pocket Atlas of Sectional Anatomy, Vol 2, 3rd ed. New York, NY: Thieme; 2007.)

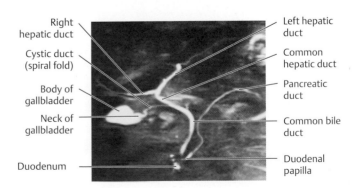

Right hepatic duct — Cystic duct (spiral fold) — Body of gallbladder — Neck of gallbladder — Duodenum

Left hepatic duct — Common hepatic duct — Pancreatic duct — Common bile duct — Duodenal papilla

Clinical box 15.7

Obstruction of the bile duct

As bile is stored and concentrated in the gallbladder, certain substances, such as cholesterol, may crystallize, resulting in the formation of gallstones. Migration of gallstones into the bile duct causes severe pain (colic). Gallstones may also block the pancreatic duct in the papillary regions, causing highly acute or even life-threatening pancreatitis.

Gallstones

Ultrasound appearance of two gallstones. Black arrows mark the echo-free area behind the stones.

Pancreas & Spleen

Fig. 15.30 Pancreas and spleen: Location

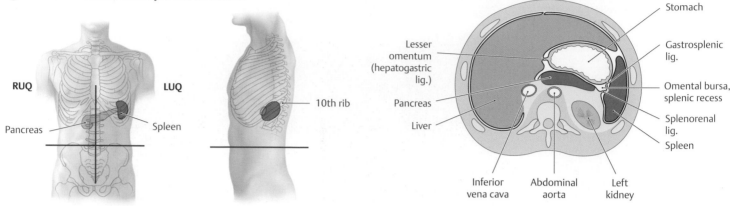

RUQ

LUQ

Pancreas

Spleen

10th rib

A Anterior view.

B Left lateral view.

Lesser omentum (hepatogastric lig.)

Pancreas

Liver

Inferior vena cava

Abdominal aorta

Left kidney

Stomach

Gastrosplenic lig.

Omental bursa, splenic recess

Splenorenal lig.

Spleen

C Transverse section through L1 vertebra, inferior view.

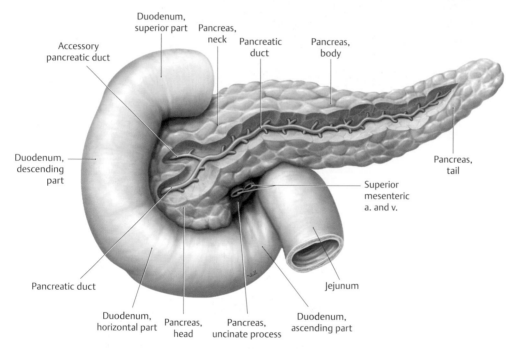

Duodenum, superior part

Pancreas, neck

Pancreatic duct

Pancreas, body

Accessory pancreatic duct

Duodenum, descending part

Pancreatic duct

Duodenum, horizontal part

Pancreas, head

Pancreas, uncinate process

Duodenum, ascending part

Superior mesenteric a. and v.

Jejunum

Pancreas, tail

Fig. 15.31 Pancreas
Anterior view with dissection of the pancreatic duct.

Fig. 15.32 Spleen

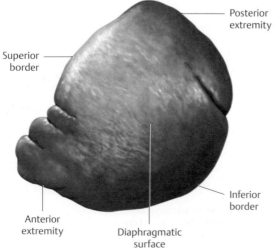

Superior border

Anterior extremity

Diaphragmatic surface

Posterior extremity

Inferior border

A Costal surface.

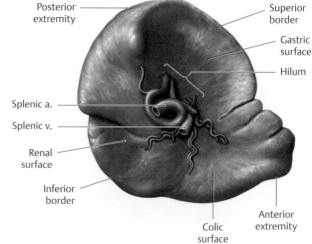

Posterior extremity

Splenic a.

Splenic v.

Renal surface

Inferior border

Colic surface

Superior border

Gastric surface

Hilum

Anterior extremity

B Visceral surface.

Fig. 15.33 Pancreas and spleen in situ

Anterior view. *Removed:* Liver, stomach, small intestine, and large intestine. The pancreas is retroperitoneal, whereas the spleen is intraperitoneal.

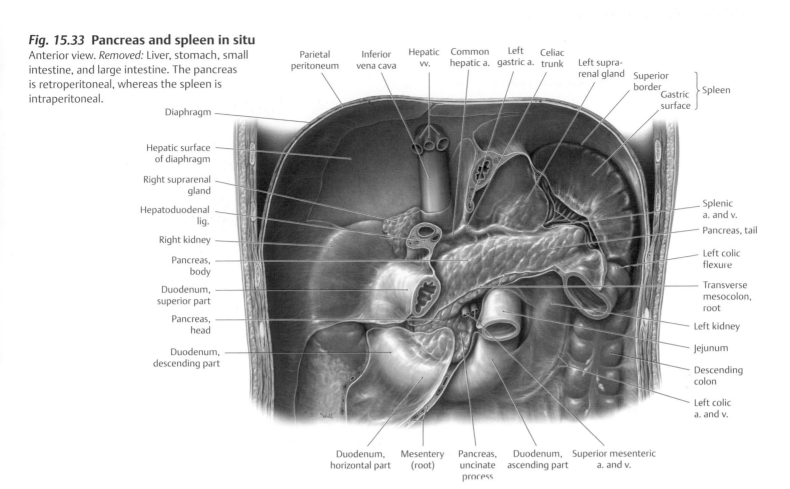

Fig. 15.34 Pancreas and spleen: Transverse section

Superior view. Section through L1 vertebra.

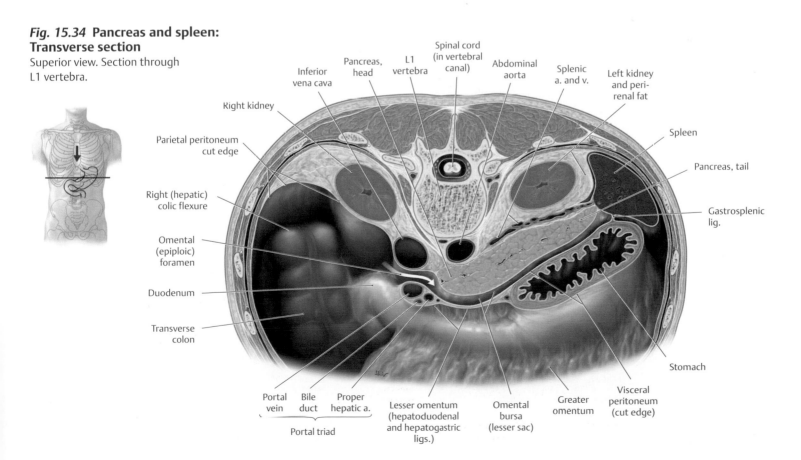

Kidneys & Suprarenal Glands (I)

Fig. 15.35 Kidneys and suprarenal glands: Location

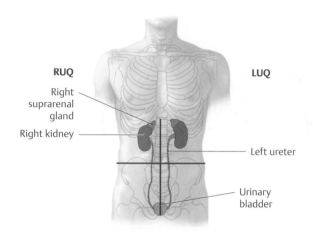

RUQ

LUQ

Right suprarenal gland

Right kidney

Left ureter

Urinary bladder

A Anterior view.

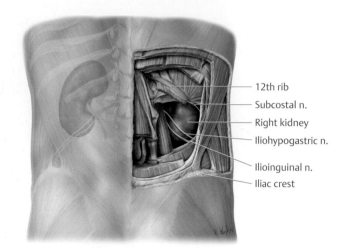

12th rib

Subcostal n.

Right kidney

Iliohypogastric n.

Ilioinguinal n.

Iliac crest

B Posterior view. Right side windowed.

Fig. 15.36 Relations of the kidneys: areas of organ contact.
Anterior view.

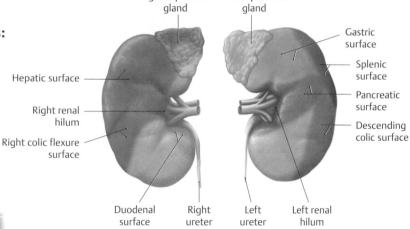

Right suprarenal gland

Left suprarenal gland

Gastric surface

Hepatic surface

Splenic surface

Right renal hilum

Pancreatic surface

Right colic flexure surface

Descending colic surface

Duodenal surface

Right ureter

Left ureter

Left renal hilum

Fig. 15.37 Right kidney in the renal bed

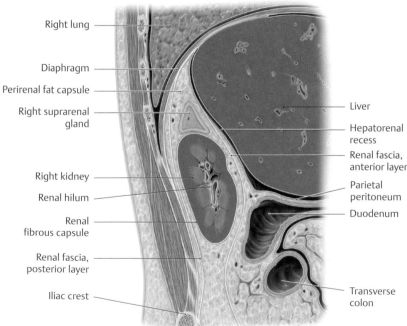

Right lung

Diaphragm

Perirenal fat capsule

Right suprarenal gland

Right kidney

Renal hilum

Renal fibrous capsule

Renal fascia, posterior layer

Iliac crest

Liver

Hepatorenal recess

Renal fascia, anterior layer

Parietal peritoneum

Duodenum

Transverse colon

A Sagittal section at approximately the level of the renal hilum, viewed from the right side.

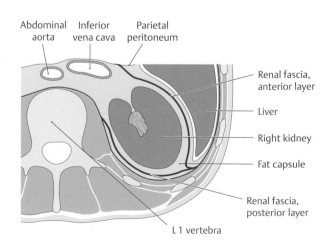

Abdominal aorta

Inferior vena cava

Parietal peritoneum

Renal fascia, anterior layer

Liver

Right kidney

Fat capsule

Renal fascia, posterior layer

L 1 vertebra

B Transverse section through the abdomen at approximately the L1/L2 level, viewed from above.

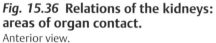

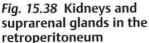

Fig. 15.38 Kidneys and suprarenal glands in the retroperitoneum

Anterior view. Both the kidneys and suprarenal glands are retroperitoneal.

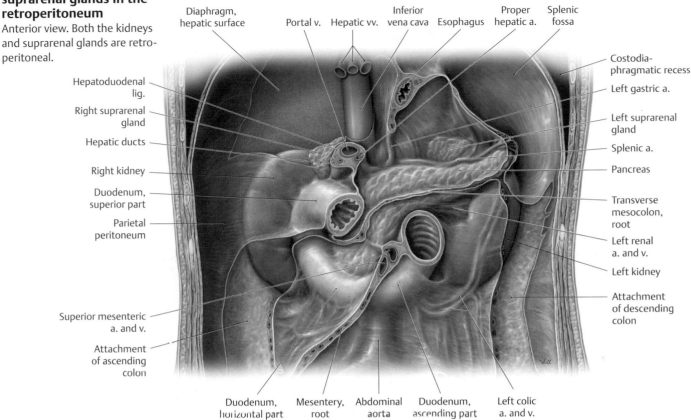

Diaphragm, hepatic surface — Portal v. — Hepatic vv. — Inferior vena cava — Esophagus — Proper hepatic a. — Splenic fossa

Hepatoduodenal lig.

Right suprarenal gland

Hepatic ducts

Right kidney

Duodenum, superior part

Parietal peritoneum

Costodiaphragmatic recess

Left gastric a.

Left suprarenal gland

Splenic a.

Pancreas

Transverse mesocolon, root

Left renal a. and v.

Left kidney

Attachment of descending colon

Superior mesenteric a. and v.

Attachment of ascending colon

Duodenum, horizontal part — Mesentery, root — Abdominal aorta — Duodenum, ascending part — Left colic a. and v.

A *Removed:* Intraperitoneal organs, along with portions of the ascending and descending colon.

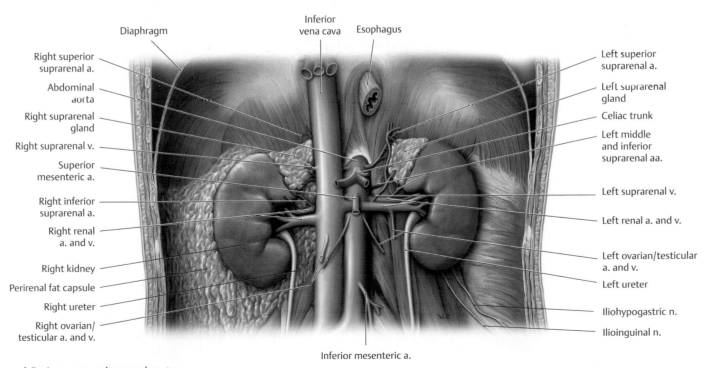

Diaphragm — Inferior vena cava — Esophagus

Right superior suprarenal a.

Abdominal aorta

Right suprarenal gland

Right suprarenal v.

Superior mesenteric a.

Right inferior suprarenal a.

Right renal a. and v.

Right kidney

Perirenal fat capsule

Right ureter

Right ovarian/testicular a. and v.

Left superior suprarenal a.

Left suprarenal gland

Celiac trunk

Left middle and inferior suprarenal aa.

Left suprarenal v.

Left renal a. and v.

Left ovarian/testicular a. and v.

Left ureter

Iliohypogastric n.

Ilioinguinal n.

Inferior mesenteric a.

B *Removed:* Peritoneum, spleen and gastrointestinal organs, along with fat capsule (left side) *Retracted:* Esophagus

Kidneys & Suprarenal Glands (II)

***Fig. 15.39* Kidney: Structure**
Right kidney with suprarenal gland.

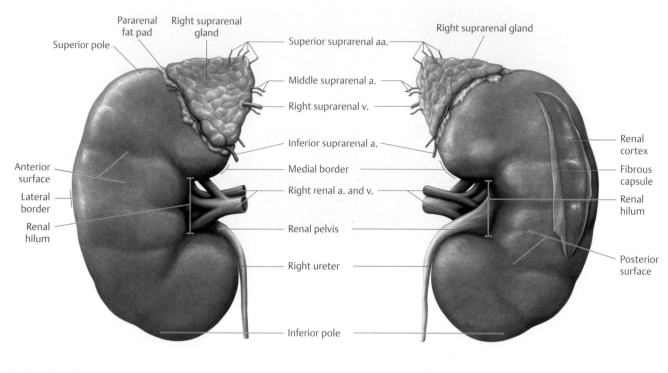

Pararenal fat pad
Right suprarenal gland
Superior pole
Superior suprarenal aa.
Middle suprarenal a.
Right suprarenal v.
Inferior suprarenal a.
Anterior surface
Medial border
Right renal a. and v.
Lateral border
Renal pelvis
Renal hilum
Right ureter
Inferior pole

A Anterior view.

Right suprarenal gland
Renal cortex
Fibrous capsule
Renal hilum
Posterior surface

B Posterior view.

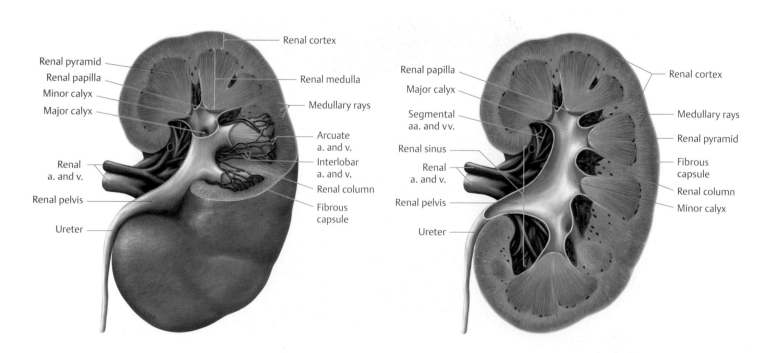

Renal cortex
Renal pyramid
Renal papilla
Renal medulla
Minor calyx
Major calyx
Medullary rays
Arcuate a. and v.
Renal a. and v.
Interlobar a. and v.
Renal column
Renal pelvis
Fibrous capsule
Ureter

C Posterior view with upper half partially removed.

Renal papilla
Renal cortex
Major calyx
Segmental aa. and vv.
Medullary rays
Renal pyramid
Renal sinus
Renal a. and v.
Fibrous capsule
Renal column
Renal pelvis
Minor calyx
Ureter

D Posterior view, midsagittal section.

Fig. 15.40 Right kidney and suprarenal gland

Anterior view. *Removed:* Perirenal fat capsule.
Retracted: Inferior vena cava.

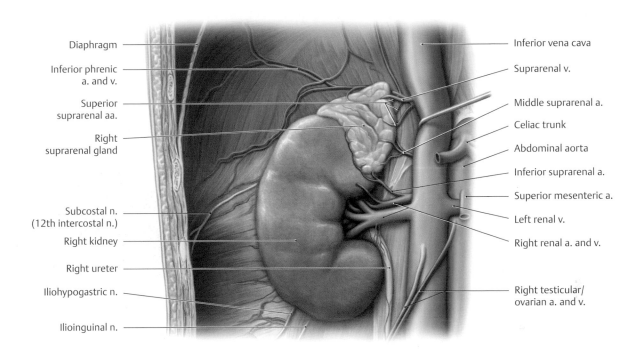

Diaphragm

Inferior phrenic
a. and v.

Superior
suprarenal aa.

Right
suprarenal gland

Subcostal n.
(12th intercostal n.)

Right kidney

Right ureter

Iliohypogastric n.

Ilioinguinal n.

Inferior vena cava

Suprarenal v.

Middle suprarenal a.

Celiac trunk

Abdominal aorta

Inferior suprarenal a.

Superior mesenteric a.

Left renal v.

Right renal a. and v.

Right testicular/
ovarian a. and v.

Fig. 15.41 Left kidney and suprarenal gland

Anterior view. *Removed:* Perirenal fat capsule.
Retracted: Pancreas.

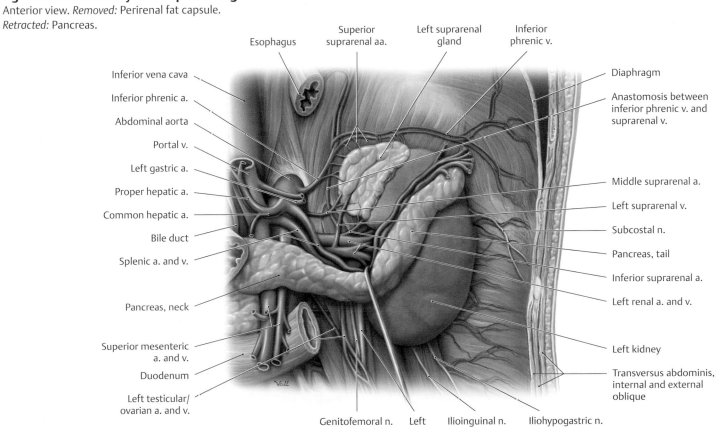

Esophagus

Superior
suprarenal aa.

Left suprarenal
gland

Inferior
phrenic v.

Inferior vena cava

Inferior phrenic a.

Abdominal aorta

Portal v.

Left gastric a.

Proper hepatic a.

Common hepatic a.

Bile duct

Splenic a. and v.

Pancreas, neck

Superior mesenteric
a. and v.

Duodenum

Left testicular/
ovarian a. and v.

Genitofemoral n.   Left
ureter

Ilioinguinal n.   Iliohypogastric n.

Diaphragm

Anastomosis between
inferior phrenic v. and
suprarenal v.

Middle suprarenal a.

Left suprarenal v.

Subcostal n.

Pancreas, tail

Inferior suprarenal a.

Left renal a. and v.

Left kidney

Transversus abdominis,
internal and external
oblique

16 Neurovasculature

Arteries of the Abdominal Wall & Organs

Fig 16.1 Arteries of the abdominal wall

In addition to thoracic and abdominal aortic branches, the abdominal wall is supplied by branches of the subclavian, external iliac and femoral arteries. Numerous potential anastomoses exist between these vessels, which allows the potential for blood to bypass the abdominal aorta.

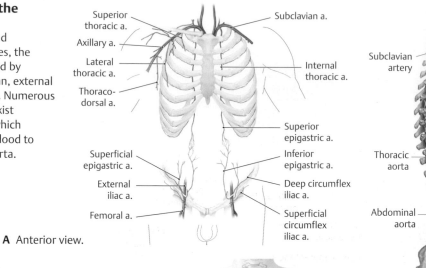

A Anterior view.

B Lateral view.

Fig. 16.2 Abdominal aorta and major branches

Anterior view. The abdominal aorta extends from T12 to its bifurcation at L4. It gives off visceral branches to the kidneys, suprarenal glands, gonads, and organs of the gastrointestinal system, and parietal branches to the body wall.

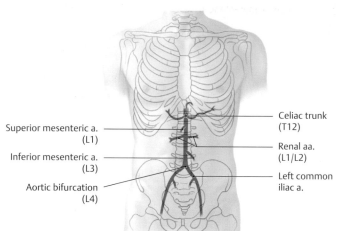

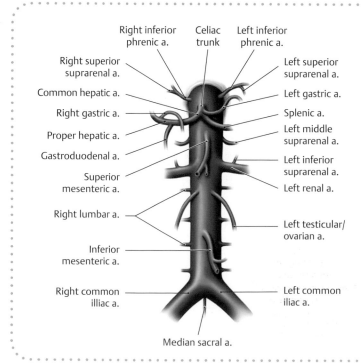

Table 16.1	Branches of the abdominal aorta		
The abdominal aorta gives rise to three major unpaired trunks (bold) and the unpaired median sacral artery, as well as six paired branches.			
Branch from abdominal aorta	**Branches**		
Inferior phrenic aa. (paired)	Superior suprarenal aa.		
Celiac trunk	Left gastric a.		
	Splenic a.		
	Common hepatic a.	Proper hepatic a.
			Right gastric a.
			Gastroduodenal a.
Middle suprarenal aa. (paired)			
Superior mesenteric a.			
Renal aa. (paired)	Inferior suprarenal aa.		
Lumbar aa. (1st through 4th, paired)			
Testicular/ovarian aa. (paired)			
Inferior mesenteric a.			
Common iliac aa. (paired)	External iliac a.		
	Internal iliac a.		
Median sacral a.			

Fig. 16.3 Celiac trunk

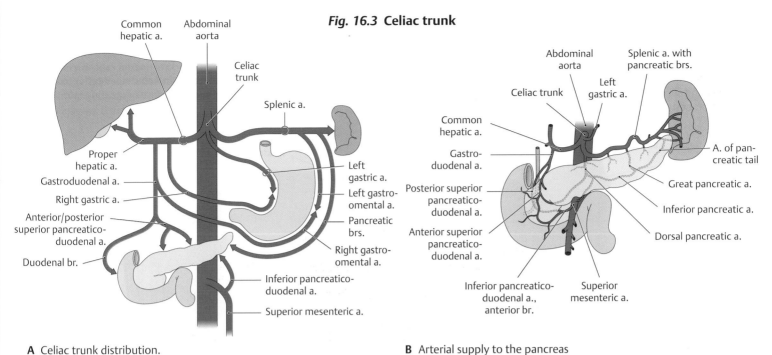

A Celiac trunk distribution.

B Arterial supply to the pancreas

Fig. 16.4 Superior mesenteric artery

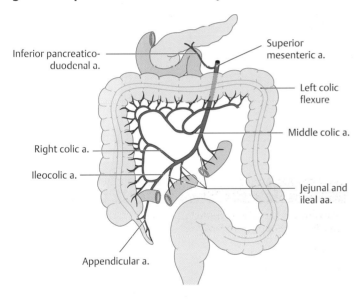

Fig. 16.5 Inferior mesenteric artery

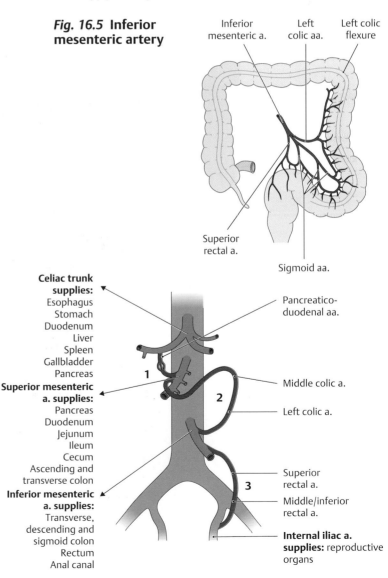

Celiac trunk
supplies:
Esophagus
Stomach
Duodenum
Liver
Spleen
Gallbladder
Pancreas
Superior mesenteric
a. supplies:
Pancreas
Duodenum
Jejunum
Ileum
Cecum
Ascending and
transverse colon
Inferior mesenteric
a. supplies:
Transverse,
descending and
sigmoid colon
Rectum
Anal canal

Fig. 16.6 Abdominal arterial anastomoses

Three major anastomoses provide overlap in the arterial supply to abdominal areas to ensure adequate blood flow. Between the:
1–celiac trunk and the superior mesenteric artery via the pancreaticoduodenal arteries.
2–superior and inferior mesenteric arteries via the middle and left colic arteries.
3–inferior mesenteric and the internal iliac arteries via the superior and middle or inferior rectal arteries.

Superior & Inferior Mesenteric Arteries

Fig. 16.11 Superior mesenteric artery

Anterior view. *Partially removed:* Stomach, duodenum, and peritoneum. *Reflected:* Liver and gallbladder. *Note:* The middle colic artery has been truncated (see **Fig. 16.12**). The superior mesenteric artery arises from the aorta opposite L1. It supplies the structures of the midgut: the duodenum (distal half), jejunum and ileum, cecum and appendix, ascending colon, right colic flexure, and the proximal two thirds of the transverse colon.

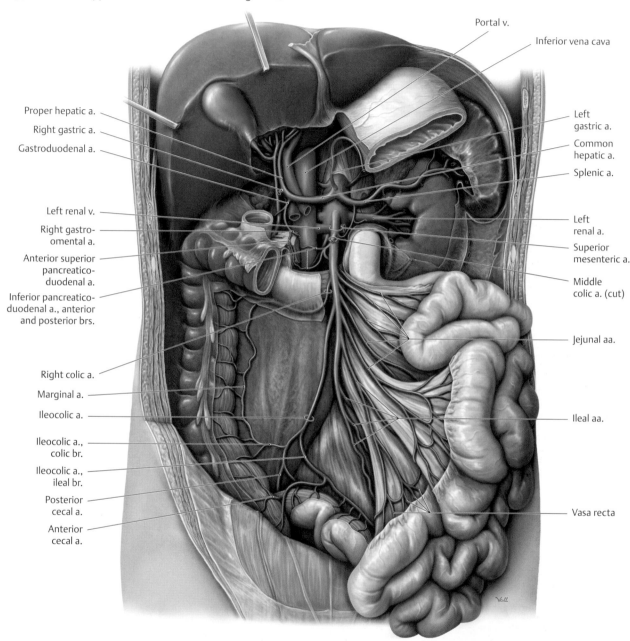

Portal v.
Inferior vena cava
Proper hepatic a.
Right gastric a.
Gastroduodenal a.
Left gastric a.
Common hepatic a.
Splenic a.
Left renal v.
Right gastro-omental a.
Anterior superior pancreatico-duodenal a.
Inferior pancreatico-duodenal a., anterior and posterior brs.
Left renal a.
Superior mesenteric a.
Middle colic a. (cut)
Jejunal aa.
Right colic a.
Marginal a.
Ileocolic a.
Ileocolic a., colic br.
Ileocolic a., ileal br.
Posterior cecal a.
Anterior cecal a.
Ileal aa.
Vasa recta

🏥 Clinical box 16.3

Mesenteric ischemia

A decrease in blood flow to the intestine (ischemia) can result from occlusion of the superior mesenteric artery (SMA) by a thrombus or embolus (acute) or may be secondary to severe atherosclerosis (chronic). In the acute condition, the embolus can obstruct the SMA at its origin or, if small enough, may travel further to obstruct a more peripheral branch. Acute ischemia results in necrosis of the affected part of the intestine. Chronic ischemia is less threatening since obstruction of the vessels occurs gradually, allowing the formation of collateral vessels that will supply the affected intestine. Because of the extensive anastomoses between intestinal arteries, chronic vascular ischemia is rare. Symptoms occur only if two of the three major vessels (celiac trunk or superior or inferior mesenteric arteries) are compromised.

Fig. 16.12 Inferior mesenteric artery

Anterior view. *Removed:* Jejunum and ileum.
Reflected: Transverse colon.

The inferior mesenteric artery arises from the aorta opposite L3. It supplies structures of the hindgut: the transverse colon (distal third), left colic flexure, descending and sigmoid colons, rectum, and anal canal (upper part).

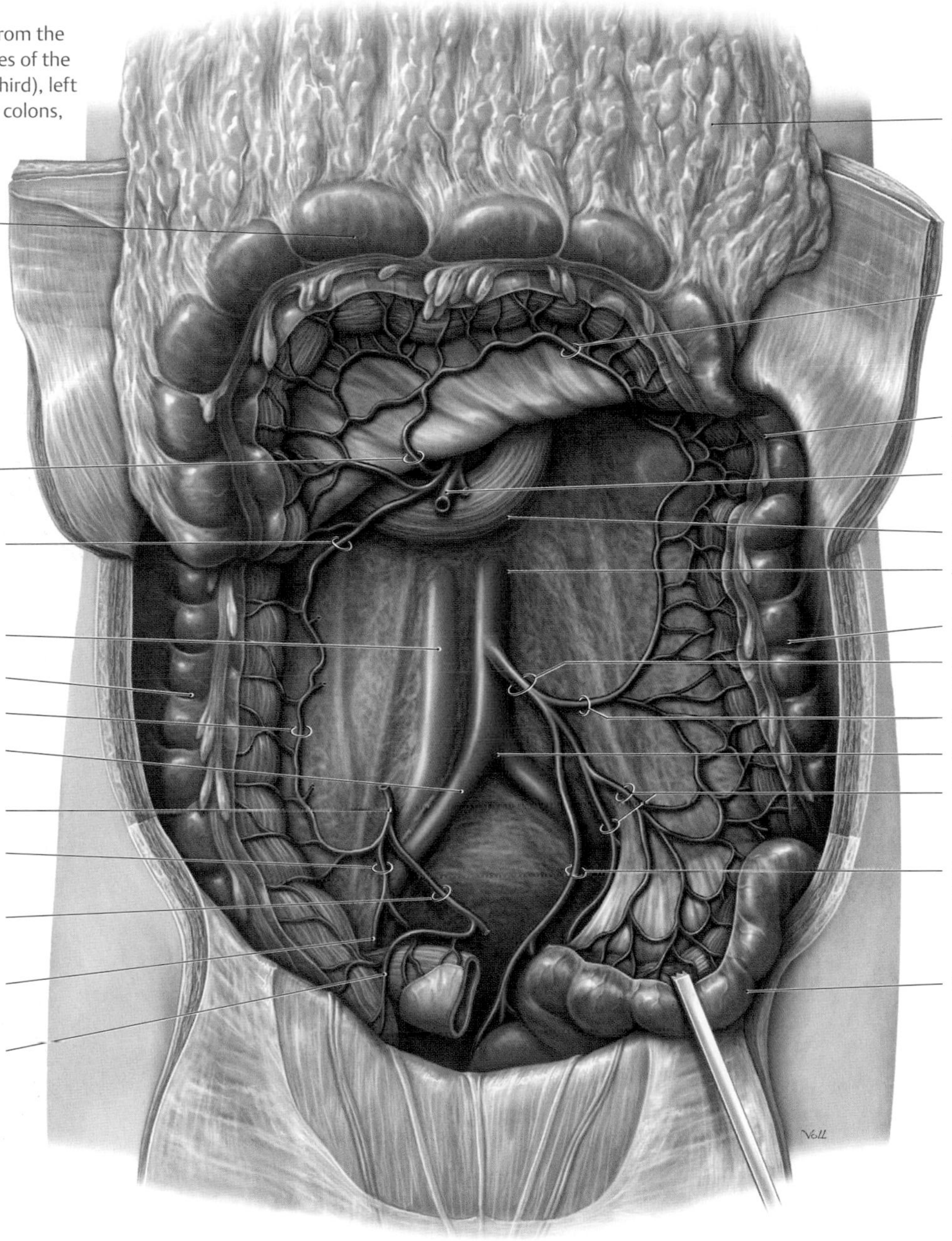

Greater omentum
Transverse colon
Marginal a.
Left colic (splenic) flexure
Middle colic a.
Superior mesenteric a. (cut)
Right colic a.
Duodenum
Abdominal aorta
Inferior vena cava
Descending colon
Ascending colon
Inferior mesenteric a.
Marginal a.
Left colic a.
Right common iliac a.
Aortic bifurcation
Sigmoid aa.
Ileocolic a. (cut)
Ileocolic a., colic br.
Superior rectal a.
Ileocolic a., ileal br.
Posterior cecal a.
Sigmoid colon
Anterior cecal a.

Clinical box 16.4

Anatomoses between arteries of the large intestine

Anastomoses between branches of the superior mesenteric and inferior mesenteric arteries can compensate for abnormally low blood flow in either of the arteries. Two of these anastomoses, although variable, are of significant value:

Riolan's arcade (arc of Riolan) – a connection between the middle colic artery and the left colic artery that arises close to their origins from the superior and inferior mesenteric arteries, respectively.

Marginal artery (of Drummond) – a connection between all arteries of the colon that runs along the periphery of the mesentery close to the intestinal tube.

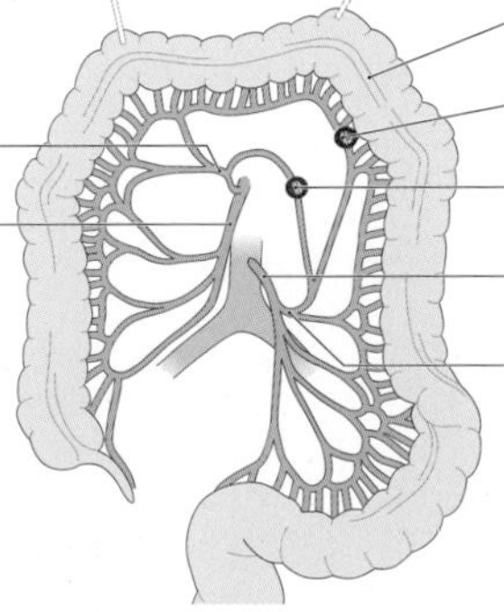

Left colic flexure
Marginal a. (of Drummond)
Middle colic a.
Arc of Riolan
Superior mesenteric a.
Inferior mesenteric a.
Left colic a.

Veins of the Abdominal Wall & Organs

Fig 16.13 **Veins of the abdominal wall**

The abdominal wall is drained by veins that accompany the arteries and are tributaries of the azygos system and inferior vena cava. Additionally, a large thoracoepigastric vein connects the femoral and axillary veins.

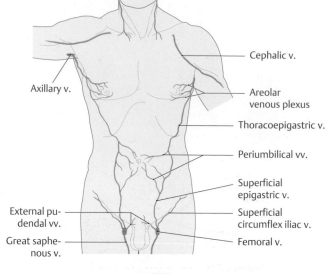

A Anterior view.

Fig. 16.14 **Inferior vena cava**

Anterior view. The inferior vena cava arises at L5 with the convergence of the common iliac veins. It ascends along the right side of the vertebral column, passes through the caval opening in the diaphragm at T8 and terminates in the thorax in the right atrium of the heart.

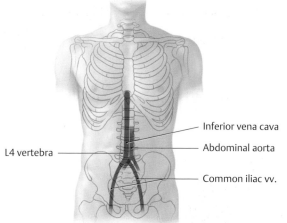

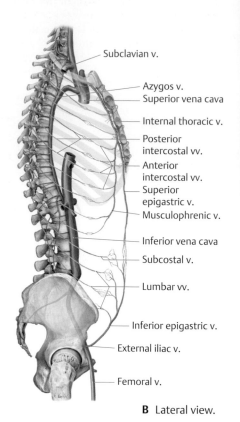

B Lateral view.

Table 16.2		Tributaries of the inferior vena cava
①R	①L	Inferior phrenic vv. (paired)
	②	Hepatic vv. (3)
③R	③L	Suprarenal vv. (the right vein is a direct tributary)
④R	④L	Renal vv. (paired)
⑤R	⑤L	Testicular/ovarian vv. (the right vein is a direct tributary)
⑥R	⑥L	Ascending lumbar vv. (paired), not direct tributaries
⑦R	⑦L	Lumbar vv.
⑧R	⑧L	Common iliac vv. (paired)
	⑨	Median sacral v.

Fig. 16.15 Portal vein

The portal vein (see **p. 198**) drains venous blood from the abdominopelvic organs supplied by the celiac trunk and superior and inferior mesenteric arteries.

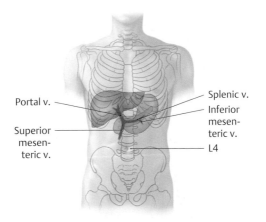

A Location, anterior view.

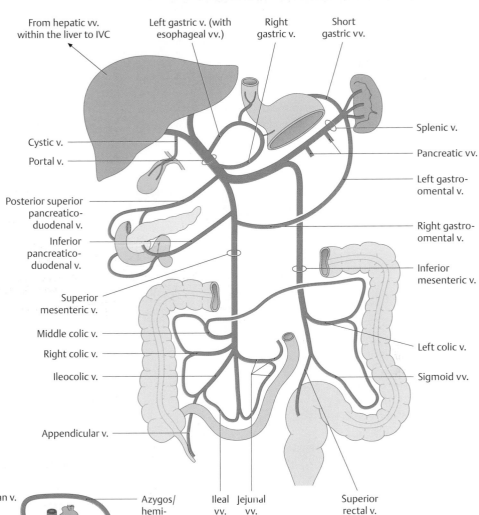

B Portal vein distribution.

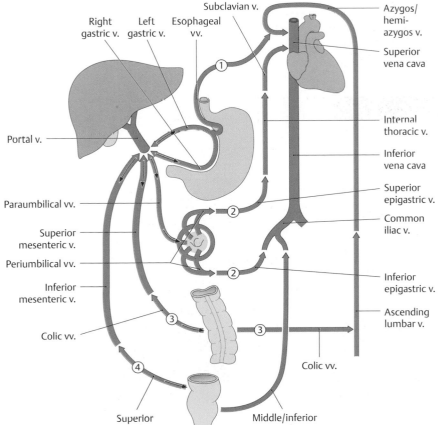

Clinical box 16.5

Cancer metastases

Tumors in the region drained by the superior rectal vein may spread through the portal venous system to the capillary bed of the liver (hepatic metastasis). Tumors drained by the middle or inferior rectal veins may metastasize to the capillary bed of the lung (pulmonary metastasis) via the inferior vena cava and right heart.

C Portocaval anastomotic collateral pathways between the portal and systemic systems. When the portal system is compromised, the portal vein can divert blood away from the liver back to its supplying veins, which return this nutrient-rich blood to the heart via the venae cavae. The red arrows indicate the flow reversal in the (1) esophageal veins, (2) paraumbilical veins, (3) the colic veins, and (4) the middle and inferior rectal veins.

Inferior Vena Cava & Renal Veins

Fig. 16.16 Inferior vena cava

Anterior view of the female abdomen. *Removed:* All organs except the left kidney and suprarenal gland. The inferior vena cava courses along the right side of the vertebral bodies from its origin at L5 to the caval opening in the diaphragm at T8. Unlike the branches of the aorta, vis-ceral and parietal drainages to the inferior vena cava are asymmetrical (note drainages of the suprarenal glands, gonads and azygos veins). It communicates with the azygos system through lumbar veins and receives blood from the portal venous system via the hepatic veins.

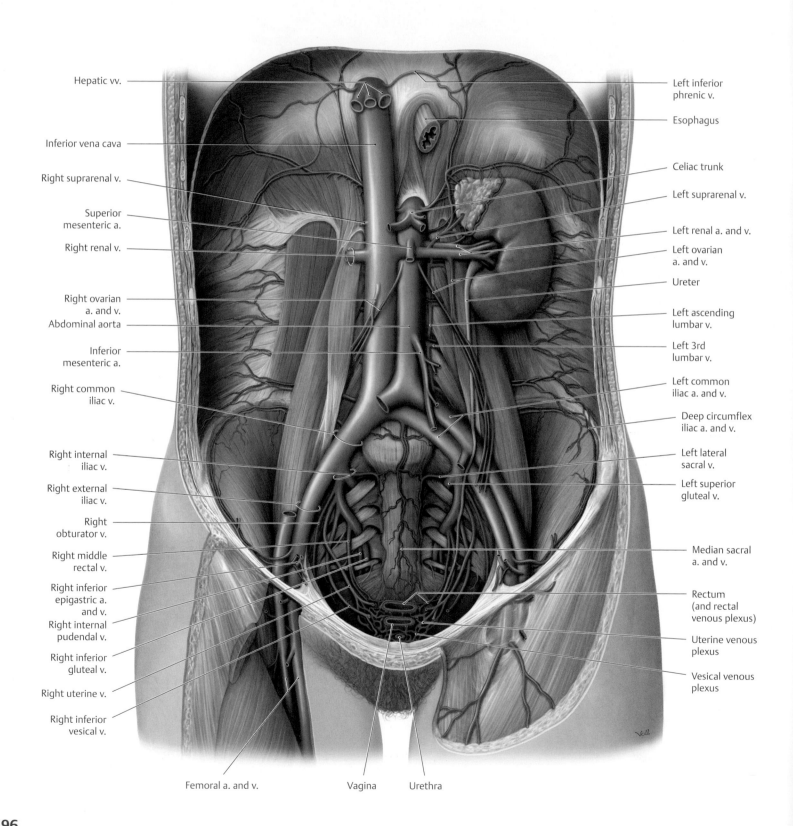

Hepatic vv.

Inferior vena cava

Right suprarenal v.

Superior mesenteric a.

Right renal v.

Right ovarian a. and v.

Abdominal aorta

Inferior mesenteric a.

Right common iliac v.

Right internal iliac v.

Right external iliac v.

Right obturator v.

Right middle rectal v.

Right inferior epigastric a. and v.

Right internal pudendal v.

Right inferior gluteal v.

Right uterine v.

Right inferior vesical v.

Femoral a. and v.

Vagina

Urethra

Left inferior phrenic v.

Esophagus

Celiac trunk

Left suprarenal v.

Left renal a. and v.

Left ovarian a. and v.

Ureter

Left ascending lumbar v.

Left 3rd lumbar v.

Left common iliac a. and v.

Deep circumflex iliac a. and v.

Left lateral sacral v.

Left superior gluteal v.

Median sacral a. and v.

Rectum (and rectal venous plexus)

Uterine venous plexus

Vesical venous plexus

Fig. 16.17 Renal veins

Anterior view. See **p. 189** for the renal arteries in isolation.
Removed: All organs except kidneys and suprarenal glands.

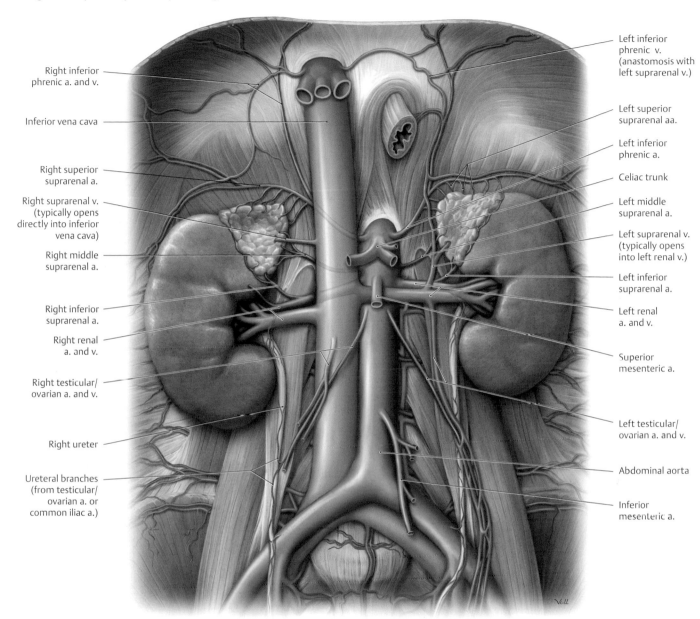

Right inferior phrenic a. and v.

Inferior vena cava

Right superior suprarenal a.

Right suprarenal v. (typically opens directly into inferior vena cava)

Right middle suprarenal a.

Right inferior suprarenal a.

Right renal a. and v.

Right testicular/ ovarian a. and v.

Right ureter

Ureteral branches (from testicular/ ovarian a. or common iliac a.)

Left inferior phrenic v. (anastomosis with left suprarenal v.)

Left superior suprarenal aa.

Left inferior phrenic a.

Celiac trunk

Left middle suprarenal a.

Left suprarenal v. (typically opens into left renal v.)

Left inferior suprarenal a.

Left renal a. and v.

Superior mesenteric a.

Left testicular/ ovarian a. and v.

Abdominal aorta

Inferior mesenteric a.

Clinical box 16.6

Tributaries of the left renal vein

On the right side, the suprarenal and testicular/ovarian veins drain directly into the inferior vena cava. The corresponding veins on the left side, however, drain into the left renal vein. (This is a remnant from early development when there were both right and left sided venae cave.) It is believed that this asymmetrical drainage pattern is the cause of the varicose dilations of the veins in the spermatic cord (varicoceles) that occur more commonly on the left side.

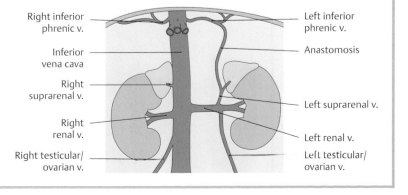

Right inferior phrenic v.

Inferior vena cava

Right suprarenal v.

Right renal v.

Right testicular/ ovarian v.

Left inferior phrenic v.

Anastomosis

Left suprarenal v.

Left renal v.

Left testicular/ ovarian v.

Superior & Inferior Mesenteric Veins

Fig. 16.20 Superior mesenteric vein

Anterior view. *Partially removed*: Stomach, duodenum, and peritoneum. *Removed*: Pancreas, greater omentum, and transverse colon. *Reflected*: Liver and gallbladder. *Displaced*: Small intestine. The superior mesenteric vein receives tributaries from the entire small intestine as well as the cecum, appendix, ascending colon, and two thirds of the transverse colon. It normally lies to the right of the superior mesenteric artery then joins with the splenic vein posterior to the neck of the pancreas to form the portal vein.

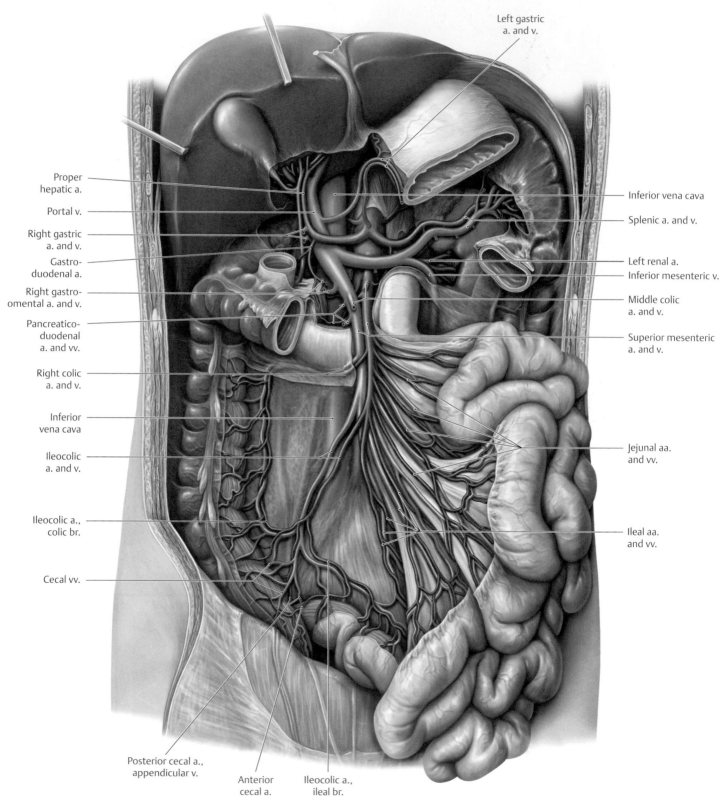

Left gastric a. and v.

Proper hepatic a.

Portal v.

Right gastric a. and v.

Gastro-duodenal a.

Right gastro-omental a. and v.

Pancreatico-duodenal a. and vv.

Right colic a. and v.

Inferior vena cava

Ileocolic a. and v.

Ileocolic a., colic br.

Cecal vv.

Posterior cecal a., appendicular v.

Anterior cecal a.

Ileocolic a., ileal br.

Inferior vena cava

Splenic a. and v.

Left renal a.

Inferior mesenteric v.

Middle colic a. and v.

Superior mesenteric a. and v.

Jejunal aa. and vv.

Ileal aa. and vv.

Fig. 16.21 Inferior mesenteric vein

Anterior view. *Partially removed*: Stomach, duodenum, and peritoneum. *Removed*: Pancreas, greater omentum, transverse colon, and small intestine. *Reflected*: Liver and gallbladder. The inferior mesenteric vein drains a smaller territory than the superior mesenteric vein. It receives tributaries from the distal transverse colon, descending and sigmoid colons and upper rectum. It ascends in the retroperitoneum, separate from the artery, and generally joins with the splenic vein posterior to the stomach and pancreas. Note that the ascending and descending colons may also be drained by lumbar veins in the retroperitoneum, which empty into the inferior vena cava, constituting a portocaval collateral pathway.

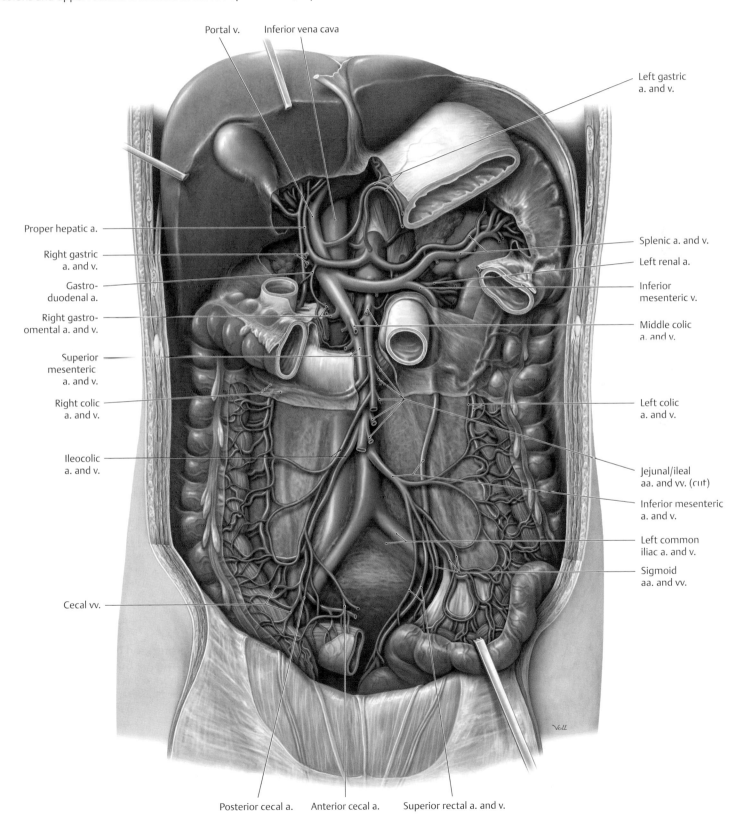

Portal v.

Inferior vena cava

Left gastric a. and v.

Proper hepatic a.

Right gastric a. and v.

Gastro-duodenal a.

Right gastro-omental a. and v.

Superior mesenteric a. and v.

Right colic a. and v.

Ileocolic a. and v.

Cecal vv.

Splenic a. and v.

Left renal a.

Inferior mesenteric v.

Middle colic a. and v.

Left colic a. and v.

Jejunal/ileal aa. and vv. (cut)

Inferior mesenteric a. and v.

Left common iliac a. and v.

Sigmoid aa. and vv.

Posterior cecal a.   Anterior cecal a.   Superior rectal a. and v.

Lymph Nodes of the Posterior Abdominal Wall

Lymph nodes in the abdomen and pelvis may be classified as either parietal or visceral. The majority of the parietal lymph nodes are located on the posterior abdominal wall.

Fig. 16.25 Parietal lymph nodes in the abdomen and pelvis
Anterior view. *Removed:* All visceral structures except vessels.

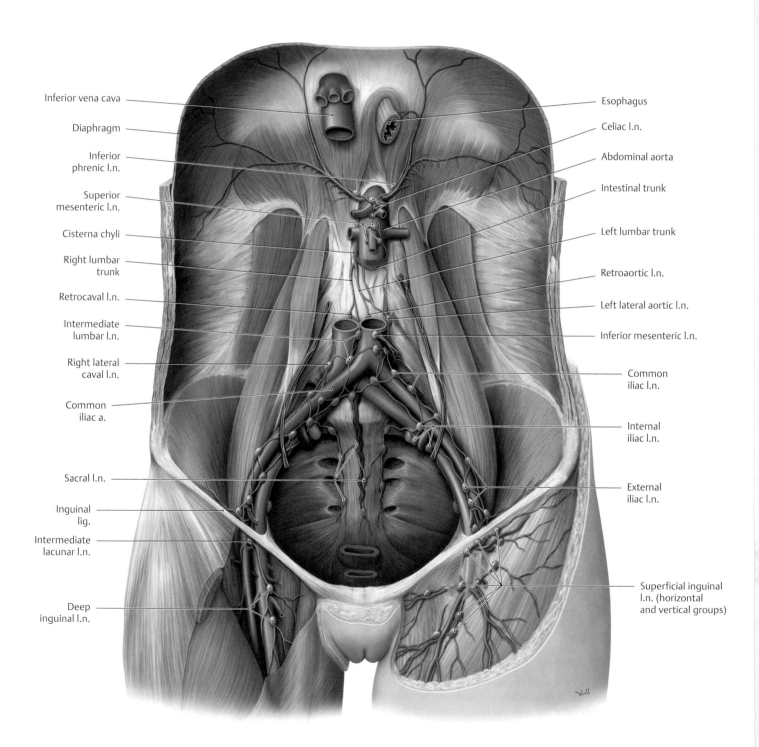

Inferior vena cava

Diaphragm

Inferior phrenic l.n.

Superior mesenteric l.n.

Cisterna chyli

Right lumbar trunk

Retrocaval l.n.

Intermediate lumbar l.n.

Right lateral caval l.n.

Common iliac a.

Sacral l.n.

Inguinal lig.

Intermediate lacunar l.n.

Deep inguinal l.n.

Esophagus

Celiac l.n.

Abdominal aorta

Intestinal trunk

Left lumbar trunk

Retroaortic l.n.

Left lateral aortic l.n.

Inferior mesenteric l.n.

Common iliac l.n.

Internal iliac l.n.

External iliac l.n.

Superficial inguinal l.n. (horizontal and vertical groups)

Fig. 16.26 Lymph nodes of the kidneys, ureters, and suprarenal glands

Anterior view.

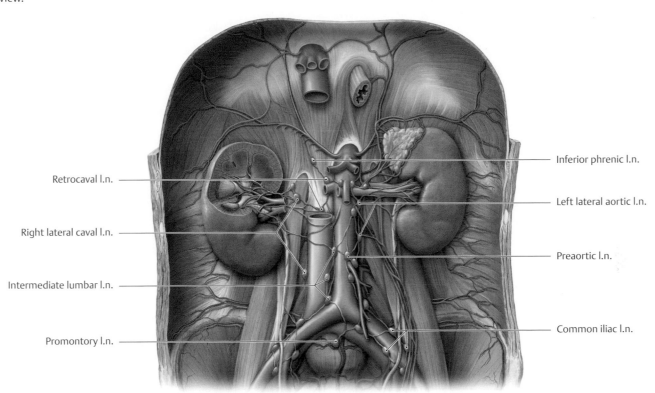

Retrocaval l.n.

Right lateral caval l.n.

Intermediate lumbar l.n.

Promontory l.n.

Inferior phrenic l.n.

Left lateral aortic l.n.

Preaortic l.n.

Common iliac l.n.

Fig. 16.27 Lymphatic drainage of the kidneys and gonads (with pelvic organs)

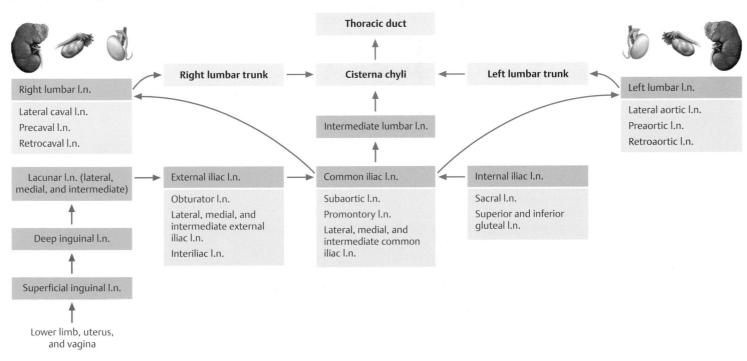

Lymph Nodes of the Supracolic Organs

**Fig. 16.28 Lymph nodes
of the stomach and liver**
Anterior view. *Removed:* Lesser omentum.
Opened: Greater omentum. Arrows show
direction of lymphatic drainage.

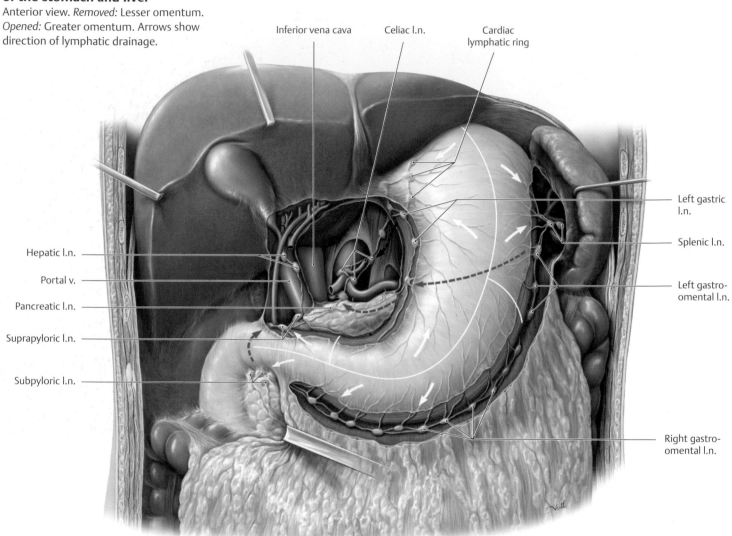

**Fig. 16.29 Lymphatic drainage of the liver
and biliary tract**
Anterior view. In the region of the liver, the major lymph-producing
organ, the important pathways are:

- *Liver and intrahepatic bile ducts:* Most lymph drains inferiorly through
  the hepatic nodes to the celiac nodes and then to the
  intestinal trunk and cisterna chyli, but it may take a more direct
  route bypassing the celiac nodes. A small amount drains cranially
  through the inferior phrenic nodes to the lumbar trunk. It also can
  drain through the diaphragm to the superior phrenic nodes and on
  to the bronchomediastinal trunk.
- *Gallbladder:* Lymph drains initially to the cystic node, then follows
  one of the pathways described above.
- *Common bile duct:* Lymph drains through the pyloric nodes
  (supra-, sub-, and retropyloric) and the foraminal node to the
  celiac nodes, then to the intestinal trunk.

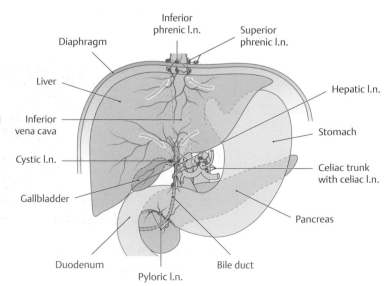

Fig. 16.30 Lymph nodes of the spleen, pancreas, and duodenum

Anterior view. *Removed:* Stomach and colon.

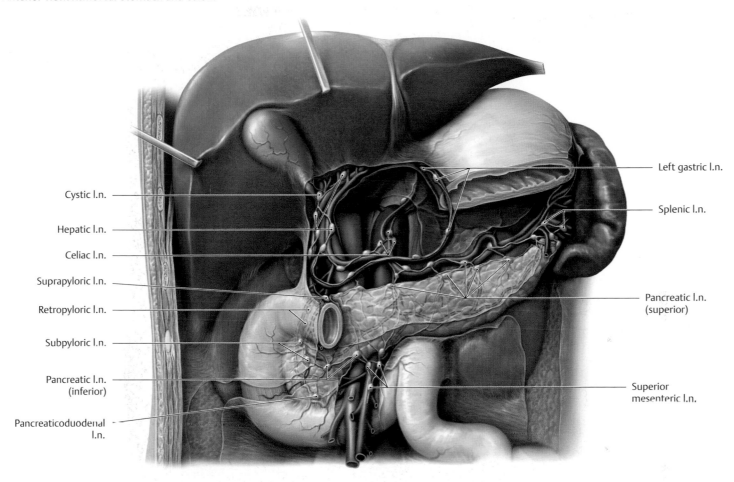

Cystic l.n.

Hepatic l.n.

Celiac l.n.

Suprapyloric l.n.

Retropyloric l.n.

Subpyloric l.n.

Pancreatic l.n. (inferior)

Pancreaticoduodenal l.n.

Left gastric l.n.

Splenic l.n.

Pancreatic l.n. (superior)

Superior mesenteric l.n.

Fig. 16.31 Lymphatic drainage of the stomach, liver, spleen, pancreas, and duodenum

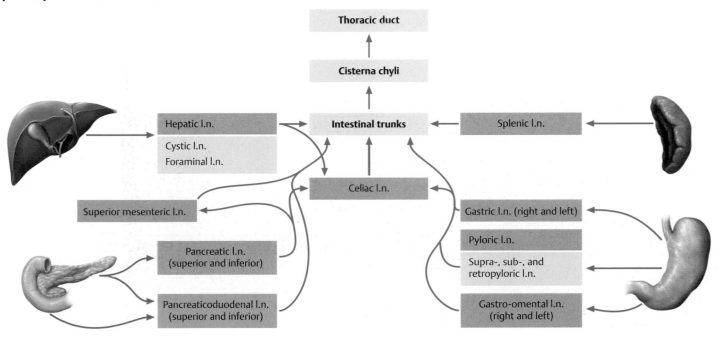

Thoracic duct

Cisterna chyli

Intestinal trunks

Hepatic l.n.

Cystic l.n.
Foraminal l.n.

Splenic l.n.

Celiac l.n.

Superior mesenteric l.n.

Gastric l.n. (right and left)

Pancreatic l.n. (superior and inferior)

Pyloric l.n.

Supra-, sub-, and retropyloric l.n.

Pancreaticoduodenal l.n. (superior and inferior)

Gastro-omental l.n. (right and left)

Lymph Nodes of the Infracolic Organs

***Fig. 16.32* Lymph nodes of the jejunum and ileum**
Anterior view. *Removed:* Stomach, liver, pancreas, and colon.

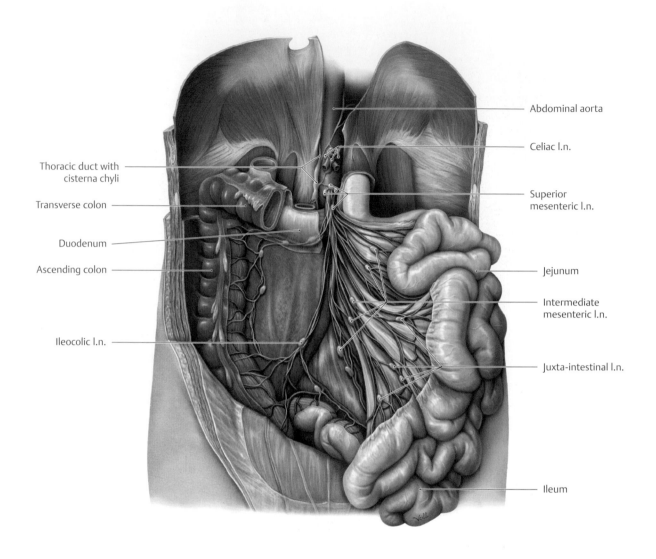

- Abdominal aorta
- Celiac l.n.
- Superior mesenteric l.n.
- Jejunum
- Intermediate mesenteric l.n.
- Juxta-intestinal l.n.
- Ileum

- Thoracic duct with cisterna chyli
- Transverse colon
- Duodenum
- Ascending colon
- Ileocolic l.n.

***Fig. 16.33* Lymphatic drainage of the intestines**

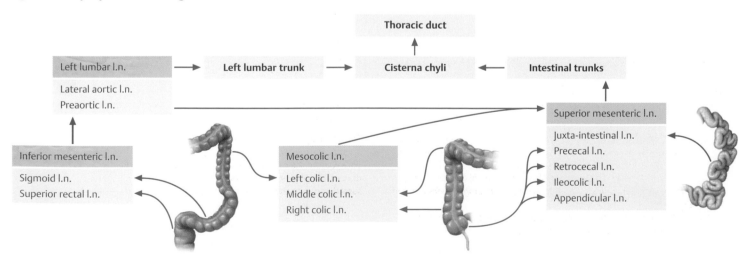

Fig. 16.34 Lymph nodes of the large intestine

Anterior view. *Reflected:* Transverse colon and greater omentum.

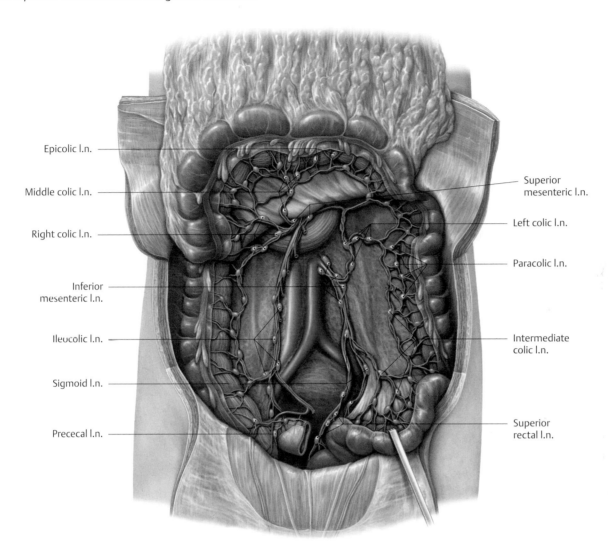

Epicolic l.n.

Middle colic l.n.

Right colic l.n.

Inferior mesenteric l.n.

Ileocolic l.n.

Sigmoid l.n.

Prececal l.n.

Superior mesenteric l.n.

Left colic l.n.

Paracolic l.n.

Intermediate colic l.n.

Superior rectal l.n.

 Clinical box 16.8

Lymphatic drainage of the large intestine

Regional lymphatic pathways in the large intestine have important clinical affects.

- **Ascending colon, cecum, and transverse colon**: Lymph drains initially to the *right and middle colic nodes*, then to the *superior mesenteric nodes*, and finally to the *intestinal trunk*.
- **Descending colon**: Lymph drains initially to the regional *left colic nodes*, then to the *inferior mesenteric nodes*, then via the *left lumbar nodes* into the *left lumbar trunk*.
- **Sigmoid colon**: Lymph drains initially to *sigmoid nodes* then follows the pathway described above for the descending colon.

- **Upper rectum**: Lymph drains initially to the *superior rectal nodes* then follows the pathway described above for the sigmoid colon.

Thus, a malignant tumor undergoing lymphogenous spread must negotiate several lymph node groups (all of which should be removed in tumor resections) before the malignant cells can reach the intestinal trunk and thoracic duct and finally enter the bloodstream. This long route of lymphogenous spread improves the prospects for a cure.

Nerves of the Abdominal Wall

Fig. 16.35 Somatic nerves of the abdomen and pelvis

Anterior view. The abdominal wall is innervated by somatic nerves that include the lower intercostal nerves and branches of the lumbar plexus.

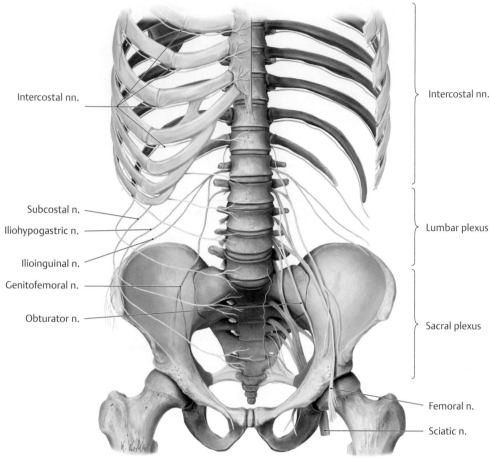

Intercostal nn.

Intercostal nn.

Subcostal n.

Iliohypogastric n.

Lumbar plexus

Ilioinguinal n.

Genitofemoral n.

Obturator n.

Sacral plexus

Femoral n.

Sciatic n.

Fig. 16.36 Cutaneous innervation of the anterior trunk
Anterior view.

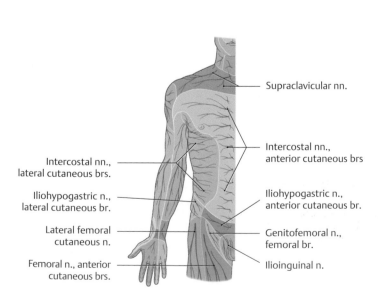

Supraclavicular nn.

Intercostal nn., lateral cutaneous brs.

Intercostal nn., anterior cutaneous brs

Iliohypogastric n., lateral cutaneous br.

Iliohypogastric n., anterior cutaneous br.

Lateral femoral cutaneous n.

Genitofemoral n., femoral br.

Femoral n., anterior cutaneous brs.

Ilioinguinal n.

Fig. 16.37 Dermatomes of the anterior trunk
Anterior view.

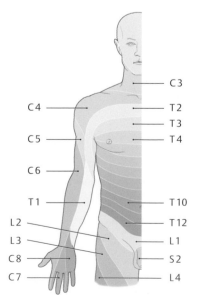

C 3

C 4

T 2

T 3

C 5

T 4

C 6

T 1

T 10

L 2

T 12

L 3

L 1

C 8

S 2

C 7

L 4

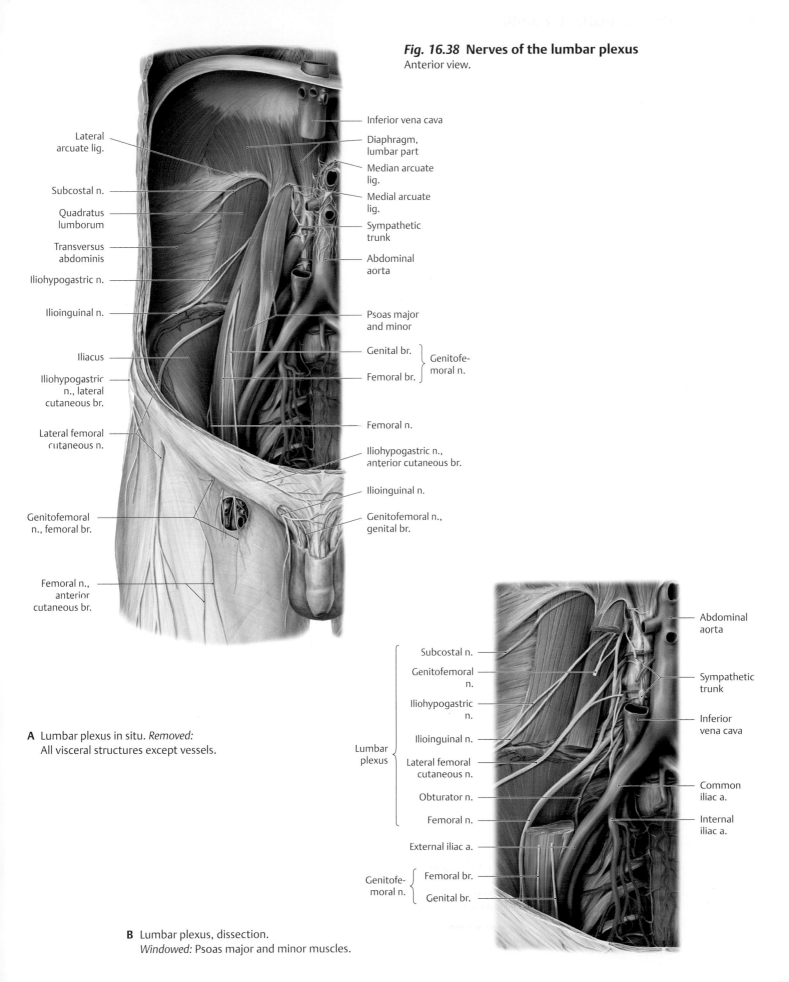

Fig. 16.38 Nerves of the lumbar plexus
Anterior view.

Lateral arcuate lig.

Subcostal n.

Quadratus lumborum

Transversus abdominis

Iliohypogastric n.

Ilioinguinal n.

Iliacus

Iliohypogastric n., lateral cutaneous br.

Lateral femoral cutaneous n.

Genitofemoral n., femoral br.

Femoral n., anterior cutaneous br.

Inferior vena cava

Diaphragm, lumbar part

Median arcuate lig.

Medial arcuate lig.

Sympathetic trunk

Abdominal aorta

Psoas major and minor

Genital br. ⎱ Genitofe-
Femoral br. ⎰ moral n.

Femoral n.

Iliohypogastric n., anterior cutaneous br.

Ilioinguinal n.

Genitofemoral n., genital br.

A Lumbar plexus in situ. *Removed:*
All visceral structures except vessels.

Subcostal n.

Genitofemoral n.

Iliohypogastric n.

Ilioinguinal n.

Lumbar plexus

Lateral femoral cutaneous n.

Obturator n.

Femoral n.

External iliac a.

Genitofe-moral n. ⎰ Femoral br.
⎱ Genital br.

Abdominal aorta

Sympathetic trunk

Inferior vena cava

Common iliac a.

Internal iliac a.

B Lumbar plexus, dissection.
Windowed: Psoas major and minor muscles.

Autonomic Innervation: Overview

Fig. 16.39 Sympathetic and parasympathetic nervous systems in the abdomen and pelvis

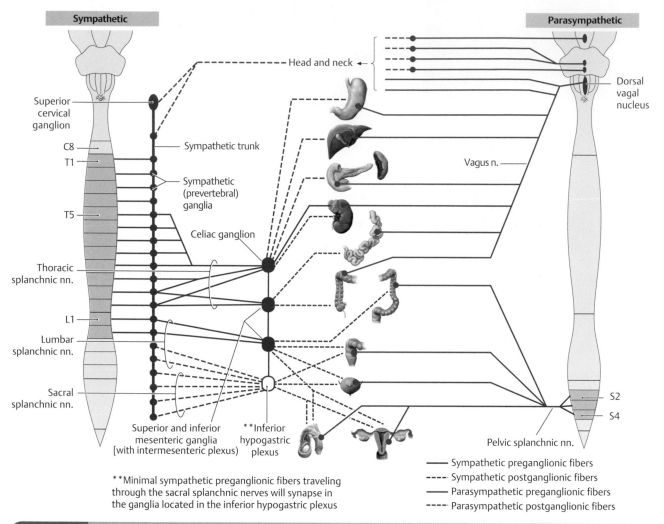

Sympathetic

Superior cervical ganglion

C8
T1

Sympathetic trunk

Sympathetic (prevertebral) ganglia

T5

Celiac ganglion

Thoracic splanchnic nn.

L1

Lumbar splanchnic nn.

Sacral splanchnic nn.

Superior and inferior mesenteric ganglia (with intermesenteric plexus)

**Inferior hypogastric plexus

Head and neck

Parasympathetic

Dorsal vagal nucleus

Vagus n.

S2
S4

Pelvic splanchnic nn.

**Minimal sympathetic preganglionic fibers traveling through the sacral splanchnic nerves will synapse in the ganglia located in the inferior hypogastric plexus

— Sympathetic preganglionic fibers
---- Sympathetic postganglionic fibers
— Parasympathetic preganglionic fibers
---- Parasympathetic postganglionic fibers

Table 16.4	Effects of the autonomic nervous system in the abdomen and pelvis		
Organ (organ system)		**Sympathetic effect**	**Parasympathetic effect**
Gastrointestinal tract	Longitudinal and circular muscle fibers	↓ motility	↑ motility
	Sphincter muscles	Contraction	Relaxation
	Glands	↓ secretions	↑ secretions
Splenic capsule		Contraction	
Liver		↑ glycogenolysis/gluconeogenesis	No effect
Pancreas	Endocrine pancreas	↓ insulin secretion	
	Exocrine pancreas	↓ secretion	↑ secretion
Urinary bladder	Detrusor vesicae	Relaxation	Contraction
	Functional bladder sphincter	Contraction	Inhibits contraction
Seminal glands and ductus deferens		Contraction (ejaculation)	
Uterus		Contraction or relaxation, depending on hormonal status	No effect
Arteries		Vasoconstriction	Vasodilation of the arteries of the penis and clitoris (erection)
Suprarenal glands (medulla)		Release of adrenalin	No effect
Urinary tract	Kidney	Vasoconstriction (↓ urine formation)	Vasodilation

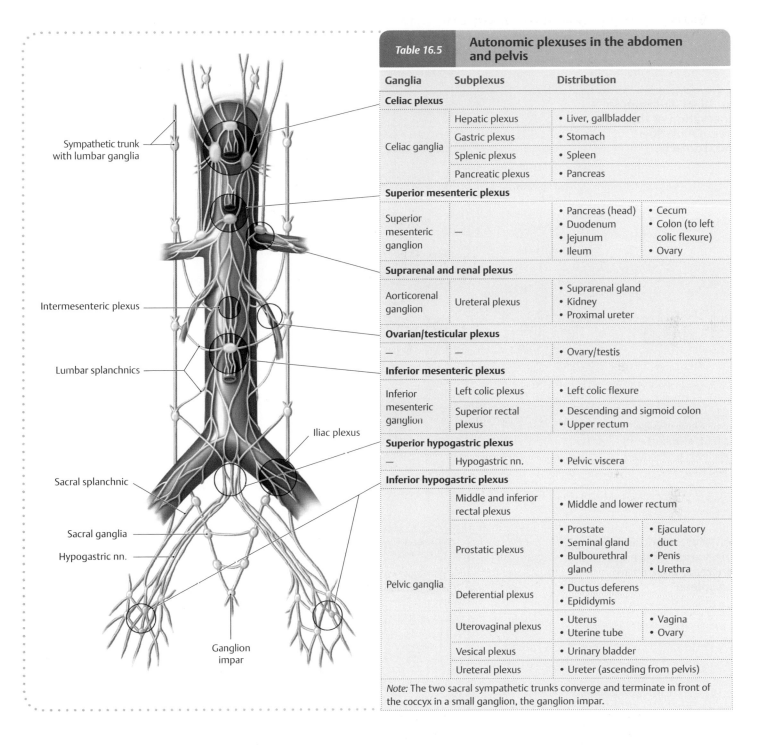

Sympathetic trunk with lumbar ganglia

Intermesenteric plexus

Lumbar splanchnics

Iliac plexus

Sacral splanchnic

Sacral ganglia

Hypogastric nn.

Ganglion impar

Table 16.5	**Autonomic plexuses in the abdomen and pelvis**		
Ganglia	**Subplexus**	**Distribution**	
Celiac plexus			
Celiac ganglia	Hepatic plexus	• Liver, gallbladder	
	Gastric plexus	• Stomach	
	Splenic plexus	• Spleen	
	Pancreatic plexus	• Pancreas	
Superior mesenteric plexus			
Superior mesenteric ganglion	—	• Pancreas (head) • Duodenum • Jejunum • Ileum	• Cecum • Colon (to left colic flexure) • Ovary
Suprarenal and renal plexus			
Aorticorenal ganglion	Ureteral plexus	• Suprarenal gland • Kidney • Proximal ureter	
Ovarian/testicular plexus			
—	—	• Ovary/testis	
Inferior mesenteric plexus			
Inferior mesenteric ganglion	Left colic plexus	• Left colic flexure	
	Superior rectal plexus	• Descending and sigmoid colon • Upper rectum	
Superior hypogastric plexus			
—	Hypogastric nn.	• Pelvic viscera	
Inferior hypogastric plexus			
Pelvic ganglia	Middle and inferior rectal plexus	• Middle and lower rectum	
	Prostatic plexus	• Prostate • Seminal gland • Bulbourethral gland	• Ejaculatory duct • Penis • Urethra
	Deferential plexus	• Ductus deferens • Epididymis	
	Uterovaginal plexus	• Uterus • Uterine tube	• Vagina • Ovary
	Vesical plexus	• Urinary bladder	
	Ureteral plexus	• Ureter (ascending from pelvis)	

Note: The two sacral sympathetic trunks converge and terminate in front of the coccyx in a small ganglion, the ganglion impar.

Autonomic Innervation & Referred Pain

Pain afferents from the viscera (visceral pain) and dermatomes (somatic pain) terminate at the same processing neurons in the posterior horn of the spinal cord. The convergence of these visceral and somatic afferent fibers confuses the relationship between the pain's origin and its perception. This phenomenon is called *referred pain*. The pain impulses from a particular internal organ are consistently projected to the same well-defined skin area. Thus, the area of skin that the pain is projected to provides crucial information regarding what organ is affected.

Fig. 16.40 Autonomic innervation of the liver, gallbladder, and stomach

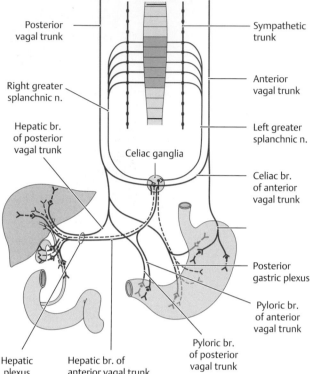

A Schematic of celiac plexus distribution to the liver, gallbladder, and stomach.

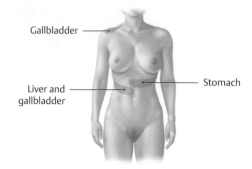

B Zones of referred pain from the liver, gallbladder, and stomach.

——— Sympathetic preganglionic fibers
----- Sympathetic postganglionic fibers
——— Parasympathetic preganglionic fibers
----- Parasympathetic postganglionic fibers

Fig. 16.41 Autonomic innervation of the pancreas, duodenum, and spleen

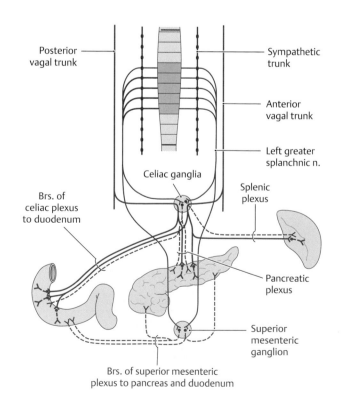

A Schematic of celiac plexus distribution to the pancreas, duodenum, and spleen.

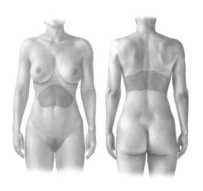

B Zones of referred pain from the pancreas. There are no zones associated with the duodenum and spleen.

——— Sympathetic preganglionic fibers
----- Sympathetic postganglionic fibers
——— Parasympathetic preganglionic fibers
----- Parasympathetic postganglionic fibers

Fig. 16.42 Autonomic innervation of the midgut and hindgut

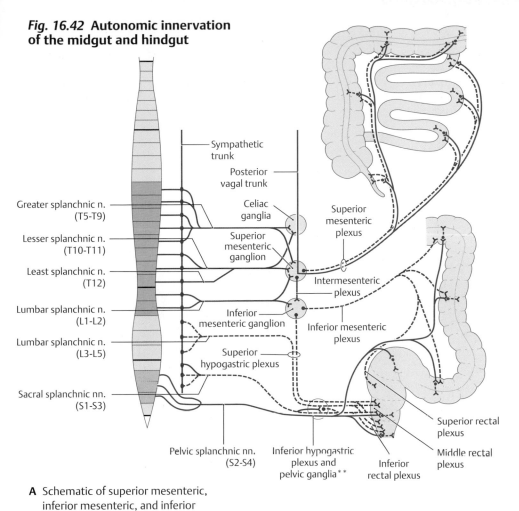

Sympathetic trunk

Posterior vagal trunk

Greater splanchnic n. (T5–T9)

Celiac ganglia

Superior mesenteric plexus

Lesser splanchnic n. (T10–T11)

Superior mesenteric ganglion

Least splanchnic n. (T12)

Intermesenteric plexus

Lumbar splanchnic n. (L1–L2)

Inferior mesenteric ganglion

Inferior mesenteric plexus

Lumbar splanchnic n. (L3–L5)

Superior hypogastric plexus

Sacral splanchnic nn. (S1–S3)

Superior rectal plexus

Middle rectal plexus

Pelvic splanchnic nn. (S2–S4)

Inferior hypogastric plexus and pelvic ganglia**

Inferior rectal plexus

A Schematic of superior mesenteric, inferior mesenteric, and inferior hypogastric plexuses distribution.

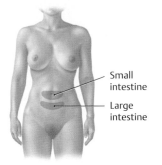

Small intestine

Large intestine

B Zones of referred pain from the small and large intestine.

—— Sympathetic preganglionic fibers
- - - Sympathetic postganglionic fibers
—— Parasympathetic preganglionic fibers
- - - Parasympathetic postganglionic fibers

**Minimal sympathetic preganglionic fibers traveling through the sacral splanchnic nerves will synapse in the ganglia located in the inferior hypogastric plexus.

Fig. 16.43 Autonomic innervation of the kidneys and upper ureters

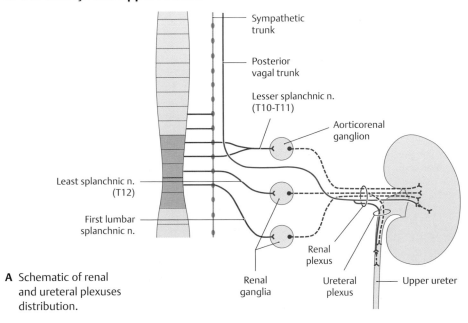

Sympathetic trunk

Posterior vagal trunk

Lesser splanchnic n. (T10–T11)

Aorticorenal ganglion

Least splanchnic n. (T12)

First lumbar splanchnic n.

Renal plexus

Renal ganglia

Ureteral plexus

Upper ureter

A Schematic of renal and ureteral plexuses distribution.

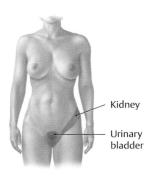

Kidney

Urinary bladder

B Zones of referred pain from the left kidney and bladder.

—— Sympathetic preganglionic fibers
- - - Sympathetic postganglionic fibers
—— Parasympathetic preganglionic fibers
- - - Parasympathetic postganglionic fibers

Innervation of the Foregut & Urinary Organs

Fig. 16.44 Innervation of the foregut and spleen

Anterior view. *Removed:* Lesser omentum, ascending colon, and parts of the transverse colon. *Opened:* Omental bursa. The anterior and posterior vagal trunks each produce a celiac, hepatic, and pyloric branch, and a gastric plexus. See **p. 214** for schematic.

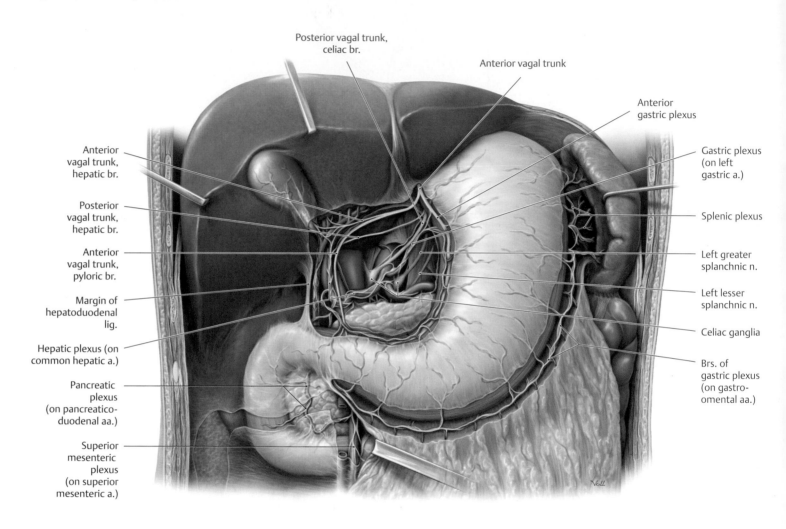

Posterior vagal trunk, celiac br.

Anterior vagal trunk

Anterior gastric plexus

Anterior vagal trunk, hepatic br.

Posterior vagal trunk, hepatic br.

Anterior vagal trunk, pyloric br.

Margin of hepatoduodenal lig.

Hepatic plexus (on common hepatic a.)

Pancreatic plexus (on pancreatico-duodenal aa.)

Superior mesenteric plexus (on superior mesenteric a.)

Gastric plexus (on left gastric a.)

Splenic plexus

Left greater splanchnic n.

Left lesser splanchnic n.

Celiac ganglia

Brs. of gastric plexus (on gastro-omental aa.)

✳ Clinical box 16.9

Organization of the enteric plexus

The enteric plexus is the portion of the autonomic nervous system that specifically serves *all the organs of the gastrointestinal tract*. Located within the wall of the digestive tube (intramural nervous system), it is subject to both sympathetic and parasympathetic influences. Congenital absence of the enteric plexus leads to severe disturbances of gastrointestinal transit (e.g., Hirschsprung disease). The enteric plexus has basically the same organization throughout the gastrointestinal tract, although there is an area in the wall of the lower rectum that is devoid of ganglion cells. Three subsystems are distinguished in the enteric plexus:

- Submucosal plexus (Meissner's plexus)
- Myenteric plexus (Auerbach's plexus)
- Subserosal plexus

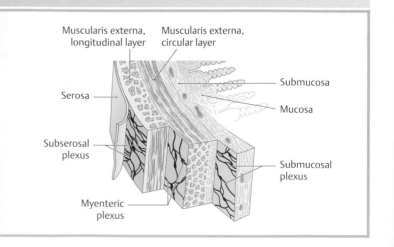

Muscularis externa, longitudinal layer

Muscularis externa, circular layer

Submucosa

Mucosa

Serosa

Subserosal plexus

Submucosal plexus

Myenteric plexus

Fig. 16.45 **Innervation of the urinary organs**

Anterior view of the male abdomen and pelvis. *Removed:* Peritoneum, majority of stomach, and abdominal organs except kidneys, suprarenal glands, and bladder. See **pp. 215 and 282** for schematic.

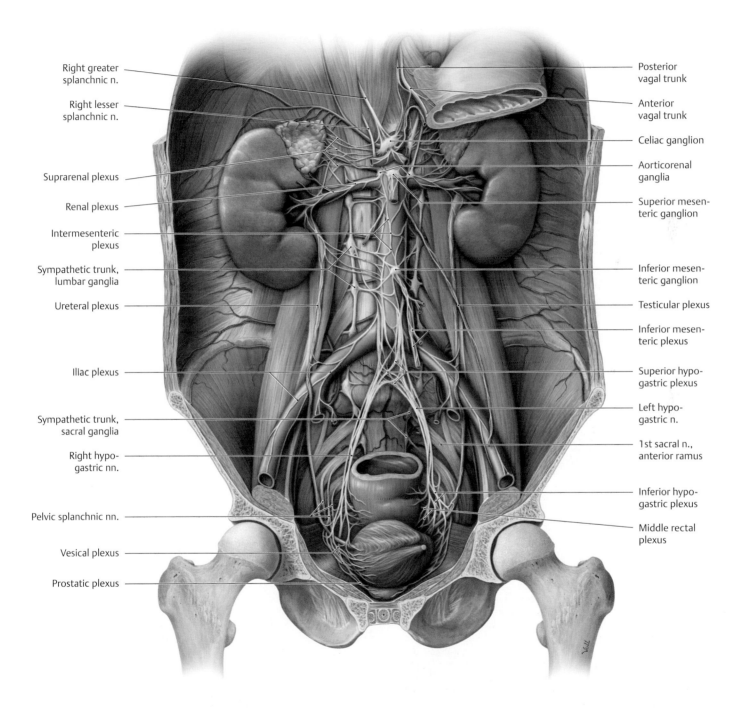

Right greater splanchnic n.

Right lesser splanchnic n.

Suprarenal plexus

Renal plexus

Intermesenteric plexus

Sympathetic trunk, lumbar ganglia

Ureteral plexus

Iliac plexus

Sympathetic trunk, sacral ganglia

Right hypo-gastric nn.

Pelvic splanchnic nn.

Vesical plexus

Prostatic plexus

Posterior vagal trunk

Anterior vagal trunk

Celiac ganglion

Aorticorenal ganglia

Superior mesen-teric ganglion

Inferior mesen-teric ganglion

Testicular plexus

Inferior mesen-teric plexus

Superior hypo-gastric plexus

Left hypo-gastric n.

1st sacral n., anterior ramus

Inferior hypo-gastric plexus

Middle rectal plexus

Innervation of the Intestines

Fig. 16.46 Innervation of the small intestine
Anterior view. *Partially removed:* Stomach, pancreas,
and transverse colon (distal part). See **p. 215** for schematic.

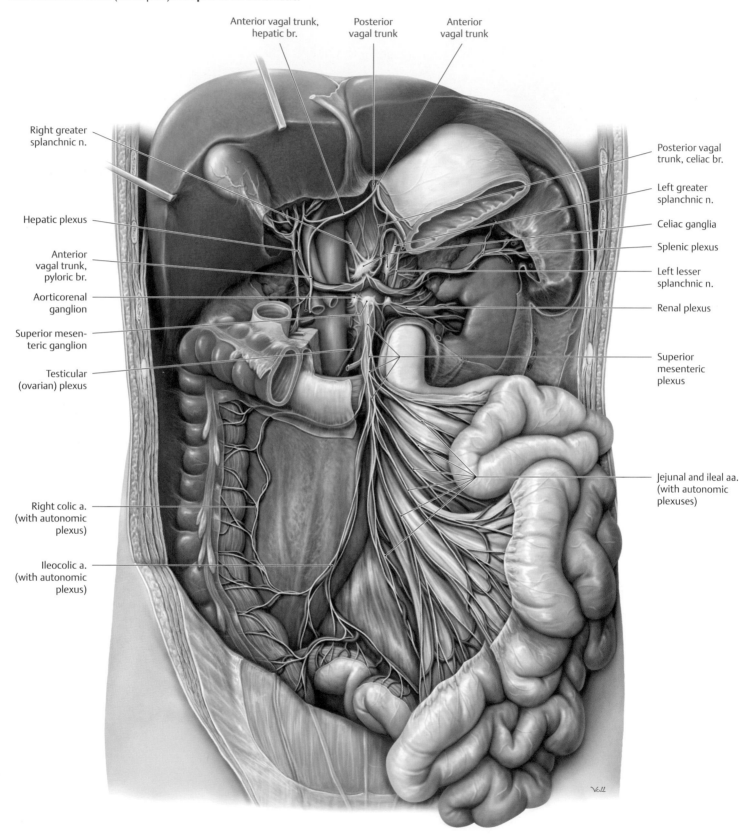

Anterior vagal trunk,
hepatic br.

Posterior
vagal trunk

Anterior
vagal trunk

Right greater
splanchnic n.

Hepatic plexus

Anterior
vagal trunk,
pyloric br.

Aorticorenal
ganglion

Superior mesen-
teric ganglion

Testicular
(ovarian) plexus

Right colic a.
(with autonomic
plexus)

Ileocolic a.
(with autonomic
plexus)

Posterior vagal
trunk, celiac br.

Left greater
splanchnic n.

Celiac ganglia

Splenic plexus

Left lesser
splanchnic n.

Renal plexus

Superior
mesenteric
plexus

Jejunal and ileal aa.
(with autonomic
plexuses)

Fig. 16.47 Innervation of the large intestine

Anterior view. *Removed:* Small intestine.
Reflected: Transverse and sigmoid colons. See **p. 215** for schematic.

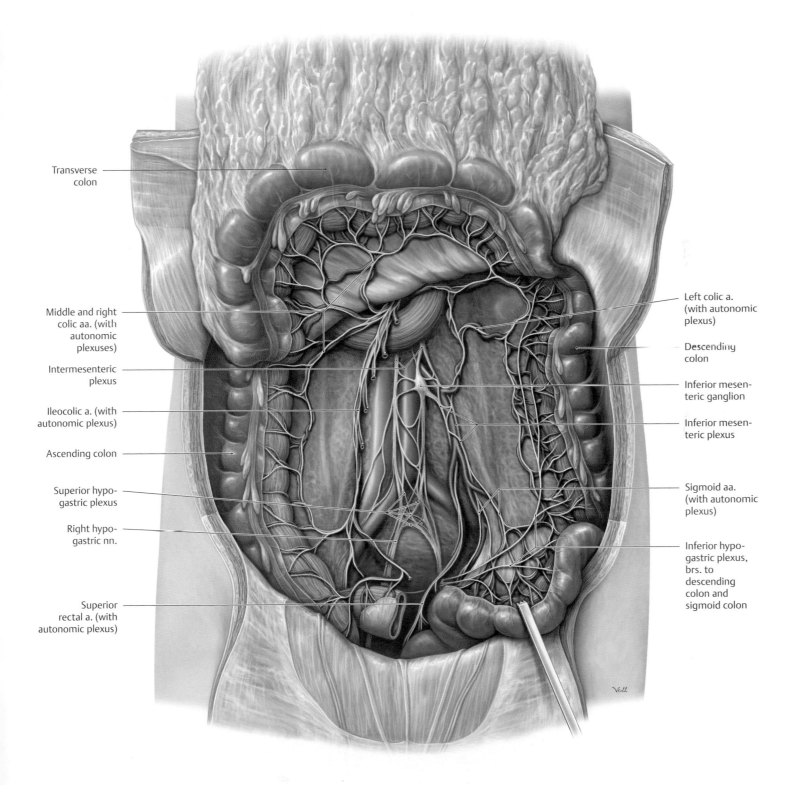

Transverse colon

Middle and right colic aa. (with autonomic plexuses)

Intermesenteric plexus

Ileocolic a. (with autonomic plexus)

Ascending colon

Superior hypogastric plexus

Right hypogastric nn.

Superior rectal a. (with autonomic plexus)

Left colic a. (with autonomic plexus)

Descending colon

Inferior mesenteric ganglion

Inferior mesenteric plexus

Sigmoid aa. (with autonomic plexus)

Inferior hypogastric plexus, brs. to descending colon and sigmoid colon

17 Sectional & Radiographic Anatomy
Sectional Anatomy of the Abdomen

Fig. 17.1 Transverse sections of the abdomen
Inferior view.

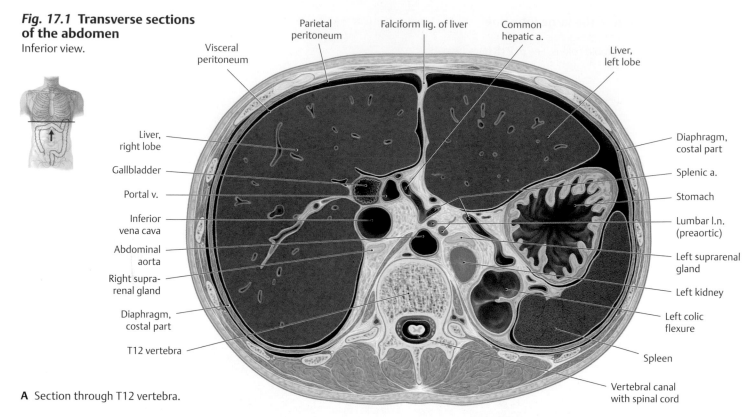

A Section through T12 vertebra.

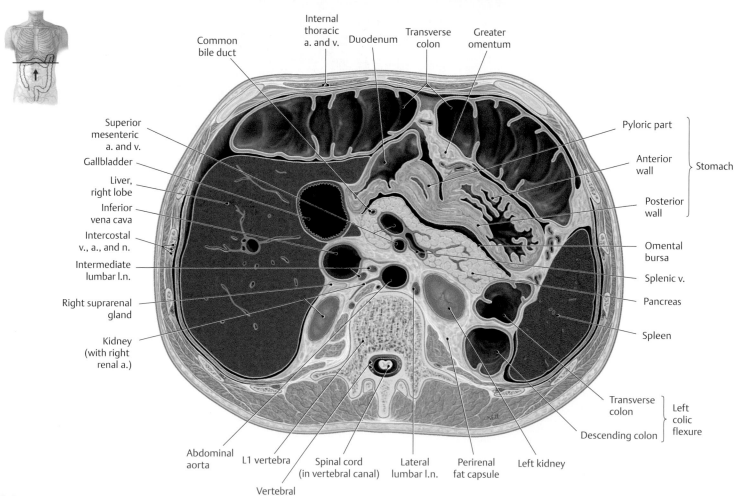

B Section through L1 vertebra.

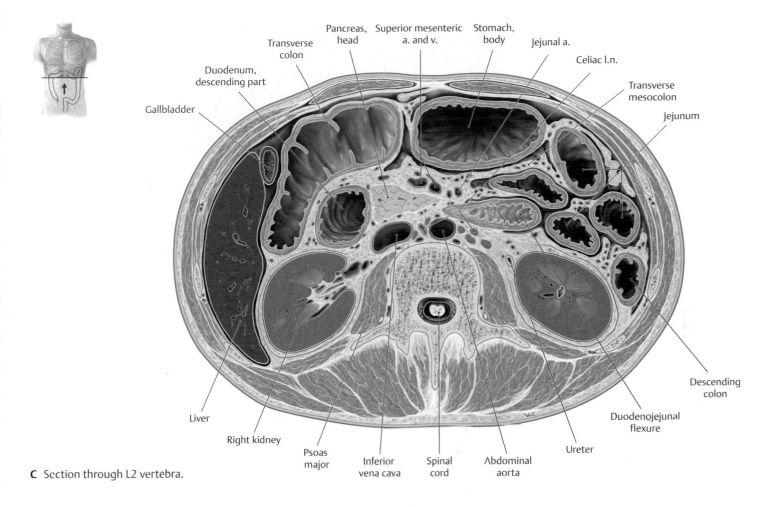

Duodenum, descending part

Transverse colon

Pancreas, head

Superior mesenteric a. and v.

Stomach, body

Jejunal a.

Celiac l.n.

Transverse mesocolon

Jejunum

Gallbladder

Descending colon

Liver

Right kidney

Psoas major

Inferior vena cava

Spinal cord

Abdominal aorta

Ureter

Duodenojejunal flexure

C Section through L2 vertebra.

Radiographic Anatomy of the Abdomen (I)

Fig. 17.2 CT of the abdomen: Transverse sections
(Reproduced from Moeller TB, Reif E. Pocket Atlas of Sectional Anatomy, Vol 2, 4th ed. New York, NY: Thieme; 2014.)

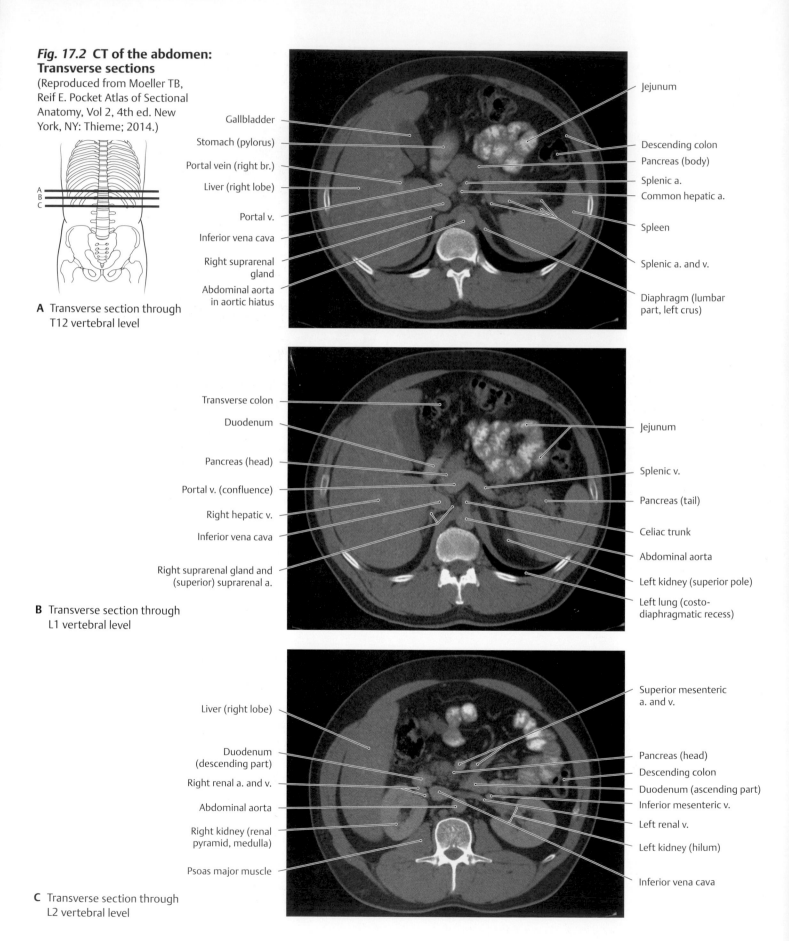

A Transverse section through T12 vertebral level

Labels on section A:
Gallbladder, Stomach (pylorus), Portal vein (right br.), Liver (right lobe), Portal v., Inferior vena cava, Right suprarenal gland, Abdominal aorta in aortic hiatus, Jejunum, Descending colon, Pancreas (body), Splenic a., Common hepatic a., Spleen, Splenic a. and v., Diaphragm (lumbar part, left crus)

B Transverse section through L1 vertebral level

Labels on section B:
Transverse colon, Duodenum, Pancreas (head), Portal v. (confluence), Right hepatic v., Inferior vena cava, Right suprarenal gland and (superior) suprarenal a., Jejunum, Splenic v., Pancreas (tail), Celiac trunk, Abdominal aorta, Left kidney (superior pole), Left lung (costo-diaphragmatic recess)

C Transverse section through L2 vertebral level

Labels on section C:
Liver (right lobe), Duodenum (descending part), Right renal a. and v., Abdominal aorta, Right kidney (renal pyramid, medulla), Psoas major muscle, Superior mesenteric a. and v., Pancreas (head), Descending colon, Duodenum (ascending part), Inferior mesenteric v., Left renal v., Left kidney (hilum), Inferior vena cava

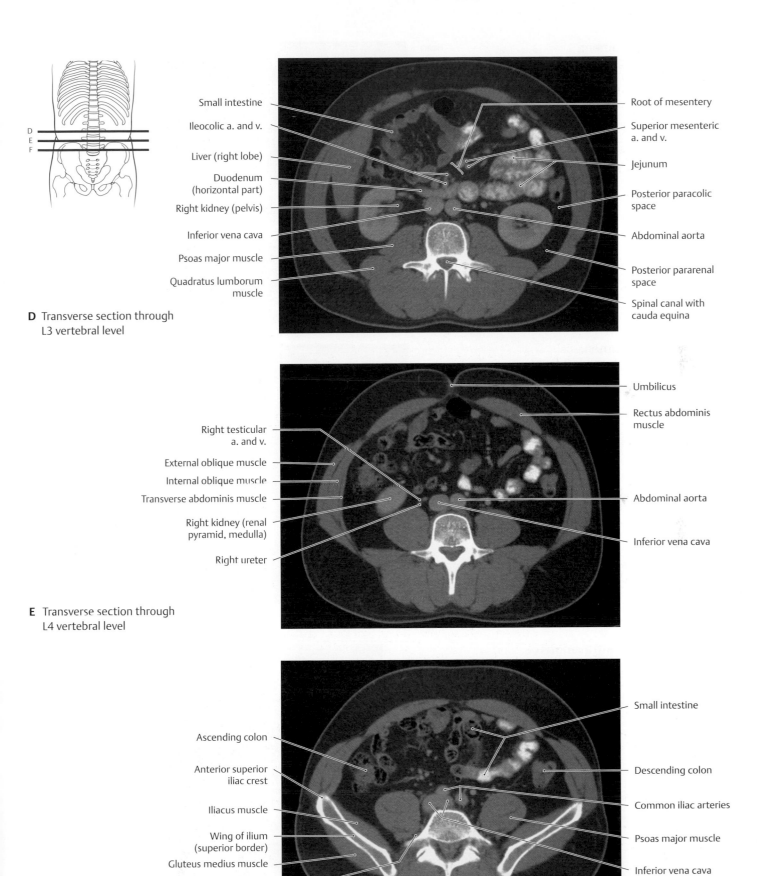

Small intestine

Ileocolic a. and v.

Liver (right lobe)

Duodenum (horizontal part)

Right kidney (pelvis)

Inferior vena cava

Psoas major muscle

Quadratus lumborum muscle

Root of mesentery

Superior mesenteric a. and v.

Jejunum

Posterior paracolic space

Abdominal aorta

Posterior pararenal space

Spinal canal with cauda equina

D Transverse section through L3 vertebral level

Umbilicus

Rectus abdominis muscle

Right testicular a. and v.

External oblique muscle

Internal oblique muscle

Transverse abdominis muscle

Right kidney (renal pyramid, medulla)

Right ureter

Abdominal aorta

Inferior vena cava

E Transverse section through L4 vertebral level

Small intestine

Ascending colon

Anterior superior iliac crest

Iliacus muscle

Wing of ilium (superior border)

Gluteus medius muscle

Lumbar plexus

Descending colon

Common iliac arteries

Psoas major muscle

Inferior vena cava (confluence)

F Transverse section through L5 vertebral level

Radiographic Anatomy of the Abdomen (II)

Fig. 17.3 **CT of the abdomen:**
Sagittal section through the aorta
(Reproduced from Moeller TB, Reif E. Pocket
Atlas of Sectional Anatomy, Vol 2, 4th ed.
New York, NY: Thieme; 2014.)

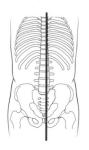

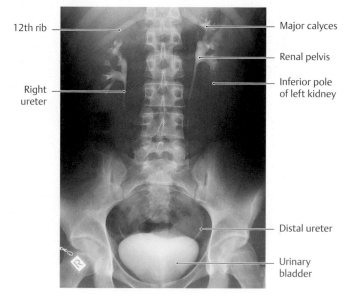

Heart
Liver (left lobe)
Stomach
Pancreas
Transverse colon
Jejunum
Celiac trunk
Superior mesenteric a.
Right renal v.
Lumbar vertebral body (L2)
Abdominal aorta
Promontory of sacrum
Duodenum (horizontal part)
Urinary bladder
Rectum

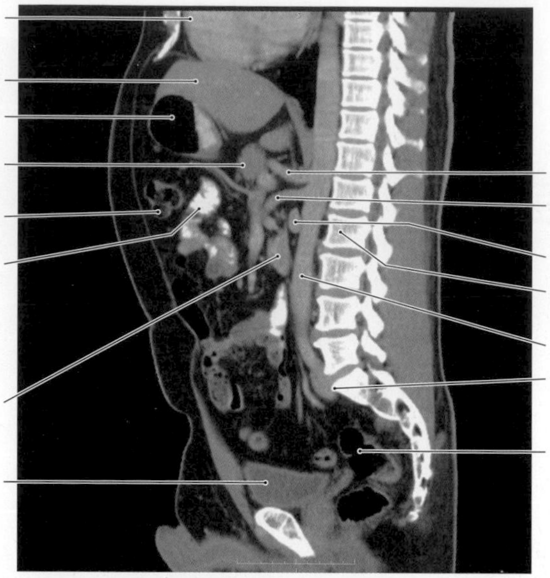

Fig. 17.4 **CT of the Abdomen:**
Coronal section through the kidneys
(Reproduced from Moeller TB, Reif E. Pocket
Atlas of Sectional Anatomy, Vol 2, 4th ed. New
York, NY: Thieme; 2014.)

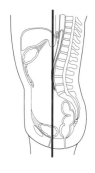

Liver (right lobe)
Inferior vena cava
Right kidney, superior pole, and right renal a.
Renal pelvis
Psoas muscle
Iliacus muscle
Gluteus medius muscle
Stomach (fundus)
Spleen with splenic a. and v.
Pancreas (tail)
Left renal v. and a.
Left kidney (renal cortex)
Inferior mesenteric v.
Common iliac a. and v. (left)

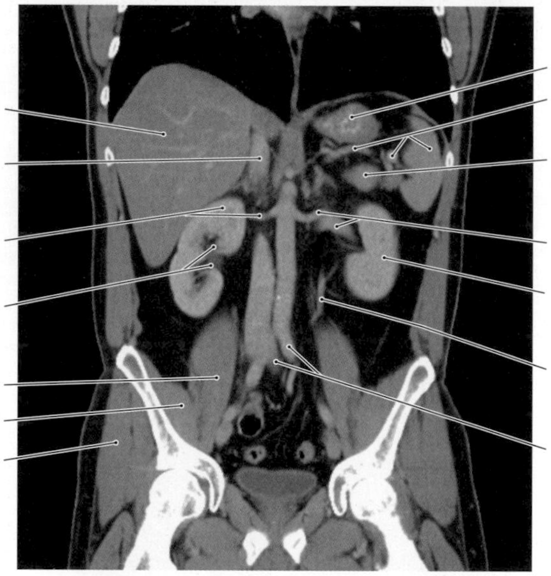

Fig. 17.5 **Radiograph of intravenous**
pylegram
Anterior view.

12th rib
Right ureter
Major calyces
Renal pelvis
Inferior pole of left kidney
Distal ureter
Urinary bladder

Fig. 17.6 Radiographs of double contrast barium enema.

Anterior view.

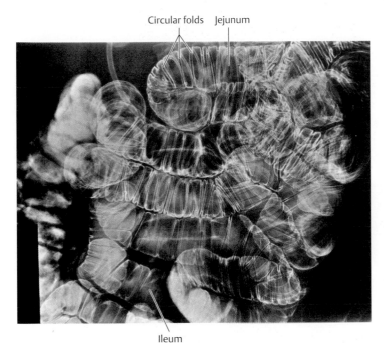

Circular folds · Jejunum

Ileum

A Small intestine. (Reproduced courtesy of Universitätsmedizin Mainz, Klinik und Poliklinik für Diagnostische und Interventionelle Radiologie.)

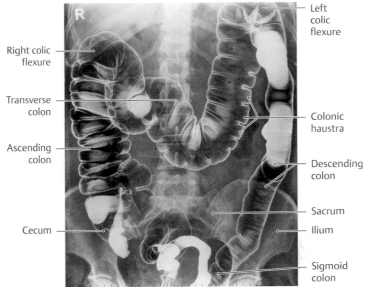

Left colic flexure

Right colic flexure

Transverse colon

Ascending colon

Colonic haustra

Descending colon

Sacrum

Cecum

Ilium

Sigmoid colon

B Large intestine. (Reproduced courtesy of Klinik für Diagnostische Radiologie, Universitätsklinikum Schleswig Holstein, Campus Kiel: Prof. Dr. Med. S. Müller-Huelsbeck.)

Fig. 17.7 MRI of the intestines

Coronal view. Sectional imaging modalities like CT and MR have mostly replaced conventional radiographs in the evaluation of gastrointestinal disease. (Reproduced from Krombach GA, Mahnken AH. Body Imaging: Thorax and Abdomen. New York, NY: Thieme; 2018.)

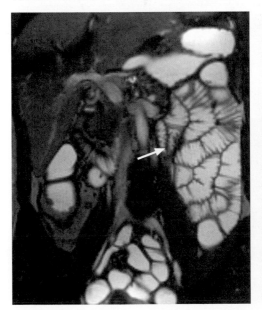

A Jejunum *(arrow)*

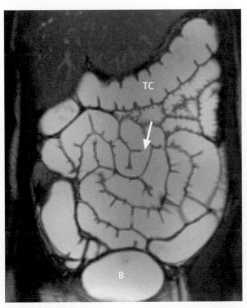

B Ileum *(arrow)*, transverse colon (TC), urinary bladder (B)

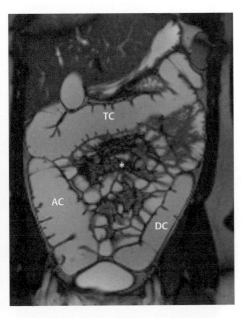

C Ascending colon (AC), descending colon (DC), transverse colon (TC), * small bowel and mesenteric structures.

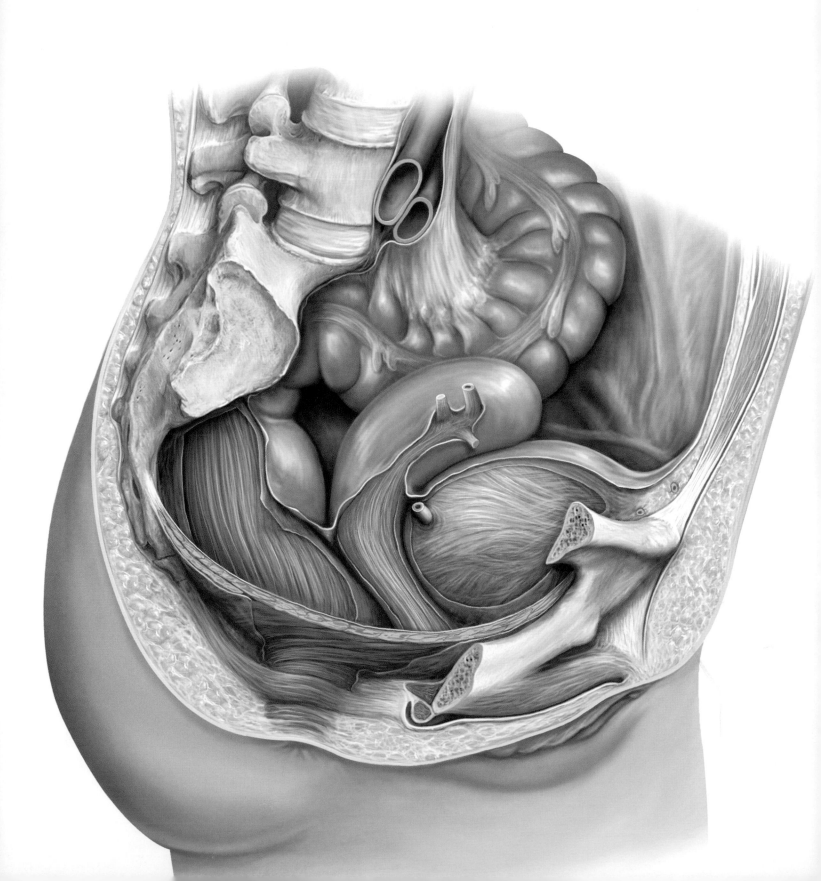

Pelvis & Perineum

18 Surface Anatomy

Surface Anatomy

Fig. 18.1 Palpable structures of the pelvis
Anterior view. The structures are common to both male and female. See **pp. 2–3** for structures of the back.

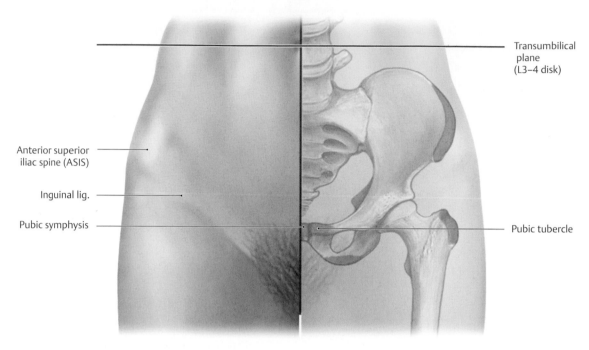

Transumbilical plane (L3–4 disk)

Anterior superior iliac spine (ASIS)

Inguinal lig.

Pubic symphysis

Pubic tubercle

A Bony prominences, female pelvis.

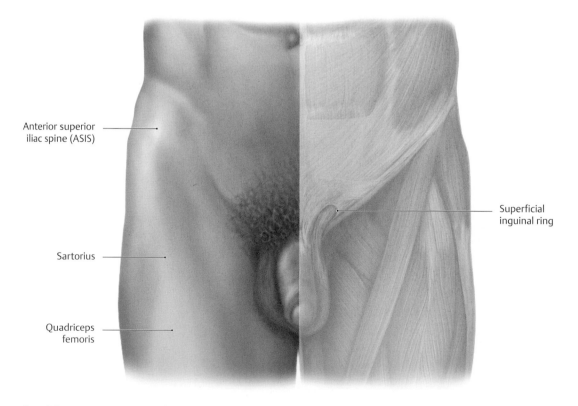

Anterior superior iliac spine (ASIS)

Superficial inguinal ring

Sartorius

Quadriceps femoris

B Musculature, male pelvis.

The *perineum* is the inferiormost portion of the trunk, between the thighs and buttocks, extending from the pubis to the coccyx and superiorly to the inferior fascia of the pelvic diaphragm, including all of the structures of the anal and urogenital triangles (**Fig. 18.2A**). The bilateral boundaries of the perineum are the pubic symphysis, ischiopubic ramus, ischial tuberosity, sacrotuberous ligament, and coccyx.

Fig. 18.2 Regions of the female perineum
Lithotomy position.

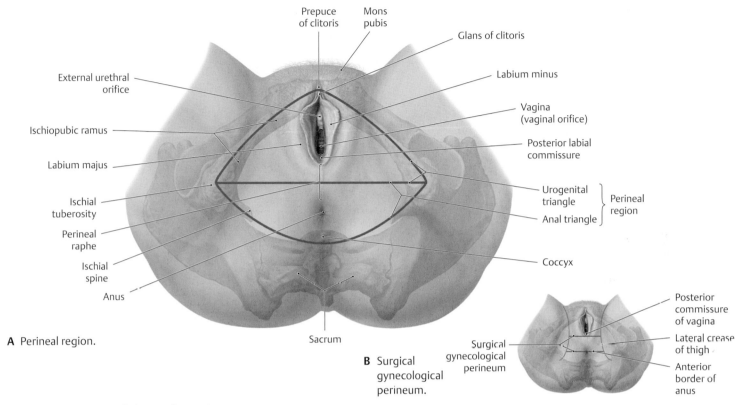

A Perineal region.

B Surgical gynecological perineum.

Fig. 18.3 Regions of the male perineum
Lithotomy position.

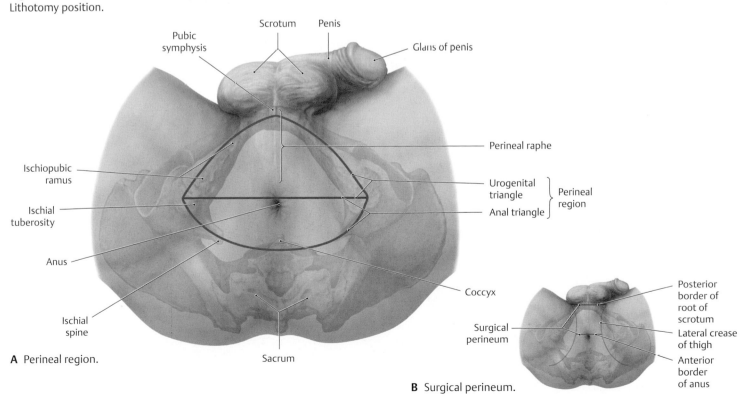

A Perineal region.

B Surgical perineum.

19 Bones, Ligaments & Muscles
Pelvic Girdle

The pelvis is the region of the body inferior to the abdomen and surrounded by the pelvic girdle, which is the two coxal (hip) bones and the sacrum that connect the vertebral column to the femur. The two coxal bones are connected to each other at the cartilaginous pubic symphysis and to the sacrum via the sacroiliac joints, creating the pelvic brim (red, **Fig. 19.1**). The stability of the pelvic girdle is necessary for the transfer of trunk loads to the lower limb, which occurs in normal gait.

Fig. 19.1 **Pelvic girdle**
Anterosuperior view. The pelvic girdle consists of the two coxal bones and the sacrum.

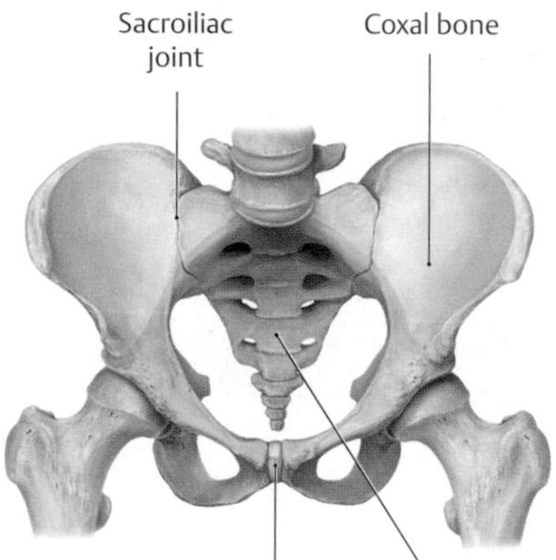

Fig. 19.2 **Coxal bone**
Right side (male).

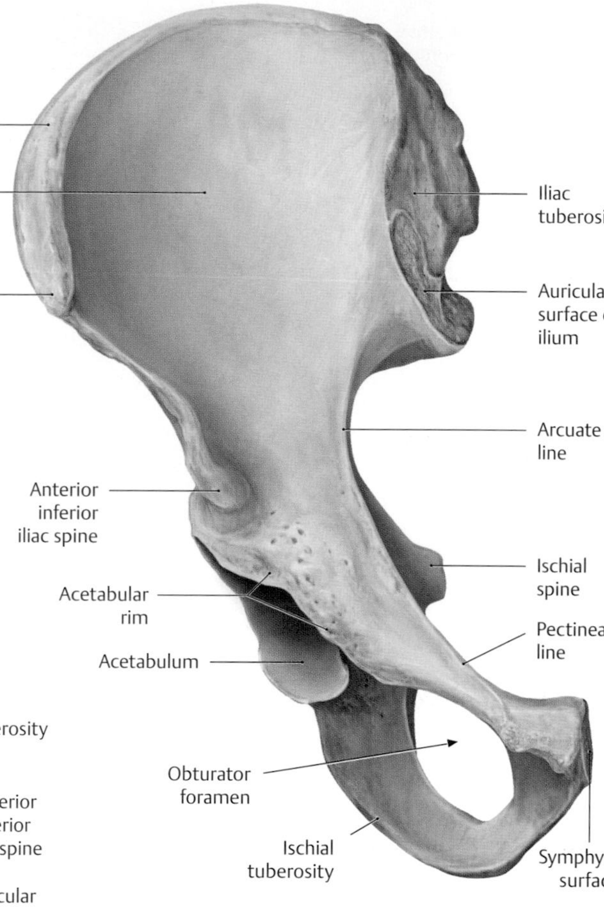

A Anterior view.

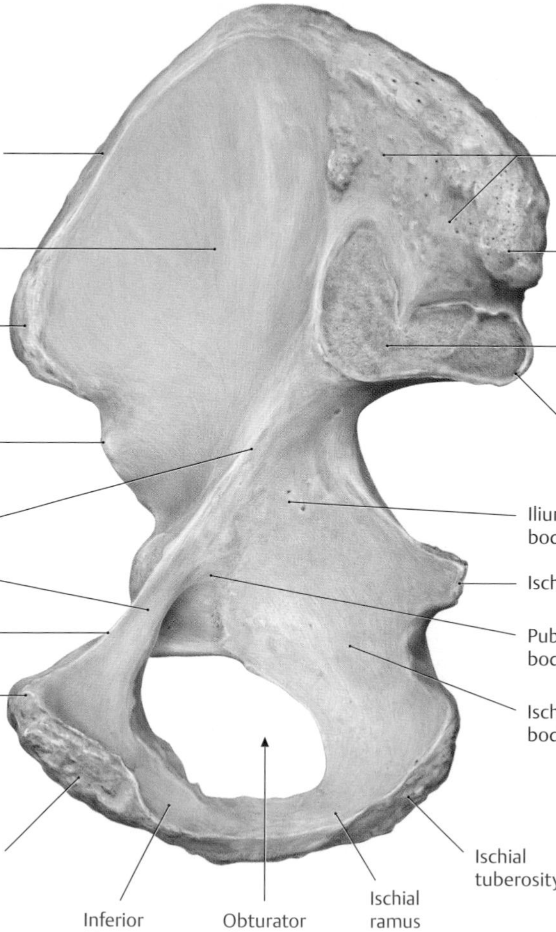

B Medial view.

Fig. 19.3 Triradiate cartilage of the coxal bone

Right coxal bone, lateral view. The coxal bone consists of the ilium, ischium, and pubis.

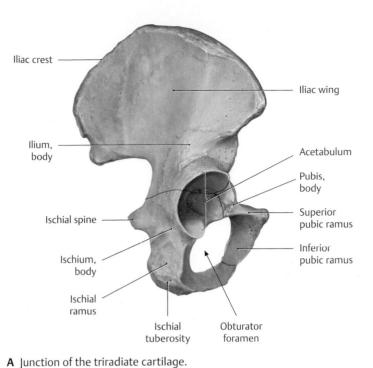

A Junction of the triradiate cartilage.

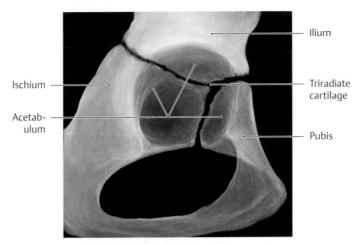

B Radiograph of a child's acetabulum.

Fig. 19.4 Coxal bone

Right side (male), lateral view.

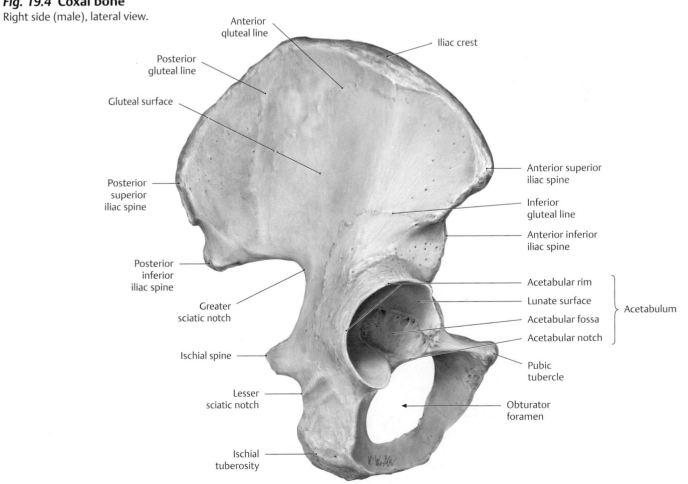

Female & Male Pelvis

Fig. 19.5 Female pelvis

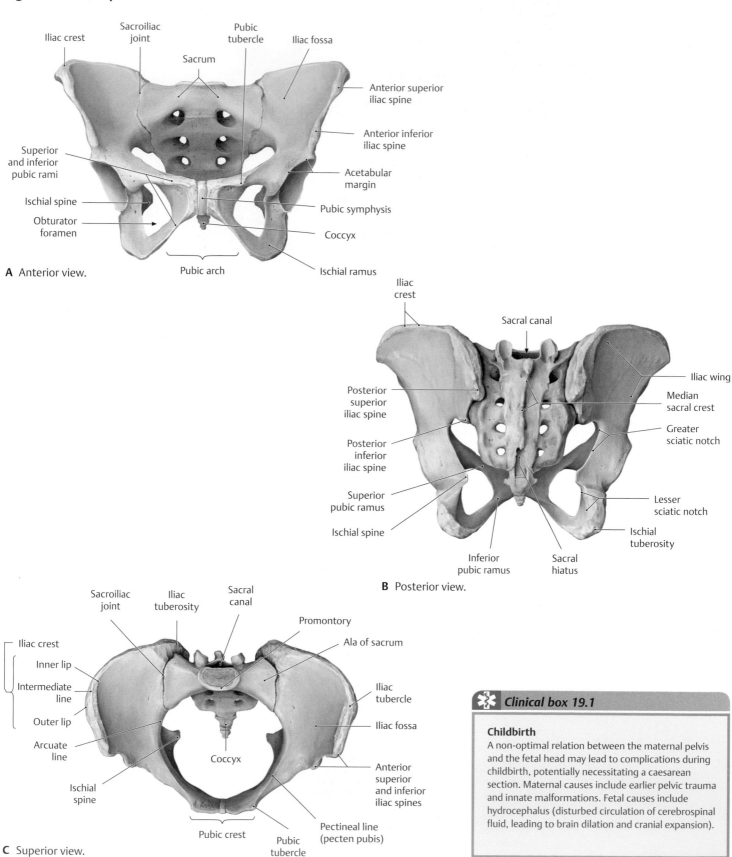

A Anterior view.

Iliac crest — Sacroiliac joint — Sacrum — Pubic tubercle — Iliac fossa

Anterior superior iliac spine

Anterior inferior iliac spine

Superior and inferior pubic rami

Acetabular margin

Ischial spine

Pubic symphysis

Obturator foramen

Coccyx

Pubic arch

Ischial ramus

B Posterior view.

Iliac crest — Sacral canal

Iliac wing

Posterior superior iliac spine

Median sacral crest

Greater sciatic notch

Posterior inferior iliac spine

Superior pubic ramus

Lesser sciatic notch

Ischial spine

Ischial tuberosity

Inferior pubic ramus — Sacral hiatus

C Superior view.

Sacroiliac joint — Iliac tuberosity — Sacral canal — Promontory

Ala of sacrum

Iliac crest — Inner lip — Intermediate line — Outer lip

Iliac tubercle

Iliac fossa

Arcuate line

Coccyx

Ischial spine

Anterior superior and inferior iliac spines

Pectineal line (pecten pubis)

Pubic crest — Pubic tubercle

Clinical box 19.1

Childbirth

A non-optimal relation between the maternal pelvis and the fetal head may lead to complications during childbirth, potentially necessitating a caesarean section. Maternal causes include earlier pelvic trauma and innate malformations. Fetal causes include hydrocephalus (disturbed circulation of cerebrospinal fluid, leading to brain dilation and cranial expansion).

Fig. 19.6 **Male pelvis**

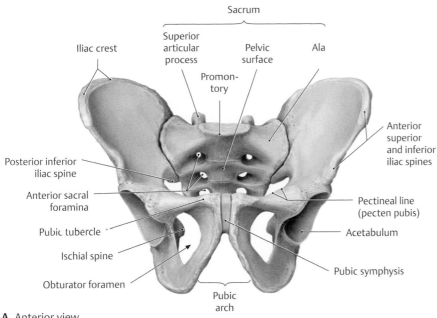

Sacrum

Iliac crest

Superior articular process

Promontory

Pelvic surface

Ala

Posterior inferior iliac spine

Anterior sacral foramina

Pubic tubercle

Ischial spine

Obturator foramen

Pubic arch

Anterior superior and inferior iliac spines

Pectineal line (pecten pubis)

Acetabulum

Pubic symphysis

A Anterior view.

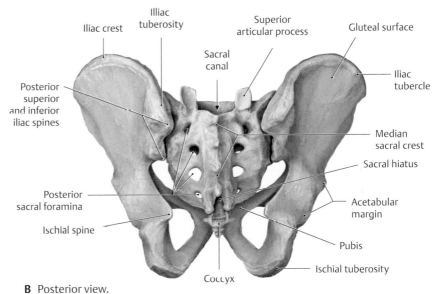

Iliac crest

Iliac tuberosity

Sacral canal

Superior articular process

Gluteal surface

Posterior superior and inferior iliac spines

Iliac tubercle

Median sacral crest

Sacral hiatus

Posterior sacral foramina

Acetabular margin

Ischial spine

Pubis

Coccyx

Ischial tuberosity

B Posterior view.

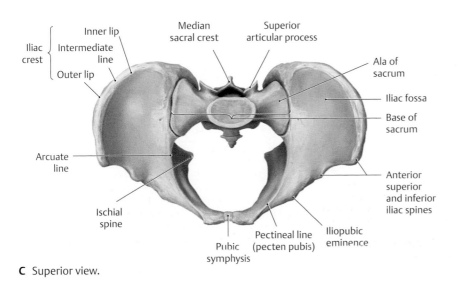

Iliac crest

Inner lip

Intermediate line

Outer lip

Median sacral crest

Superior articular process

Ala of sacrum

Iliac fossa

Base of sacrum

Arcuate line

Anterior superior and inferior iliac spines

Ischial spine

Pubic symphysis

Pectineal line (pecten pubis)

Iliopubic eminence

C Superior view.

233

Female & Male Pelvic Measurements

The *pelvic inlet*, the superior aperture of the pelvis, is the boundary between the abdominal and pelvic cavities. It is defined by the plane that passes through its edge, the *pelvic brim*, which is the prominence of the sacrum, the arcuate and pectineal lines, and the upper margin of the pubic symphysis. Occasionally, the terms *pelvic inlet* and *pelvic brim* are used interchangeably. The *pelvic outlet* is the plane of the inferior aperture, passing through the pubic arch, the ischial tuberosities, the inferior margin of the sacrotuberous ligament, and the tip of the coccyx.

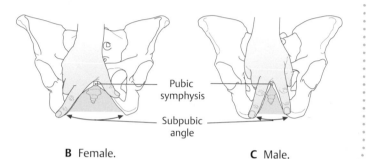

Table 19.1	Gender-specific features of the pelvis	
Structure	♀	♂
False pelvis	Wide and shallow	Narrow and deep
Pelvic inlet	Transversely oval	Heart-shaped
Pelvic outlet	Roomy and round	Narrow and oblong
Ischial tuberosities	Everted	Inverted
Pelvic cavity	Roomy and shallow	Narrow and deep
Sacrum	Short, wide, and flat	Long, narrow, and convex
Subpubic angle	90–100 degrees	70 degrees

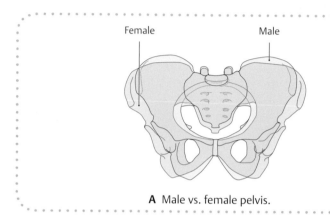

A Male vs. female pelvis.

B Female. **C** Male.

Fig. 19.7 True and false pelvis

The pelvis is the region of the body inferior to the abdomen, surrounded by the pelvic girdle. The *false pelvis* is immediately inferior to the abdominal cavity, between the iliac alae, and superior to the pelvic inlet. The *true pelvis* is the bony-walled space between the pelvic inlet and the pelvic outlet. It is bounded inferiorly by the pelvic diaphragm, also called the pelvic floor.

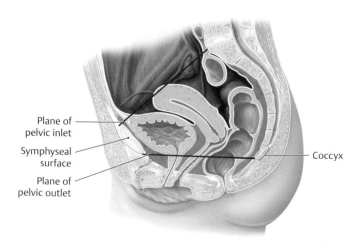

A Female. Midsagittal section, viewed from left side.

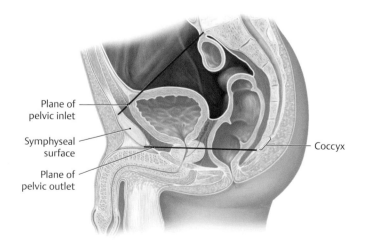

B Male. Midsagittal section, viewed from left side.

Fig. 19.8 Narrowest diameter of female pelvic canal

The true conjugate, the distance between the promontory and the most posterosuperior point of the pubic symphysis, is the narrowest AP (anteroposterior) diameter of the pelvic (birth) canal. This diameter is difficult to measure due to the viscera, so the diagonal conjugate, the distance between the promontory and the inferior border of the pubic symphysis, is used to estimate it. The linea terminalis is part of the border defining the pelvic inlet (pelvic brim).

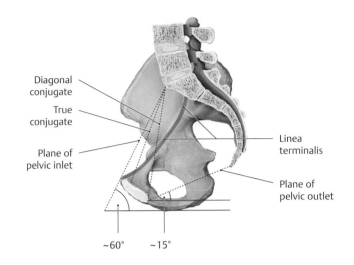

Fig. 19.9 Pelvic inlet and outlet

The measurements shown are applicable to both male and female. The transverse and oblique diameters of the female pelvic inlet are obstetrically important, as they are the measure of the diameter of the pelvic (birth) canal. The interspinous distance is the narrowest diameter of the pelvic outlet.

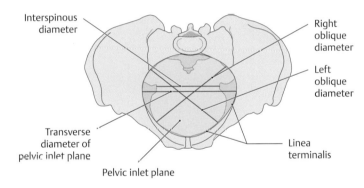

A Female pelvis, superior view.
Pelvic inlet outlined in red.

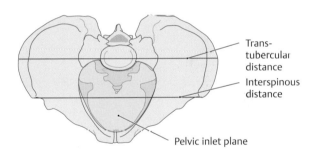

B Male pelvis, superior view.
Pelvic inlet outlined in red.

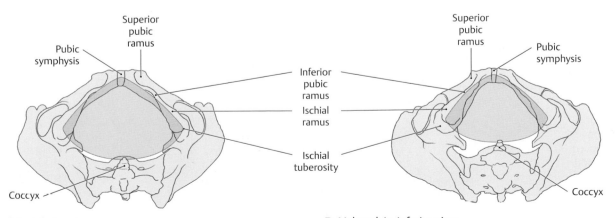

C Female pelvis, inferior view.
Pelvic outlet outlined in red.

D Male pelvis, inferior view.
Pelvic outlet outlined in red.

Pelvic Ligaments

Fig. 19.10 **Ligaments of the pelvis**
Male pelvis.

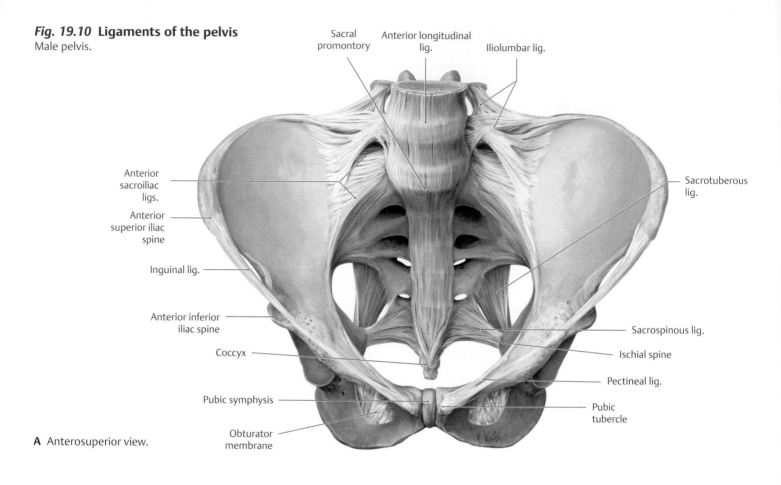

Sacral promontory — Anterior longitudinal lig. — Iliolumbar lig.

Anterior sacroiliac ligs.

Anterior superior iliac spine

Inguinal lig.

Anterior inferior iliac spine

Coccyx

Pubic symphysis

Obturator membrane

Sacrotuberous lig.

Sacrospinous lig.

Ischial spine

Pectineal lig.

Pubic tubercle

A Anterosuperior view.

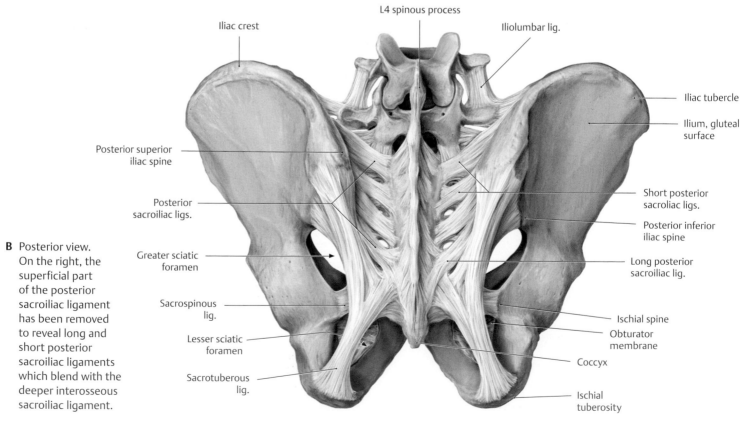

Iliac crest — L4 spinous process — Iliolumbar lig.

Posterior superior iliac spine

Posterior sacroiliac ligs.

Iliac tubercle

Ilium, gluteal surface

Short posterior sacroiliac ligs.

Posterior inferior iliac spine

B Posterior view.
On the right, the superficial part of the posterior sacroiliac ligament has been removed to reveal long and short posterior sacroiliac ligaments which blend with the deeper interosseous sacroiliac ligament.

Greater sciatic foramen

Sacrospinous lig.

Lesser sciatic foramen

Sacrotuberous lig.

Long posterior sacroiliac lig.

Ischial spine

Obturator membrane

Coccyx

Ischial tuberosity

Fig. 19.11 Ligaments of the sacroiliac joint
Male pelvis, midsagittal section.

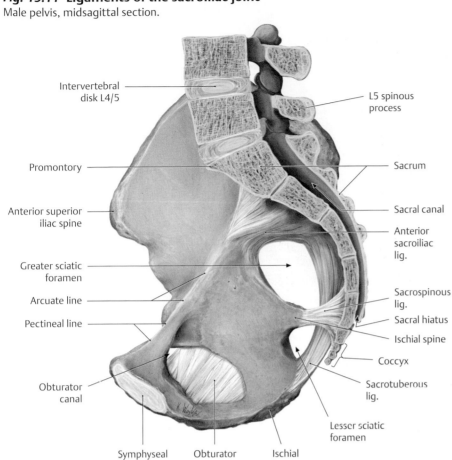

Intervertebral disk L4/5

L5 spinous process

Promontory

Sacrum

Anterior superior iliac spine

Sacral canal

Anterior sacroiliac lig.

Greater sciatic foramen

Sacrospinous lig.

Arcuate line

Sacral hiatus

Pectineal line

Ischial spine

Obturator canal

Coccyx

Sacrotuberous lig.

Lesser sciatic foramen

Symphyseal surface

Obturator membrane

Ischial tuberosity

A Right half of pelvis, medial view.

Fig. 19.12 Pelvic ligament attachment sites on the coxal bone
Left coxal bone, medial view. Ligament attachments are shown in green.

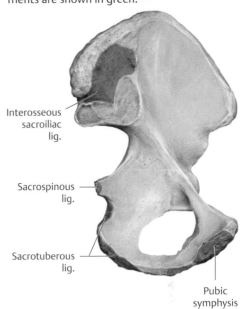

Interosseous sacroiliac lig.

Sacrospinous lig.

Sacrotuberous lig.

Pubic symphysis

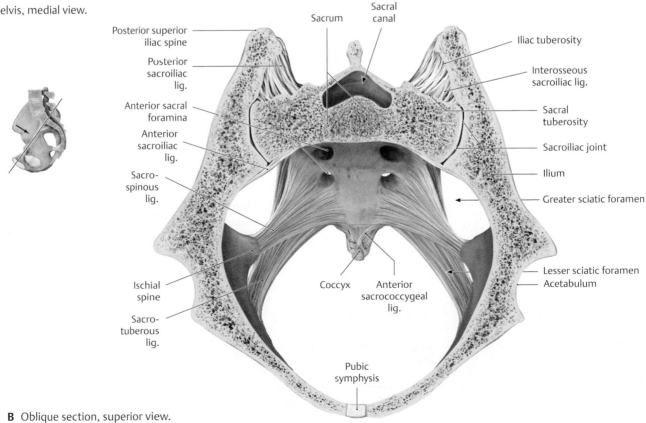

Posterior superior iliac spine

Sacrum

Sacral canal

Iliac tuberosity

Posterior sacroiliac lig.

Interosseous sacroiliac lig.

Anterior sacral foramina

Sacral tuberosity

Anterior sacroiliac lig.

Sacroiliac joint

Sacro- spinous lig.

Ilium

Greater sciatic foramen

Ischial spine

Lesser sciatic foramen

Acetabulum

Sacro- tuberous lig.

Coccyx

Anterior sacrococcygeal lig.

Pubic symphysis

B Oblique section, superior view.

237

Muscles of the Pelvic Floor & Perineum

Fig. 19.13 Muscles of the pelvic floor

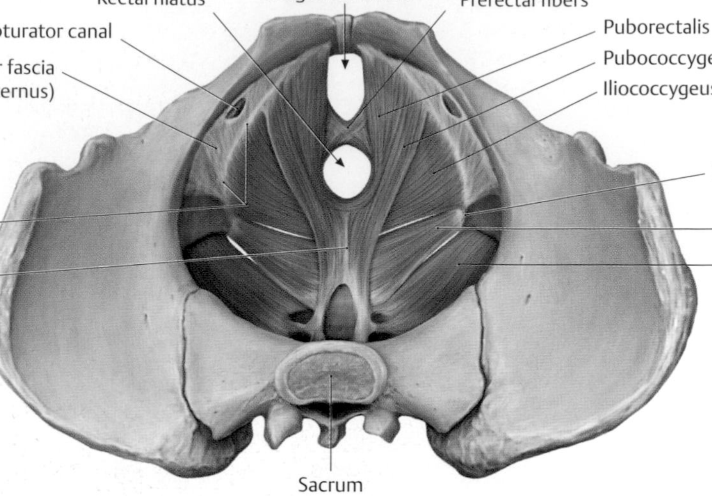

Rectal hiatus
Urogenital hiatus
Prerectal fibers
Obturator canal
Obturator fascia (obturator internus)
Puborectalis
Pubococcygeus — Levator ani
Iliococcygeus
Ischial spine
Tendinous arch of levator ani
Coccygeus
Anococcygeal raphe
Piriformis
Sacrum

A Superior view.

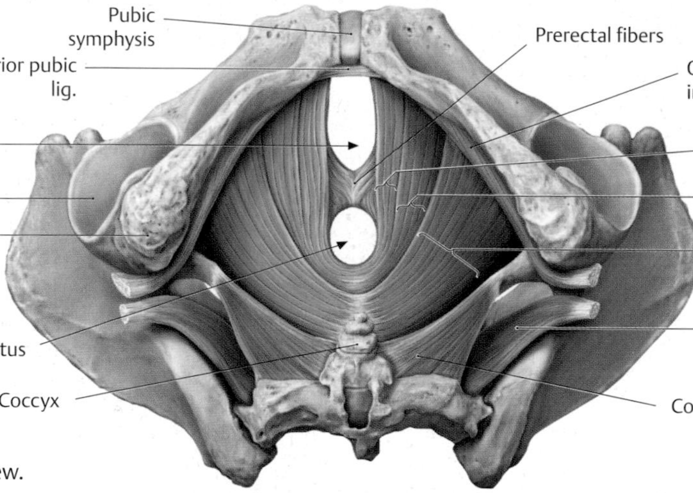

Pubic symphysis
Prerectal fibers
Inferior pubic lig.
Obturator internus
Urogenital hiatus
Pubo-rectalis
Acetabulum
Pubo-coccygeus — Levator ani
Ischial tuberosity
Ilio-coccygeus
Piriformis
Rectal hiatus
Coccyx
Coccygeus

B Inferior view.

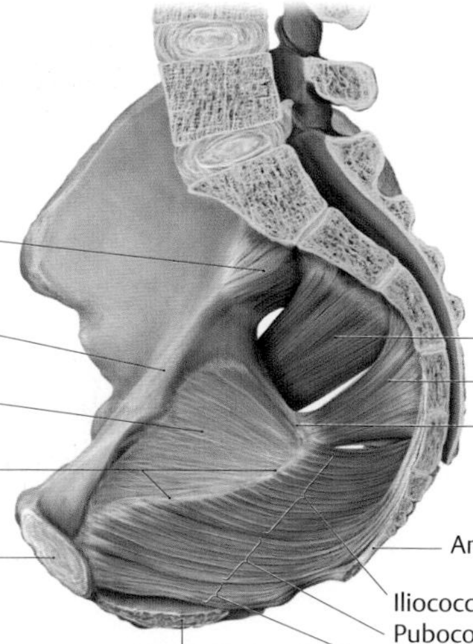

Anterior sacroiliac lig.
Arcuate line
Piriformis
Coccygeus
Obturator internus fascia
Ischial spine
Tendinous arch of levator ani
Pubic symphysis
Anococcygeal lig.
Iliococcygeus
Pubococcygeus — Levator ani
Deep transverse perineal
Puborectalis

C Medial view of right hemipelvis.

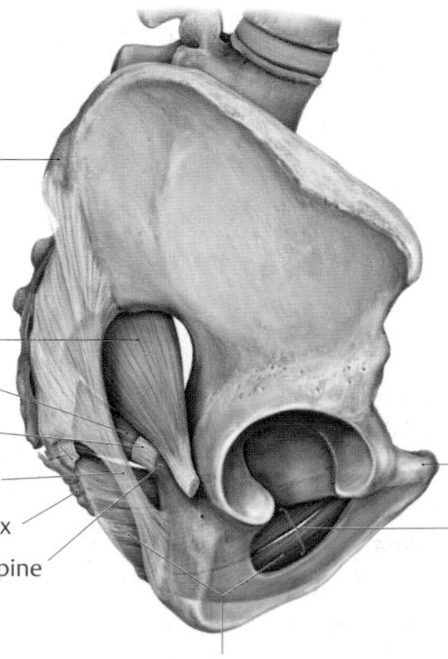

Posterior superior iliac spine
Piriformis
Coccygeus
Sacrospinous lig.
Sacrotuberous lig.
Coccyx
Pubic tubercle
Ischial spine
Obturator foramen
Levator ani

D Right lateral view.

Fig. 19.14 Muscles and fascia of the pelvic floor and perineum, in situ

Lithotomy position. Removed on left side: Superficial perineal (Colles') fascia, inferior fascia of the pelvic diaphragm, and obturator fascia.

Note: The green arrows are pointing forward to the anterior recess of the ischioanal fossa.

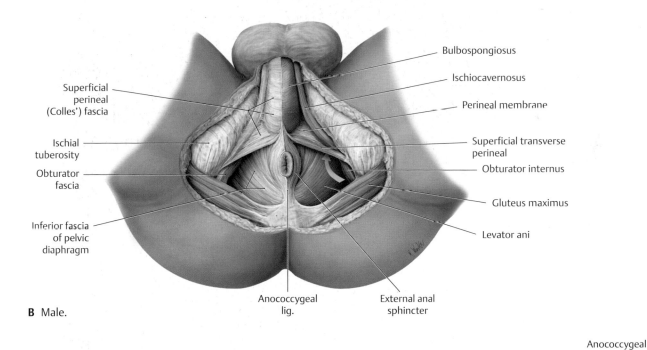

Bulbospongiosus
Ischiocavernosus
Perineal membrane
Superficial transverse perineal
Obturator internus
Gluteus maximus
Levator ani

Superficial perineal (Colles') fascia
Perineal body
Ischial tuberosity
Obturator fascia
Inferior fascia of pelvic diaphragm
Anococcygeal lig.
Coccyx   Anal cleft   External anal sphincter

A Female.

Bulbospongiosus
Ischiocavernosus
Perineal membrane
Superficial transverse perineal
Obturator internus
Gluteus maximus
Levator ani
External anal sphincter

Superficial perineal (Colles') fascia
Ischial tuberosity
Obturator fascia
Inferior fascia of pelvic diaphragm
Anococcygeal lig.

B Male.

Fig. 19.15 Gender-related differences in structure of the levator ani

Posterior view. Note the connective tissue gaps between muscular parts of the levator ani in the female.

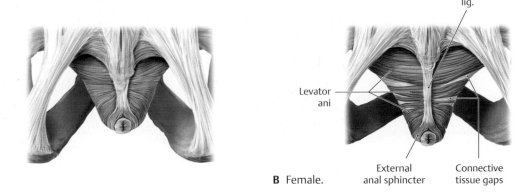

Anococcygeal lig.
Levator ani
External anal sphincter   Connective tissue gaps

A Male.

B Female.

Pelvic Floor & Perineal Muscle Facts

Fig. 19.16 **Muscles of the pelvic floor**
Superior view.

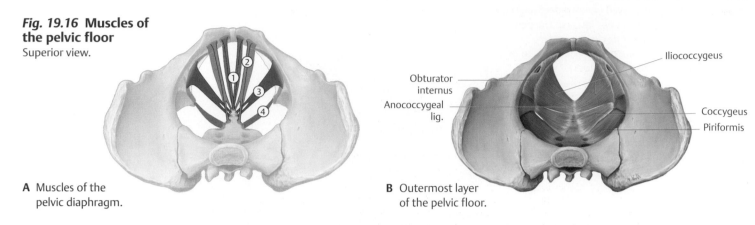

A Muscles of the pelvic diaphragm.

B Outermost layer of the pelvic floor.

Table 19.2		Muscles of the pelvic floor			
Muscle		**Origin**	**Insertion**	**Innervation**	**Action**
Muscles of the pelvic diaphragm					
Levator ani	① Puborectalis	Superior pubic ramus (both sides of pubic symphysis)	Anococcygeal lig.	Nerve to levator ani (S4), inferior rectal n.	Pelvic diaphragm: Supports pelvic viscera
	② Pubococcygeus	Pubis (lateral to origin of puborectalis)	Anococcygeal lig., coccyx		
	③ Iliococcygeus	Internal obturator fascia of levator ani (tendinous arch)			
④ Coccygeus		Lateral surface of coccyx and S5 segment	Ischial spine	Direct branches from sacral plexus (S4–S5)	Supports pelvic viscera, flexes coccyx
Muscles of the pelvic wall (parietal muscles)					
Piriformis*		Sacrum (pelvic surface)	Femur (apex of greater trochanter)	Direct branches from sacral plexus (S1–S2)	Hip joint: External rotation, stabilization, and abduction of flexed hip
Obturator internus*		Obturator membrane and bony boundaries (inner surface)	Femur (greater trochanter, medial surface)	Direct branches from sacral plexus (L5–S1)	Hip joint: External rotation and abduction of flexed hip

*The piriformis and obturator internus are considered muscles of the hip (see **p. 426**).
The female and male external genitalia are shown on **pp. 262–265.**

Fig. 19.17 **Muscles of the perineum**
Inferior view.

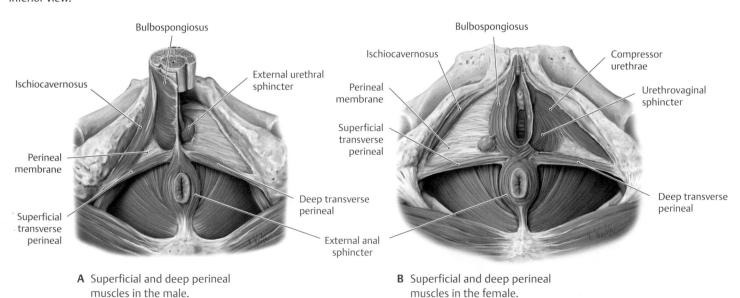

A Superficial and deep perineal muscles in the male.

B Superficial and deep perineal muscles in the female.

Table 19.3   Muscles of the perineum

Muscle	Origin	Insertion	Innervation	Action
① Ischiocavernosus	Ischial ramus	Crus of clitoris or penis	Pudendal n. (S2–S4)	Maintains erection by squeezing blood into corpus cavernosum of clitoris or penis
② Bulbospongiosus	Runs anteriorly from perineal body to clitoris (females) or penile raphe (males)			Females: Compresses greater vestibular gland Males: Assists in erection
③ Superficial transverse perineal	Ischiopubic ramus	Perineal body		Helps hold perineal body in median plane, holds the pelvic organs in place, and supports visceral canals through the muscles of the perineum
④ Deep transverse perineal*	Ishiopubic ramus	Perineal body and external anal sphincter		
⑤ External urethral sphincter	Encircles urethra (division of deep transverse perineal muscle), in males ascends anteriorly to neck of the bladder; in females, some fibers surround the vagina as the **urethrovaginal sphincter**, others extend laterally as the **compressor urethrae** (See **Figs. 21.9 and 21.11**)			Closes urethra
⑥ External anal sphincter	Encircles anus (runs posteriorly from perineal body to anococcygeal lig.)			Closes anus

* Typically, this muscle is not developed in females and is replaced by smooth muscle tissue. When developed, it provides dynamic support to the pelvic organs.

Fig. 19.18 Muscles of the male perineum

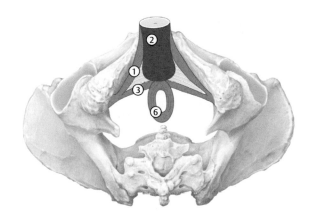

A Muscles of the superficial pouch in the male.

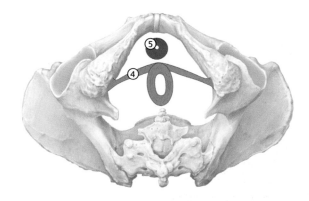

B Muscles of the deep pouch in the male.

Fig. 19.19 Muscles of the female perineum

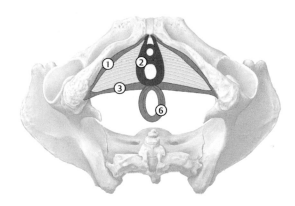

A Muscles of the superficial pouch in the female.

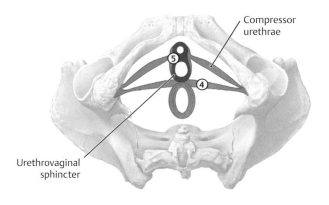

Compressor urethrae

Urethrovaginal sphincter

B Muscles of the deep pouch in the female.

20 Spaces
Contents of the Pelvis

Fig. 20.1 **Male pelvis**
Parasagittal section, viewed from the right side.

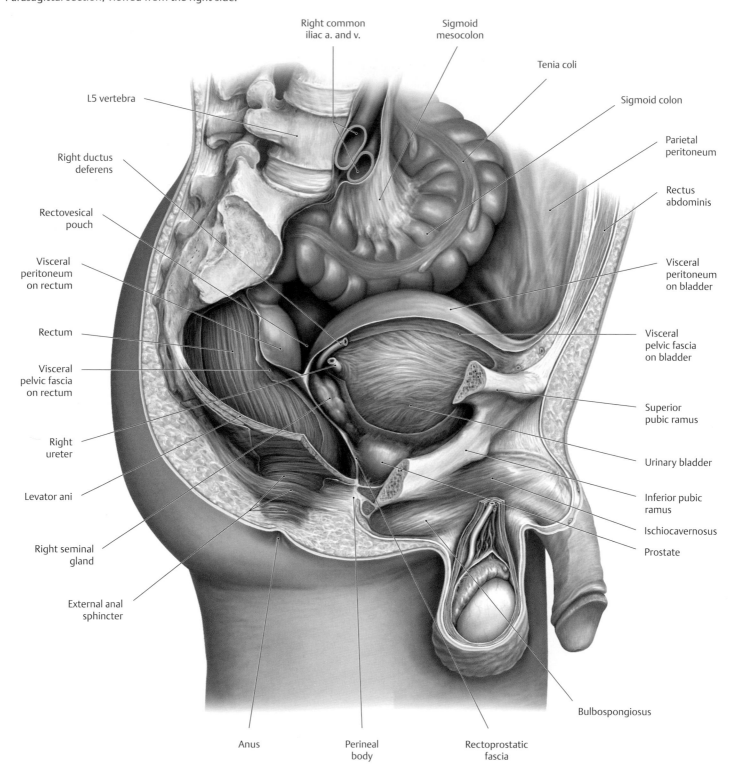

Right common iliac a. and v.

Sigmoid mesocolon

Tenia coli

Sigmoid colon

Parietal peritoneum

Rectus abdominis

Visceral peritoneum on bladder

Visceral pelvic fascia on bladder

Superior pubic ramus

Urinary bladder

Inferior pubic ramus

Ischiocavernosus

Prostate

Bulbospongiosus

L5 vertebra

Right ductus deferens

Rectovesical pouch

Visceral peritoneum on rectum

Rectum

Visceral pelvic fascia on rectum

Right ureter

Levator ani

Right seminal gland

External anal sphincter

Anus

Perineal body

Rectoprostatic fascia

Fig. 20.2 **Female pelvis**
Parasagittal section, viewed from the right side.

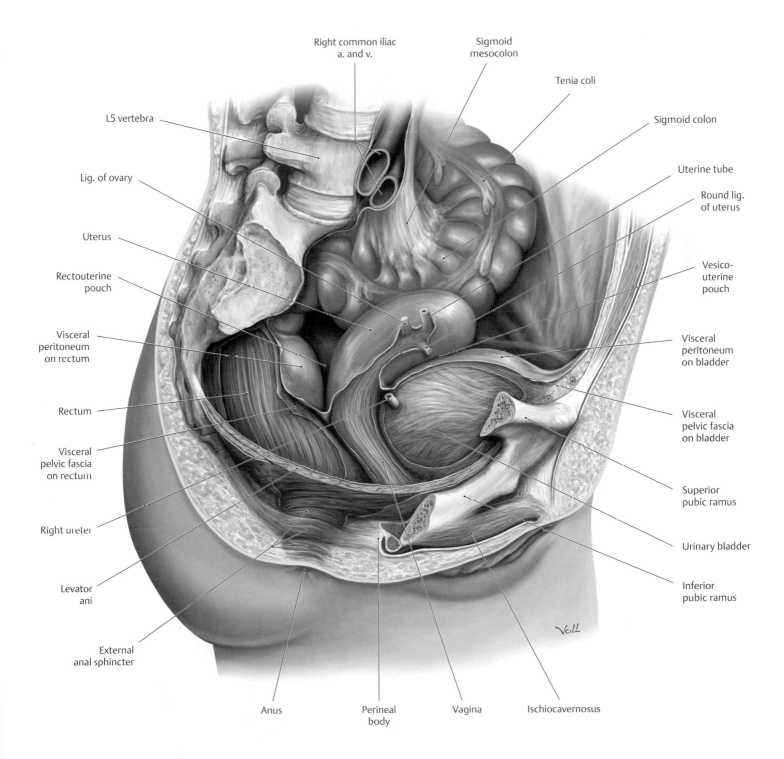

Right common iliac a. and v.

Sigmoid mesocolon

Tenia coli

Sigmoid colon

L5 vertebra

Uterine tube

Lig. of ovary

Round lig. of uterus

Uterus

Vesico-uterine pouch

Rectouterine pouch

Visceral peritoneum on rectum

Visceral peritoneum on bladder

Rectum

Visceral pelvic fascia on bladder

Visceral pelvic fascia on rectum

Superior pubic ramus

Right ureter

Urinary bladder

Levator ani

Inferior pubic ramus

External anal sphincter

Anus

Perineal body

Vagina

Ischiocavernosus

Peritoneal Relationships

Fig. 20.3 **Peritoneal relationships in the pelvis: Female**
Superior view.

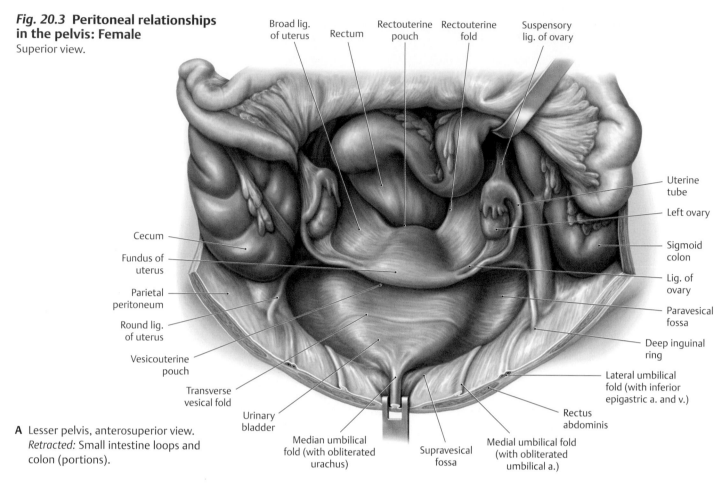

A Lesser pelvis, anterosuperior view.
Retracted: Small intestine loops and colon (portions).

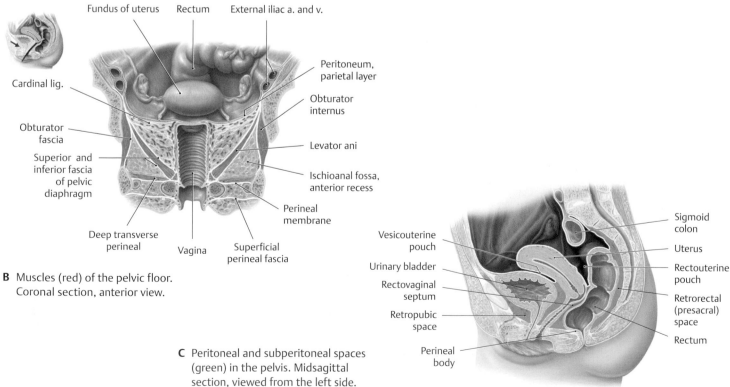

B Muscles (red) of the pelvic floor.
Coronal section, anterior view.

C Peritoneal and subperitoneal spaces (green) in the pelvis. Midsagittal section, viewed from the left side.

Fig. 20.4 **Peritoneal relationships in the pelvis: Male**

Superior view.

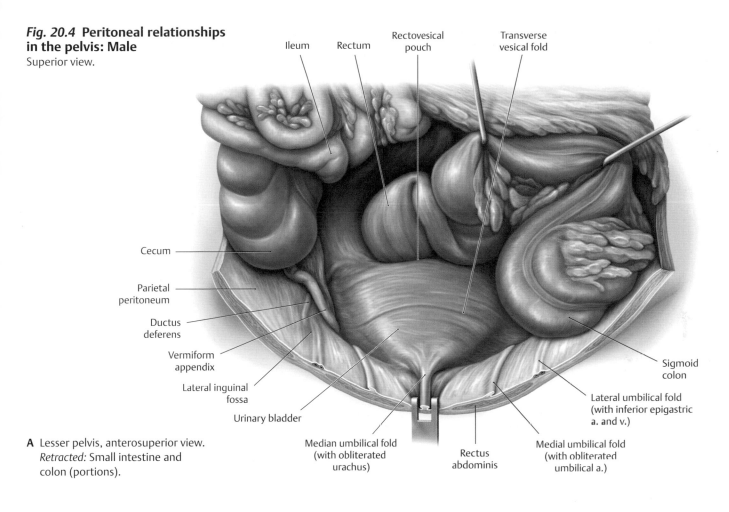

A Lesser pelvis, anterosuperior view.
Retracted: Small intestine and colon (portions).

Ileum · Rectum · Rectovesical pouch · Transverse vesical fold · Cecum · Parietal peritoneum · Ductus deferens · Vermiform appendix · Lateral inguinal fossa · Urinary bladder · Median umbilical fold (with obliterated urachus) · Rectus abdominis · Medial umbilical fold (with obliterated umbilical a.) · Lateral umbilical fold (with inferior epigastric a. and v.) · Sigmoid colon

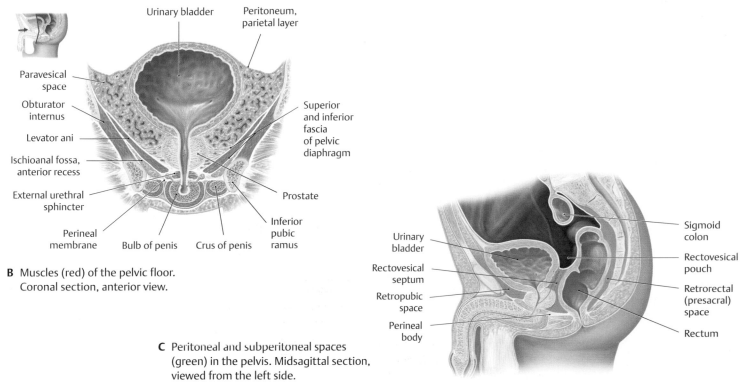

B Muscles (red) of the pelvic floor. Coronal section, anterior view.

Urinary bladder · Peritoneum, parietal layer · Paravesical space · Obturator internus · Levator ani · Ischioanal fossa, anterior recess · External urethral sphincter · Perineal membrane · Bulb of penis · Crus of penis · Inferior pubic ramus · Prostate · Superior and inferior fascia of pelvic diaphragm

C Peritoneal and subperitoneal spaces (green) in the pelvis. Midsagittal section, viewed from the left side.

Urinary bladder · Rectovesical septum · Retropubic space · Perineal body · Sigmoid colon · Rectovesical pouch · Retrorectal (presacral) space · Rectum

Pelvis & Perineum

The *pelvis* is the region of the body inferior to the abdomen, surrounded by the pelvic girdle. The *false*, or greater, *pelvis* is immediately inferior to the abdominal cavity, between the iliac alae, and superior to the pelvic inlet. The *true*, or lesser, *pelvis* is found between the pelvic inlet and the pelvic outlet and extends inferiorly to the pelvic diaphragm (levator ani and coccygeus), a muscular sling attached to the boundaries of the pelvic outlet. The *perineum* is the inferior most portion of the trunk, between the thighs and buttocks, extending from the pubis to the coccyx and superiorly to the pelvic diaphragm. The *superficial perineal* pouch lies between the membranous layer of the subcutaneous tissue (Colles' fascia) and the perineal membrane. The *deep perineal* pouch lies between the perineal membrane and the inferior fascia of the pelvic diaphragm.

Table 20.1	Divisions of the pelvis and perineum	
The levels of the pelvis are determined by bony landmarks (iliac alae and pelvic inlet/brim). The contents of the perineum are separated from the true pelvis by the pelvic diaphragm and two fascial layers.		

Iliac crest		
Pelvis	False pelvis	• Ileum (coils)
		• Cecum and appendix
		• Sigmoid colon
		• Common and external iliac aa. and vv.
		• Lumbar plexus (brs.)
	Pelvic inlet	
	True pelvis	• Distal ureters
		• Urinary bladder
		• Rectum
		♀: Vagina, uterus, uterine tubes, and ovaries
		♂: Ductus deferens, seminal gland, and prostate
		• Internal iliac a. and v. and brs.
		• Sacral plexus
		• Inferior hypogastric plexus
Pelvic diaphragm (levator ani & coccygeus)		
Perineum	Deep pouch	• Sphincter urethrae and deep transverse perineal mm.
		• Urethra (membranous)
		• Vagina
		• Rectum
		• Bulbourethral gland
		• Ischioanal fossa
		• Internal pudendal a. and v., pudendal n. and brs.
	Perineal membrane	
	Superficial pouch	• Ischiocavernosus, bulbospongiosus, and superficial transverse perineal mm.
		• Urethra (penile)
		• Clitoris and penis
		• Internal pudendal a. and v., pudendal n. and branches
	Superficial perineal (Colles') fascia	
	Subcutaneous perineal space	• Fat
Skin		

Fig. 20.5 Pelvis and urogenital triangle

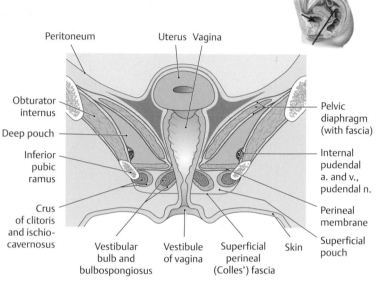

A Female. Oblique section.

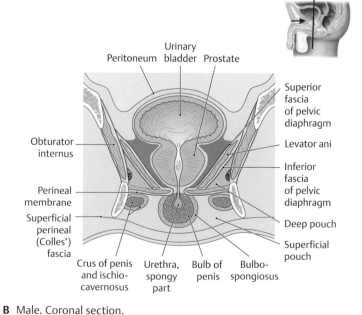

B Male. Coronal section.

Legend:
- ☐ Peritoneal cavity
- ☐ Subperitoneal space
- ☐ Ischioanal fossa
- — Visceral pelvic fascia
- — Parietal pelvic fascia

Fig. 20.6 Pelvis: Oblique section
Anterior view.

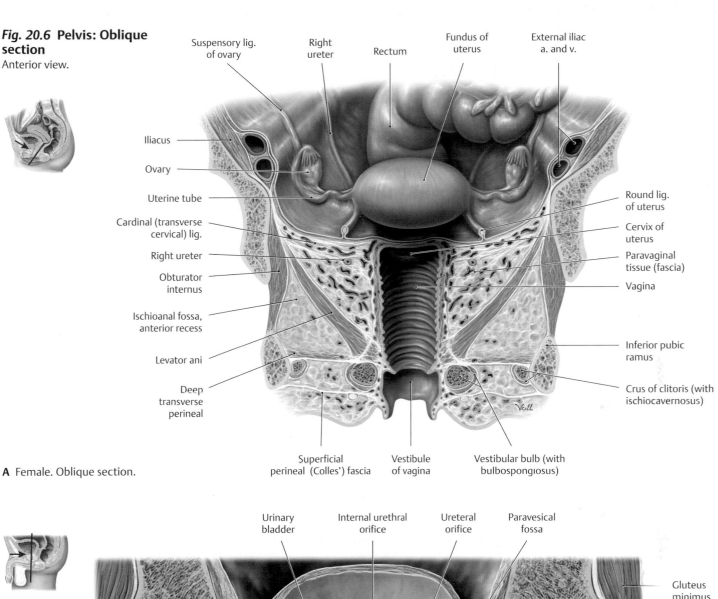

Suspensory lig. of ovary

Right ureter

Rectum

Fundus of uterus

External iliac a. and v.

Iliacus

Ovary

Uterine tube

Cardinal (transverse cervical) lig.

Right ureter

Obturator internus

Ischioanal fossa, anterior recess

Levator ani

Deep transverse perineal

Round lig. of uterus

Cervix of uterus

Paravaginal tissue (fascia)

Vagina

Inferior pubic ramus

Crus of clitoris (with ischiocavernosus)

Superficial perineal (Colles') fascia

Vestibule of vagina

Vestibular bulb (with bulbospongiosus)

A Female. Oblique section.

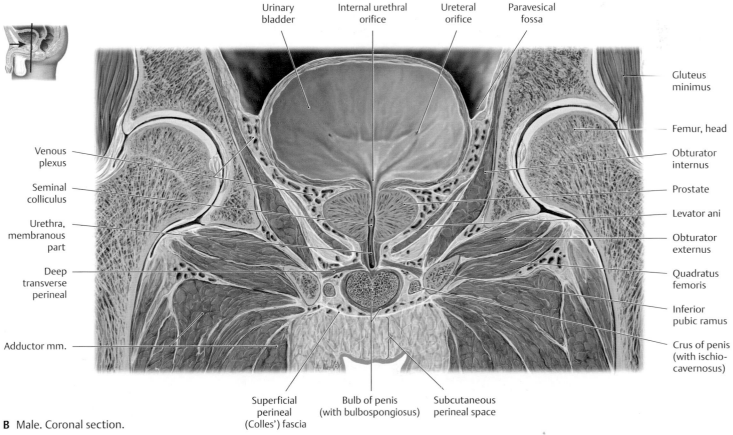

Urinary bladder

Internal urethral orifice

Ureteral orifice

Paravesical fossa

Venous plexus

Seminal colliculus

Urethra, membranous part

Deep transverse perineal

Adductor mm.

Gluteus minimus

Femur, head

Obturator internus

Prostate

Levator ani

Obturator externus

Quadratus femoris

Inferior pubic ramus

Crus of penis (with ischio-cavernosus)

Superficial perineal (Colles') fascia

Bulb of penis (with bulbospongiosus)

Subcutaneous perineal space

B Male. Coronal section.

21 Internal Organs
Rectum & Anal Canal

Fig. 21.1 Rectum: Location

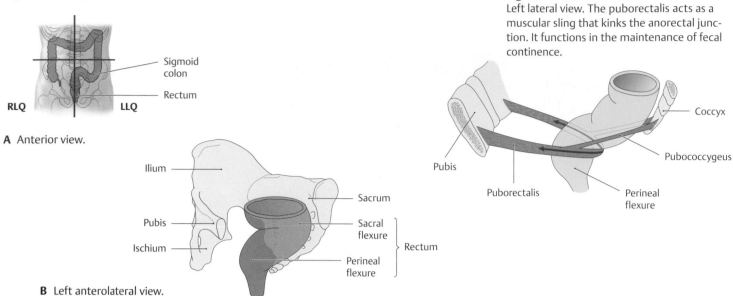

Sigmoid colon

Rectum

RLQ   LLQ

A Anterior view.

Ilium

Sacrum

Pubis

Sacral flexure

Ischium

Rectum

Perineal flexure

B Left anterolateral view.

Fig. 21.2 Closure of the rectum

Left lateral view. The puborectalis acts as a muscular sling that kinks the anorectal junction. It functions in the maintenance of fecal continence.

Coccyx

Pubis

Pubococcygeus

Puborectalis

Perineal flexure

Fig. 21.3 Rectum in situ

Coronal section, anterior view of the female pelvis. The upper third of the rectum is covered with visceral peritoneum on its anterior and lateral sides. The middle third is covered only anteriorly and the lower third is inferior to the parietal peritoneum.

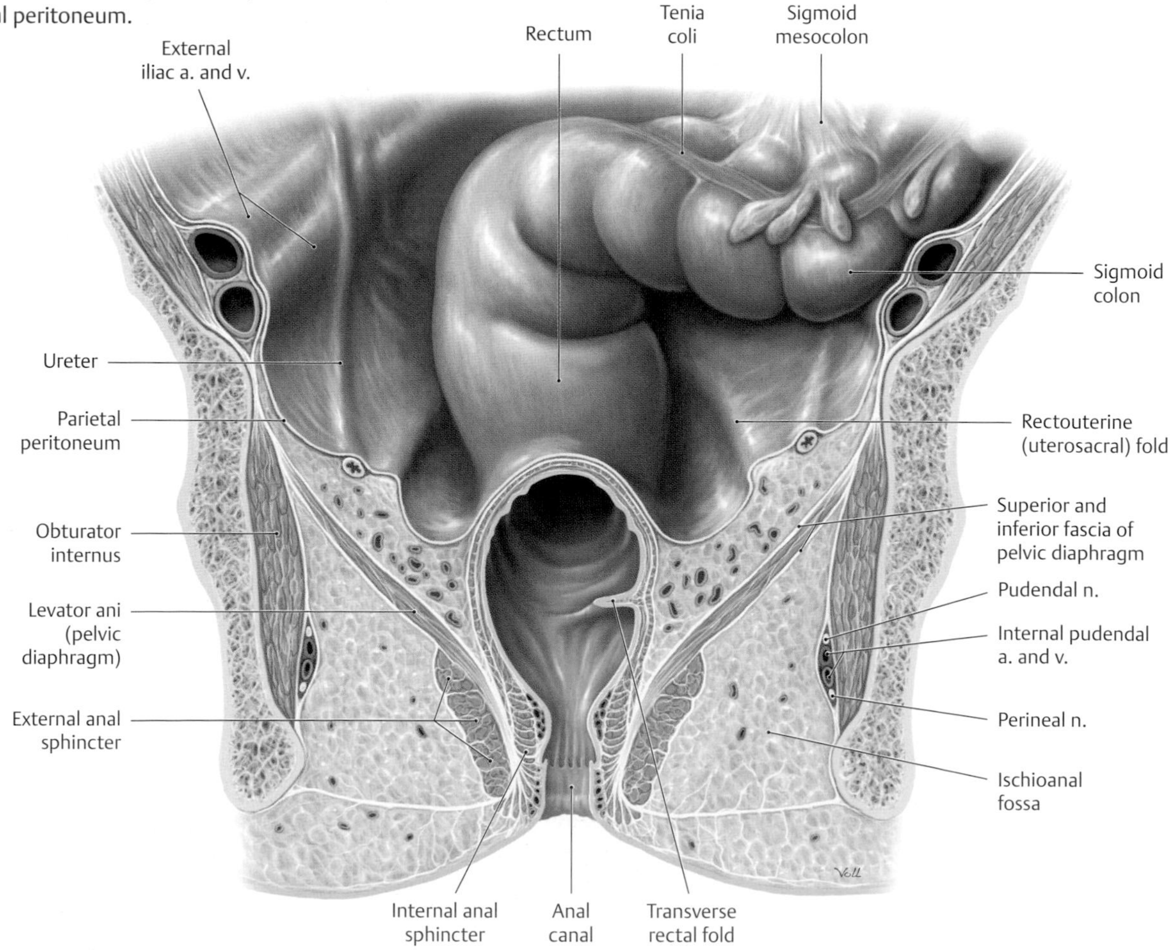

External iliac a. and v.

Rectum

Tenia coli

Sigmoid mesocolon

Ureter

Sigmoid colon

Parietal peritoneum

Rectouterine (uterosacral) fold

Obturator internus

Superior and inferior fascia of pelvic diaphragm

Levator ani (pelvic diaphragm)

Pudendal n.

Internal pudendal a. and v.

External anal sphincter

Perineal n.

Ischioanal fossa

Internal anal sphincter

Anal canal

Transverse rectal fold

Fig. 21.4 Rectum and anal canal

Coronal section, anterior view with the anterior wall removed.

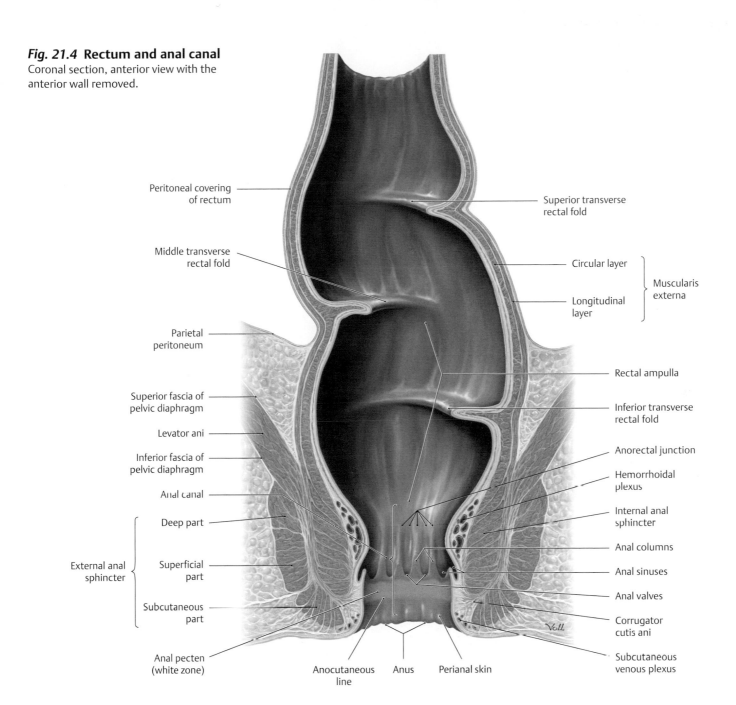

Peritoneal covering of rectum

Middle transverse rectal fold

Parietal peritoneum

Superior fascia of pelvic diaphragm

Levator ani

Inferior fascia of pelvic diaphragm

Anal canal

External anal sphincter
- Deep part
- Superficial part
- Subcutaneous part

Anal pecten (white zone)

Anocutaneous line

Anus

Perianal skin

Superior transverse rectal fold

Circular layer
Longitudinal layer
} Muscularis externa

Rectal ampulla

Inferior transverse rectal fold

Anorectal junction

Hemorrhoidal plexus

Internal anal sphincter

Anal columns

Anal sinuses

Anal valves

Corrugator cutis ani

Subcutaneous venous plexus

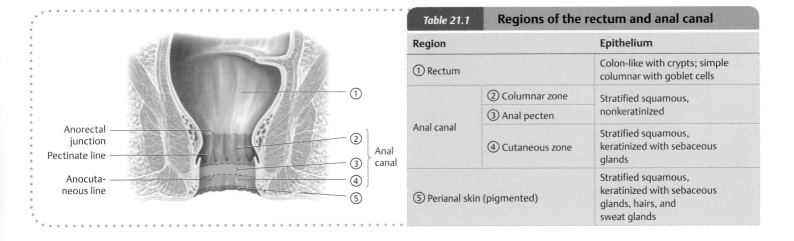

Anorectal junction

Pectinate line

Anocutaneous line

① ② ③ ④ ⑤ } Anal canal

Table 21.1		Regions of the rectum and anal canal
Region		**Epithelium**
① Rectum		Colon-like with crypts; simple columnar with goblet cells
Anal canal	② Columnar zone	Stratified squamous, nonkeratinized
	③ Anal pecten	
	④ Cutaneous zone	Stratified squamous, keratinized with sebaceous glands
⑤ Perianal skin (pigmented)		Stratified squamous, keratinized with sebaceous glands, hairs, and sweat glands

Ureters

Fig. 21.5 Ureters in situ

Anterior view, male abdomen. *Removed:* Nonurinary organs and rectal stump. The ureters descend along the posterior abdominal wall in the retroperitoneal space. On each side, they enter the pelvis after crossing the common iliac artery at its bifurcation into the external and internal arteries.

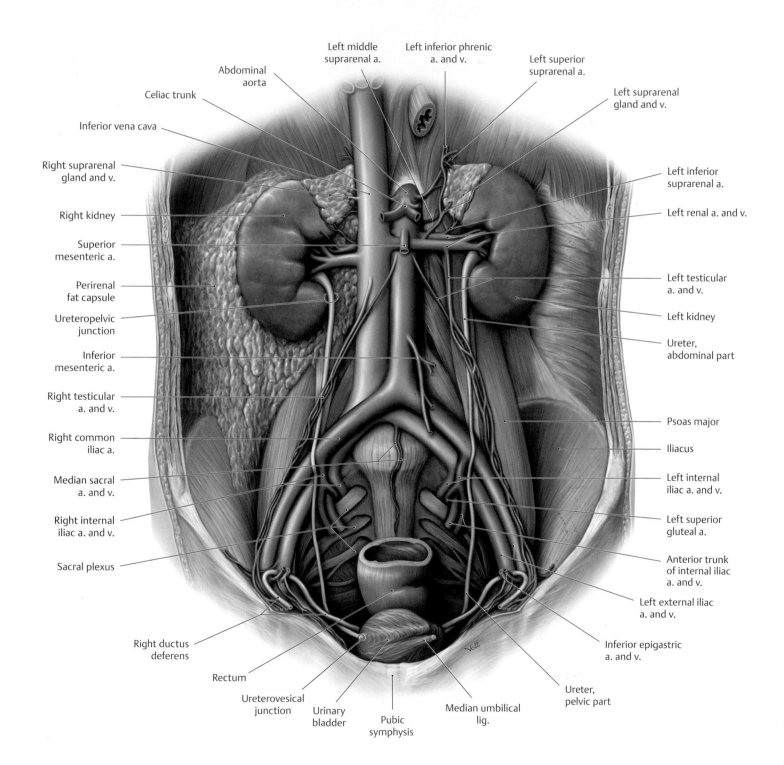

Fig. 21.6 Ureter in the male pelvis
Superior view with peritoneum removed.

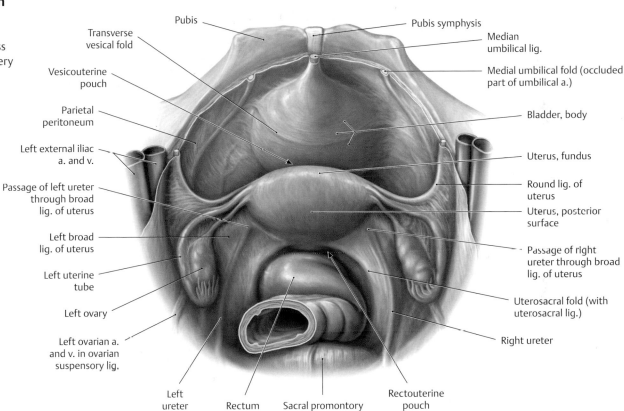

Pubic symphysis — Pubis

Inferior (arcuate) pubic lig. — Tendinous arch of levator ani

Pubovesical muscles — Pelvic diaphragm, superior fascia

Bladder, body — Bladder, apex

Median umbilical lig. — Right ductus deferens

Left ductus deferens — Tendinous arch of pelvic fascia

Left ureter

Rectum with peritoneal covering on anterior wall — Right ureter

Fig. 21.7 Ureter in the female pelvis
Superior view.
The pelvic ureters pass under the uterine artery approximately 2 cm lateral to the cervix.

Pubis — Pubis symphysis

Transverse vesical fold — Median umbilical lig.

Vesicouterine pouch — Medial umbilical fold (occluded part of umbilical a.)

Parietal peritoneum — Bladder, body

Left external iliac a. and v. — Uterus, fundus

Passage of left ureter through broad lig. of uterus — Round lig. of uterus

Left broad lig. of uterus — Uterus, posterior surface

Left uterine tube — Passage of right ureter through broad lig. of uterus

Left ovary — Uterosacral fold (with uterosacral lig.)

Left ovarian a. and v. in ovarian suspensory lig. — Right ureter

Left ureter — Rectum — Sacral promontory — Rectouterine pouch

---

🚑 Clinical box 21.1

Anatomical constrictions of the ureter

There are three normal *anatomical constrictions* where a pain-causing kidney stone from the renal pelvis is apt to become lodged:

- Narrowing at the origin of the ureter from the renal pelvis (ureteropelvic junction)
- Site where the ureter crosses over the external or common iliac vessels
- Passage of the ureter through the bladder wall (ureterovesical junction).

Occasionally a *fourth constriction* can be identified where the testicular or ovarian artery and vein pass anterior to the ureter.

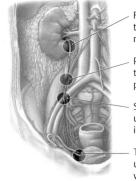

First constriction: narrowing of the ureter as it passes over inferior renal pole (abdominal part)

Possible constriction where the testicular or ovarian vessels pass anterior to the ureter

Second constriction: ureter crosses over external iliac vessels (pelvic part)

Third constriction: ureter traverses the bladder wall (intramural part)

Urinary Bladder & Urethra

Fig. 21.8 Female urinary bladder and urethra

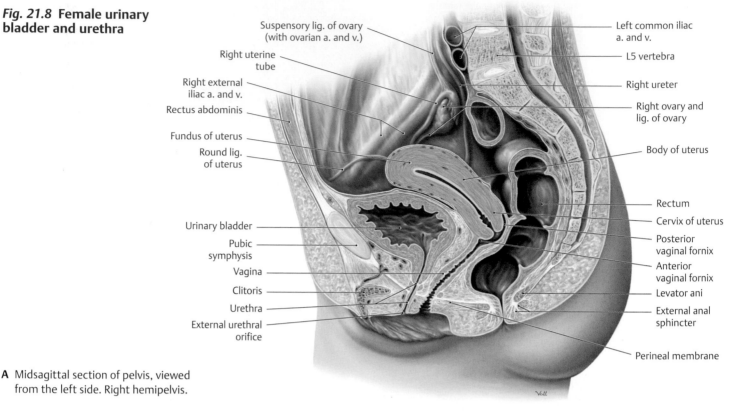

Suspensory lig. of ovary (with ovarian a. and v.)

Right uterine tube

Right external iliac a. and v.

Rectus abdominis

Fundus of uterus

Round lig. of uterus

Urinary bladder

Pubic symphysis

Vagina

Clitoris

Urethra

External urethral orifice

Left common iliac a. and v.

L5 vertebra

Right ureter

Right ovary and lig. of ovary

Body of uterus

Rectum

Cervix of uterus

Posterior vaginal fornix

Anterior vaginal fornix

Levator ani

External anal sphincter

Perineal membrane

A Midsagittal section of pelvis, viewed from the left side. Right hemipelvis.

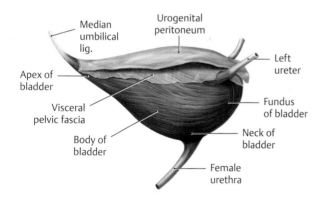

Median umbilical lig.

Urogenital peritoneum

Apex of bladder

Visceral pelvic fascia

Body of bladder

Left ureter

Fundus of bladder

Neck of bladder

Female urethra

B Bladder and urethra, left lateral view.

Fig. 21.9 Urethral sphincter mechanism in the female
Anterolateral view.

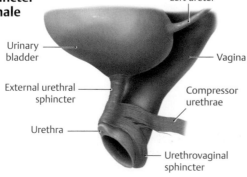

Left ureter

Urinary bladder

External urethral sphincter

Urethra

Vagina

Compressor urethrae

Urethrovaginal sphincter

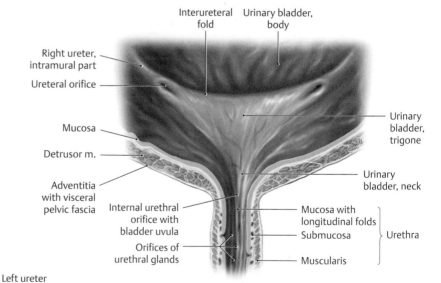

Interureteral fold

Urinary bladder, body

Right ureter, intramural part

Ureteral orifice

Mucosa

Detrusor m.

Adventitia with visceral pelvic fascia

Internal urethral orifice with bladder uvula

Orifices of urethral glands

Urinary bladder, trigone

Urinary bladder, neck

Mucosa with longitudinal folds

Submucosa

Muscularis

Urethra

C Trigone and urethra, coronal section, anterior view.

Fig. 21.10 Male urinary bladder and urethra

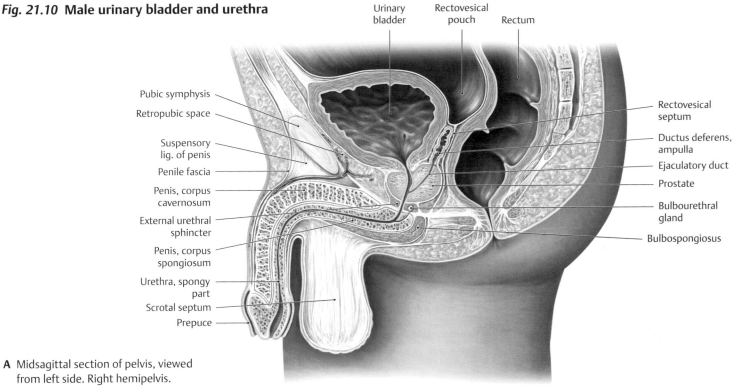

A Midsagittal section of pelvis, viewed from left side. Right hemipelvis.

Labels (Fig. 21.10 A): Urinary bladder, Rectovesical pouch, Rectum, Pubic symphysis, Retropubic space, Suspensory lig. of penis, Penile fascia, Penis, corpus cavernosum, External urethral sphincter, Penis, corpus spongiosum, Urethra, spongy part, Scrotal septum, Prepuce, Rectovesical septum, Ductus deferens, ampulla, Ejaculatory duct, Prostate, Bulbourethral gland, Bulbospongiosus

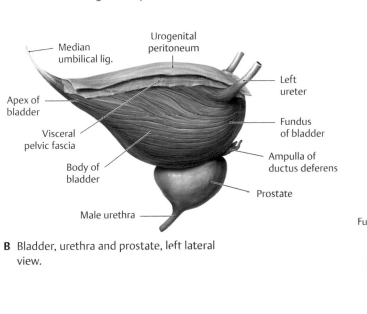

Labels (Fig. 21.10 B): Median umbilical lig., Urogenital peritoneum, Left ureter, Apex of bladder, Visceral pelvic fascia, Fundus of bladder, Body of bladder, Ampulla of ductus deferens, Male urethra, Prostate

B Bladder, urethra and prostate, left lateral view.

Labels (Fig. 21.10 C): Ureteral orifice, Interureteric crest, Detrusor muscle, Fundus of bladder, trigone, Internal urethral sphincter, Neck of bladder, internal urethral orifice, Seminal colliculus, Prostatic urethra, Prostatic utricle, Openings of ejaculatory ducts, Prostate

C Trigone, urethra and prostate, coronal section, anterior view.

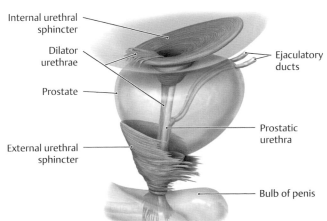

Labels (Fig. 21.11): Internal urethral sphincter, Dilator urethrae, Prostate, External urethral sphincter, Ejaculatory ducts, Prostatic urethra, Bulb of penis

Fig. 21.11 Urethral sphincter mechanism in the male
Lateral view.

Uterus & Ovaries

Fig. 21.14 The broad ligament

Regions of the broad ligament, sagittal section. The uterus and ovaries are suspended by the broad ligament of the uterus, which is composed of a double layer of peritoneum, arranged as a combination of mesenteries: the mesosalpinx, mesovarium, and mesometrium.

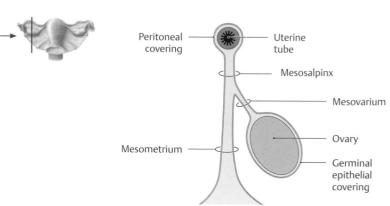

Peritoneal covering
Uterine tube
Mesosalpinx
Mesovarium
Mesometrium
Ovary
Germinal epithelial covering

Fig. 21.15 Ovary

Right ovary, posterior view.

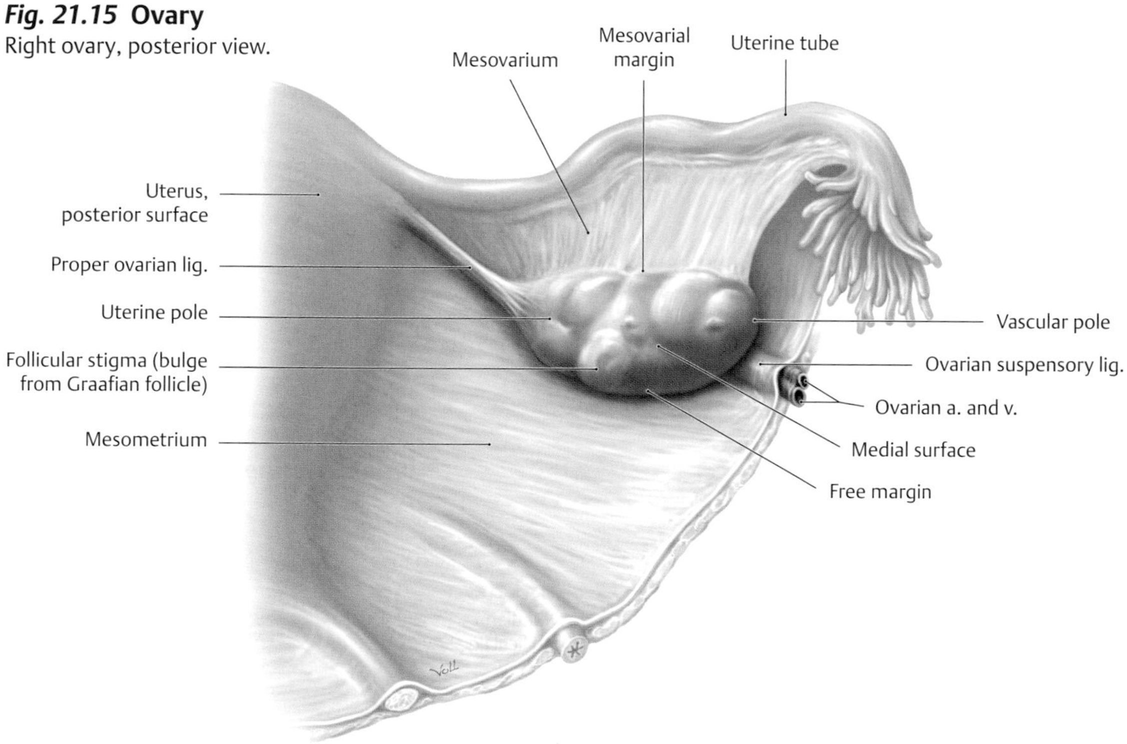

Mesovarium
Mesovarial margin
Uterine tube
Uterus, posterior surface
Proper ovarian lig.
Uterine pole
Follicular stigma (bulge from Graafian follicle)
Mesometrium
Vascular pole
Ovarian suspensory lig.
Ovarian a. and v.
Medial surface
Free margin

Fig. 21.16 Normal curvature and position of the uterus

Midsagittal section, left lateral view. The position of the uterus can be described in terms of:

① Flexion, the angle between the longitudinal cervical axis and the longitudinal uterine axis; the normal position is anteflexion.

② Version, the angle between the longitudinal cervical axis and longitudinal vaginal axis; the normal position is anteversion.

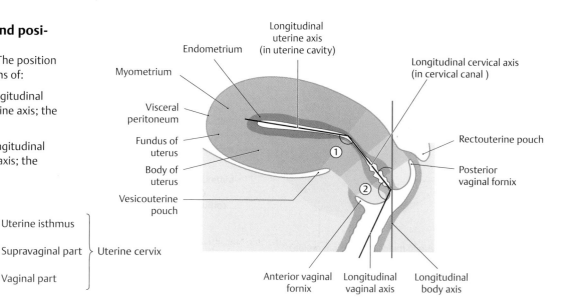

Longitudinal uterine axis (in uterine cavity)
Endometrium
Myometrium
Longitudinal cervical axis (in cervical canal)
Visceral peritoneum
Fundus of uterus
Rectouterine pouch
Body of uterus
Posterior vaginal fornix
Vesicouterine pouch
Anterior vaginal fornix
Longitudinal vaginal axis
Longitudinal body axis

Uterine isthmus
Supravaginal part } Uterine cervix
Vaginal part

Fig. 21.17 Uterus and uterine tube

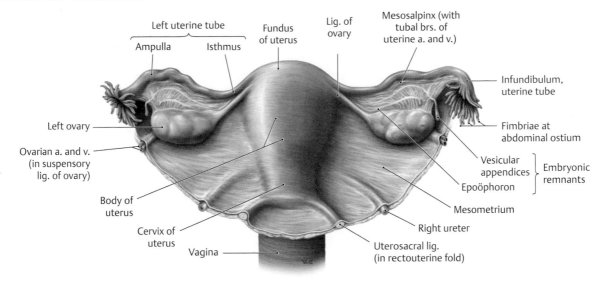

A Posterosuperior view.

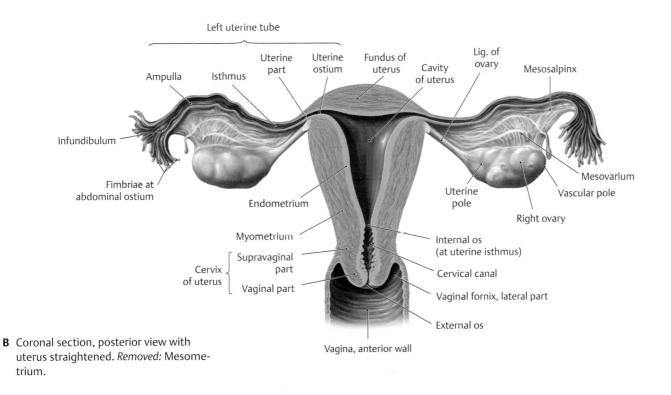

B Coronal section, posterior view with uterus straightened. *Removed:* Mesometrium.

✳ Clinical box 21.2

Ectopic pregnancy

After fertilization in the ampulla of the uterine tube, the ovum usually implants in the wall of the uterine cavity. However, it may become implanted at other sites (e.g., the uterine tube or even the peritoneal cavity). Tubal pregnancies, the most common type of ectopic pregnancy, pose the risk of tubal wall rupture and potentially life-threatening bleeding into the peritoneal cavity. Tubal pregnancies are promoted by adhesion of the tubal mucosa, mostly due to inflammation.

Ligaments & Fascia of the Deep Pelvis

Fig. 21.18 **Ligaments of the female pelvis**

Superior view. *Removed:* Peritoneum, neurovasculature, and superior portion of the bladder to demonstrate only the fascial condensations (ligaments). Deep pelvic ligaments support the uterus within the pelvic cavity and prevent uterine prolapse, the downward displacement of the uterus into the vagina.

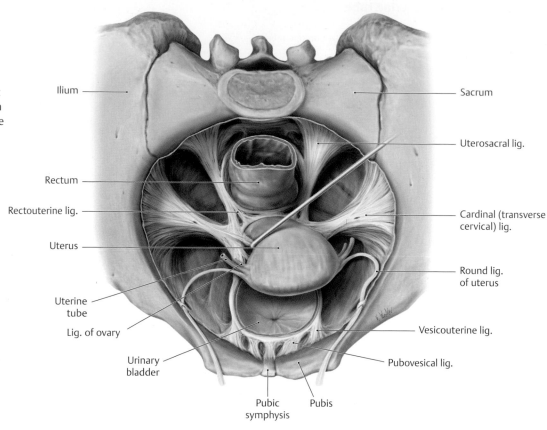

Ilium — Sacrum

Uterosacral lig.

Rectum

Rectouterine lig. — Cardinal (transverse cervical) lig.

Uterus

Round lig. of uterus

Uterine tube

Lig. of ovary — Vesicouterine lig.

Urinary bladder — Pubovesical lig.

Pubic symphysis | Pubis

Fig. 21.19 **Ligaments of the deep pelvis in the female**

Superior view. *Removed:* peritoneum, neurovasculature, uterus and bladder. Uterosacral ligaments and the paracolpium support and help maintain the positions of the cervix and vagina in the pelvis.

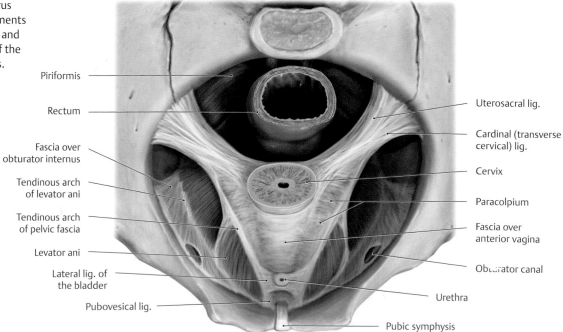

Piriformis

Rectum — Uterosacral lig.

Cardinal (transverse cervical) lig.

Fascia over obturator internus

Tendinous arch of levator ani — Cervix

Tendinous arch of pelvic fascia — Paracolpium

Levator ani — Fascia over anterior vagina

Lateral lig. of the bladder — Obturator canal

Pubovesical lig. — Urethra

Pubic symphysis

Fascia of the pelvis plays an important role in the support of pelvic viscera. On either side of the pelvic floor, where the visceral fascia of the pelvic organs is continuous with the parietal fascia of the muscular walls, thickenings called tendinous arches of the pelvic fascia are formed. In females, the paracolpium—lateral connections between the visceral fascia and the tendinous arches—suspends and supports the vagina. Pubovesical ligaments (and puboprostatic ligaments in the male) are extensions of the tendinous arches that support the bladder and prostate. Endopelvic fascia, a loose areolar (fatty) tissue that fills the spaces between pelvic viscera, condenses to form "ligaments" (cardinal, lateral visceral, and lateral rectal ligaments; see **Fig. 21.20**) that provide passage for the ureters and neurovascular elements within the pelvis.

Fig. 21.20 **Fascia and ligaments of the female pelvis**

Transverse section, through cervix, superior view.

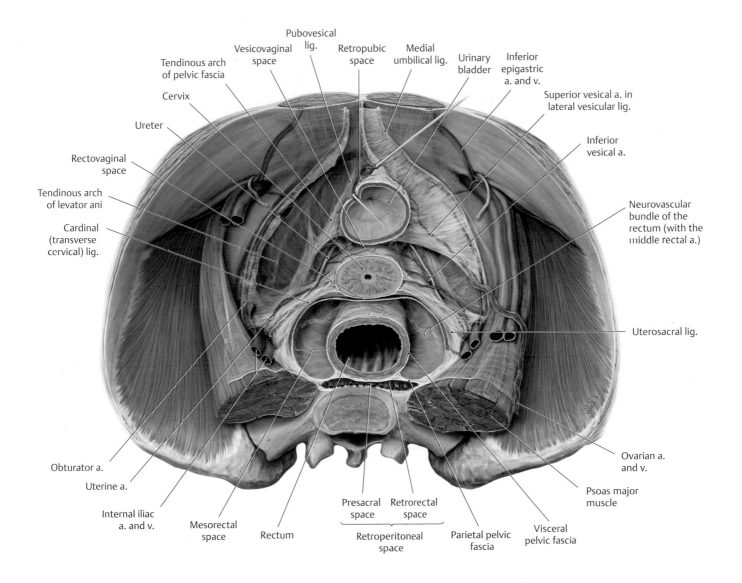

Vagina

Fig. 21.21 Location of vagina
Midsagittal section, left lateral view.

Vesicouterine pouch

Visceral peritoneum on uterus

Body of uterus

Rectouterine pouch

Cervix of uterus, supravaginal part

Cervix of uterus, vaginal part

Posterior part

Vaginal fornix

Urinary bladder

Anterior part

Vagina, anterior wall

Vagina, posterior wall

Urethra

Rectum

Vesicovaginal septum (clinical term)

Rectovaginal septum

Vaginal orifice

Deep transverse perineal

External urethral orifice

Urethrovaginal sphincter

Vaginal vestibule with labium minus

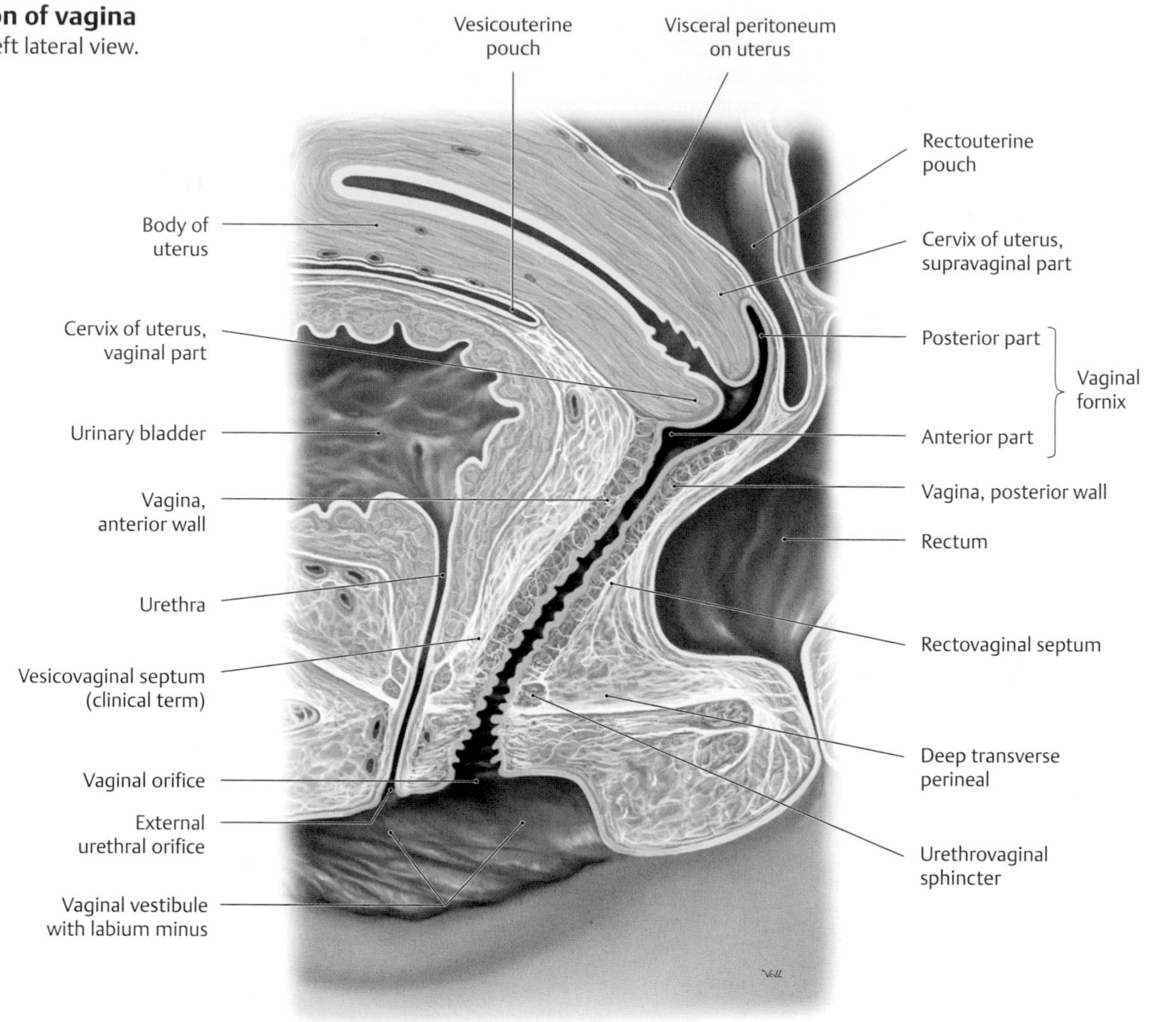

Fig 21.22 Relationship of the vagina to the peritoneum and pelvic organs
Midsagittal section, left lateral view. The vagina lies almost completely in the subperitoneal space. However, drainage of peritoneal fluid or pus from an abcess in the rectouterine space, a procedure known as culdocentesis, can be achieved through an incision in the posterior fornix.

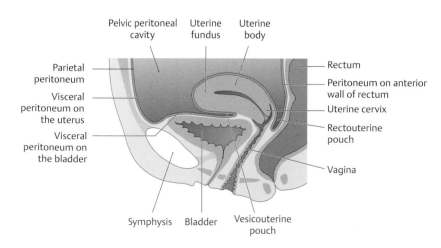

Pelvic peritoneal cavity

Uterine fundus

Uterine body

Parietal peritoneum

Rectum

Visceral peritoneum on the uterus

Peritoneum on anterior wall of rectum

Uterine cervix

Visceral peritoneum on the bladder

Rectouterine pouch

Vagina

Symphysis   Bladder   Vesicouterine pouch

Fig. 21.23 Structure of vagina
Posteriorly angled coronal section, posterior view.

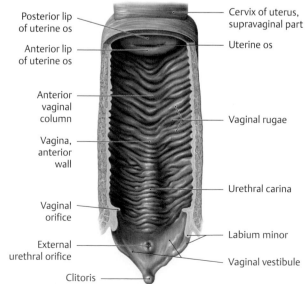

Posterior lip of uterine os

Cervix of uterus, supravaginal part

Anterior lip of uterine os

Uterine os

Anterior vaginal column

Vaginal rugae

Vagina, anterior wall

Urethral carina

Vaginal orifice

External urethral orifice

Labium minor

Clitoris

Vaginal vestibule

Fig. 21.24 **Female genital organs: Coronal section**

Anterior view. The vagina is both pelvic and perineal in location.
It is also retroperitoneal.

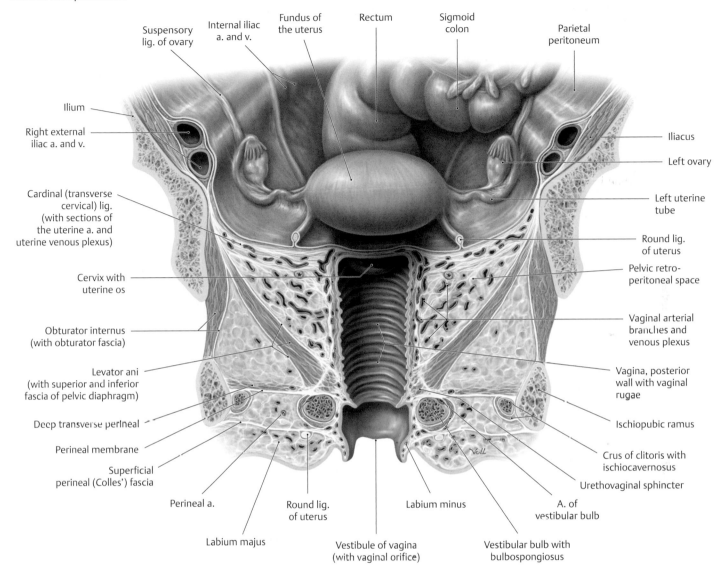

Suspensory lig. of ovary
Internal iliac a. and v.
Fundus of the uterus
Rectum
Sigmoid colon
Parietal peritoneum

Ilium
Right external iliac a. and v.
Cardinal (transverse cervical) lig. (with sections of the uterine a. and uterine venous plexus)
Cervix with uterine os
Obturator internus (with obturator fascia)
Levator ani (with superior and inferior fascia of pelvic diaphragm)
Deep transverse perineal
Perineal membrane
Superficial perineal (Colles') fascia

Iliacus
Left ovary
Left uterine tube
Round lig. of uterus
Pelvic retro-peritoneal space
Vaginal arterial branches and venous plexus
Vagina, posterior wall with vaginal rugae
Ischiopubic ramus
Crus of clitoris with ischiocavernosus
Urethovaginal sphincter

Perineal a.
Round lig. of uterus
Labium majus
Vestibule of vagina (with vaginal orifice)
Labium minus
Vestibular bulb with bulbospongiosus
A. of vestibular bulb

Fig. 21.25 **Vagina: Location in the perineum**

Inferior view.

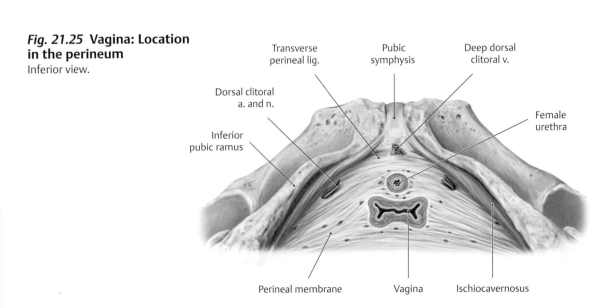

Transverse perineal lig.
Pubic symphysis
Deep dorsal clitoral v.
Dorsal clitoral a. and n.
Inferior pubic ramus
Female urethra

Perineal membrane
Vagina
Ischiocavernosus

Female External Genitalia

Fig. 21.26 Female external genitalia
Lithotomy position with labia minora separated.

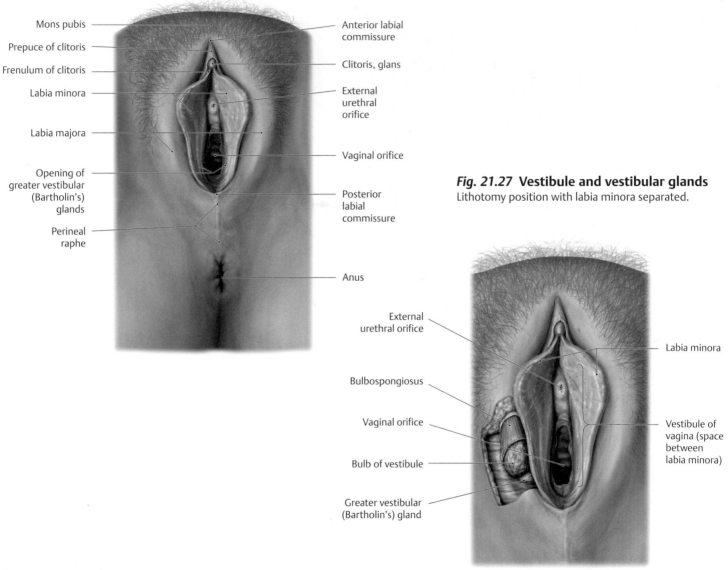

Mons pubis

Prepuce of clitoris

Frenulum of clitoris

Labia minora

Labia majora

Opening of greater vestibular (Bartholin's) glands

Perineal raphe

Anterior labial commissure

Clitoris, glans

External urethral orifice

Vaginal orifice

Posterior labial commissure

Anus

Fig. 21.27 Vestibule and vestibular glands
Lithotomy position with labia minora separated.

External urethral orifice

Bulbospongiosus

Vaginal orifice

Bulb of vestibule

Greater vestibular (Bartholin's) gland

Labia minora

Vestibule of vagina (space between labia minora)

Fig. 21.28 Erectile tissue in the female perineum

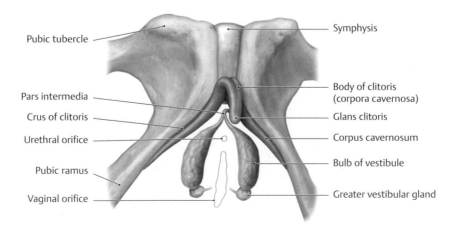

Pubic tubercle

Pars intermedia

Crus of clitoris

Urethral orifice

Pubic ramus

Vaginal orifice

Symphysis

Body of clitoris (corpora cavernosa)

Glans clitoris

Corpus cavernosum

Bulb of vestibule

Greater vestibular gland

Fig. 21.29 Erectile tissue and muscles of the female

Lithotomy position. *Removed:* Labia and skin. *Removed from left side:* Ischiocavernosus and bulbospongiosus muscles.

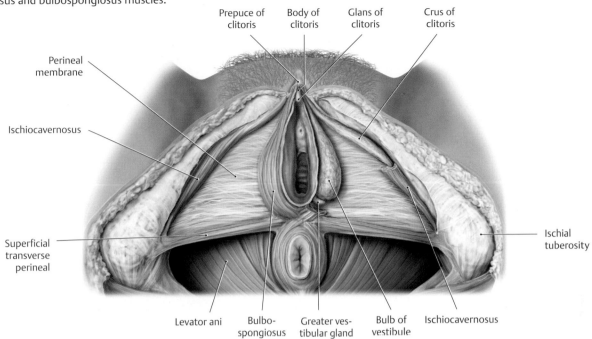

Prepuce of clitoris · Body of clitoris · Glans of clitoris · Crus of clitoris

Perineal membrane

Ischiocavernosus

Superficial transverse perineal

Ischial tuberosity

Levator ani · Bulbo-spongiosus · Greater vestibular gland · Bulb of vestibule · Ischiocavernosus

---

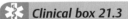 **Clinical box 21.3**

Episiotomy

Episiotomy is a common obstetric procedure used to enlarge the birth canal during the expulsive stage of labor. The procedure is generally used to expedite the delivery of a baby at risk for hypoxia during the expulsive stage. Alternately, if the perineal skin turns white (indicating diminished blood flow), there is imminent danger of perineal laceration, and an episiotomy is often performed. More lateral incisions gain more room, but they are more difficult to repair.

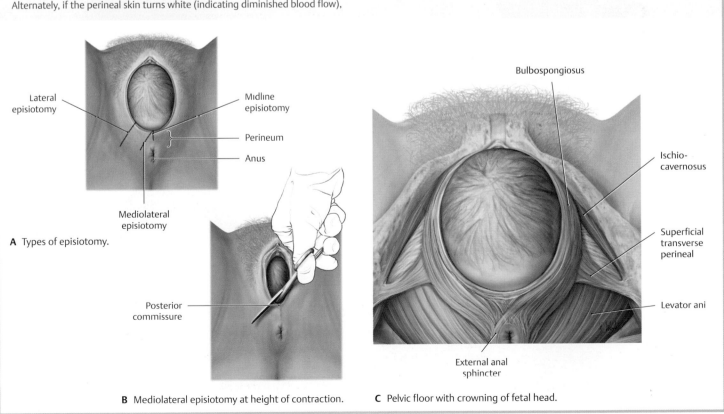

Lateral episiotomy · Midline episiotomy · Perineum · Anus · Mediolateral episiotomy

A Types of episiotomy.

Posterior commissure

B Mediolateral episiotomy at height of contraction.

Bulbospongiosus · Ischio-cavernosus · Superficial transverse perineal · Levator ani · External anal sphincter

C Pelvic floor with crowning of fetal head.

Penis, Testis & Epididymis

Fig. 21.30 **Penis**

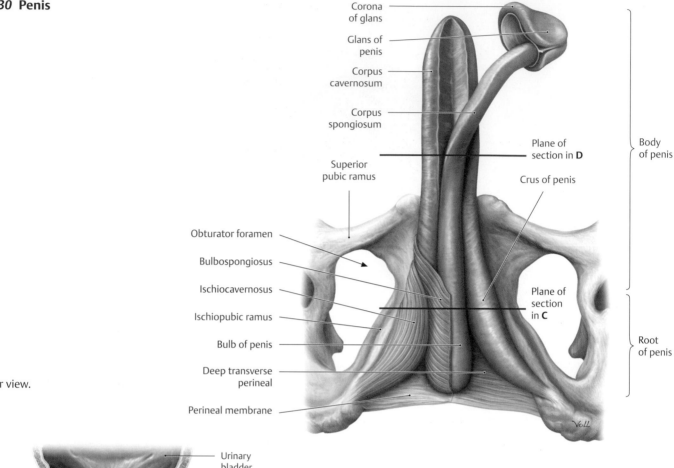

Corona
of glans

Glans of
penis

Corpus
cavernosum

Corpus
spongiosum

Superior
pubic ramus

Plane of
section in **D**

Crus of penis

Obturator foramen

Bulbospongiosus

Ischiocavernosus

Ischiopubic ramus

Bulb of penis

Deep transverse
perineal

Perineal membrane

Plane of
section
in **C**

Body
of penis

Root
of penis

A Inferior view.

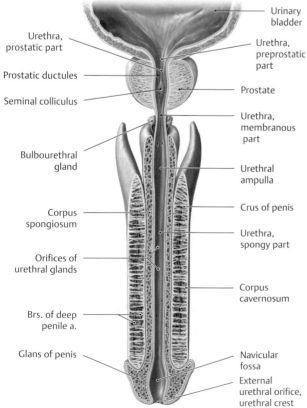

Urinary
bladder

Urethra,
prostatic part

Prostatic ductules

Seminal colliculus

Bulbourethral
gland

Corpus
spongiosum

Orifices of
urethral glands

Brs. of deep
penile a.

Glans of penis

Urethra,
preprostatic
part

Prostate

Urethra,
membranous
part

Urethral
ampulla

Crus of penis

Urethra,
spongy part

Corpus
cavernosum

Navicular
fossa

External
urethral orifice,
urethral crest

B Longitudinal section.

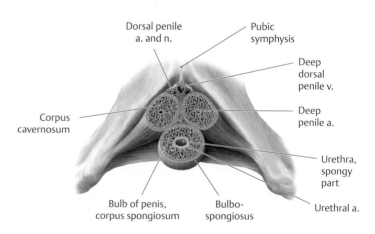

Dorsal penile
a. and n.

Pubic
symphysis

Corpus
cavernosum

Deep
dorsal
penile v.

Deep
penile a.

Urethra,
spongy
part

Bulb of penis,
corpus spongiosum

Bulbo-
spongiosus

Urethral a.

C Cross section through the root of the penis.

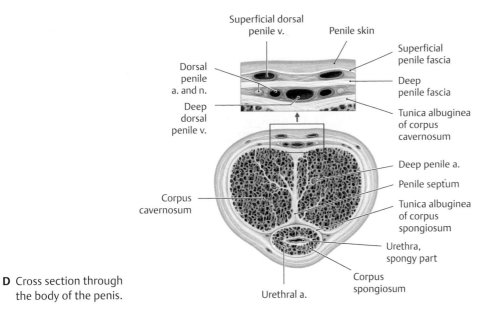

Superficial dorsal penile v.

Penile skin

Superficial penile fascia

Deep penile fascia

Tunica albuginea of corpus cavernosum

Dorsal penile a. and n.

Deep dorsal penile v.

Deep penile a.

Penile septum

Tunica albuginea of corpus spongiosum

Corpus cavernosum

Urethra, spongy part

Corpus spongiosum

Urethral a.

D Cross section through the body of the penis.

Fig. 21.31 **Testis and epididymis**
Left lateral view.

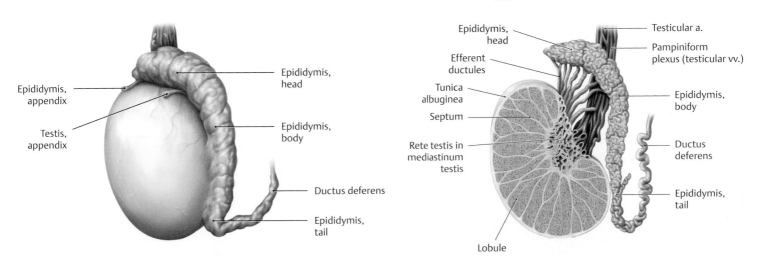

Superficial fascia, deep layer

External spermatic fascia

Cremaster m. and cremasteric fascia

Pampiniform plexus (testicular vv.)

Tunica dartos

Epididymis, body

Tunica vaginalis, visceral layer (on testis)

Scrotum

Internal spermatic fascia

Testicular a.

Tunica vaginalis, parietal layer

Epididymis, head

Glans of penis

A Testis and epididymis in situ.

Epididymis, appendix

Testis, appendix

Epididymis, head

Epididymis, body

Ductus deferens

Epididymis, tail

B Surface anatomy of the testis and epididymis.

Epididymis, head

Efferent ductules

Tunica albuginea

Septum

Rete testis in mediastinum testis

Lobule

Testicular a.

Pampiniform plexus (testicular vv.)

Epididymis, body

Ductus deferens

Epididymis, tail

C Sagittal section of the testis and epididymis.

Male Accessory Sex Glands

The accessory male sex glands consist of the seminal, prostate, and bulbourethral glands, which contribute fluid to the ejaculate that provides nourishment for the spermatozoa as well as neutralizes the pH of the male urethra and the vaginal environment.

Fig. 21.32 Accessory sex glands

Posterior view.
The ducts of the seminal gland and ductus deferens combine to form the ejaculatory duct.

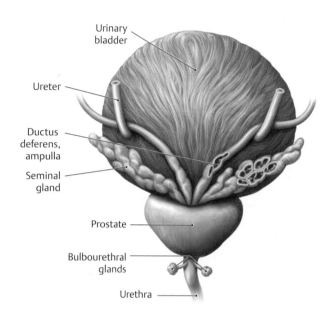

Fig. 21.33 Anatomic divisions of the prostate

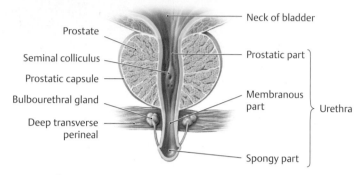

A Coronal section, anterior view.

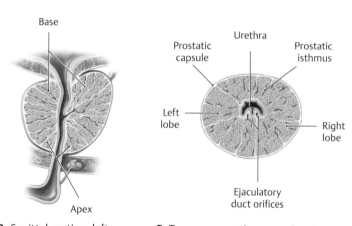

B Sagittal section, left lateral view.

C Transverse section, superior view.

Fig. 21.34 Clinical divisions of the prostate

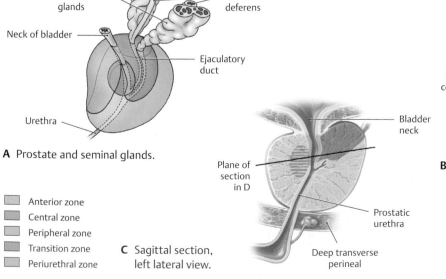

A Prostate and seminal glands.

Anterior zone
Central zone
Peripheral zone
Transition zone
Periurethral zone

C Sagittal section, left lateral view.

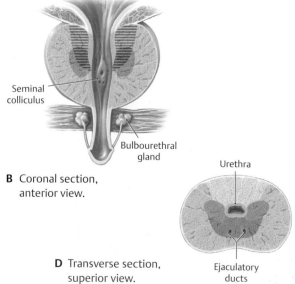

B Coronal section, anterior view.

D Transverse section, superior view.

Fig. 21.35 **Prostate in situ**
Sagittal section through the male pelvis, left lateral view.

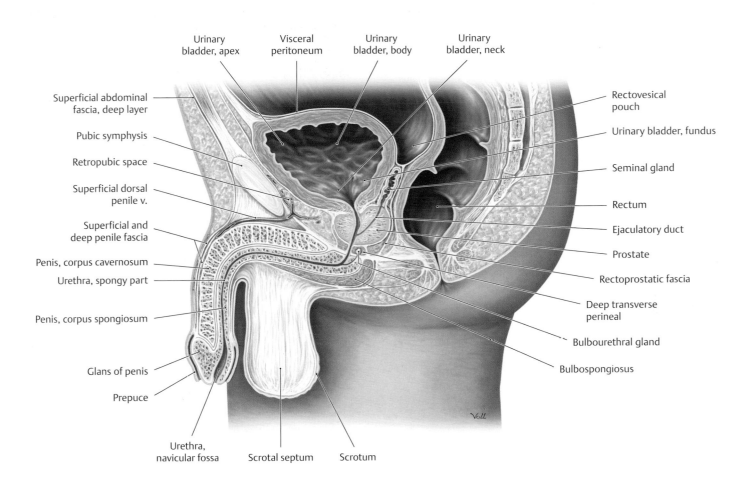

Urinary bladder, apex — Visceral peritoneum — Urinary bladder, body — Urinary bladder, neck

Superficial abdominal fascia, deep layer

Pubic symphysis

Retropubic space

Superficial dorsal penile v.

Superficial and deep penile fascia

Penis, corpus cavernosum

Urethra, spongy part

Penis, corpus spongiosum

Glans of penis

Prepuce

Urethra, navicular fossa — Scrotal septum — Scrotum

Rectovesical pouch

Urinary bladder, fundus

Seminal gland

Rectum

Ejaculatory duct

Prostate

Rectoprostatic fascia

Deep transverse perineal

Bulbourethral gland

Bulbospongiosus

 Clinical box 21.4

Prostatic carcinoma and hypertrophy

Prostatic carcinoma is one of the most common malignant tumors in older men, often growing at a subcapsular location (deep to the prostatic capsule) in the peripheral zone of the prostate. Unlike benign prostatic hyperplasia, which begins in the central part of the gland, prostatic carcinoma does not cause urinary outflow obstruction in its early stages. Being in the peripheral zone, the tumor is palpable as a firm mass through the anterior wall of the rectum during rectal examination. In certain prostate diseases, especially cancer, increased amounts of a protein, prostate-specific antigen or PSA, appear in the blood. This protein can be measured by a simple blood test.

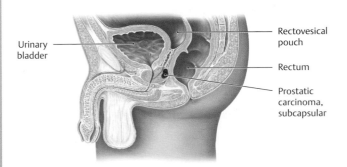

Urinary bladder

Rectovesical pouch

Rectum

Prostatic carcinoma, subcapsular

A Most common site of prostatic carcinoma.

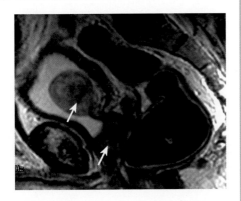

B Prostatic carcinoma (*arrows*) with bladder infiltration.

22 Neurovasculature

Overview of the Blood Supply to Pelvic Organs & Wall

Fig 22.1 Branches of the right internal iliac artery

Side wall of the male pelvis, left lateral view. The internal iliac artery arises from the common iliac artery. Its anterior trunk gives off visceral branches to pelvic organs and parietal branches to the pelvic wall. The posterior trunk gives off only parietal branches. Branches to the uterus and vagina in the female are the principal differences from the male vasculature.

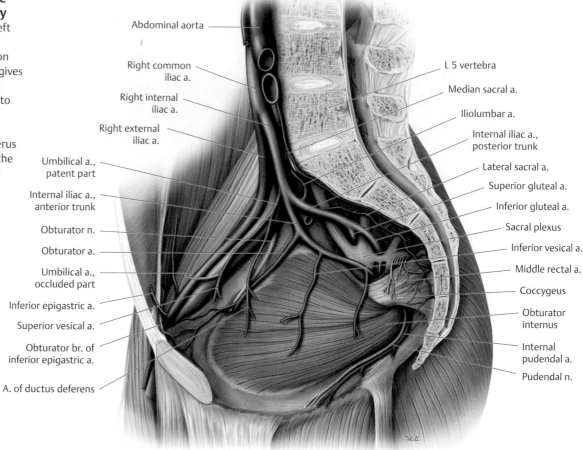

Abdominal aorta

Right common iliac a.

Right internal iliac a.

Right external iliac a.

Umbilical a., patent part

Internal iliac a., anterior trunk

Obturator n.

Obturator a.

Umbilical a., occluded part

Inferior epigastric a.

Superior vesical a.

Obturator br. of inferior epigastric a.

A. of ductus deferens

L 5 vertebra

Median sacral a.

Iliolumbar a.

Internal iliac a., posterior trunk

Lateral sacral a.

Superior gluteal a.

Inferior gluteal a.

Sacral plexus

Inferior vesical a.

Middle rectal a.

Coccygeus

Obturator internus

Internal pudendal a.

Pudendal n.

Table 22.1	Neurovascular pathways in the pelvis

There are six major neurovascular tracts on the pelvic walls, four of which (*) contain branches from the internal iliac artery.

Tract	Neurovascular structures transmitted
Posterior	
① Greater sciatic foramen, suprapiriform part* (above the piriformis)	Superior gluteal a. and v., superior gluteal n.
② Greater sciatic foramen, infrapiriform part* (below the piriformis)	Inferior gluteal a. and v., inferior gluteal n., sciatic n., internal pudendal a. and v., pudendal n., posterior femoral cutaneous n.
On pelvic floor	
③ Lesser sciatic foramen through pudendal canal*	Internal pudendal a. and v., pudendal n.
Lateral	
④ Obturator canal*	Obturator a. and v., obturator n.
Anterior	
⑤ Muscular lacuna (posterior to inguinal lig., lateral to iliopectineal arch)	Femoral n., lateral femoral cutaneous n.
⑥ Vascular lacuna (posterior to inguinal lig., medial to iliopectineal arch)	Femoral a. and v., lymphatic vessels (the femoral a. is a branch of the external iliac a.), femoral branch of genito-femoral n.

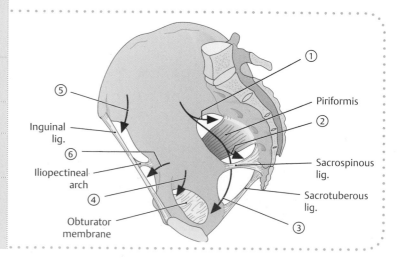

Inguinal lig.

Iliopectineal arch

Obturator membrane

Piriformis

Sacrospinous lig.

Sacrotuberous lig.

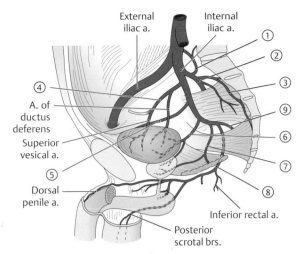

A Male pelvis.

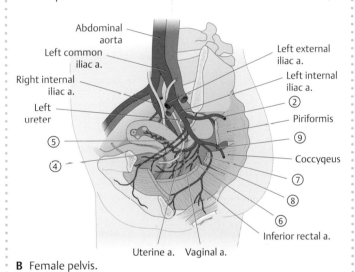

B Female pelvis.

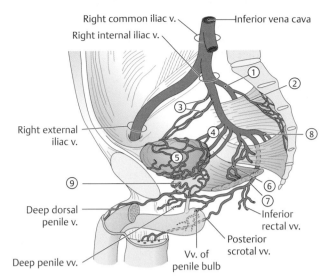

A Male pelvis.

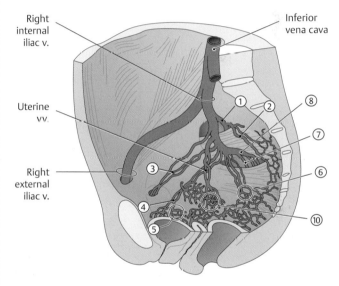

B Female pelvis.

Table 22.2	Branches of the internal iliac artery

The internal iliac artery gives off five parietal (pelvic wall) and four visceral (pelvic organs) branches.* Parietal branches are shown in italics.

Branches		
①	*Iliolumbar a.*	
②	*Superior gluteal a.*	
③	*Lateral sacral a.*	
④	Umbilical a.	A. of ductus deferens
		Superior vesical a.
⑤	*Obturator a.*	
⑥	Inferior vesical a.	
⑦	Middle rectal a.	
⑧	Internal pudendal a.	Inferior rectal a.
		Dorsal penile a.
		Posterior scrotal aa.
⑨	*Inferior gluteal a.*	

* In the female pelvis, the origin of the uterine and vaginal arteries is highly variable.

Table 22.3	Venous drainage of the pelvis

Tributaries	
①	Superior gluteal v.
②	Lateral sacral v.
③	Obturator vv.
④	Vesical vv.
⑤	Vesical venous plexus
⑥	Middle rectal vv. (rectal venous plexus) (also superior and inferior rectal vv., not shown)
⑦	Internal pudendal v.
⑧	Inferior gluteal vv.
⑨	Prostatic venous plexus
⑩	Uterine and vaginal venous plexus

The male pelvis also contains veins draining the penis and scrotum.

Arteries & Veins of the Male Pelvis

Fig 22.2 Blood vessels of the male pelvis
Right hemipelvis, left lateral view.

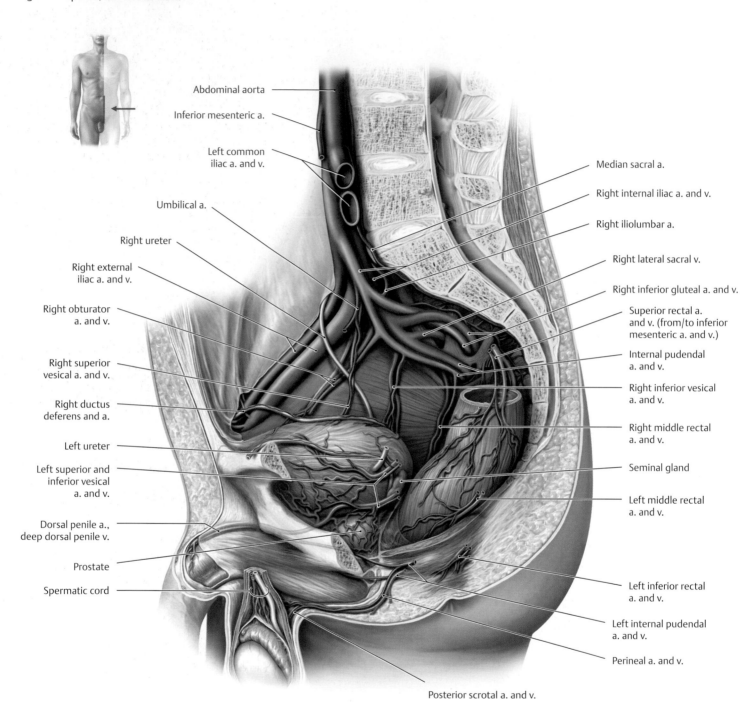

Abdominal aorta

Inferior mesenteric a.

Left common iliac a. and v.

Umbilical a.

Right ureter

Right external iliac a. and v.

Right obturator a. and v.

Right superior vesical a. and v.

Right ductus deferens and a.

Left ureter

Left superior and inferior vesical a. and v.

Dorsal penile a., deep dorsal penile v.

Prostate

Spermatic cord

Median sacral a.

Right internal iliac a. and v.

Right iliolumbar a.

Right lateral sacral v.

Right inferior gluteal a. and v.

Superior rectal a. and v. (from/to inferior mesenteric a. and v.)

Internal pudendal a. and v.

Right inferior vesical a. and v.

Right middle rectal a. and v.

Seminal gland

Left middle rectal a. and v.

Left inferior rectal a. and v.

Left internal pudendal a. and v.

Perineal a. and v.

Posterior scrotal a. and v.

Fig 22.3 Blood vessels of the male genitalia
Opened: Inguinal canal and coverings of the spermatic cord

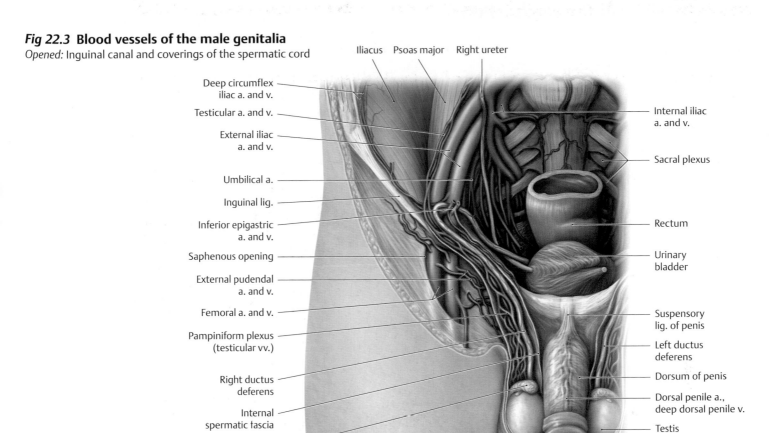

Iliacus Psoas major Right ureter

Deep circumflex iliac a. and v.

Testicular a. and v.

External iliac a. and v.

Umbilical a.

Inguinal lig.

Inferior epigastric a. and v.

Saphenous opening

External pudendal a. and v.

Femoral a. and v.

Pampiniform plexus (testicular vv.)

Right ductus deferens

Internal spermatic fascia

Epididymis

Internal iliac a. and v.

Sacral plexus

Rectum

Urinary bladder

Suspensory lig. of penis

Left ductus deferens

Dorsum of penis

Dorsal penile a., deep dorsal penile v.

Testis

Glans of penis

Fig 22.4 Blood vessels of the testis
Left lateral view.

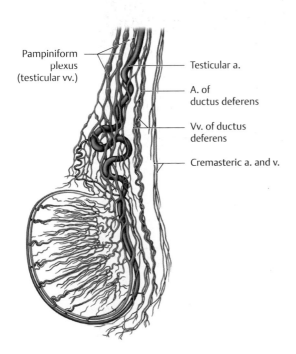

Pampiniform plexus (testicular vv.)

Testicular a.

A. of ductus deferens

Vv. of ductus deferens

Cremasteric a. and v.

⚕ **Clinical box 22.1**

Asymmetric venous drainage of the testes

The pampiniform plexus has an important cooling affect on the testis. Because drainage of the left testicular vein into the left renal vein is at a right angle, a physiological constriction may occur that can obstruct outflow from the testicular vein. This can result in enlargements, or "varicoceles," of the left testicular vein and pampiniform plexus, which can disrupt the cooling function of the plexus and the fertility of the testis.

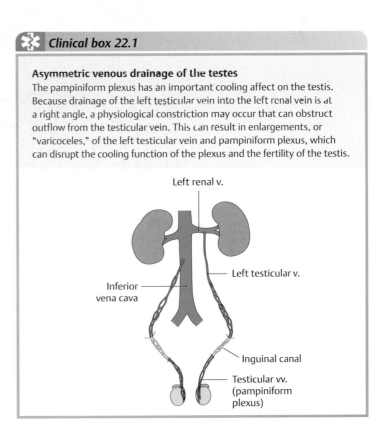

Left renal v.

Inferior vena cava

Left testicular v.

Inguinal canal

Testicular vv. (pampiniform plexus)

Arteries & Veins of the Female Pelvis

Fig 22.5 Blood vessels of the female pelvis
Right hemipelvis, left lateral view.

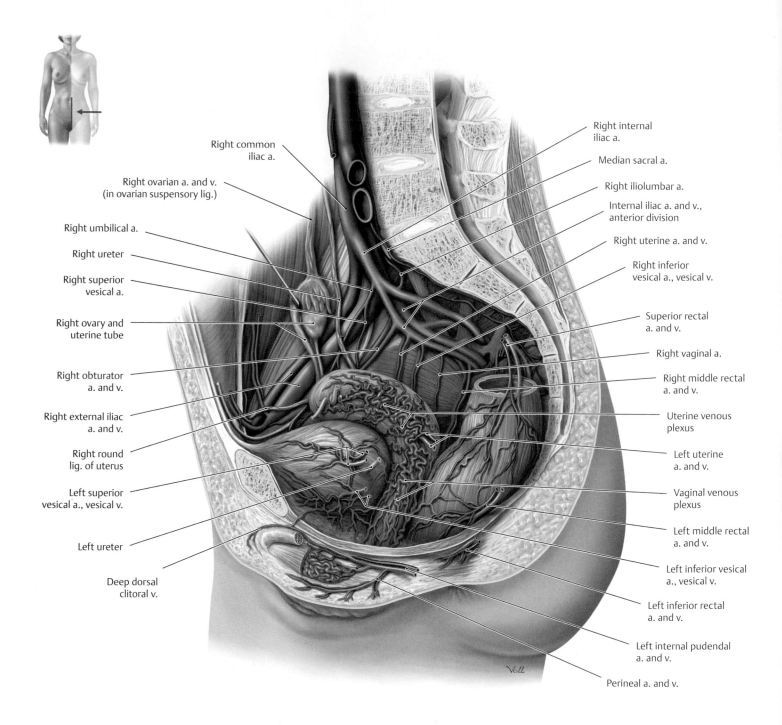

Right common iliac a.

Right ovarian a. and v. (in ovarian suspensory lig.)

Right umbilical a.

Right ureter

Right superior vesical a.

Right ovary and uterine tube

Right obturator a. and v.

Right external iliac a. and v.

Right round lig. of uterus

Left superior vesical a., vesical v.

Left ureter

Deep dorsal clitoral v.

Right internal iliac a.

Median sacral a.

Right iliolumbar a.

Internal iliac a. and v., anterior division

Right uterine a. and v.

Right inferior vesical a., vesical v.

Superior rectal a. and v.

Right vaginal a.

Right middle rectal a. and v.

Uterine venous plexus

Left uterine a. and v.

Vaginal venous plexus

Left middle rectal a. and v.

Left inferior vesical a., vesical v.

Left inferior rectal a. and v.

Left internal pudendal a. and v.

Perineal a. and v.

Fig 22.6 Blood vessels of the female genitalia

Removed: peritoneum on left side; *Retracted:* uterus.

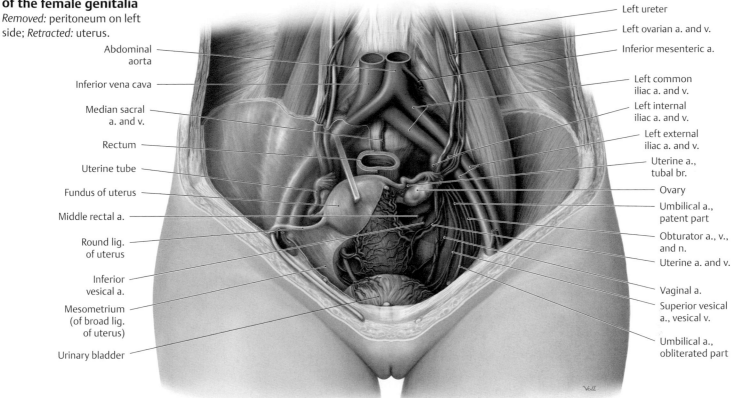

Abdominal aorta

Inferior vena cava

Median sacral a. and v.

Rectum

Uterine tube

Fundus of uterus

Middle rectal a.

Round lig. of uterus

Inferior vesical a.

Mesometrium (of broad lig. of uterus)

Urinary bladder

Left ureter

Left ovarian a. and v.

Inferior mesenteric a.

Left common iliac a. and v.

Left internal iliac a. and v.

Left external iliac a. and v.

Uterine a., tubal br.

Ovary

Umbilical a., patent part

Obturator a., v., and n.

Uterine a. and v.

Vaginal a.

Superior vesical a., vesical v.

Umbilical a., obliterated part

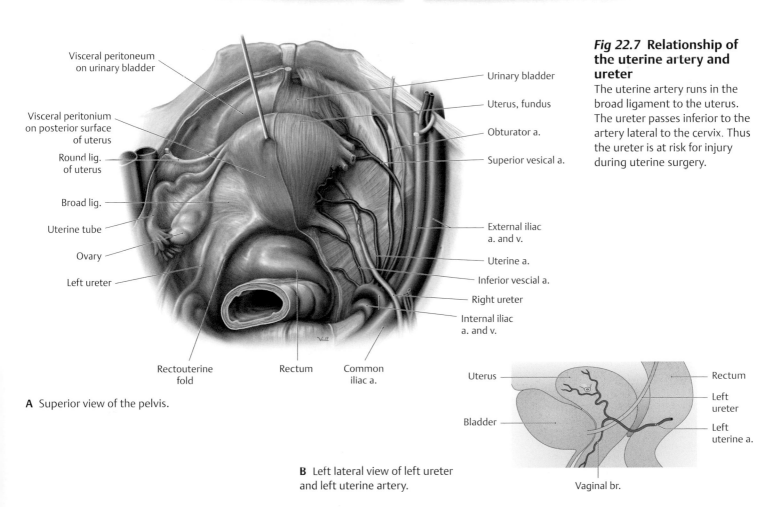

Visceral peritoneum on urinary bladder

Visceral peritonium on posterior surface of uterus

Round lig. of uterus

Broad lig.

Uterine tube

Ovary

Left ureter

Rectouterine fold

Rectum

Common iliac a.

A Superior view of the pelvis.

Urinary bladder

Uterus, fundus

Obturator a.

Superior vesical a.

External iliac a. and v.

Uterine a.

Inferior vescial a.

Right ureter

Internal iliac a. and v.

Fig 22.7 Relationship of the uterine artery and ureter

The uterine artery runs in the broad ligament to the uterus. The ureter passes inferior to the artery lateral to the cervix. Thus the ureter is at risk for injury during uterine surgery.

Uterus

Bladder

Rectum

Left ureter

Left uterine a.

Vaginal br.

B Left lateral view of left ureter and left uterine artery.

Arteries & Veins of the Rectum & External Genitalia

Fig. 22.8 **Blood vessels of the rectum**

Posterior view. The superior rectal arteries are the main blood supply to the rectum; the middle rectal arteries serve as an anastomosis between the superior and inferior rectal arteries. Similarly, the middle rectal veins provide an important portocaval collateral pathway between the superior and inferior rectal veins.

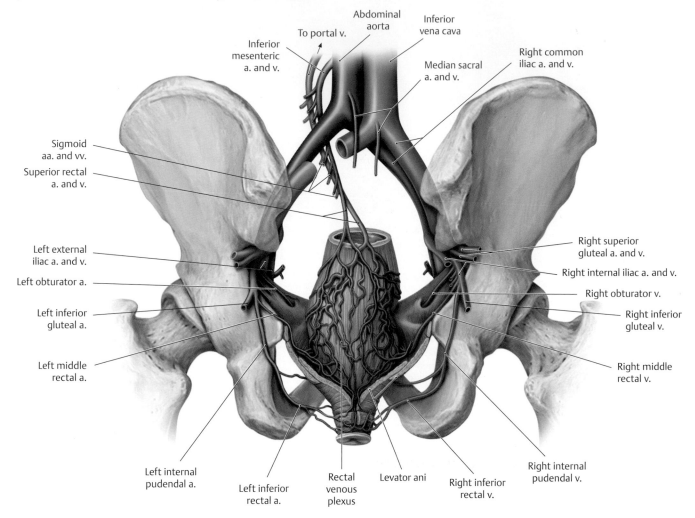

Fig. 22.9 **The hemorrhoidal plexus**

Longitudinal section of the anal canal with the hemorrhoidal plexus windowed.

The hemorrhoidal plexus, supplied by branches of the superior rectal artery, is a permanently distended cavernous body that forms circular cushions in the area of the anal columns. When filled with blood, these cushions serve as an effective continence mechanism that ensures liquid and gas-tight closure. The sustained contraction of the muscular sphincter apparatus inhibits venous drainage, but when the sphincter relaxes during defecation, blood is allowed to drain via arteriovenous anatomoses to the inferior mesenteric vein and middle and inferior rectal veins.

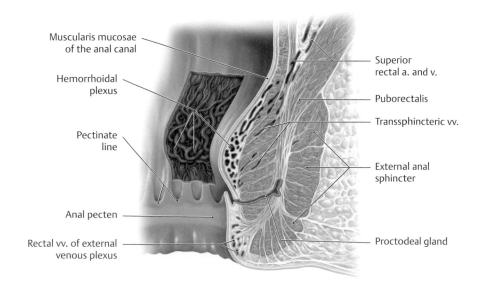

Fig. 22.10 Neurovasculature of the penis and scrotum

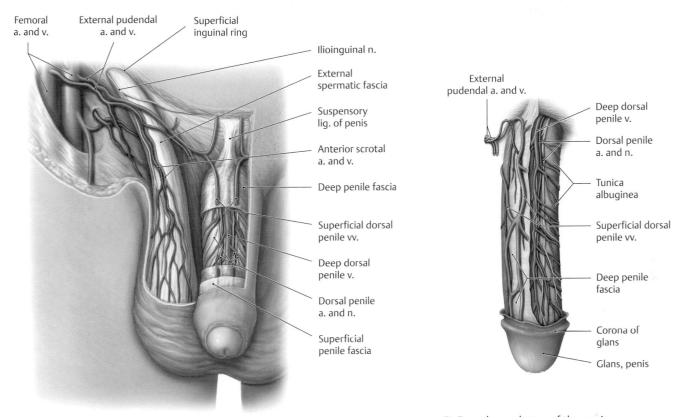

Femoral a. and v.
External pudendal a. and v.
Superficial inguinal ring
Ilioinguinal n.
External spermatic fascia
Suspensory lig. of penis
Anterior scrotal a. and v.
Deep penile fascia
Superficial dorsal penile vv.
Deep dorsal penile v.
Dorsal penile a. and n.
Superficial penile fascia

External pudendal a. and v.
Deep dorsal penile v.
Dorsal penile a. and n.
Tunica albuginea
Superficial dorsal penile vv.
Deep penile fascia
Corona of glans
Glans, penis

A Anterior view. *Partially removed:* Skin and fascia.

B Dorsal vasculature of the penis.
Removed from left side: Deep penile fascia.

Fig. 22.11 Blood vessels of the female external genitalia
Inferior view.

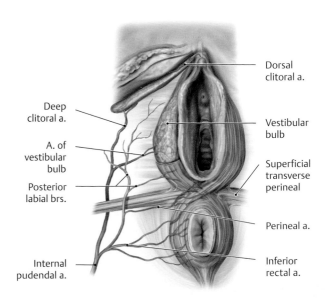

Deep clitoral a.
A. of vestibular bulb
Posterior labial brs.
Internal pudendal a.
Dorsal clitoral a.
Vestibular bulb
Superficial transverse perineal
Perineal a.
Inferior rectal a.

A Arterial supply.

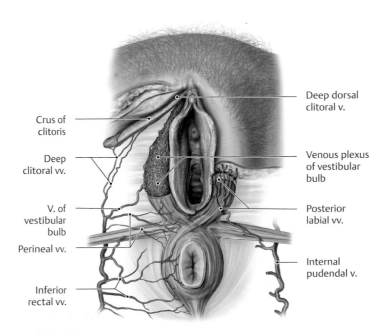

Crus of clitoris
Deep clitoral vv.
V. of vestibular bulb
Perineal vv.
Inferior rectal vv.
Deep dorsal clitoral v.
Venous plexus of vestibular bulb
Posterior labial vv.
Internal pudendal v.

B Venous drainage.

Lymphatics of the Pelvis

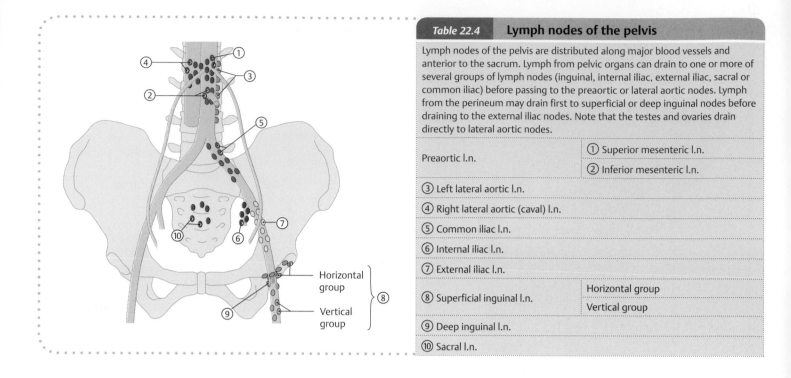

Table 22.4	Lymph nodes of the pelvis	
Lymph nodes of the pelvis are distributed along major blood vessels and anterior to the sacrum. Lymph from pelvic organs can drain to one or more of several groups of lymph nodes (inguinal, internal iliac, external iliac, sacral or common iliac) before passing to the preaortic or lateral aortic nodes. Lymph from the perineum may drain first to superficial or deep inguinal nodes before draining to the external iliac nodes. Note that the testes and ovaries drain directly to lateral aortic nodes.		
Preaortic l.n.	① Superior mesenteric l.n.	
	② Inferior mesenteric l.n.	
③ Left lateral aortic l.n.		
④ Right lateral aortic (caval) l.n.		
⑤ Common iliac l.n.		
⑥ Internal iliac l.n.		
⑦ External iliac l.n.		
⑧ Superficial inguinal l.n.	Horizontal group	
	Vertical group	
⑨ Deep inguinal l.n.		
⑩ Sacral l.n.		

Fig 22.12 Lymphatic drainage of the rectum

Anterior view. Three zones of the rectum drain to different groups of lymph nodes. The upper zone drains to inferior mesenteric nodes. The middle zone and columnar part of the lower zone drains to internal iliac nodes. The cutaneous part of the lower zone drains to superficial inguinal nodes.

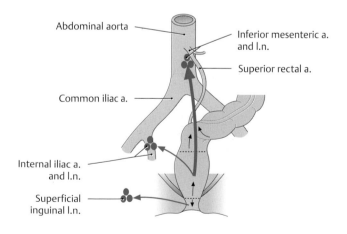

Fig 22.13 Lymphatic drainage of the bladder and urethra

Anterior view. Different parts of the bladder drain to internal iliac or external iliac nodes or directly to the common iliac nodes. The urethra, as well as the penis in the male, is drained by superficial and deep inguinal nodes.

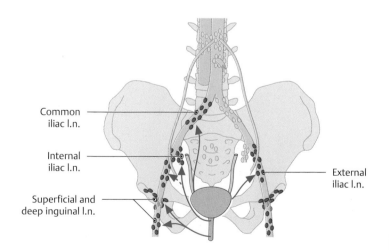

Fig 22.14 Lymphatic drainage of the male genitalia

Male pelvis, anterior view. Male genitalia drain to the lumbar lymph nodes via several pathways:

Testis and epididymis – drain via a direct pathway along the testicular vessels to the right and left lumbar lymph nodes. Some lymph from the epididymis may drain first to internal iliac nodes.

Ductus deferens and seminal glands – drain to external iliac (primarily) and internal iliac nodes.

Prostate – drain along multiple pathways including to external iliac, internal iliac, and sacral nodes

Scrotum and coverings of the testes – drain to superficial inguinal nodes

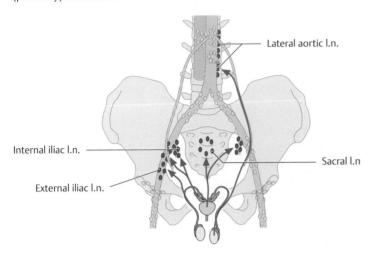

A Lymphatic drainage of the prostate, epididymis, ductus deferens and testes.

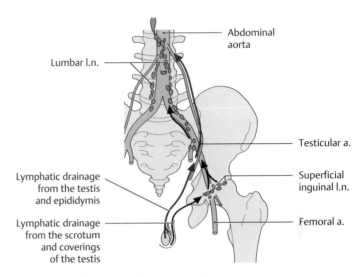

B Lymphatic drainage of the testes and scrotum.

Fig 22.15 Lymphatic drainage of the female genitalia

Female pelvis, anterior view. Female genitalia drain to the lumbar lymph nodes via several pathways:

Ovary, uterine fundus and distal part of uterine tube – drain via a direct pathway along the ovarian vessels to right and left lumbar lymph nodes.

Uterine fundus and body, and proximal part of uterine tube – drain to internal iliac, external iliac, and sacral nodes.

Uterine cervix, middle and upper part of vagina – drain to deep inguinal nodes

External genitalia (except anterior clitoris) – drain to superficial inguinal nodes

Body and glans of the clitoris – drain to deep inguinal and internal iliac nodes

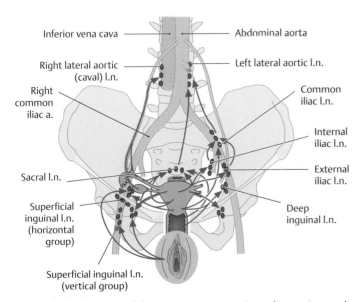

A Lymphatic drainage of the ovary, uterus, uterine tube, vagina, and labia.

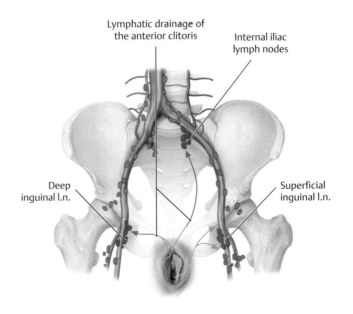

B Lymphatic drainage of the clitoris.

Lymph Nodes of the Genitalia

Fig. 22.16 Lymph nodes of the male genitalia
Anterior view. *Removed:* Gastrointestinal tract (except rectal stump) and peritoneum.

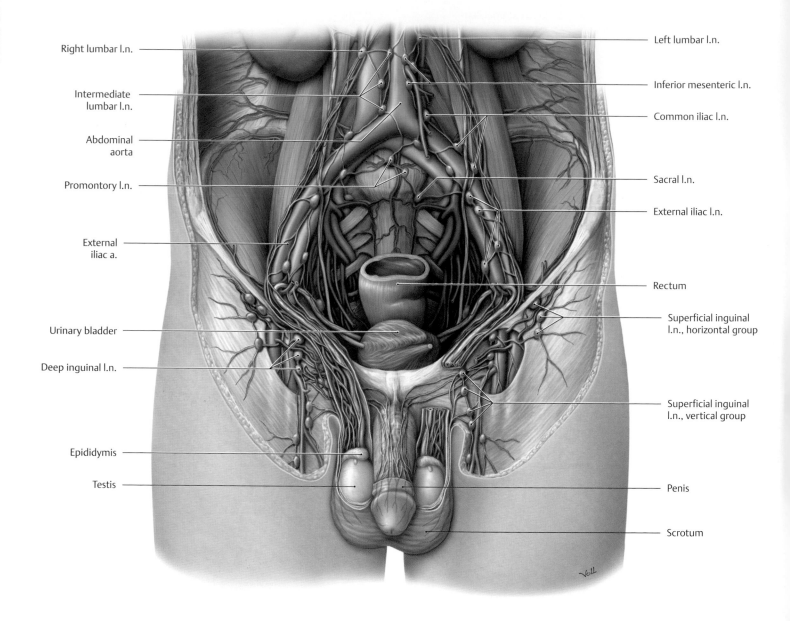

Right lumbar l.n.

Intermediate lumbar l.n.

Abdominal aorta

Promontory l.n.

External iliac a.

Urinary bladder

Deep inguinal l.n.

Epididymis

Testis

Left lumbar l.n.

Inferior mesenteric l.n.

Common iliac l.n.

Sacral l.n.

External iliac l.n.

Rectum

Superficial inguinal l.n., horizontal group

Superficial inguinal l.n., vertical group

Penis

Scrotum

Fig. 22.17 Lymph nodes of the female genitalia

Anterior view. *Removed:* Gastrointestinal tract (except rectal stump) and peritoneum. *Retracted:* Uterus.

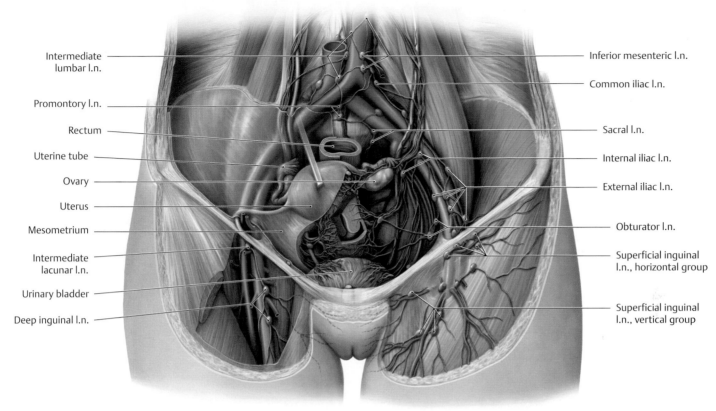

Intermediate lumbar l.n.

Promontory l.n.

Rectum

Uterine tube

Ovary

Uterus

Mesometrium

Intermediate lacunar l.n.

Urinary bladder

Deep inguinal l.n.

Inferior mesenteric l.n.

Common iliac l.n.

Sacral l.n.

Internal iliac l.n.

External iliac l.n.

Obturator l.n.

Superficial inguinal l.n., horizontal group

Superficial inguinal l.n., vertical group

Fig. 22.18 Lymphatic drainage of the pelvic organs

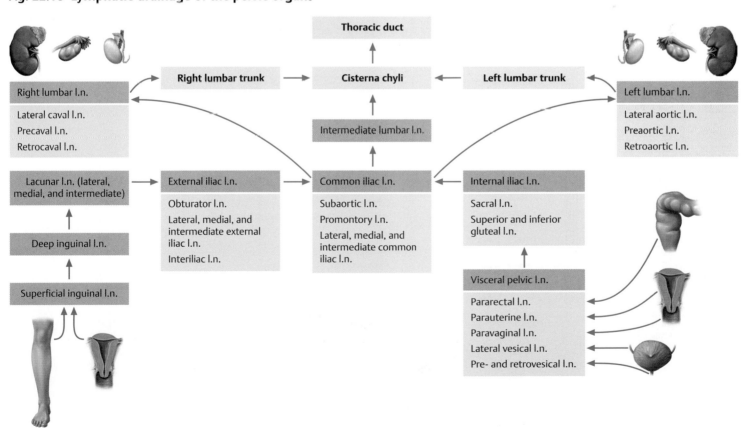

Thoracic duct

Right lumbar trunk → Cisterna chyli ← Left lumbar trunk

Right lumbar l.n.
Lateral caval l.n.
Precaval l.n.
Retrocaval l.n.

Left lumbar l.n.
Lateral aortic l.n.
Preaortic l.n.
Retroaortic l.n.

Intermediate lumbar l.n.

Lacunar l.n. (lateral, medial, and intermediate)

External iliac l.n.
Obturator l.n.
Lateral, medial, and intermediate external iliac l.n.
Interiliac l.n.

Common iliac l.n.
Subaortic l.n.
Promontory l.n.
Lateral, medial, and intermediate common iliac l.n.

Internal iliac l.n.
Sacral l.n.
Superior and inferior gluteal l.n.

Deep inguinal l.n.

Superficial inguinal l.n.

Visceral pelvic l.n.
Pararectal l.n.
Parauterine l.n.
Paravaginal l.n.
Lateral vesical l.n.
Pre- and retrovesical l.n.

Autonomic Innervation of the Genital Organs

Fig 22.19 Innervation of the male pelvis

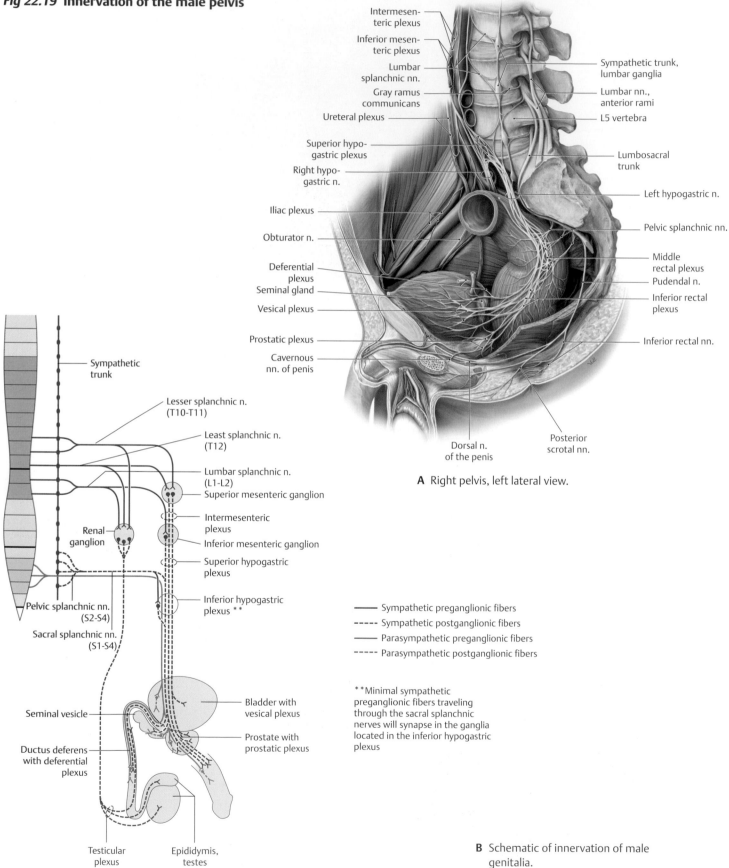

Intermesen-
teric plexus
Inferior mesen-
teric plexus
Lumbar
splanchnic nn.
Gray ramus
communicans
Ureteral plexus
Superior hypo-
gastric plexus
Right hypo-
gastric n.
Iliac plexus
Obturator n.
Deferential
plexus
Seminal gland
Vesical plexus
Prostatic plexus
Cavernous
nn. of penis
Dorsal n.
of the penis

Sympathetic trunk,
lumbar ganglia
Lumbar nn.,
anterior rami
L5 vertebra
Lumbosacral
trunk
Left hypogastric n.
Pelvic splanchnic nn.
Middle
rectal plexus
Pudendal n.
Inferior rectal
plexus
Inferior rectal nn.
Posterior
scrotal nn.

A Right pelvis, left lateral view.

Sympathetic
trunk
Lesser splanchnic n.
(T10-T11)
Least splanchnic n.
(T12)
Lumbar splanchnic n.
(L1-L2)
Superior mesenteric ganglion
Intermesenteric
plexus
Inferior mesenteric ganglion
Superior hypogastric
plexus
Inferior hypogastric
plexus **
Renal
ganglion
Pelvic splanchnic nn.
(S2-S4)
Sacral splanchnic nn.
(S1-S4)
Seminal vesicle
Bladder with
vesical plexus
Prostate with
prostatic plexus
Ductus deferens
with deferential
plexus
Testicular
plexus
Epididymis,
testes

——— Sympathetic preganglionic fibers
------- Sympathetic postganglionic fibers
——— Parasympathetic preganglionic fibers
------- Parasympathetic postganglionic fibers

**Minimal sympathetic
preganglionic fibers traveling
through the sacral splanchnic
nerves will synapse in the ganglia
located in the inferior hypogastric
plexus

B Schematic of innervation of male
genitalia.

Fig 22.20 Innervation of the female pelvis

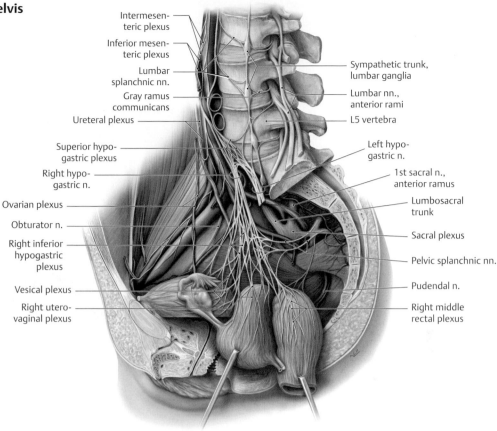

Intermesen-
teric plexus

Inferior mesen-
teric plexus

Lumbar
splanchnic nn.

Gray ramus
communicans

Ureteral plexus

Superior hypo-
gastric plexus

Right hypo-
gastric n.

Ovarian plexus

Obturator n.

Right inferior
hypogastric
plexus

Vesical plexus

Right utero-
vaginal plexus

Sympathetic trunk,
lumbar ganglia

Lumbar nn.,
anterior rami

L5 vertebra

Left hypo-
gastric n.

1st sacral n.,
anterior ramus

Lumbosacral
trunk

Sacral plexus

Pelvic splanchnic nn.

Pudendal n.

Right middle
rectal plexus

A Right pelvis, left lateral view.

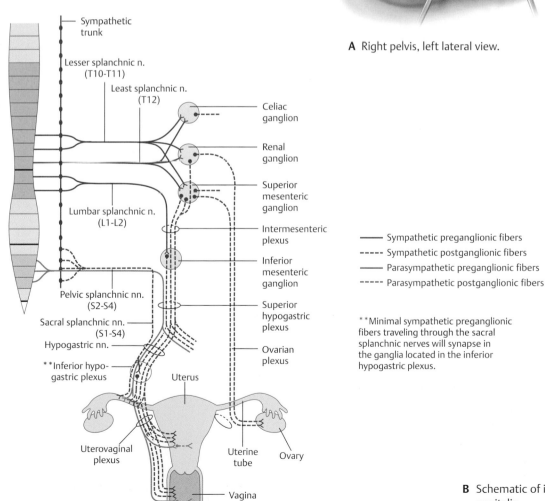

Sympathetic
trunk

Lesser splanchnic n.
(T10-T11)

Least splanchnic n.
(T12)

Lumbar splanchnic n.
(L1-L2)

Pelvic splanchnic nn.
(S2-S4)

Sacral splanchnic nn.
(S1-S4)

Hypogastric nn.

**Inferior hypo-
gastric plexus

Uterovaginal
plexus

Uterus

Uterine
tube

Ovary

Vagina

Celiac
ganglion

Renal
ganglion

Superior
mesenteric
ganglion

Intermesenteric
plexus

Inferior
mesenteric
ganglion

Superior
hypogastric
plexus

Ovarian
plexus

——— Sympathetic preganglionic fibers
- - - - Sympathetic postganglionic fibers
——— Parasympathetic preganglionic fibers
- - - - Parasympathetic postganglionic fibers

**Minimal sympathetic preganglionic
fibers traveling through the sacral
splanchnic nerves will synapse in
the ganglia located in the inferior
hypogastric plexus.

B Schematic of innervation of female
genitalia.

Autonomic Innervation of the Urinary Organs & Rectum

Fig 22.21 Innervation of the pelvic urinary organs
See **pp. 215 and 217** for innervation of the kidneys and upper ureters.

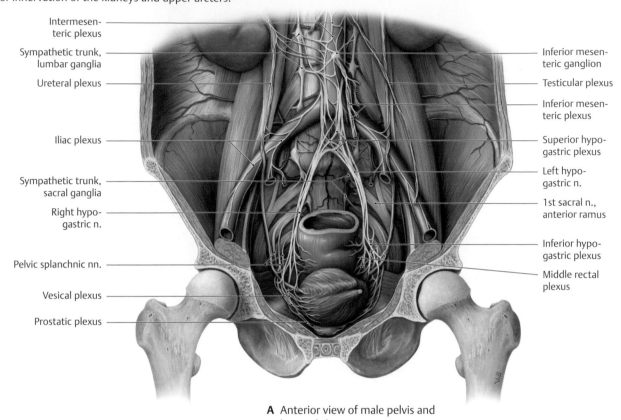

Intermesen-
teric plexus

Sympathetic trunk,
lumbar ganglia

Ureteral plexus

Iliac plexus

Sympathetic trunk,
sacral ganglia

Right hypo-
gastric n.

Pelvic splanchnic nn.

Vesical plexus

Prostatic plexus

Inferior mesen-
teric ganglion

Testicular plexus

Inferior mesen-
teric plexus

Superior hypo-
gastric plexus

Left hypo-
gastric n.

1st sacral n.,
anterior ramus

Inferior hypo-
gastric plexus

Middle rectal
plexus

A Anterior view of male pelvis and
lower abdomen.

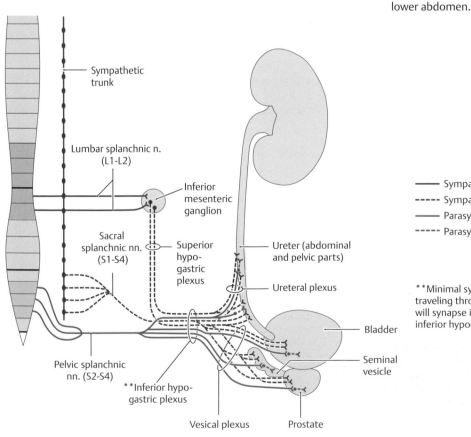

Sympathetic
trunk

Lumbar splanchnic n.
(L1–L2)

Inferior
mesenteric
ganglion

Sacral
splanchnic nn.
(S1–S4)

Superior
hypo-
gastric
plexus

Ureter (abdominal
and pelvic parts)

Ureteral plexus

Pelvic splanchnic
nn. (S2–S4)

**Inferior hypo-
gastric plexus

Bladder

Seminal
vesicle

Vesical plexus

Prostate

——— Sympathetic preganglionic fibers

- - - - Sympathetic postganglionic fibers

——— Parasympathetic preganglionic fibers

- - - - Parasympathetic postganglionic fibers

**Minimal sympathetic preganglionic fibers
traveling through the sacral splanchnic nerves
will synapse in the ganglia located in the
inferior hypogastric plexus.

B Schematic of the urinary bladder
and ureter.

Fig 22.22 Innervation of the anal sphincter mechanism

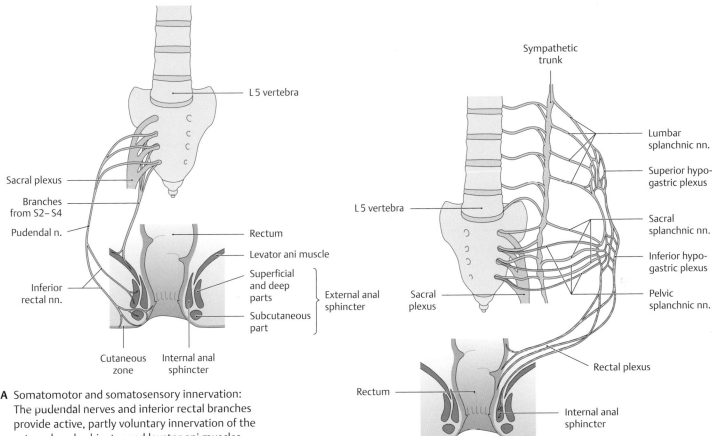

A Somatomotor and somatosensory innervation: The pudendal nerves and inferior rectal branches provide active, partly voluntary innervation of the external anal sphincter and levator ani muscles, and sensation for the anus and perianal skin.

B Visceromotor and viscerosensory innervation: Pelvic splanchnic nerves (S2-4) innervate the internal anal sphincter, which helps to maintain closure of the anal canal. They also supply sensation to the wall of the rectum, particularly the stretch receptors in the rectal ampulla, which when stretched trigger an awareness of the need to defecate.

✚ Clinical box 22.2

Mechanism of defecation (after Wedel)
Both defecation and continence are under central nervous system control involving such diverse structures as the cerebral cortex, muscles of the abdomen and pelvis and perianal skin.

Filling of the rectal ampulla and stimulation of local stretch receptors in the ampullary wall. When the fecal bolus is propelled into the ampulla, mechanoreceptors detect distension and transmit the information to the sensory cortex, which perceives the urge to defecate.

Rectoanal inhibitory reflex and relaxation of the voluntary innervated sphincters. When the ampulla fills, the intrarectal pressure increases and the internal anal sphincter relaxes. This is followed by voluntary relaxation of the puborectalis sling and the external anal sphincter, which results in the straightening of the anorectal angle and widening of the anal canal.

Propulsion of the fecal column. Rectal evacuation is assisted by a direct involuntary increase in pressure in the rectal area and by simultaneous increase in pressure by the contraction of voluntarily innervated muscles in the abdomen wall, pelvic floor, and diaphragm. With propulsion of the fecal column, the hemorrhoidal cushions are drained and pushed out.

Completion of defecation. After the sphincter apparatus allows the fecal column to pass through, it comes in contact with the highly sensitive anoderm, which perceives the volume, consistency and location of the stool. This perception initiates the voluntary process of completing defecation, which is marked by the contraction of the sphincter apparatus and filling of the hemorrhoidal plexus.

Neurovasculature of the Male & Female Perineum

Fig. 22.23 Nerves of the male perineum and genitalia
Lithotomy position.

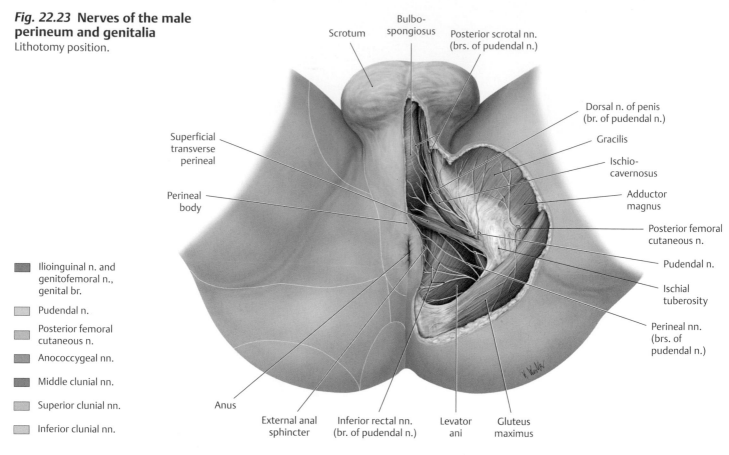

Legend:
- Ilioinguinal n. and genitofemoral n., genital br.
- Pudendal n.
- Posterior femoral cutaneous n.
- Anococcygeal nn.
- Middle clunial nn.
- Superior clunial nn.
- Inferior clunial nn.

Labels:
- Scrotum
- Bulbospongiosus
- Posterior scrotal nn. (brs. of pudendal n.)
- Dorsal n. of penis (br. of pudendal n.)
- Gracilis
- Ischiocavernosus
- Adductor magnus
- Posterior femoral cutaneous n.
- Pudendal n.
- Ischial tuberosity
- Perineal nn. (brs. of pudendal n.)
- Superficial transverse perineal
- Perineal body
- Anus
- External anal sphincter
- Inferior rectal nn. (br. of pudendal n.)
- Levator ani
- Gluteus maximus

Fig. 22.24 Neurovasculature of the male perineum
Lithotomy position.
Removed from left side: Perineal membrane, bulbospongiosus, and root of penis.

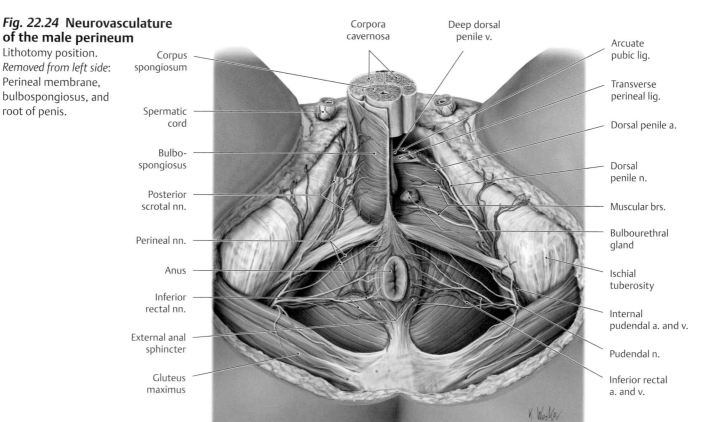

Labels:
- Corpora cavernosa
- Deep dorsal penile v.
- Arcuate pubic lig.
- Corpus spongiosum
- Transverse perineal lig.
- Spermatic cord
- Dorsal penile a.
- Bulbospongiosus
- Dorsal penile n.
- Posterior scrotal nn.
- Muscular brs.
- Perineal nn.
- Bulbourethral gland
- Anus
- Ischial tuberosity
- Inferior rectal nn.
- Internal pudendal a. and v.
- External anal sphincter
- Pudendal n.
- Gluteus maximus
- Inferior rectal a. and v.

Fig. 22.25 Nerves of the female perineum and genitalia

Sensory innervation of the female perineum. Lithotomy position.

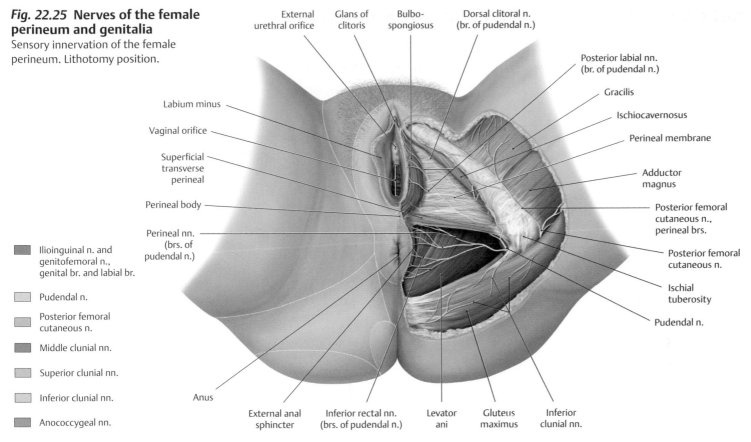

External urethral orifice

Glans of clitoris

Bulbo-spongiosus

Dorsal clitoral n. (br. of pudendal n.)

Posterior labial nn. (br. of pudendal n.)

Gracilis

Ischiocavernosus

Perineal membrane

Labium minus

Vaginal orifice

Superficial transverse perineal

Perineal body

Perineal nn. (brs. of pudendal n.)

Adductor magnus

Posterior femoral cutaneous n., perineal brs.

Posterior femoral cutaneous n.

Ischial tuberosity

Pudendal n.

- Ilioinguinal n. and genitofemoral n., genital br. and labial br.
- Pudendal n.
- Posterior femoral cutaneous n.
- Middle clunial nn.
- Superior clunial nn.
- Inferior clunial nn.
- Anococcygeal nn.

Anus

External anal sphincter

Inferior rectal nn. (brs. of pudendal n.)

Levator ani

Gluteus maximus

Inferior clunial nn.

Fig. 22.26 Neurovasculature of the female perineum

Lithotomy position.
Removed from left side: Bulbospongiosus and ischiocavernosus.

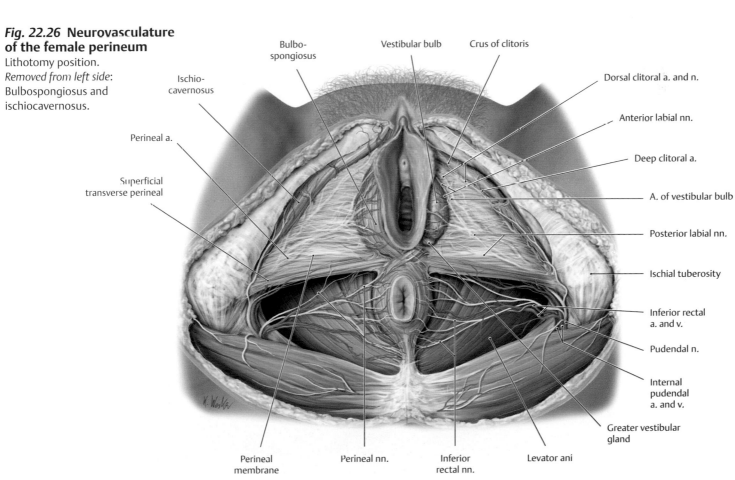

Bulbo-spongiosus

Vestibular bulb

Crus of clitoris

Ischio-cavernosus

Dorsal clitoral a. and n.

Anterior labial nn.

Perineal a.

Deep clitoral a.

Superficial transverse perineal

A. of vestibular bulb

Posterior labial nn.

Ischial tuberosity

Inferior rectal a. and v.

Pudendal n.

Internal pudendal a. and v.

Greater vestibular gland

Perineal membrane

Perineal nn.

Inferior rectal nn.

Levator ani

23 Sectional & Radiographic Anatomy
Sectional Anatomy of the Pelvis & Perineum

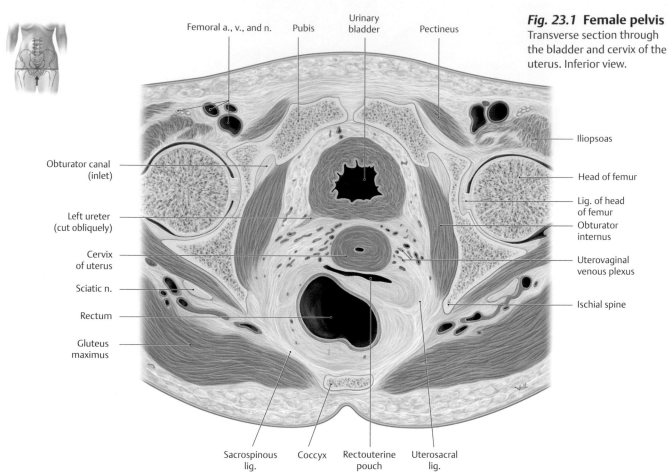

***Fig. 23.1* Female pelvis**
Transverse section through the bladder and cervix of the uterus. Inferior view.

Femoral a., v., and n. — Pubis — Urinary bladder — Pectineus

Obturator canal (inlet)

Left ureter (cut obliquely)

Cervix of uterus

Sciatic n.

Rectum

Gluteus maximus

Iliopsoas

Head of femur

Lig. of head of femur

Obturator internus

Uterovaginal venous plexus

Ischial spine

Sacrospinous lig. — Coccyx — Rectouterine pouch — Uterosacral lig.

***Fig. 23.2* Male pelvis**
Transverse section through the bladder and seminal glands. Inferior view.

Ductus deferens — Rectus abdominis — Urinary bladder — Orifice of right ureter

Femoral a., v., and n.

Obturator a., v., and n.

Seminal gland

Rectovesical septum

Rectum

Sciatic n.

Gluteus maximus

Iliopsoas

Head of femur

Inferior vesical a.

Vesicoprostatic venous plexus

Inferior hypogastric plexus

Obturator internus

Ischial spine

Sacrospinous lig.

Coccyx

Fig. 23.3 **Male pelvis**
Transverse section through the prostate gland and anal canal. Inferior view.

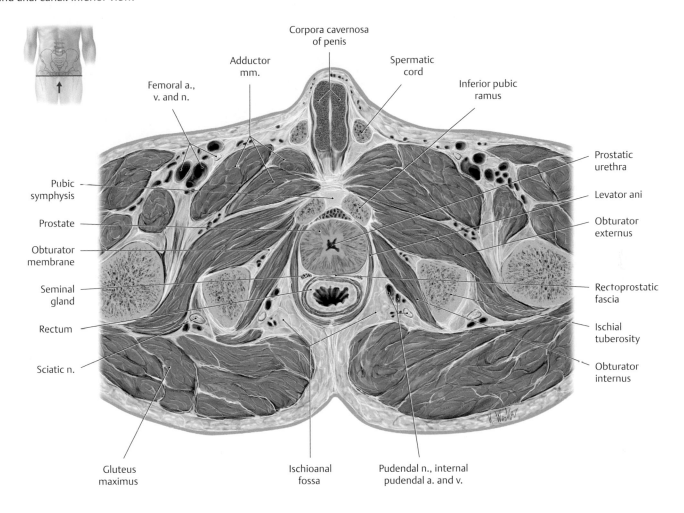

Corpora cavernosa of penis

Adductor mm.

Spermatic cord

Inferior pubic ramus

Femoral a., v. and n.

Prostatic urethra

Pubic symphysis

Levator ani

Prostate

Obturator externus

Obturator membrane

Rectoprostatic fascia

Seminal gland

Rectum

Ischial tuberosity

Sciatic n.

Obturator internus

Gluteus maximus

Ischioanal fossa

Pudendal n., internal pudendal a. and v.

Radiographic Anatomy of the Female Pelvis

Fig 23.4 **MRI of the female pelvis**
Transverse section, inferior view.

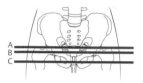

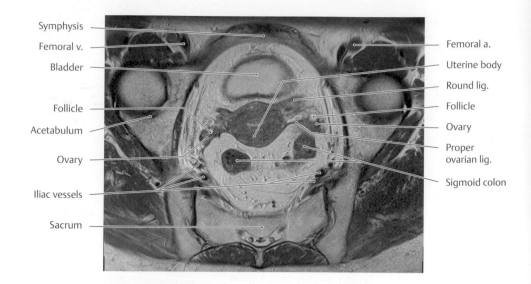

A Section through the body of the uterus. (Reproduced from Krombach GA, Mahnken AH. Body Imaging: Thorax and Abdomen. New York, NY: Thieme; 2018.)

Symphysis
Femoral v.
Bladder
Follicle
Acetabulum
Ovary
Iliac vessels
Sacrum

Femoral a.
Uterine body
Round lig.
Follicle
Ovary
Proper ovarian lig.
Sigmoid colon

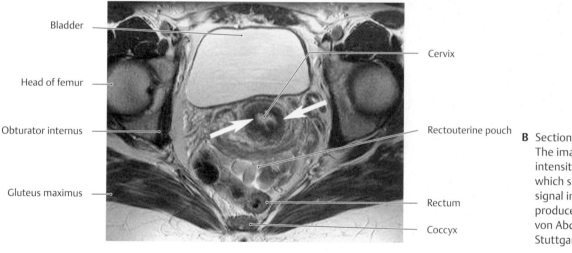

Bladder
Head of femur
Obturator internus
Gluteus maximus

Cervix
Rectouterine pouch
Rectum
Coccyx

B Section through the cervical canal. The image shows the low-signal intensity cervical stroma (arrows), which surrounds the narrow high-signal intensity cervical canal. (Reproduced from Hamm B. et al. MRT von Abdomen und Becken, 2nd ed. Stuttgart: Thieme; 2006.)

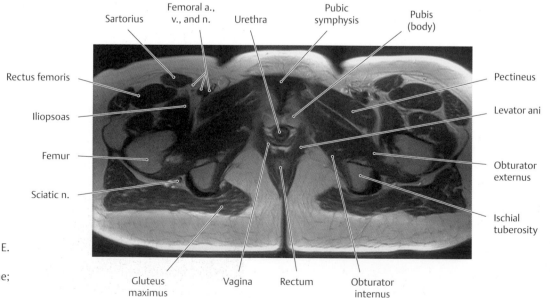

Sartorius
Femoral a., v., and n.
Urethra
Pubic symphysis
Pubis (body)
Rectus femoris
Iliopsoas
Femur
Sciatic n.

Pectineus
Levator ani
Obturator externus
Ischial tuberosity

Gluteus maximus
Vagina
Rectum
Obturator internus

C Section through the lower vagina. (Reproduced from Moeller TB, Reif E. Pocket Atlas of Sectional Anatomy, Vol 2, 4th ed. New York, NY: Thieme; 2014.)

Fig. 23.5 MRI of the female pelvis

Sagittal section, left lateral view

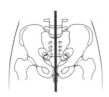

A Position of the uterus with a near empty bladder. The image shows the uterus in the first half of the menstrual cycle (proliferative phase) with narrow endometrium and relatively low-signal intensity of the mymoetrium. (Reproduced from Hamm B. et al. MRT von Abdomen und Becken, 2nd ed. Stuttgart: Thieme; 2006.)

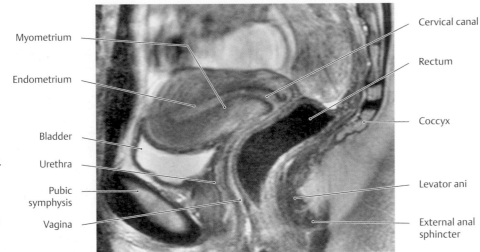

Myometrium

Endometrium

Bladder

Urethra

Pubic symphysis

Vagina

Cervical canal

Rectum

Coccyx

Levator ani

External anal sphincter

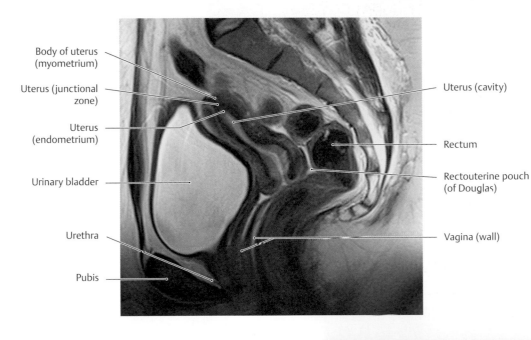

Body of uterus (myometrium)

Uterus (junctional zone)

Uterus (endometrium)

Urinary bladder

Urethra

Pubis

Uterus (cavity)

Rectum

Rectouterine pouch (of Douglas)

Vagina (wall)

B Position of the uterus with a full bladder. (Reproduced from Moeller TB, Reif E. Pocket Atlas of Sectional Anatomy, Vol 2, 4th ed. New York, NY: Thieme; 2014.)

Fig. 23.6 MRI of the female pelvis

Coronal section, anterior view. (Reproduced from Moeller TB, Reif E. Pocket Atlas of Sectional Anatomy, Vol 2, 4th ed. New York, NY: Thieme; 2014.)

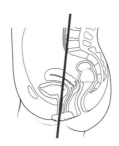

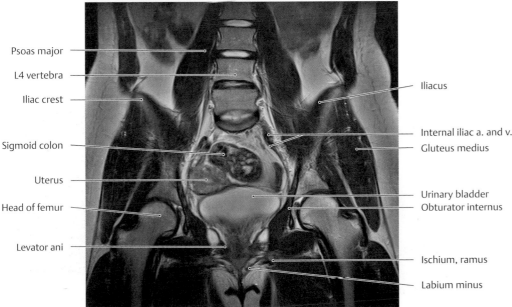

Psoas major

L4 vertebra

Iliac crest

Sigmoid colon

Uterus

Head of femur

Levator ani

Iliacus

Internal iliac a. and v.

Gluteus medius

Urinary bladder

Obturator internus

Ischium, ramus

Labium minus

Radiographic Anatomy of the Male Pelvis

Fig. 23.7 MRI of the male pelvis
Sagittal section, left lateral view. (Reproduced from Hamm B. et al. MRT von Abdomen und Becken, 2nd ed. Stuttgart: Thieme; 2006.)

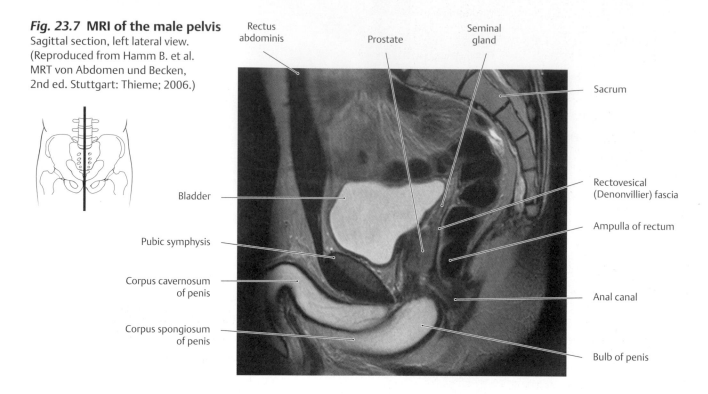

Rectus abdominis

Prostate

Seminal gland

Sacrum

Bladder

Rectovesical (Denonvillier) fascia

Pubic symphysis

Ampulla of rectum

Corpus cavernosum of penis

Anal canal

Corpus spongiosum of penis

Bulb of penis

Fig. 23.8 MRI of the testes

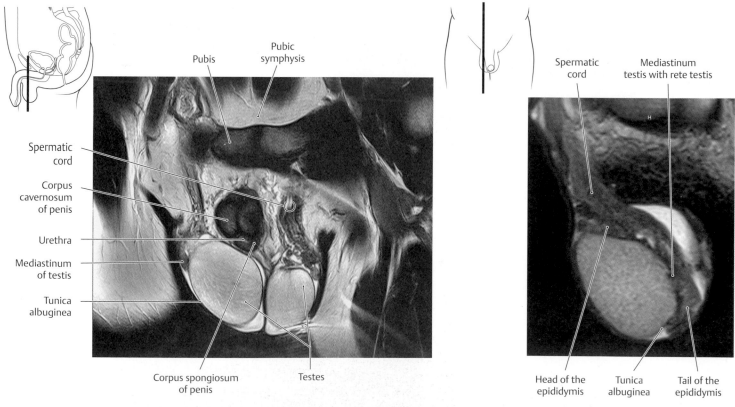

Pubis

Pubic symphysis

Spermatic cord

Corpus cavernosum of penis

Urethra

Mediastinum of testis

Tunica albuginea

Corpus spongiosum of penis

Testes

A Coronal section, anterior view. (Reproduced from Moeller TB, Reif E. Pocket Atlas of Sectional Anatomy, Vol 2, 4th ed. New York, NY: Thieme; 2014.)

Spermatic cord

Mediastinum testis with rete testis

Head of the epididymis

Tunica albuginea

Tail of the epididymis

B Parasagittal section, T2 W image. (Reproduced from Krombach GA, Mahnken AH. Body Imaging: Thorax and Abdomen. New York, NY: Thieme; 2018.)

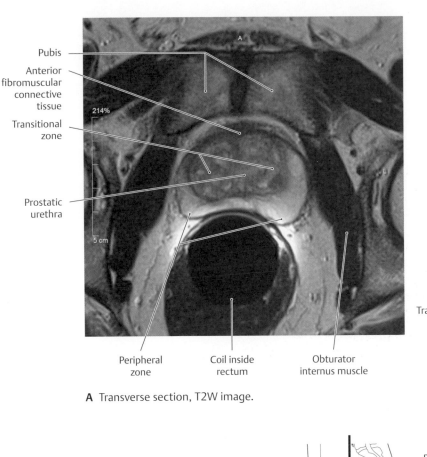

- Pubis
- Anterior fibromuscular connective tissue
- Transitional zone
- Prostatic urethra
- Peripheral zone
- Coil inside rectum
- Obturator internus muscle

A Transverse section, T2W image.

Fig. 23.9 MRI of the prostate
(Reproduced from Krombach GA, Mahnken AH. Body Imaging: Thorax and Abdomen. New York, NY: Thieme; 2018.)

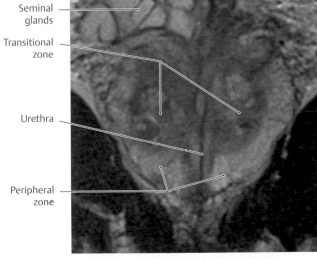

- Ductus deferens
- Seminal glands
- Transitional zone
- Urethra
- Peripheral zone

B Coronal section, T2W image.

Fig. 23.10 MRI of the male pelvis
Coronal section. (Reproduced from Moeller TB, Reif E. Pocket Atlas of Sectional Anatomy, Vol 2, 4th ed. New York, NY: Thieme; 2014.)

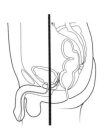

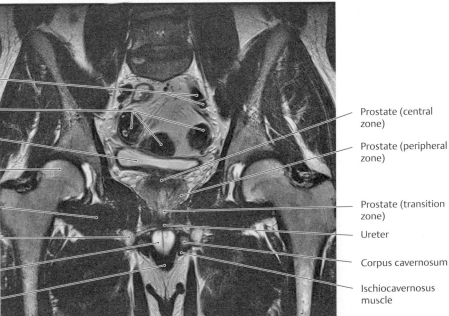

- Common iliac a. and v.
- Sigmoid colon
- Urinary bladder
- Head of femur
- Obturator externus muscle
- Pubis
- Corpus spongiosum
- Bulbospongiosus muscle
- Prostate (central zone)
- Prostate (peripheral zone)
- Prostate (transition zone)
- Ureter
- Corpus cavernosum
- Ischiocavernosus muscle

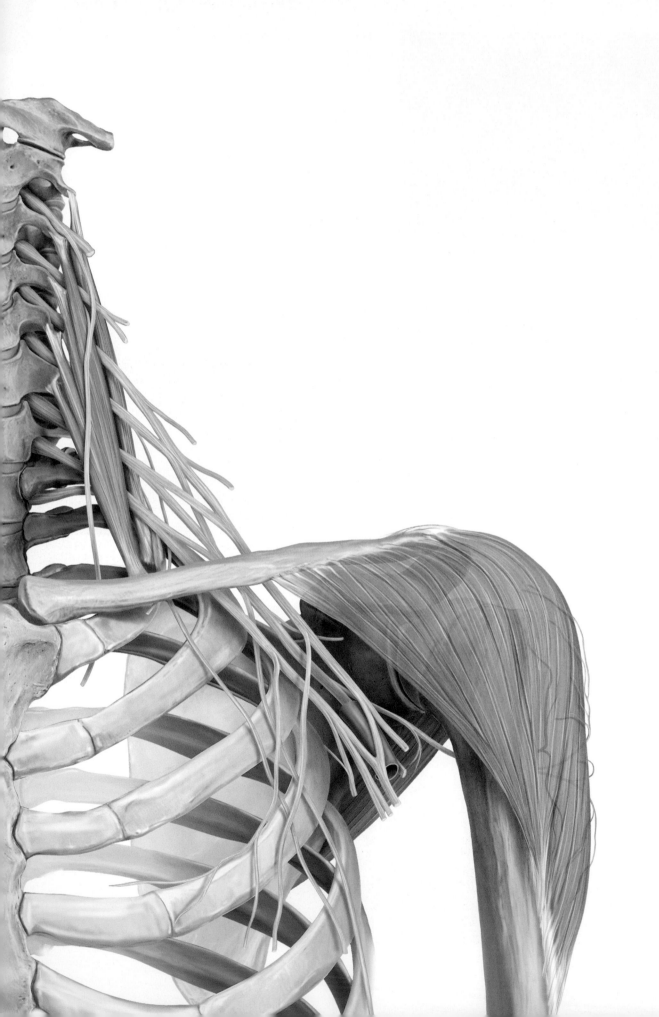

Upper Limb

25 Shoulder & Arm
Bones of the Upper Limb

***Fig. 25.1* Bones of the upper limb**

Right limb. The upper limb is subdivided into three regions: arm, forearm, and hand. The shoulder girdle (clavicle and scapula) joins the upper limb to the thorax at the sternoclavicular joint.

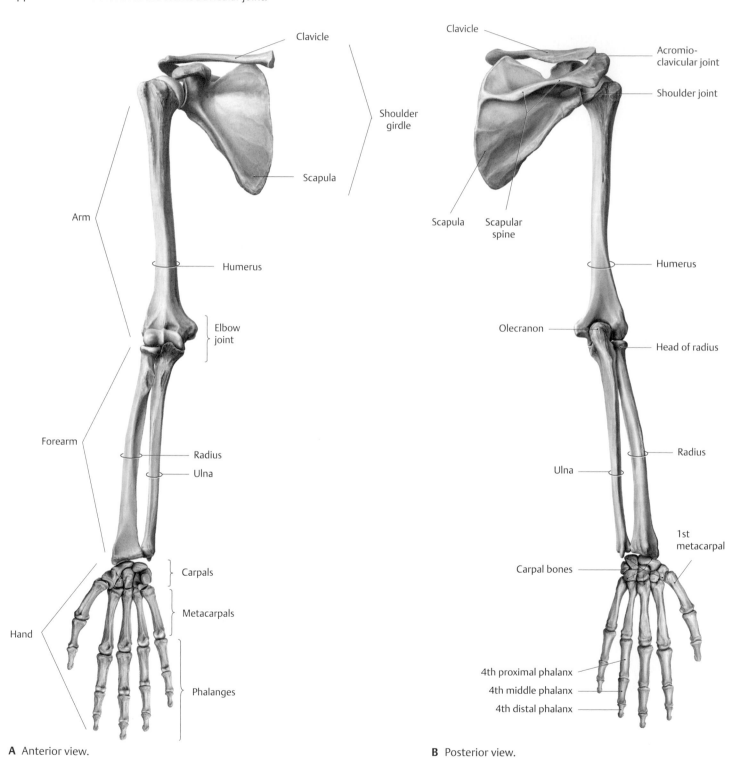

A Anterior view.

B Posterior view.

Fig. 25.2 Bones of the shoulder girdle in normal relation to those of the trunk

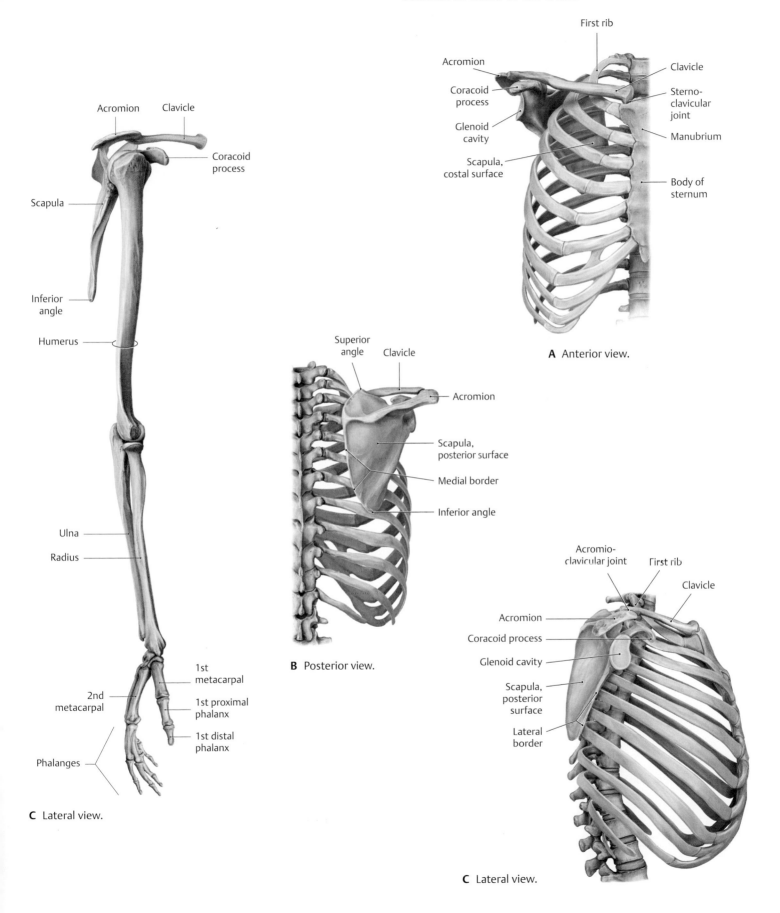

Acromion

Clavicle

Coracoid process

Scapula

Inferior angle

Humerus

Ulna

Radius

2nd metacarpal

Phalanges

1st metacarpal

1st proximal phalanx

1st distal phalanx

C Lateral view.

First rib

Acromion

Coracoid process

Glenoid cavity

Scapula, costal surface

Clavicle

Sterno-clavicular joint

Manubrium

Body of sternum

A Anterior view.

Superior angle

Clavicle

Acromion

Scapula, posterior surface

Medial border

Inferior angle

B Posterior view.

Acromio-clavicular joint

First rib

Clavicle

Acromion

Coracoid process

Glenoid cavity

Scapula, posterior surface

Lateral border

C Lateral view.

Clavicle & Scapula

The shoulder girdle (clavicle and scapula) connects the bones of the upper limb to the thoracic cage. Whereas the pelvic girdle (paired hip bones) is firmly integrated into the axial skeleton (see **p. 230**), the shoulder girdle is extremely mobile.

Fig. 25.3 **Shoulder girdle in situ**
Right shoulder, superior view.

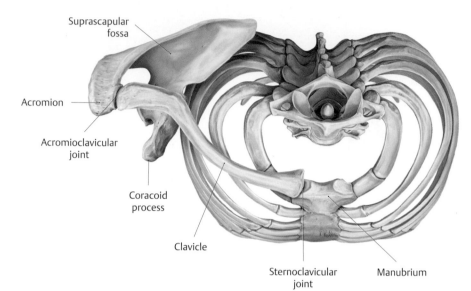

- Suprascapular fossa
- Acromion
- Acromioclavicular joint
- Coracoid process
- Clavicle
- Sternoclavicular joint
- Manubrium

Fig. 25.4 **Clavicle**
Right clavicle. The S-shaped clavicle is visible and palpable along its entire length (generally 12 to 15 cm). Its medial end articulates with the sternum at the sternoclavicular joint. Its lateral end articulates with the scapula at the acromioclavicular joint (see **Fig. 25.3**).

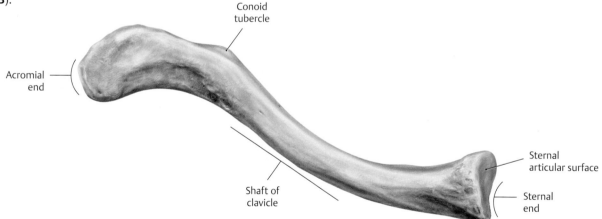

- Conoid tubercle
- Acromial end
- Sternal articular surface
- Sternal end
- Shaft of clavicle

A Superior view.

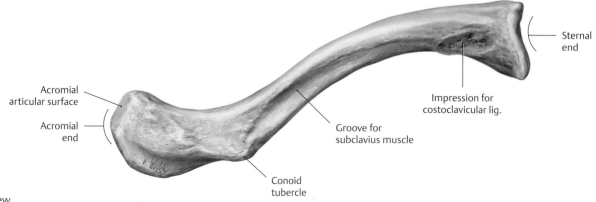

- Sternal end
- Impression for costoclavicular lig.
- Acromial articular surface
- Acromial end
- Groove for subclavius muscle
- Conoid tubercle

B Inferior view.

Fig. 25.5 Scapula

Right scapula. In its normal anatomical position, the scapula extends from the 2nd to the 7th rib.

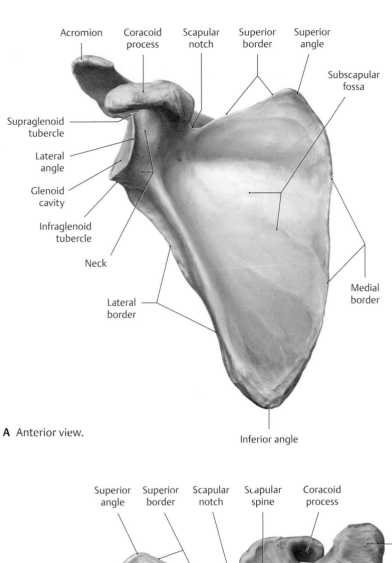

A Anterior view.

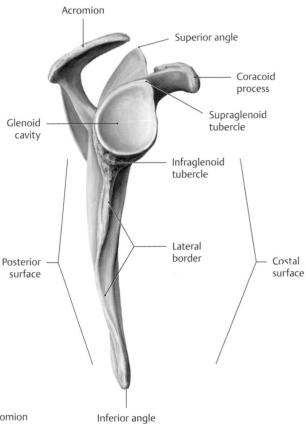

B Right lateral view.

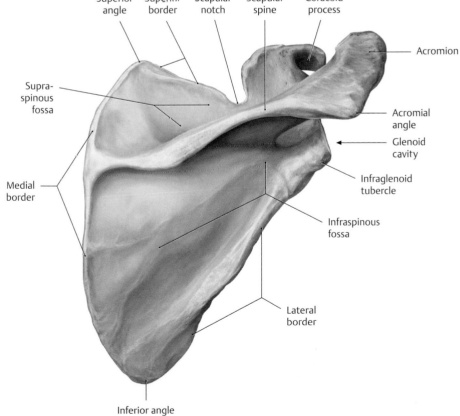

C Posterior view.

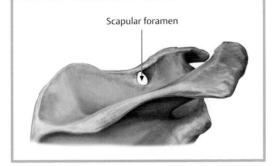

Clinical box 25.1

Scapular foramen

The superior transverse ligament of the scapula (see **Fig. 25.14**) may become ossified, transforming the scapular notch into an anomalous bony canal, the scapular foramen. This can lead to compression of the suprascapular nerve as it passes through the canal (see **p. 381**).

Scapular foramen

Humerus

Fig. 25.6 **Humerus**
Right humerus. The head of the humerus articulates with the scapula at the glenohumeral joint (see **p. 302**). The capitulum and trochlea of the humerus articulate with the radius and ulna, respectively, at the elbow (cubital) joint (see **p. 326**).

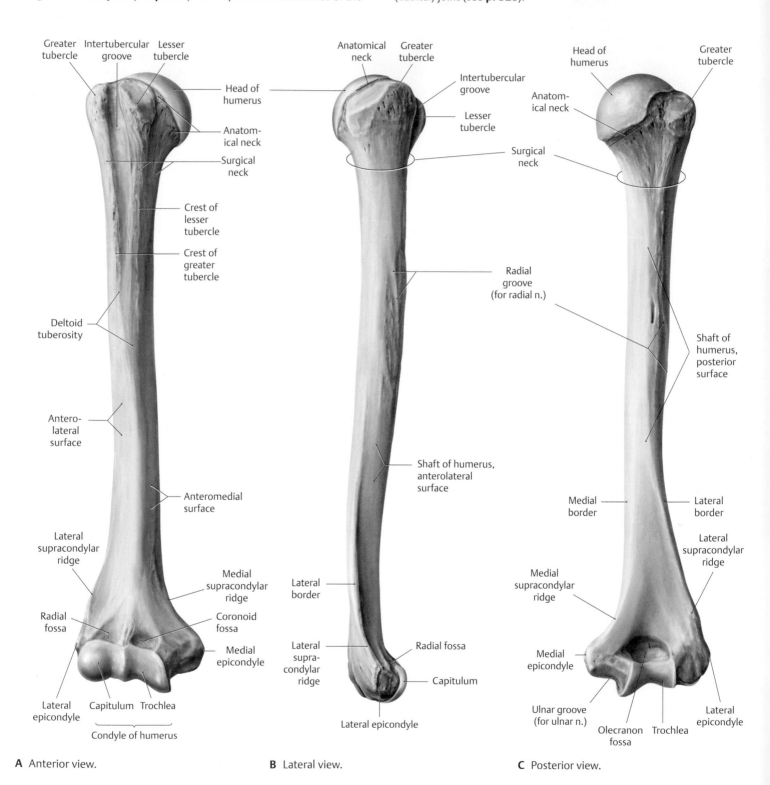

A Anterior view.

B Lateral view.

C Posterior view.

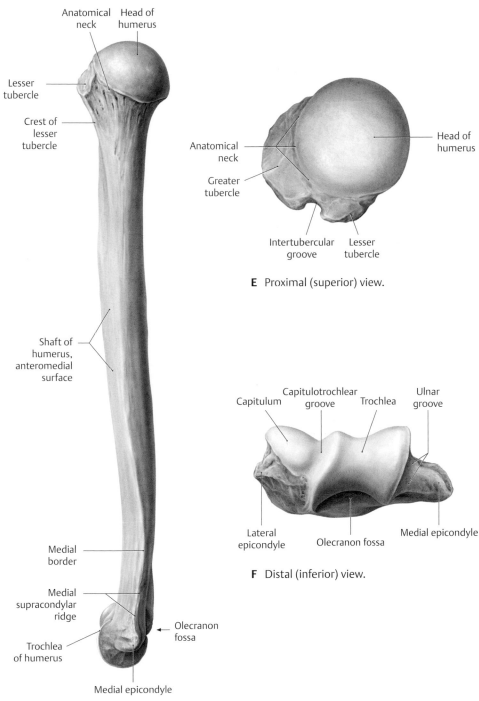

Anatomical neck
Head of humerus
Lesser tubercle
Crest of lesser tubercle
Shaft of humerus, anteromedial surface
Medial border
Medial supracondylar ridge
Trochlea of humerus
Medial epicondyle
Olecranon fossa

D Medial view.

Anatomical neck
Head of humerus
Greater tubercle
Intertubercular groove
Lesser tubercle

E Proximal (superior) view.

Capitulum
Capitulotrochlear groove
Trochlea
Ulnar groove
Lateral epicondyle
Olecranon fossa
Medial epicondyle

F Distal (inferior) view.

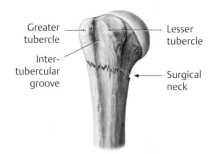

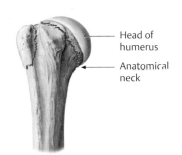

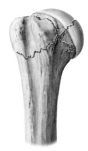

Clinical box 25.2

Fractures of the humerus

Anterior view. Fractures of the proximal humerus are very common and occur predominantly in older patients who sustain a fall onto the outstretched arm or directly onto the shoulder. Three main types are distinguished.

Greater tubercle
Inter-tubercular groove
Lesser tubercle
Surgical neck

A Extra-articular fracture.

Head of humerus
Anatomical neck

B Intra-articular fracture.

C Comminuted fracture.

Extra-articular fractures and intra-articular fractures are often accompanied by injuries of the blood vessels that supply the humeral head (anterior and posterior circumflex humeral arteries), with an associated risk of post-traumatic avascular necrosis.

Fractures of the surgical neck can damage the axillary nerve and fractures of the humeral shaft and distal humerus are frequently associated with damage to the radial nerve.

Joints of the Shoulder

Fig. 25.7 **Joints of the shoulder: Overview**
Right shoulder, anterior view.

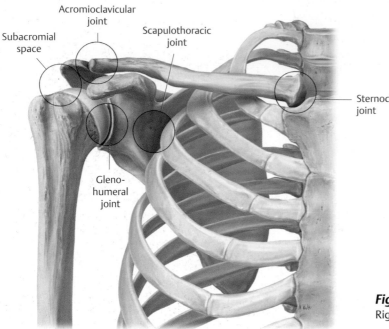

Subacromial space

Acromioclavicular joint

Scapulothoracic joint

Sternoclavicular joint

Gleno-humeral joint

Fig. 25.8 **Joints of the shoulder girdle**
Right side, superior view.

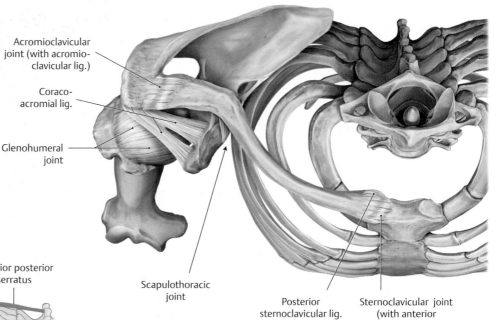

Acromioclavicular joint (with acromio-clavicular lig.)

Coraco-acromial lig.

Glenohumeral joint

Scapulothoracic joint

Posterior sternoclavicular lig.

Sternoclavicular joint (with anterior sternoclavicular lig.)

Fig. 25.9 **Scapulothoracic joint**
Right side, superior view. In all movements of the shoulder girdle, the scapula glides on a curved surface of loose connective tissue between the serratus anterior and the subscapularis muscles. This surface can be considered a scapulothoracic joint.

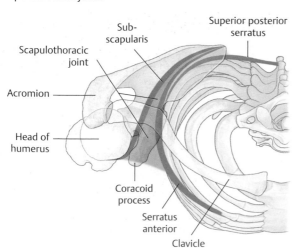

Sub-scapularis

Superior posterior serratus

Scapulothoracic joint

Acromion

Head of humerus

Coracoid process

Serratus anterior

Clavicle

Fig. 25.10 Sternoclavicular joint

Anterior view with sternum coronally sectioned (left). *Note:* A fibrocartilaginous articular disk compensates for the mismatch of surfaces between the two saddle-shaped articular facets of the clavicle and the manubrium.

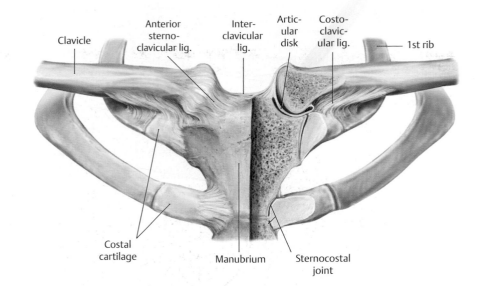

Fig. 25.11 Acromioclavicular joint

Anterior view. The acromioclavicular joint is a plane joint. Because the articulating surfaces are flat, they must be held in place by strong ligaments, greatly limiting the mobility of the joint.

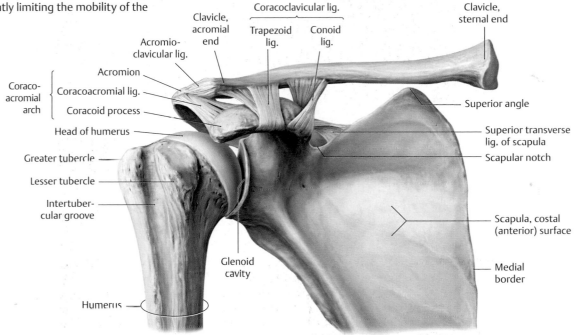

✷ Clinical box 25.3

Injuries of the acromioclavicular joint

A fall onto the outstretched arm or shoulder frequently causes dislocation of the acromioclavicular joint (often known as a "shoulder separation") and damage to the coracoclavicular ligaments.

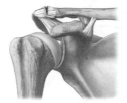
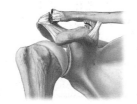
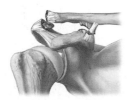

A Stretching of acromio-clavicular ligaments.

B Rupture of acromioclavicular ligament.

C Complete dislocation of acromioclavicular joint. Note rupture of acromioclavicular and coracoclavicular ligaments.

Joints of the Shoulder: Glenohumeral Joint

Fig. 25.12 Glenohumeral joint: Bony elements
Right shoulder.

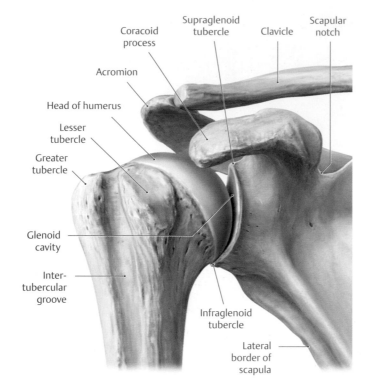

Coracoid process — Supraglenoid tubercle — Clavicle — Scapular notch
Acromion
Head of humerus
Lesser tubercle
Greater tubercle
Glenoid cavity
Inter-tubercular groove
Infraglenoid tubercle
Lateral border of scapula

A Anterior view.

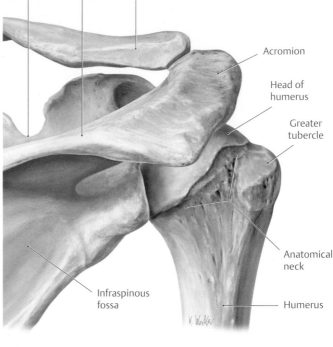

Scapular notch — Scapular spine — Clavicle
Acromion
Head of humerus
Greater tubercle
Anatomical neck
Infraspinous fossa
Humerus

B Posterior view.

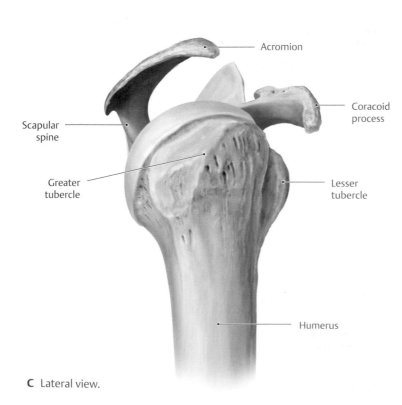

Acromion
Coracoid process
Scapular spine
Greater tubercle
Lesser tubercle
Humerus

C Lateral view.

Fig. 25.13 Glenohumeral joint cavity

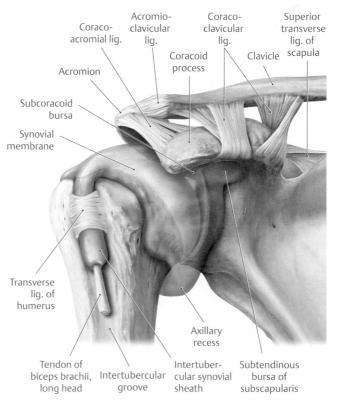

Coraco-acromial lig. — Acromio-clavicular lig. — Coraco-clavicular lig. — Superior transverse lig. of scapula
Acromion — Coracoid process — Clavicle
Subcoracoid bursa
Synovial membrane
Transverse lig. of humerus
Tendon of biceps brachii, long head
Intertubercular groove
Intertuber-cular synovial sheath
Axillary recess
Subtendinous bursa of subscapularis

Fig. 25.14 Glenohumeral joint: Capsule and ligaments

Right shoulder.

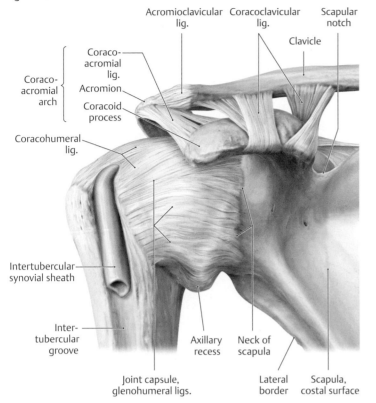

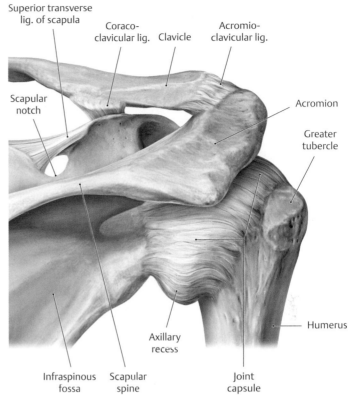

A Anterior view.

B Posterior view.

Fig. 25.15 Ligaments reinforcing capsule

Schematic representation of the ligaments reinforcing the capsule after removal of the humeral head. Right shoulder.

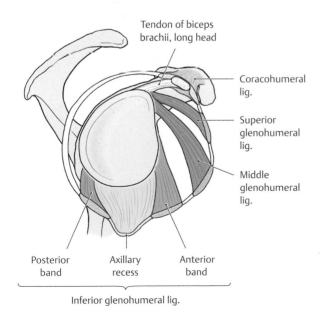

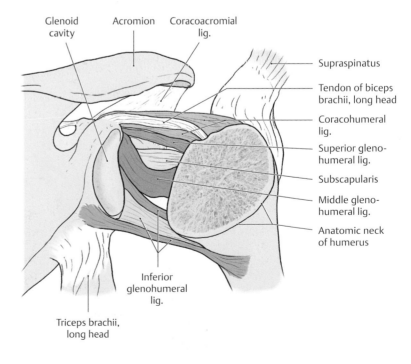

A Lateral view.

B Posterior view.

Subacromial Space & Bursae

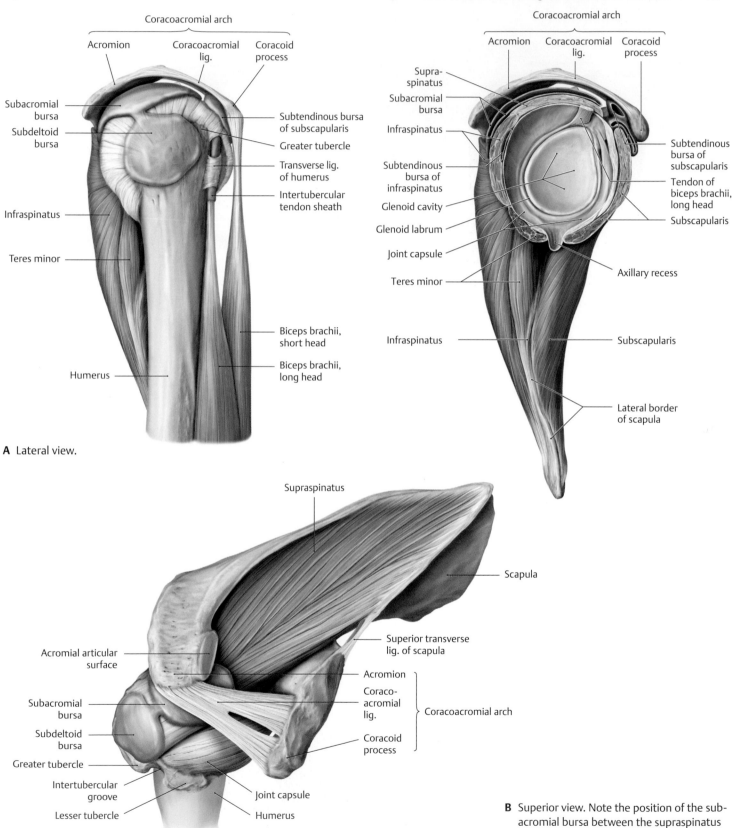

Fig. 25.16 Subacromial space
Right shoulder.

Coracoacromial arch

Acromion — Coracoacromial lig. — Coracoid process

Subacromial bursa

Subdeltoid bursa

Subtendinous bursa of subscapularis

Greater tubercle

Transverse lig. of humerus

Intertubercular tendon sheath

Infraspinatus

Teres minor

Biceps brachii, short head

Humerus

Biceps brachii, long head

A Lateral view.

Fig. 25.17 Subacromial bursa and glenoid cavity
Right shoulder, lateral view of sagittal section with humerus removed.

Coracoacromial arch

Acromion — Coracoacromial lig. — Coracoid process

Supra-spinatus

Subacromial bursa

Infraspinatus

Subtendinous bursa of infraspinatus

Glenoid cavity

Glenoid labrum

Joint capsule

Teres minor

Infraspinatus

Subtendinous bursa of subscapularis

Tendon of biceps brachii, long head

Subscapularis

Axillary recess

Subscapularis

Lateral border of scapula

Supraspinatus

Scapula

Superior transverse lig. of scapula

Acromial articular surface

Acromion

Coraco-acromial lig.

Coracoacromial arch

Coracoid process

Subacromial bursa

Subdeltoid bursa

Greater tubercle

Intertubercular groove

Joint capsule

Lesser tubercle

Humerus

B Superior view. Note the position of the sub-acromial bursa between the supraspinatus muscle and the coracoacromial arch.

Fig. 25.18 Subacromial and subdeltoid bursae

Right shoulder, anterior view.

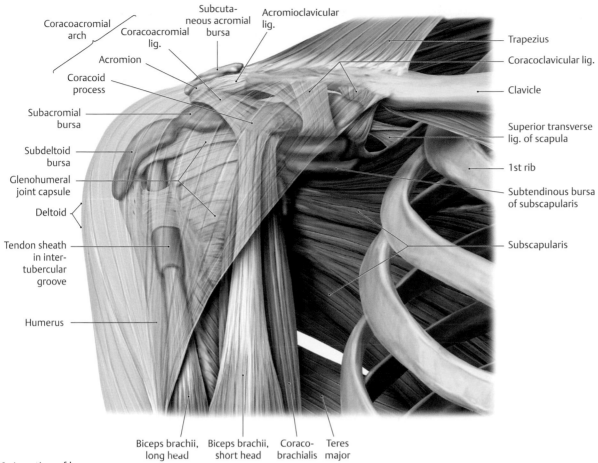

Coracoacromial arch
Coracoacromial lig.
Subcutaneous acromial bursa
Acromioclavicular lig.
Acromion
Coracoid process
Subacromial bursa
Subdeltoid bursa
Glenohumeral joint capsule
Deltoid
Tendon sheath in intertubercular groove
Humerus
Biceps brachii, long head
Biceps brachii, short head
Coracobrachialis
Teres major
Trapezius
Coracoclavicular lig.
Clavicle
Superior transverse lig. of scapula
1st rib
Subtendinous bursa of subscapularis
Subscapularis

A Location of bursae.

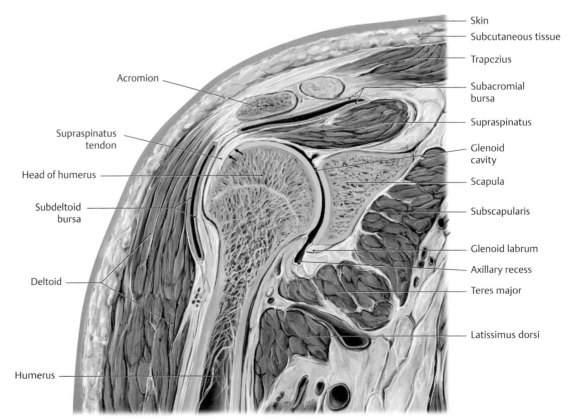

Acromion
Supraspinatus tendon
Head of humerus
Subdeltoid bursa
Deltoid
Humerus
Skin
Subcutaneous tissue
Trapezius
Subacromial bursa
Supraspinatus
Glenoid cavity
Scapula
Subscapularis
Glenoid labrum
Axillary recess
Teres major
Latissimus dorsi

B Coronal section. The arrows are pointing at the supraspinatus tendon, which is frequently injured in a "rotator cuff tear" (for rotator cuff, see **p. 317**).

Anterior Muscles of the Shoulder & Arm (I)

Fig. 25.19 Anterior muscles of the shoulder and arm
Right side, anterior view. Muscle origins are shown in red, insertions in blue.

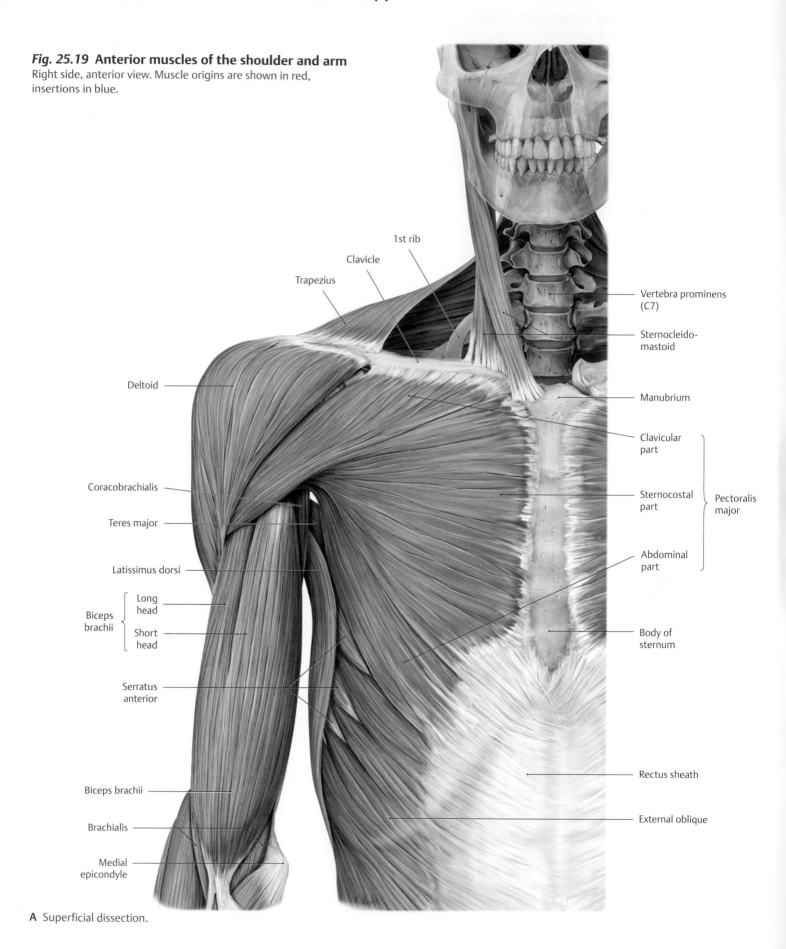

A Superficial dissection.

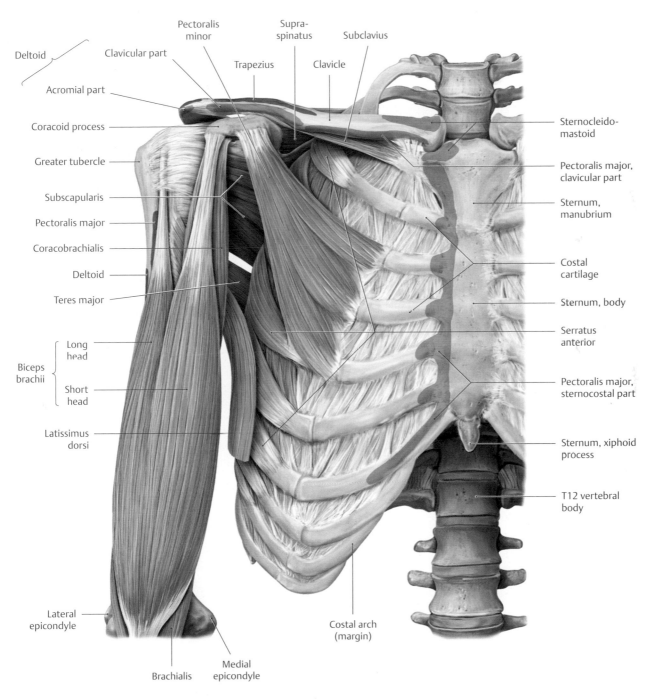

Deltoid

Clavicular part

Acromial part

Coracoid process

Greater tubercle

Subscapularis

Pectoralis major

Coracobrachialis

Deltoid

Teres major

Biceps brachii { Long head

Short head

Latissimus dorsi

Lateral epicondyle

Brachialis

Medial epicondyle

Pectoralis minor

Supra-spinatus

Subclavius

Trapezius

Clavicle

Sternocleido-mastoid

Pectoralis major, clavicular part

Sternum, manubrium

Costal cartilage

Sternum, body

Serratus anterior

Pectoralis major, sternocostal part

Sternum, xiphoid process

T12 vertebral body

Costal arch (margin)

B Deep dissection. *Removed:* Sternocleidomastoid, trapezius, pectoralis major, deltoid, and external oblique muscles.

Anterior Muscles of the Shoulder & Arm (II)

***Fig. 25.20* Anterior muscles of the shoulder and arm: Dissection**

Right arm, anterior view. Muscle origins are shown in red, insertions in blue.

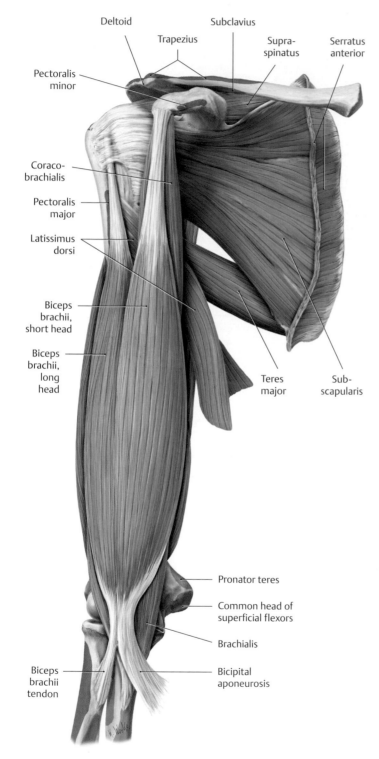

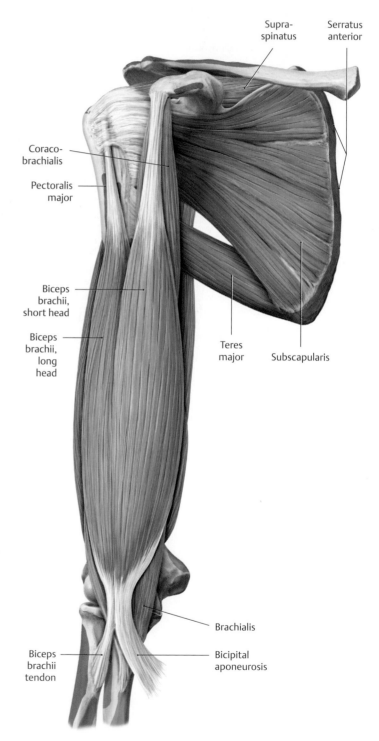

A *Removed:* Thoracic skeleton. *Partially removed:* Latissimus dorsi and serratus anterior.

B *Removed:* Latissimus dorsi and serratus anterior.

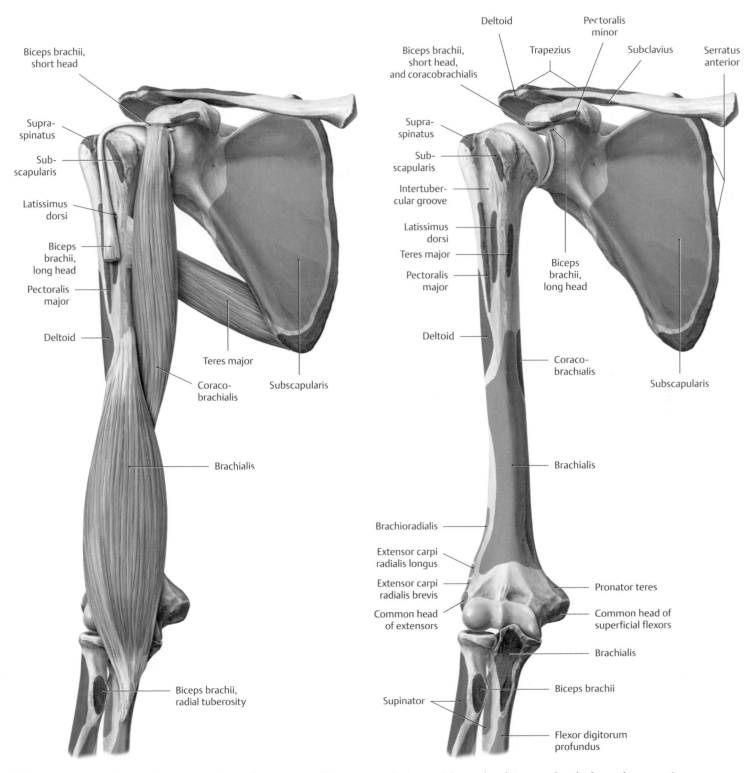

C *Removed:* Subscapularis and supraspinatus. *Partially removed:* Biceps brachii.

D *Removed:* Biceps brachii, coracobrachialis, and teres major.

Posterior Muscles of the Shoulder & Arm (I)

Fig. 25.21 **Posterior muscles of the shoulder and arm**
Right side, posterior view.

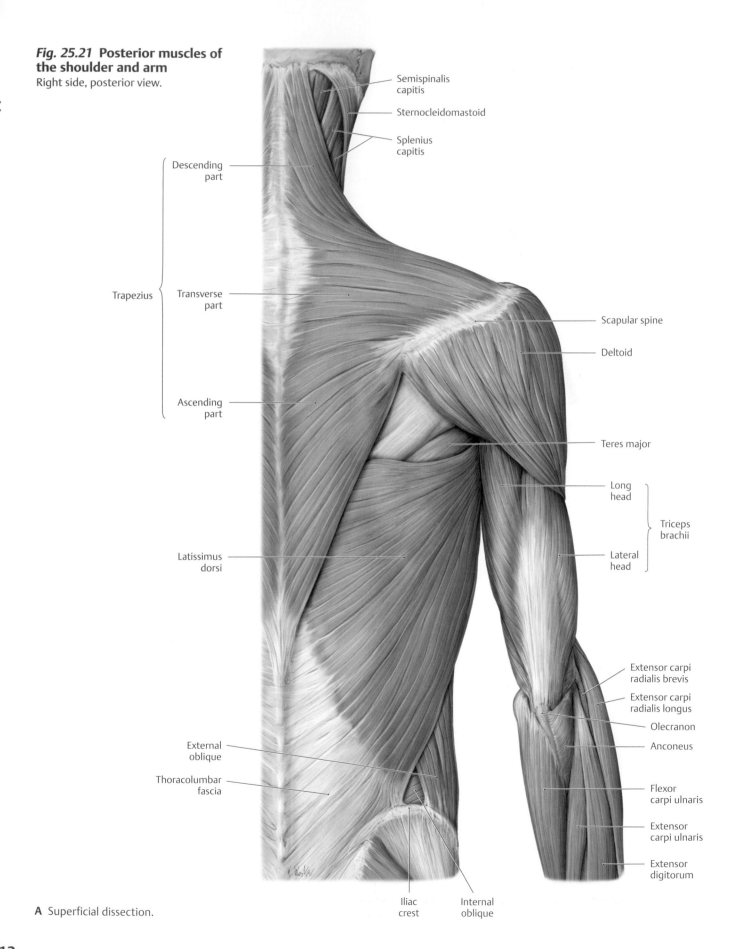

Semispinalis capitis

Sternocleidomastoid

Splenius capitis

Descending part

Trapezius

Transverse part

Scapular spine

Deltoid

Ascending part

Teres major

Long head

Triceps brachii

Lateral head

Latissimus dorsi

Extensor carpi radialis brevis

Extensor carpi radialis longus

Olecranon

Anconeus

External oblique

Thoracolumbar fascia

Flexor carpi ulnaris

Extensor carpi ulnaris

Extensor digitorum

Iliac crest

Internal oblique

A Superficial dissection.

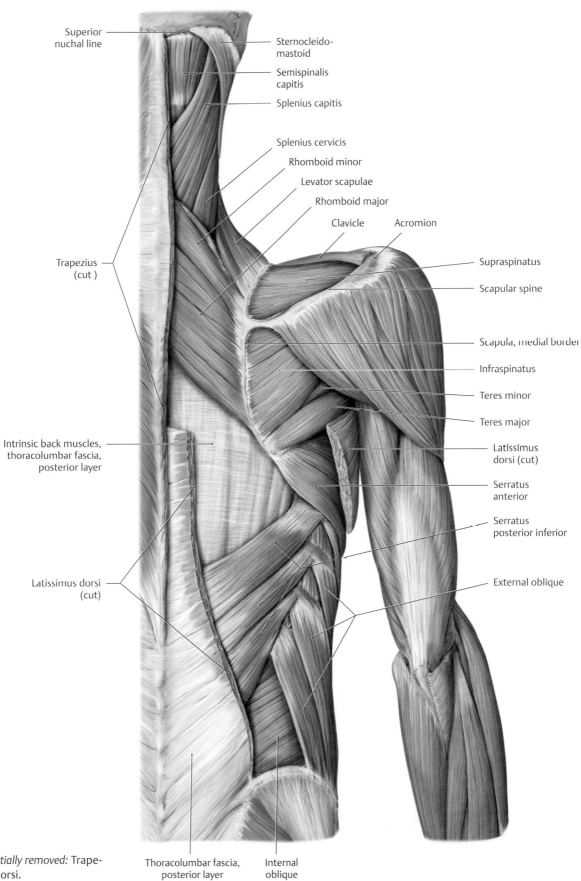

Superior
nuchal line

Sternocleido-
mastoid

Semispinalis
capitis

Splenius capitis

Splenius cervicis

Rhomboid minor

Levator scapulae

Rhomboid major

Clavicle   Acromion

Supraspinatus

Scapular spine

Trapezius
(cut)

Scapula, medial border

Infraspinatus

Teres minor

Teres major

Intrinsic back muscles,
thoracolumbar fascia,
posterior layer

Latissimus
dorsi (cut)

Serratus
anterior

Serratus
posterior inferior

Latissimus dorsi
(cut)

External oblique

B Deep dissection. *Partially removed:* Trapezius and latissimus dorsi.

Thoracolumbar fascia,
posterior layer

Internal
oblique

Posterior Muscles of the Shoulder & Arm (II)

Fig. 25.22 Posterior muscles of the shoulder and arm: Dissection

Right arm, posterior view. Muscle origins are shown in red, insertions in blue.

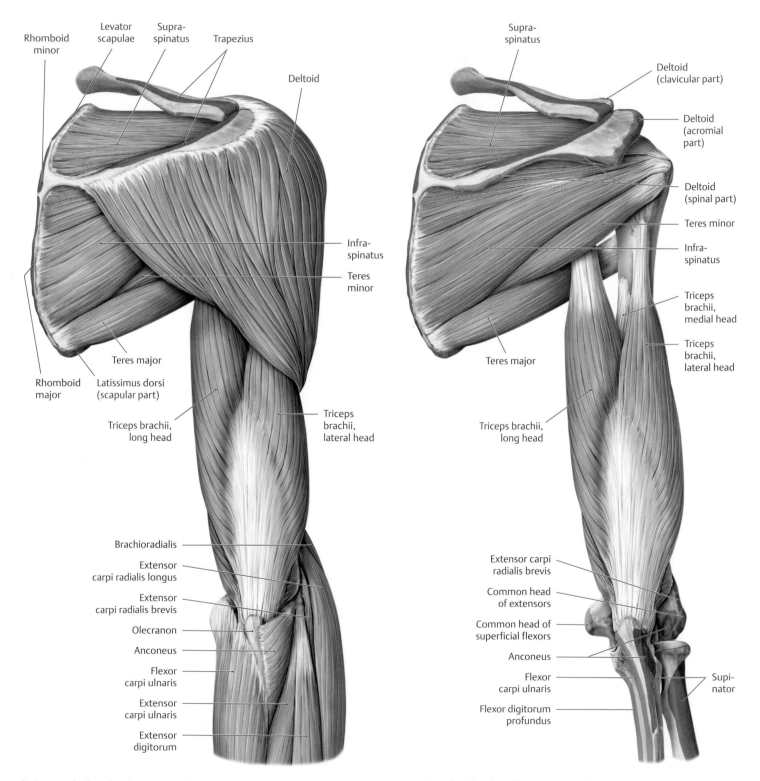

A *Removed:* Rhomboids major and minor, serratus anterior, and levator scapulae.

B *Removed:* Deltoid and forearm muscles.

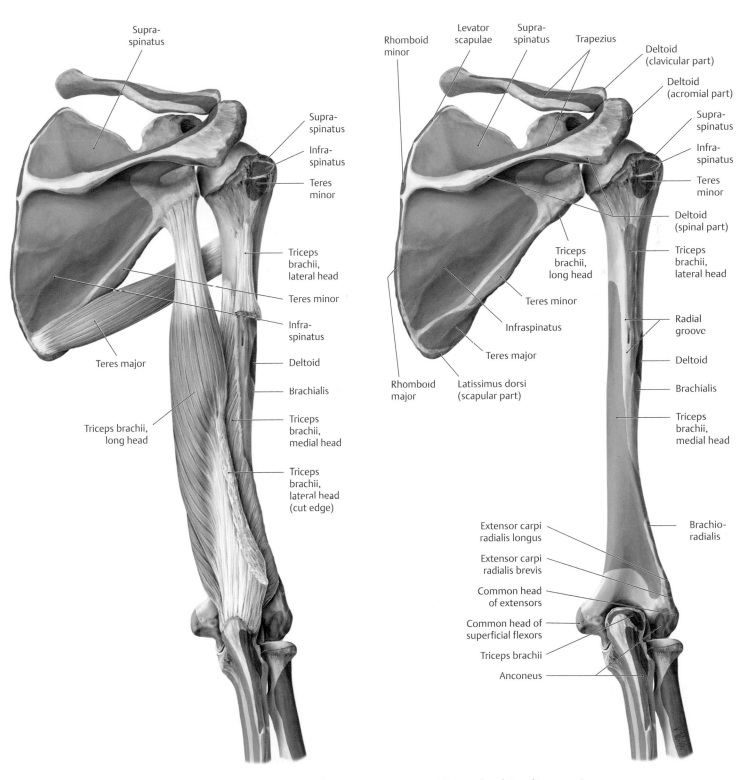

Supra-
spinatus

Supra-
spinatus

Infra-
spinatus

Teres
minor

Triceps
brachii,
lateral head

Teres minor

Infra-
spinatus

Deltoid

Brachialis

Triceps
brachii,
medial head

Triceps
brachii,
lateral head
(cut edge)

Teres major

Triceps brachii,
long head

Rhomboid
minor

Levator
scapulae

Supra-
spinatus

Trapezius

Deltoid
(clavicular part)

Deltoid
(acromial part)

Supra-
spinatus

Infra-
spinatus

Teres
minor

Deltoid
(spinal part)

Triceps
brachii,
long head

Teres minor

Infraspinatus

Teres major

Triceps
brachii,
lateral head

Radial
groove

Deltoid

Brachialis

Triceps
brachii,
medial head

Rhomboid
major

Latissimus dorsi
(scapular part)

Extensor carpi
radialis longus

Extensor carpi
radialis brevis

Common head
of extensors

Common head of
superficial flexors

Triceps brachii

Anconeus

Brachio-
radialis

C *Removed:* Supraspinatus, infraspinatus, and teres minor. *Partially removed:* Triceps brachii.

D *Removed:* Triceps brachii and teres major.

Muscle Facts (I)

The actions of the three parts of the deltoid muscle depend on their relationship to the position of the humerus and its axis of motion. At less than 60 degrees, the muscles act as adductors, but at greater than 60 degrees, they act as abductors. As a result, the parts of the deltoid can act antagonistically as well as synergistically.

Fig. 25.23 **Deltoid**
Right shoulder.

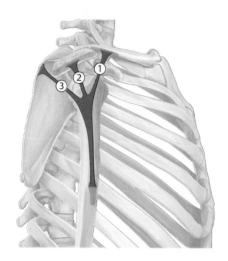

A Parts of the deltoid, right lateral view, schematic.

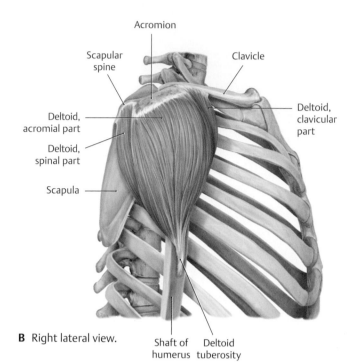

B Right lateral view.

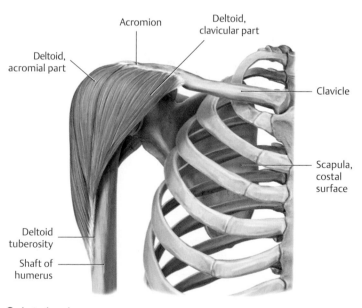

C Anterior view.

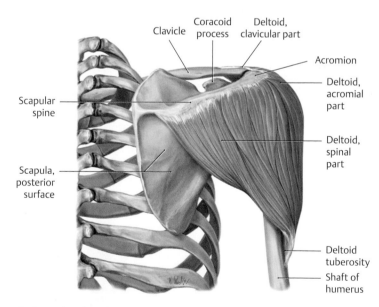

D Posterior view.

Table 25.1	Parts of the deltoid				
Muscle		**Origin**	**Insertion**	**Innervation**	**Action***
Deltoid	① Clavicular (anterior) part	Lateral one third of clavicle	Humerus (deltoid tuberosity)	Axillary n. (C5, C6)	Flexion, internal rotation, adduction
	② Acromial (lateral) part	Acromion			Abduction
	③ Spinal (posterior) part	Scapular spine			Extension, external rotation, adduction
* Between 60 and 90 degrees of abduction, the clavicular and spinal parts assist the acromial part with abduction.					

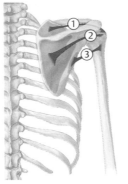

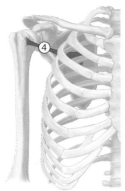

A Posterior view, schematic.

B Anterior view, schematic.

Fig. 25.24 Rotator cuff

Right shoulder. The rotator cuff consists of four muscles: supraspinatus, infraspinatus, teres minor, and subscapularis.

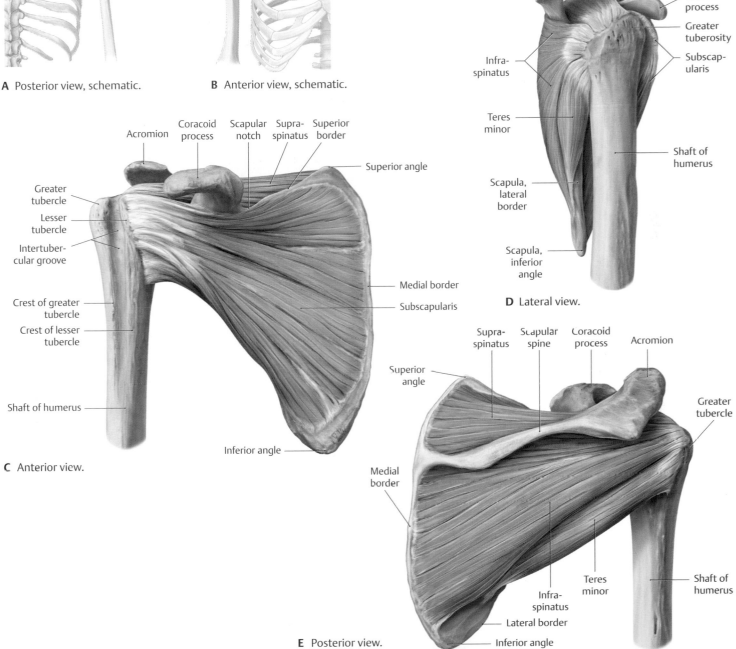

C Anterior view.

D Lateral view.

E Posterior view.

Table 25.2	Muscles of the rotator cuff				
Muscle	**Origin**		**Insertion**	**Innervation**	**Action**
① Supraspinatus	Scapula	Supraspinous fossa	Humerus (greater tuberosity)	Suprascapular n. (C4–C6)	Initiates abduction
② Infraspinatus		Infraspinous fossa			External rotation
③ Teres minor		Lateral border	Humerus	Axillary n. (C5, C6)	External rotation, weak adduction
④ Subscapularis		Subscapular fossa	Humerus (lesser tubercle)	Upper and lower subscapular nn. (C5, C6)	Internal rotation

Muscle Facts (II)

Fig. 25.25 **Pectoralis major and coracobrachialis**
Anterior view.

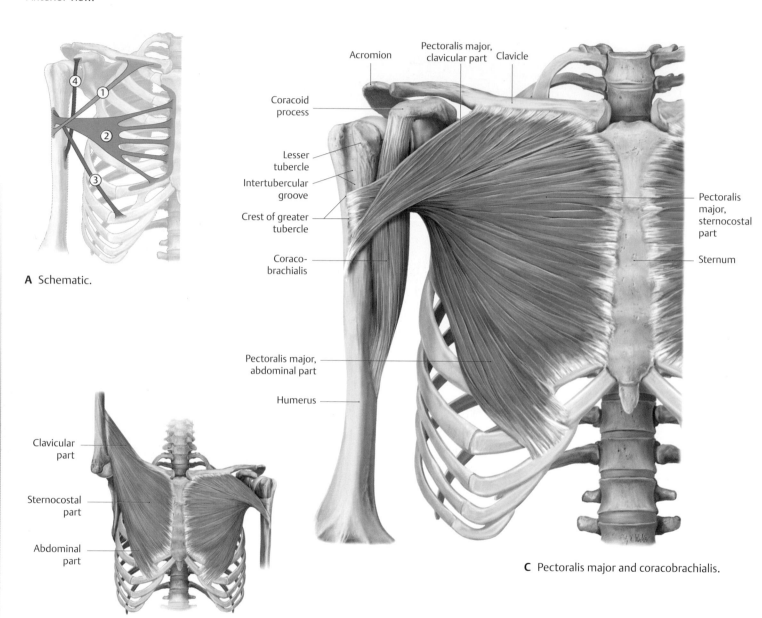

A Schematic.

Acromion

Pectoralis major, clavicular part

Clavicle

Coracoid process

Lesser tubercle

Intertubercular groove

Crest of greater tubercle

Coraco-brachialis

Pectoralis major, abdominal part

Humerus

Pectoralis major, sternocostal part

Sternum

Clavicular part

Sternocostal part

Abdominal part

B Pectoralis major in neutral position (left) and elevation (right).

C Pectoralis major and coracobrachialis.

Table 25.3		Pectoralis major and coracobrachialis			
Muscle		**Origin**	**Insertion**	**Innervation**	**Action**
Pectoralis major	① Clavicular part	Clavicle (medial half)	Humerus (crest of greater tubercle)	Medial and lateral pectoral nn. (C5–T1)	Entire muscle: adduction, internal rotation
	② Sternocostal part	Sternum and costal cartilages 1–6			Clavicular and sternocostal parts: flexion; assist in respiration when shoulder is fixed
	③ Abdominal part	Rectus sheath (anterior layer)			
④ Coracobrachialis		Scapula (coracoid process)	Humerus (in line with crest of lesser tubercle)	Musculocutaneous n. (C5–C7)	Flexion, adduction, internal rotation

Fig. 25.26 **Subclavius and pectoralis minor**
Right side, anterior view.

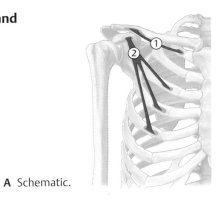

A Schematic.

Fig. 25.27 **Serratus anterior**
Right lateral view.

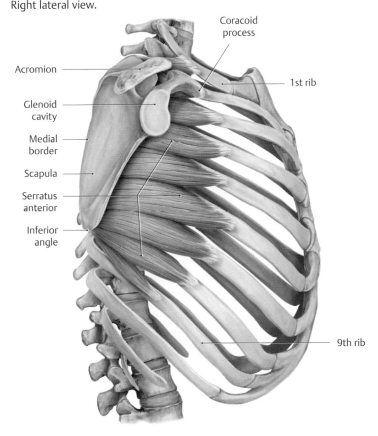

A Serratus anterior.

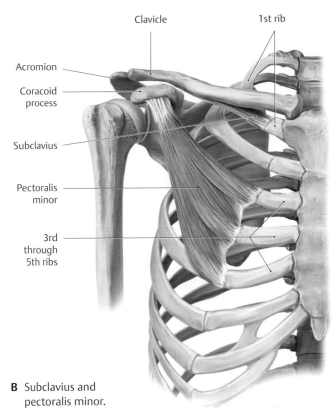

B Subclavius and pectoralis minor.

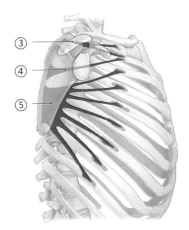

B Schematic.

Table 25.4		Subclavius, pectoralis minor, and serratus anterior			
Muscle		**Origin**	**Insertion**	**Innervation**	**Action**
① Subclavius		1st rib	Clavicle (inferior surface)	N. to subclavius (C5, C6)	Steadies the clavicle in the sternoclavicular joint
② Pectoralis minor		3rd to 5th ribs	Coracoid process	Medial pectoral n. (C8, T1)	Draws scapula downward, causing inferior angle to move posteromedially; rotates glenoid inferiorly; assists in respiration
Serratus anterior	③ Superior part	1st to 9th ribs	Scapula (costal and dorsal surfaces of superior angle)	Long thoracic n. (C5–C7)	Superior part: lowers the raised arm
	④ Intermediate part		Scapula (costal surface of medial border)		Entire muscle: draws scapula laterally forward; elevates ribs when shoulder is fixed
	⑤ Inferior part		Scapula (costal surface of medial border and costal and dorsal surfaces of inferior angle)		Inferior part: rotates inferior angle of scapula laterally forward (allows elevation of arm above 90°)

Muscle Facts (III)

Fig. 25.28 **Trapezius**
Posterior view.

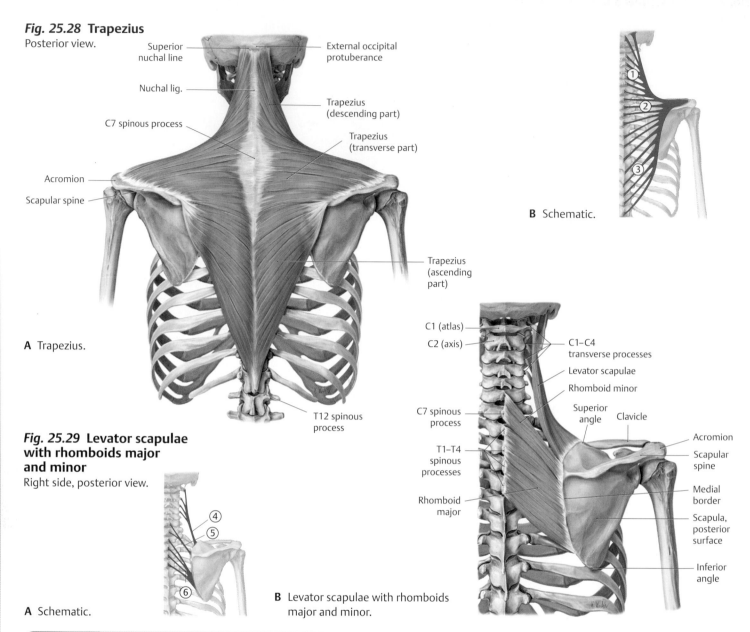

Superior
nuchal line

External occipital
protuberance

Nuchal lig.

Trapezius
(descending part)

C7 spinous process

Trapezius
(transverse part)

Acromion

Scapular spine

Trapezius
(ascending
part)

A Trapezius.

T12 spinous
process

B Schematic.

C1 (atlas)

C2 (axis)

C1–C4
transverse processes

Levator scapulae

Rhomboid minor

Superior
angle

Clavicle

C7 spinous
process

Acromion

Scapular
spine

T1–T4
spinous
processes

Medial
border

Rhomboid
major

Scapula,
posterior
surface

Inferior
angle

Fig. 25.29 **Levator scapulae
with rhomboids major
and minor**
Right side, posterior view.

A Schematic.

B Levator scapulae with rhomboids
major and minor.

Table 25.5		Trapezius, levator scapulae, and rhomboids major and minor			
Muscle		**Origin**	**Insertion**	**Innervation**	**Action**
Trapezius	① Descending part	Occipital bone; spinous processes of C1–C7	Clavicle (lateral one third)	Accessory n. (CN XI); C3–C4 of cervical plexus	Draws scapula obliquely upward; rotates glenoid cavity superiorly; tilts head to same side and rotates it to opposite
	② Transverse part	Aponeurosis at T1–T4 spinous processes	Acromion		Draws scapula medially
	③ Ascending part	Spinous processes of T5–T12	Scapular spine		Draws scapula medially downward
					Entire muscle: steadies scapula on thorax
④ Levator scapulae		Transverse processes of C1–C4	Scapula (superior angle)	Dorsal scapular n. and cervical spinal nn. (C3–C4)	Draws scapula medially upward while moving inferior angle medially; inclines neck to same side
⑤ Rhomboid minor		Spinous processes of C6, C7	Medial border of scapula above (minor) and below (major) scapular spine	Dorsal scapular n. (C4–C5)	Steadies scapula; draws scapula medially upward
⑥ Rhomboid major		Spinous processes of T1–T4 vertebrae			
CN, cranial nerve.					

Fig. 25.30 Latissimus dorsi and teres major
Posterior view.

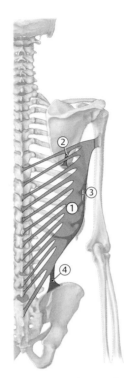

A Latissimus dorsi, schematic.

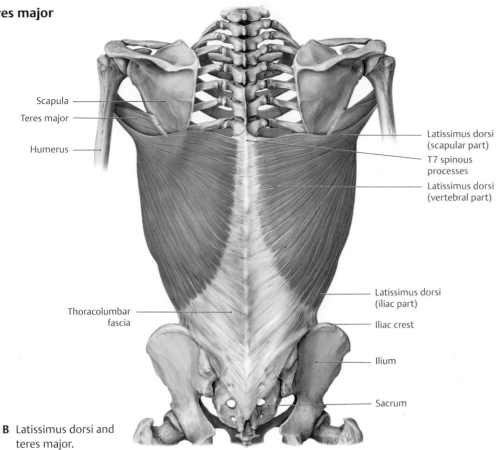

Scapula
Teres major
Humerus

Latissimus dorsi (scapular part)
T7 spinous processes
Latissimus dorsi (vertebral part)

Thoracolumbar fascia

Latissimus dorsi (iliac part)
Iliac crest

Ilium

Sacrum

B Latissimus dorsi and teres major.

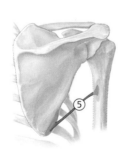

C Teres major, schematic.

D Insertion of the latissimus dorsi on the floor of the intertubercular groove and the teres major on the crest of the lesser tubercle of the humerus.

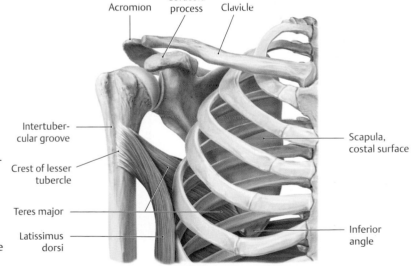

Acromion
Coracoid process
Clavicle

Intertubercular groove

Crest of lesser tubercle

Teres major

Latissimus dorsi

Scapula, costal surface

Inferior angle

Table 25.6		Latissimus dorsi and teres major			
Muscle		**Origin**	**Insertion**	**Innervation**	**Action**
Latissimus dorsi	① Vertebral part	Spinous processes of T7–T12 vertebrae; thoracolumbar fascia	Floor of the intertubercular groove of the humerus	Thoracodorsal n. (C6–C8)	Internal rotation, adduction, extension, respiration ("cough muscle")
	② Scapular part	Scapula (inferior angle)			
	③ Costal part	9th to 12th ribs			
	④ Iliac part	Iliac crest (posterior one third)			
⑤ Teres major		Scapula (inferior angle)	Crest of lesser tubercle of the humerus (anterior angle)	Lower subscapular n. (C5, C6)	Internal rotation, adduction, extension

Muscle Facts (IV)

The anterior and posterior muscles of the arm may be classified respectively as flexors and extensors relative to the movement of the elbow joint. Although the coracobrachialis is topographically part of the anterior compartment, it is functionally grouped with the muscles of the shoulder (see **p. 318**).

Fig. 25.31 Biceps brachii and brachialis
Right arm, anterior view.

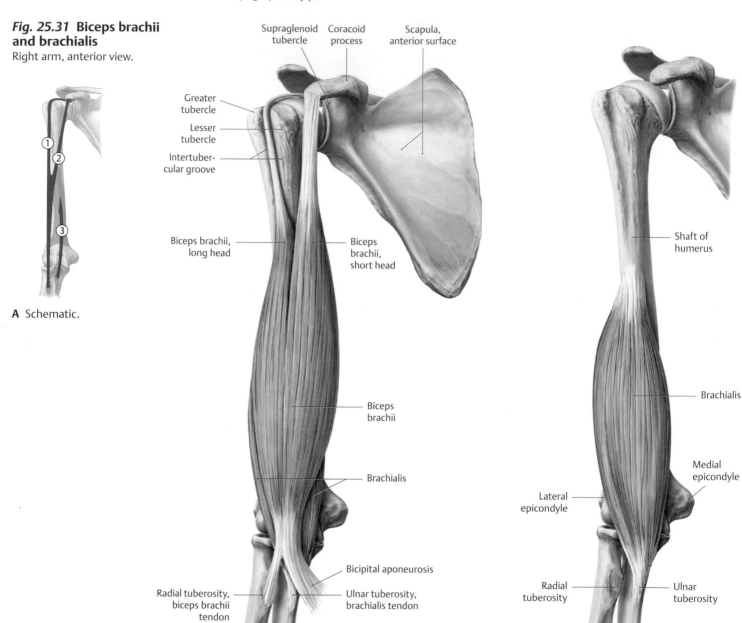

A Schematic.

B Biceps brachii and brachialis.

C Brachialis.

Table 25.7		Anterior muscles: Biceps brachii and brachialis			
Muscle		**Origin**	**Insertion**	**Innervation**	**Action**
Biceps brachii	① Long head	Supraglenoid tubercle of scapula	Radial tuberosity and bicipital aponeurosis	Musculocutaneous n. (C5–C6)	Elbow joint: flexion; supination* Shoulder joint: flexion; stabilization of humeral head during deltoid contraction; abduction and internal rotation of the humerus
	② Short head	Coracoid process of scapula			
③ Brachialis		Humerus (distal half of anterior surface)	Ulnar tuberosity	Musculocutaneous n. (C5–C6) and radial n. (C7, minor)	Flexion at the elbow joint
Note: When the elbow is flexed, the biceps brachii acts as a powerful supinator because the lever arm is almost perpendicular to the axis of pronation/supination.					

Fig. 25.32 Triceps brachii and anconeus

Right arm, posterior view.

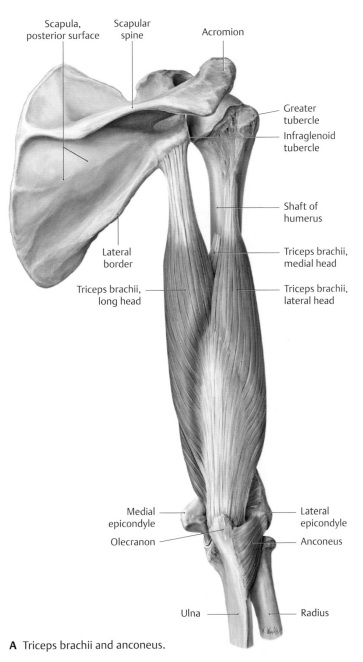

Scapula, posterior surface
Scapular spine
Acromion
Greater tubercle
Infraglenoid tubercle
Shaft of humerus
Triceps brachii, medial head
Triceps brachii, lateral head
Lateral border
Triceps brachii, long head
Medial epicondyle
Olecranon
Lateral epicondyle
Anconeus
Ulna
Radius

A Triceps brachii and anconeus.

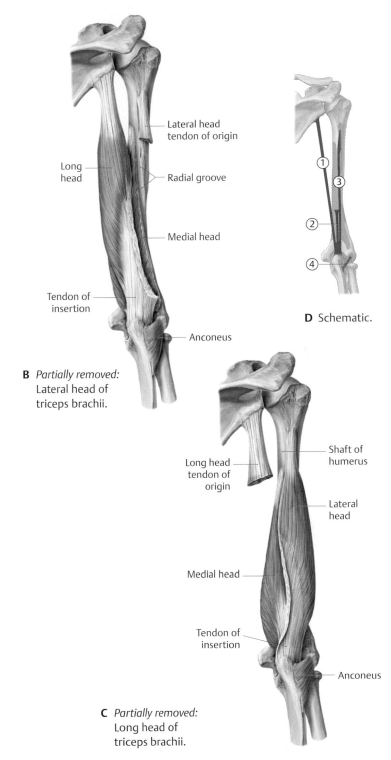

Lateral head tendon of origin
Long head
Radial groove
Medial head
Tendon of insertion
Anconeus

B *Partially removed:* Lateral head of triceps brachii.

D Schematic.

Shaft of humerus
Long head tendon of origin
Lateral head
Medial head
Tendon of insertion
Anconeus

C *Partially removed:* Long head of triceps brachii.

Table 25.8		Posterior muscles: Triceps brachii and anconeus			
Muscle		**Origin**	**Insertion**	**Innervation**	**Action**
Triceps brachii	① Long head	Scapula (infraglenoid tubercle)	Olecranon of ulna	Radial n. (C6–C8)	Elbow joint: extension Shoulder joint, long head: extension and adduction
	② Medial head	Posterior humerus, distal to radial groove; medial intermuscular septum			
	③ Lateral head	Posterior humerus, proximal to radial groove; lateral intermuscular septum			
④ Anconeus		Lateral epicondyle of humerus (variance: posterior joint capsule)	Olecranon of ulna (radial surface)		Extends the elbow and tightens its joint

26 Elbow & Forearm
Radius & Ulna

***Fig. 26.1* Radius and ulna**
Right forearm.

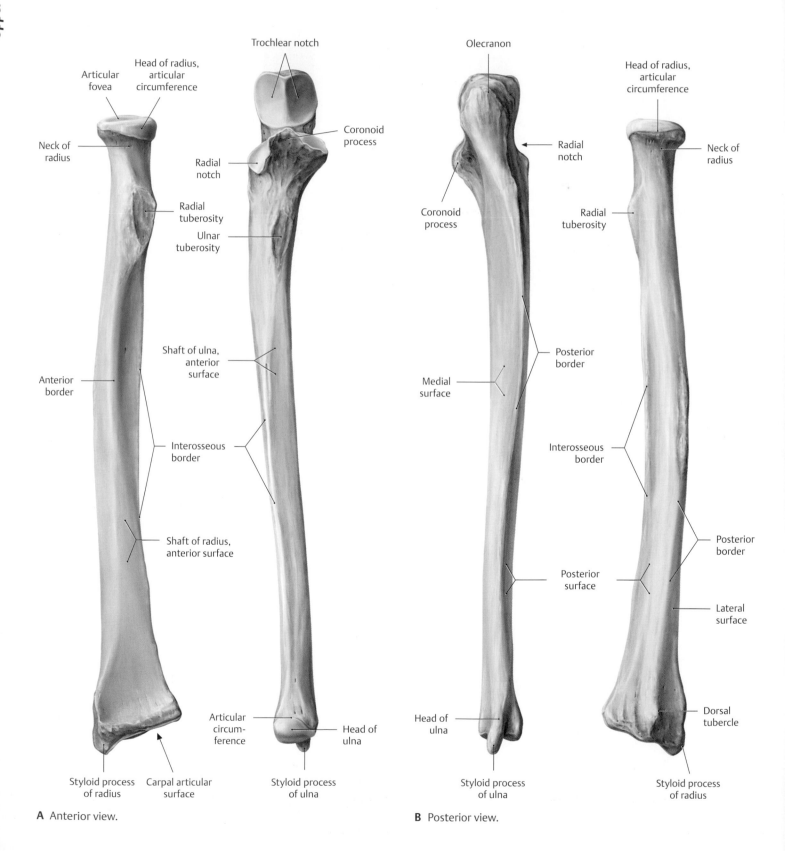

A Anterior view.

B Posterior view.

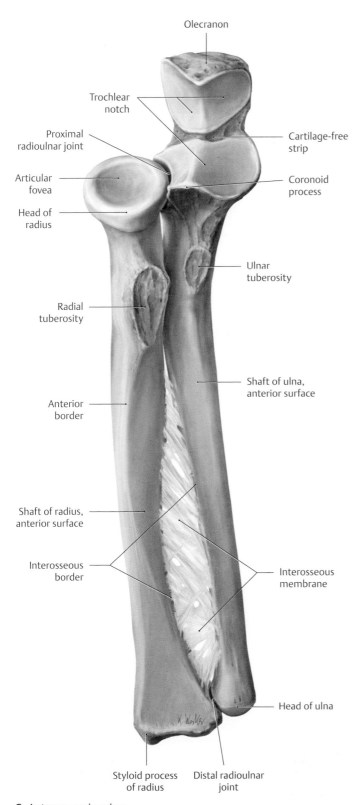

Olecranon

Trochlear
notch

Proximal
radioulnar joint

Articular
fovea

Head of
radius

Cartilage-free
strip

Coronoid
process

Ulnar
tuberosity

Radial
tuberosity

Shaft of ulna,
anterior surface

Anterior
border

Shaft of radius,
anterior surface

Interosseous
border

Interosseous
membrane

Head of ulna

Styloid process
of radius

Distal radioulnar
joint

C Anterosuperior view.

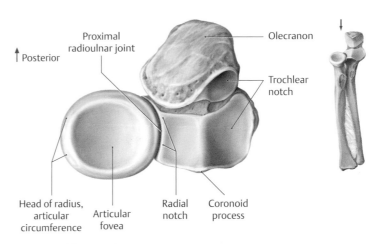

↑ Posterior

Proximal
radioulnar joint

Olecranon

Trochlear
notch

Head of radius,
articular
circumference

Articular
fovea

Radial
notch

Coronoid
process

D Proximal (superior) view.

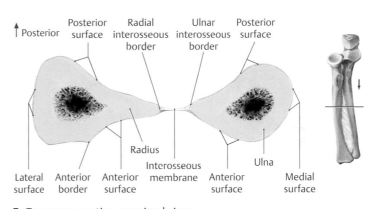

↑ Posterior

Posterior
surface

Radial
interosseous
border

Ulnar
interosseous
border

Posterior
surface

Lateral
surface

Anterior
border

Anterior
surface

Radius

Interosseous
membrane

Anterior
surface

Ulna

Medial
surface

E Transverse section, proximal view.

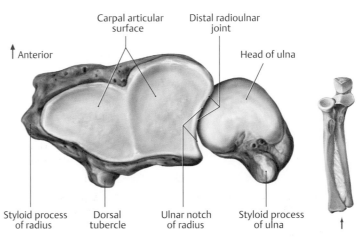

↑ Anterior

Carpal articular
surface

Distal radioulnar
joint

Head of ulna

Styloid process
of radius

Dorsal
tubercle

Ulnar notch
of radius

Styloid process
of ulna

F Distal (inferior) view.

Elbow Joint

Fig. 26.2 Elbow (cubital) joint

Right limb. The elbow consists of three articulations between the humerus, ulna, and radius: the humeroulnar, humeroradial, and proximal radioulnar joints.

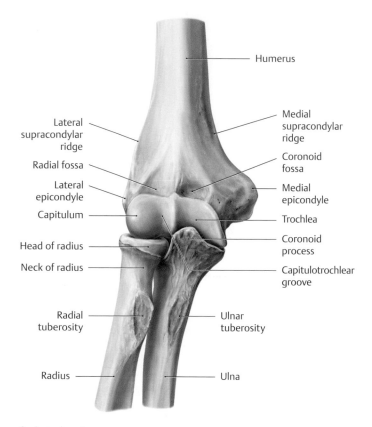

Labels (left to right, clockwise):
Humerus
Lateral supracondylar ridge
Radial fossa
Lateral epicondyle
Capitulum
Head of radius
Neck of radius
Radial tuberosity
Radius
Medial supracondylar ridge
Coronoid fossa
Medial epicondyle
Trochlea
Coronoid process
Capitulotrochlear groove
Ulnar tuberosity
Ulna

A Anterior view.

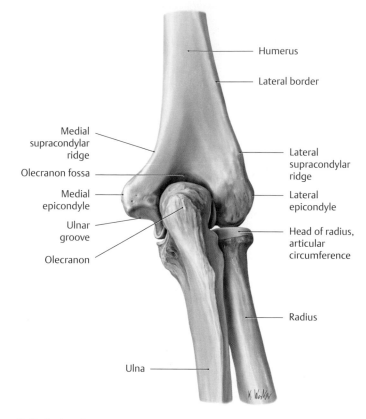

Labels:
Humerus
Lateral border
Medial supracondylar ridge
Olecranon fossa
Medial epicondyle
Ulnar groove
Olecranon
Lateral supracondylar ridge
Lateral epicondyle
Head of radius, articular circumference
Radius
Ulna

B Posterior view.

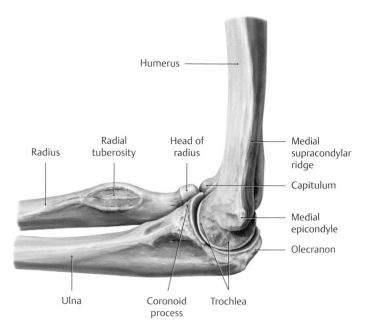

Labels:
Humerus
Radius
Radial tuberosity
Head of radius
Medial supracondylar ridge
Capitulum
Medial epicondyle
Olecranon
Ulna
Coronoid process
Trochlea

C Medial view.

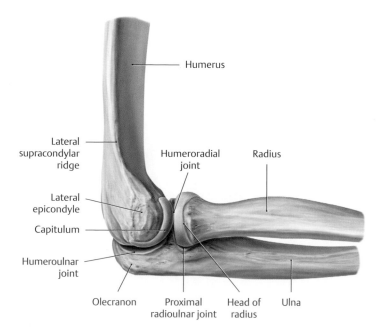

Labels:
Humerus
Lateral supracondylar ridge
Lateral epicondyle
Capitulum
Humeroulnar joint
Humeroradial joint
Radius
Olecranon
Proximal radioulnar joint
Head of radius
Ulna

D Lateral view.

Fig. 26.3 **Skeletal and soft-tissue elements of the right elbow joint**

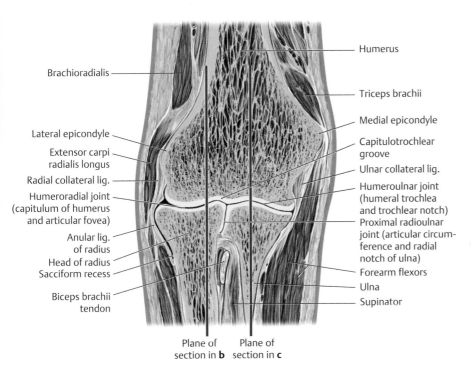
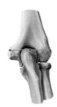

Humerus

Brachioradialis

Triceps brachii

Medial epicondyle

Lateral epicondyle

Capitulotrochlear groove

Extensor carpi radialis longus

Ulnar collateral lig.

Radial collateral lig.

Humeroradial joint (capitulum of humerus and articular fovea)

Humeroulnar joint (humeral trochlea and trochlear notch)

Proximal radioulnar joint (articular circumference and radial notch of ulna)

Anular lig. of radius

Head of radius
Sacciform recess

Forearm flexors

Ulna

Biceps brachii tendon

Supinator

Plane of section in **b**   Plane of section in **c**

A Coronal section viewed from the front (note the planes of section shown in **B** and **C**).

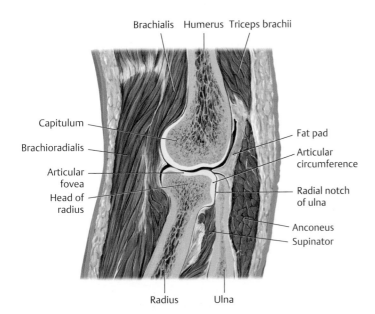

Brachialis   Humerus   Triceps brachii

Capitulum

Brachioradialis

Fat pad

Articular circumference

Articular fovea

Head of radius

Radial notch of ulna

Anconeus

Supinator

Radius   Ulna

B Sagittal section through the humeroradial joint and proximal radioulnar joint, medial view.

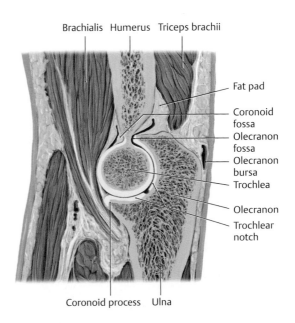

Brachialis   Humerus   Triceps brachii

Fat pad

Coronoid fossa

Olecranon fossa

Olecranon bursa

Trochlea

Olecranon

Trochlear notch

Coronoid process   Ulna

C Sagittal section through the humeroulnar joint, medial view.

Ligaments of the Elbow Joint

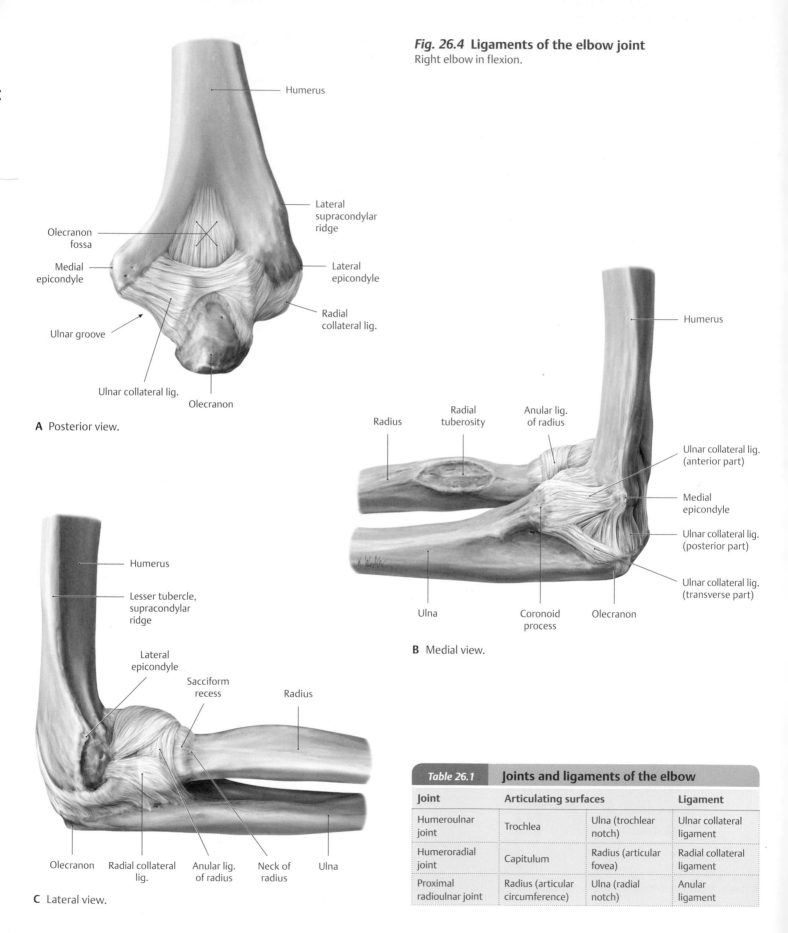

Fig. 26.4 Ligaments of the elbow joint
Right elbow in flexion.

A Posterior view.

Humerus
Lateral supracondylar ridge
Olecranon fossa
Medial epicondyle
Lateral epicondyle
Radial collateral lig.
Ulnar groove
Ulnar collateral lig.
Olecranon

B Medial view.

Radius
Radial tuberosity
Anular lig. of radius
Humerus
Ulnar collateral lig. (anterior part)
Medial epicondyle
Ulnar collateral lig. (posterior part)
Ulnar collateral lig. (transverse part)
Ulna
Coronoid process
Olecranon

C Lateral view.

Humerus
Lesser tubercle, supracondylar ridge
Lateral epicondyle
Sacciform recess
Radius
Olecranon
Radial collateral lig.
Anular lig. of radius
Neck of radius
Ulna

Table 26.1	Joints and ligaments of the elbow		
Joint	**Articulating surfaces**		**Ligament**
Humeroulnar joint	Trochlea	Ulna (trochlear notch)	Ulnar collateral ligament
Humeroradial joint	Capitulum	Radius (articular fovea)	Radial collateral ligament
Proximal radioulnar joint	Radius (articular circumference)	Ulna (radial notch)	Anular ligament

Fig. 26.5 Joint capsule of the elbow

Right elbow in extension, anterior view.

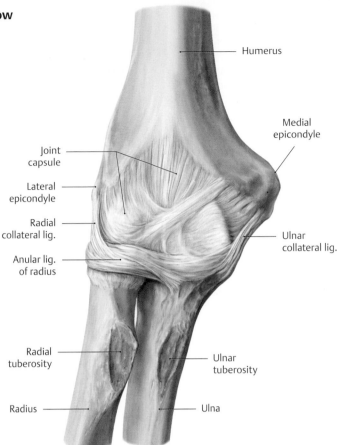

Humerus

Medial epicondyle

Joint capsule

Lateral epicondyle

Radial collateral lig.

Anular lig. of radius

Ulnar collateral lig.

Radial tuberosity

Ulnar tuberosity

Radius

Ulna

A Intact joint capsule.

Clinical box 26.2

Subluxation of the radial head (nursemaid's elbow)

A common and painful injury of small children occurs when the arm is jerked upward with the forearm pronated, tearing the anular ligament from its loose attachment on the radial neck. As the immature radial head slips out of the socket, the ligament may become trapped between the radial head and the capitulum of the humerus. Supinating the forearm and flexing the elbow usually returns the radial head to the normal position.

Humerus

Capitulum

Radial head

Ulna

Epiphyseal plates

Anular lig.

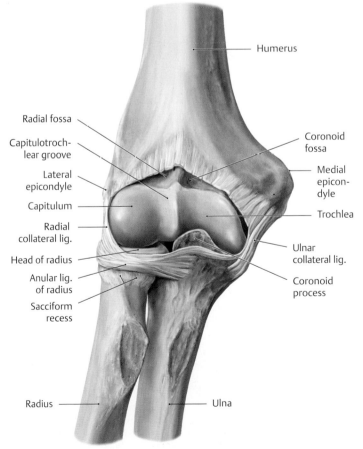

Humerus

Radial fossa

Capitulotroch-lear groove

Lateral epicondyle

Capitulum

Radial collateral lig.

Head of radius

Anular lig. of radius

Sacciform recess

Coronoid fossa

Medial epicon-dyle

Trochlea

Ulnar collateral lig.

Coronoid process

Radius

Ulna

B Windowed joint capsule.

Radioulnar Joints

The proximal and distal radioulnar joints function together to enable pronation and supination movements of the hand. The joints are functionally linked by the interosseous membrane. The axis for pronation and supination runs obliquely from the center of the humeral capitulum through the center of the radial articular fovea down to the styloid process of the ulna.

Fig. 26.6 Supination
Right forearm, anterior view.

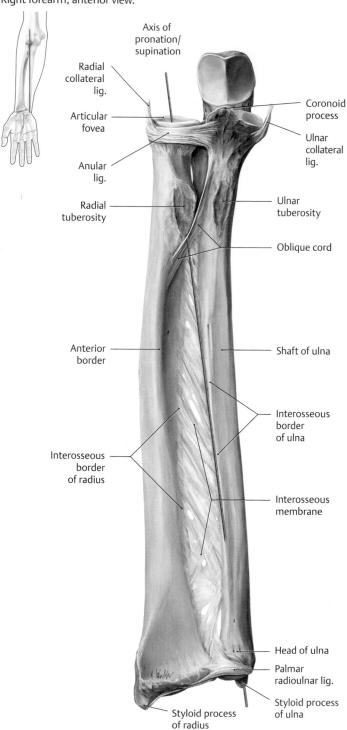

- Axis of pronation/supination
- Radial collateral lig.
- Articular fovea
- Anular lig.
- Radial tuberosity
- Coronoid process
- Ulnar collateral lig.
- Ulnar tuberosity
- Oblique cord
- Anterior border
- Shaft of ulna
- Interosseous border of ulna
- Interosseous border of radius
- Interosseous membrane
- Head of ulna
- Palmar radioulnar lig.
- Styloid process of ulna
- Styloid process of radius

Fig. 26.7 Pronation
Right forearm, anterior view.

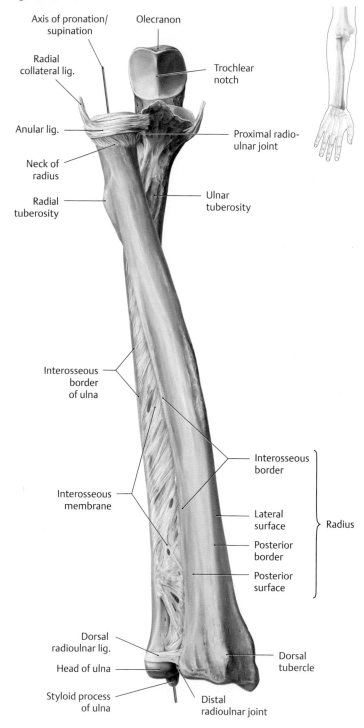

- Axis of pronation/supination
- Olecranon
- Radial collateral lig.
- Trochlear notch
- Anular lig.
- Neck of radius
- Proximal radio-ulnar joint
- Radial tuberosity
- Ulnar tuberosity
- Interosseous border of ulna
- Interosseous border
- Interosseous membrane
- Lateral surface
- Posterior border
- Posterior surface
- Radius
- Dorsal radioulnar lig.
- Head of ulna
- Dorsal tubercle
- Styloid process of ulna
- Distal radioulnar joint

Fig. 26.8 **Proximal radioulnar joint**

Right elbow, proximal (superior) view.

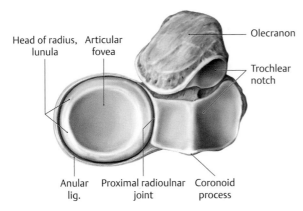

A Proximal articular surfaces of radius and ulna.

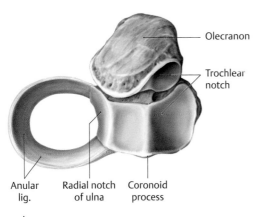

B Radius removed.

Fig. 26.9 **Distal radioulnar joint rotation**

Right forearm, distal view of articular surfaces of radius and ulna. The dorsal and palmar radioulnar ligaments stabilize the distal radioulnar joint.

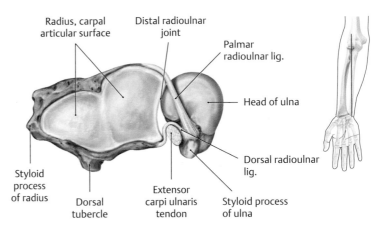

A Supination.

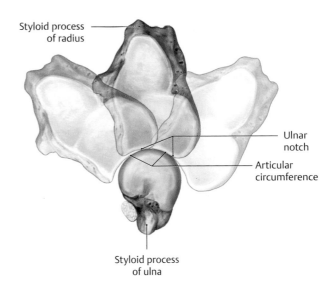

B Semipronation.

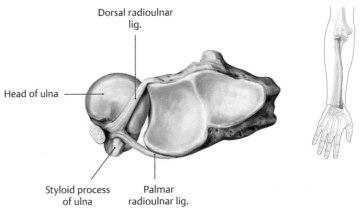

C Pronation.

> ⚕ **Clinical box 26.3**
>
> **Radius fracture**
> Falls onto the outstretched arm often result in fractures of the distal radius. In a Colles' fracture, the distal fragment is tilted dorsally.
>
> ![Radius fracture illustration]
>
> **A**   **B**
>
> Dorsal ←   ←
>
> Styloid process of radius

Muscles of the Forearm: Anterior Compartment

***Fig. 26.10* Anterior muscles of the forearm: Dissection**
Right forearm, anterior view. Muscle origins are shown in red, insertions in blue.

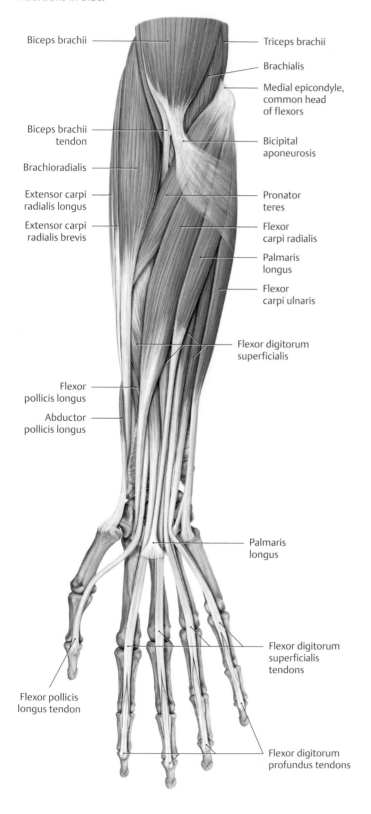

Biceps brachii
Triceps brachii
Brachialis
Medial epicondyle, common head of flexors
Biceps brachii tendon
Bicipital aponeurosis
Brachioradialis
Extensor carpi radialis longus
Pronator teres
Extensor carpi radialis brevis
Flexor carpi radialis
Palmaris longus
Flexor carpi ulnaris
Flexor digitorum superficialis
Flexor pollicis longus
Abductor pollicis longus
Palmaris longus
Flexor digitorum superficialis tendons
Flexor pollicis longus tendon
Flexor digitorum profundus tendons

A Superficial flexors and radialis muscles.

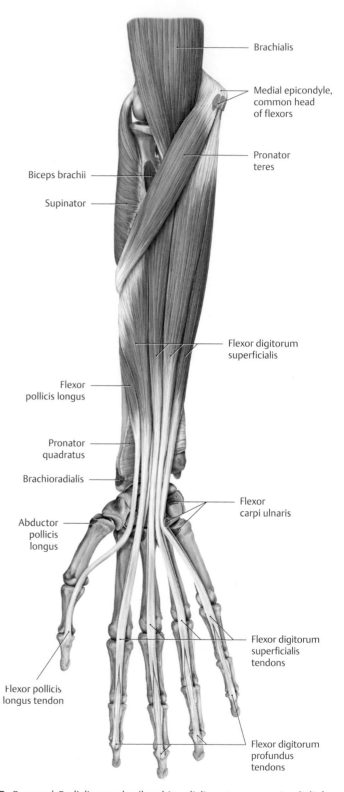

Brachialis
Medial epicondyle, common head of flexors
Biceps brachii
Pronator teres
Supinator
Flexor digitorum superficialis
Flexor pollicis longus
Pronator quadratus
Brachioradialis
Flexor carpi ulnaris
Abductor pollicis longus
Flexor digitorum superficialis tendons
Flexor pollicis longus tendon
Flexor digitorum profundus tendons

B *Removed:* Radialis muscles (brachioradialis, extensor carpi radialis longus, and extensor carpi radialis brevis), flexor carpi radialis, flexor carpi ulnaris, abductor pollicis longus, palmaris longus, and biceps brachii.

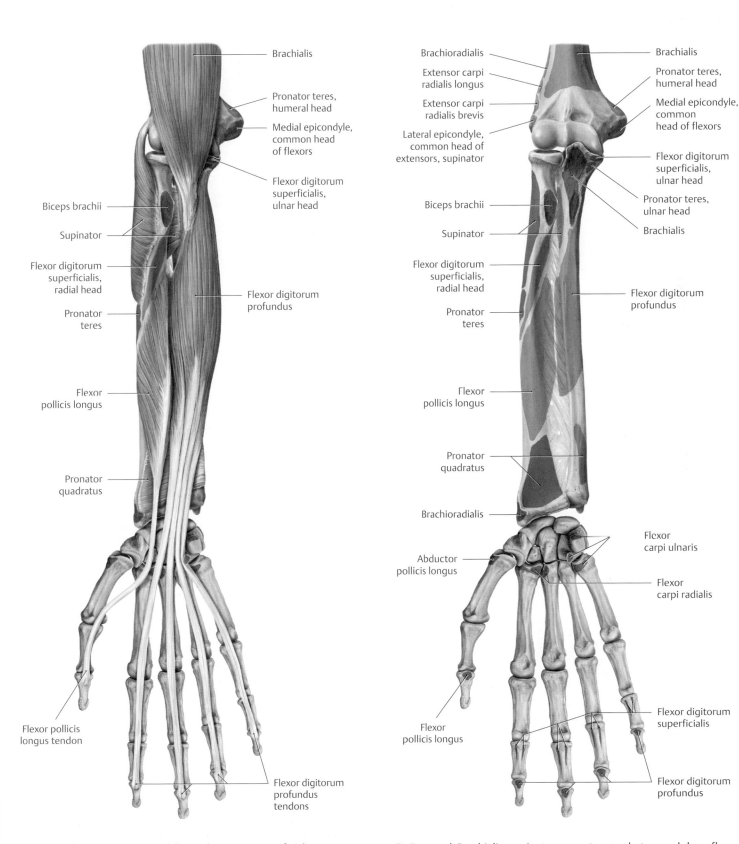

Brachialis

Pronator teres, humeral head

Medial epicondyle, common head of flexors

Flexor digitorum superficialis, ulnar head

Biceps brachii

Supinator

Flexor digitorum superficialis, radial head

Pronator teres

Flexor digitorum profundus

Flexor pollicis longus

Pronator quadratus

Flexor pollicis longus tendon

Flexor digitorum profundus tendons

Brachioradialis

Extensor carpi radialis longus

Extensor carpi radialis brevis

Lateral epicondyle, common head of extensors, supinator

Biceps brachii

Supinator

Flexor digitorum superficialis, radial head

Pronator teres

Flexor pollicis longus

Pronator quadratus

Brachioradialis

Abductor pollicis longus

Flexor pollicis longus

Brachialis

Pronator teres, humeral head

Medial epicondyle, common head of flexors

Flexor digitorum superficialis, ulnar head

Pronator teres, ulnar head

Brachialis

Flexor digitorum profundus

Flexor carpi ulnaris

Flexor carpi radialis

Flexor digitorum superficialis

Flexor digitorum profundus

C *Removed:* Pronator teres and flexor digitorum superficialis.

D *Removed:* Brachialis, supinator, pronator quadratus, and deep flexors.

Muscles of the Forearm: Posterior Compartment

Fig. 26.11 Posterior muscles of the forearm: Dissection

Right forearm, posterior view. Muscle origins are shown in red, insertions in blue.

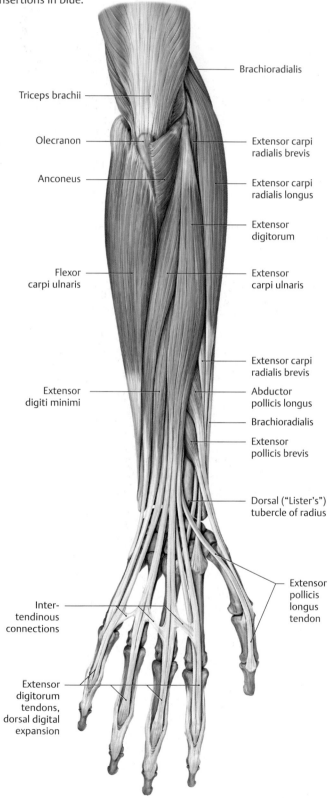

Brachioradialis

Triceps brachii

Olecranon

Anconeus

Extensor carpi radialis brevis

Extensor carpi radialis longus

Extensor digitorum

Flexor carpi ulnaris

Extensor carpi ulnaris

Extensor digiti minimi

Extensor carpi radialis brevis

Abductor pollicis longus

Brachioradialis

Extensor pollicis brevis

Dorsal ("Lister's") tubercle of radius

Inter-tendinous connections

Extensor pollicis longus tendon

Extensor digitorum tendons, dorsal digital expansion

A Superficial extensors and radialis group.

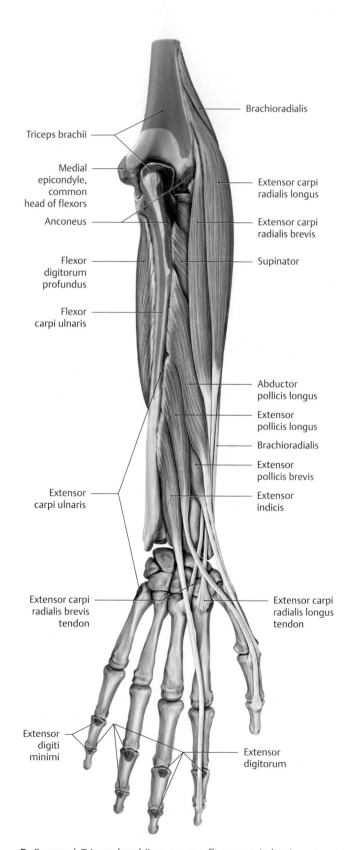

Brachioradialis

Triceps brachii

Medial epicondyle, common head of flexors

Anconeus

Extensor carpi radialis longus

Extensor carpi radialis brevis

Flexor digitorum profundus

Supinator

Flexor carpi ulnaris

Abductor pollicis longus

Extensor pollicis longus

Brachioradialis

Extensor pollicis brevis

Extensor carpi ulnaris

Extensor indicis

Extensor carpi radialis brevis tendon

Extensor carpi radialis longus tendon

Extensor digiti minimi

Extensor digitorum

B *Removed:* Triceps brachii, anconeus, flexor carpi ulnaris, extensor carpi ulnaris, and extensor digitorum.

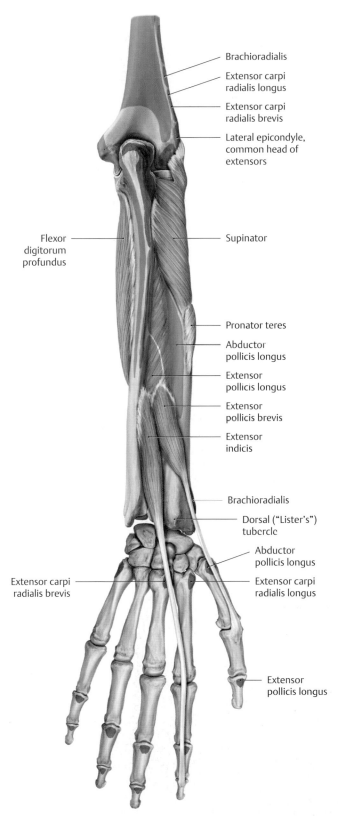

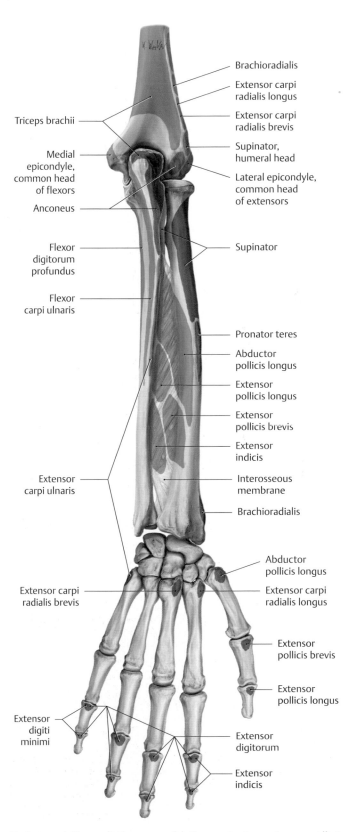

Brachioradialis

Extensor carpi radialis longus

Extensor carpi radialis brevis

Lateral epicondyle, common head of extensors

Flexor digitorum profundus

Supinator

Pronator teres

Abductor pollicis longus

Extensor pollicis longus

Extensor pollicis brevis

Extensor indicis

Brachioradialis

Dorsal ("Lister's") tubercle

Abductor pollicis longus

Extensor carpi radialis brevis

Extensor carpi radialis longus

Extensor pollicis longus

C *Removed:* Abductor pollicis longus, extensor pollicis longus, and radialis muscles.

Triceps brachii

Brachioradialis

Extensor carpi radialis longus

Extensor carpi radialis brevis

Medial epicondyle, common head of flexors

Supinator, humeral head

Lateral epicondyle, common head of extensors

Anconeus

Flexor digitorum profundus

Supinator

Flexor carpi ulnaris

Pronator teres

Abductor pollicis longus

Extensor pollicis longus

Extensor pollicis brevis

Extensor indicis

Extensor carpi ulnaris

Interosseous membrane

Brachioradialis

Abductor pollicis longus

Extensor carpi radialis brevis

Extensor carpi radialis longus

Extensor pollicis brevis

Extensor pollicis longus

Extensor digiti minimi

Extensor digitorum

Extensor indicis

D *Removed:* Flexor digitorum profundus, supinator, extensor pollicis brevis, and extensor indicis.

Muscle Facts (I)

***Fig. 26.12* Anterior compartment of the forearm**

Right forearm, anterior view.

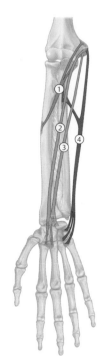
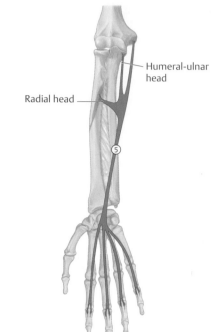
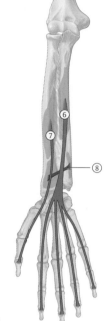

Humeral-ulnar head

Radial head

A Superficial.　　　　**B** Intermediate.　　　　**C** Deep.

Table 26.2	**Anterior compartment of the forearm**			
Muscle	**Origin**	**Insertion**	**Innervation**	**Action**
Superficial muscles				
① Pronator teres	Humeral head: medial epicondyle of humerus Ulnar head: coronoid process	Lateral radius (distal to supinator insertion)	Median n. (C6, C7)	Elbow: weak flexion Forearm: pronation
② Flexor carpi radialis	Medial epicondyle of humerus	Base of 2nd metacarpal (variance: base of 3rd metacarpal)		Wrist: flexion and abduction (radial deviation) of hand
③ Palmaris longus		Palmar aponeurosis	Median n. (C7, C8)	Elbow: weak flexion Wrist: flexion tightens palmar aponeurosis
④ Flexor carpi ulnaris	Humeral head: medial epicondyle Ulnar head: olecranon	Pisiform; hook of hamate; base of 5th metacarpal	Ulnar n. (C7–T1)	Wrist: flexion and adduction (ulnar deviation) of hand
Intermediate muscles				
⑤ Flexor digitorum superficialis	Humeral-ulnar head: medial epicondyle of humerus and coronoid process of ulna Radial head: upper half of anterior border of radius	Sides of middle phalanges of 2nd to 5th digits	Median n. (C8, T1)	Elbow: weak flexion Wrist, MCP, and PIP joints of 2nd to 5th digits: flexion
Deep muscles				
⑥ Flexor digitorum profundus	Ulna (proximal two thirds of flexor surface) and interosseous membrane	Distal phalanges of 2nd to 5th digits (palmar surface)	Median n. (C8, T1, radial half of fingers 2 and 3) Ulnar n. (C8, T1, ulnar half of fingers 4 and 5)	Wrist, MCP, PIP, and DIP joints of 2nd to 5th digits: flexion
⑦ Flexor pollicis longus	Radius (midanterior surface) and adjacent interosseous membrane	Distal phalanx of thumb (palmar surface)	Median n. (C8, T1)	Wrist: flexion and abduction (radial deviation) of hand Carpometacarpal joint of thumb: flexion MCP and IP joints of thumb: flexion
⑧ Pronator quadratus	Distal quarter of ulna (anterior surface)	Distal quarter of radius (anterior surface)		Hand: pronation Distal radioulnar joint: stabilization

DIP, distal interphalangeal; IP, interphalangeal; MCP, metacarpophalangeal; PIP, proximal interphalangeal.

Fig. 26.13 **Anterior compartment of the forearm**
Right forearm, anterior view.

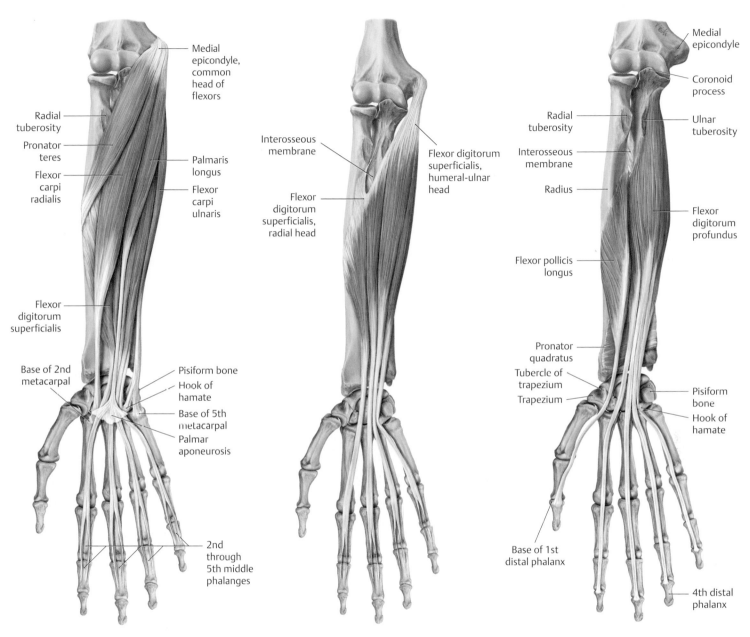

Medial
epicondyle,
common
head of
flexors

Radial
tuberosity

Pronator
teres

Flexor
carpi
radialis

Palmaris
longus

Flexor
carpi
ulnaris

Flexor
digitorum
superficialis

Base of 2nd
metacarpal

Pisiform bone

Hook of
hamate

Base of 5th
metacarpal

Palmar
aponeurosis

2nd
through
5th middle
phalanges

A Superficial muscles.

Interosseous
membrane

Flexor
digitorum
superficialis,
radial head

Flexor digitorum
superficialis,
humeral-ulnar
head

B Intermediate muscles.

Medial
epicondyle

Coronoid
process

Radial
tuberosity

Ulnar
tuberosity

Interosseous
membrane

Radius

Flexor
digitorum
profundus

Flexor pollicis
longus

Pronator
quadratus

Tubercle of
trapezium

Trapezium

Pisiform
bone

Hook of
hamate

Base of 1st
distal phalanx

4th distal
phalanx

C Deep muscles.

Muscle Facts (II)

***Fig. 26.14* Posterior compartment of the forearm: Radialis muscles**
Right forearm, posterior view, schematic.

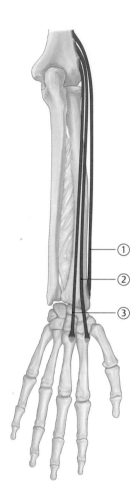

Clinical box 26.4

Lateral epicondylitis
Lateral epicondylitis, or tennis elbow, involves the extensor muscles and tendons of the forearm that attach on the lateral epicondyle. The tendon most commonly involved is that of the extensor carpi radialis brevis, a muscle that helps stabilize the wrist when the elbow is extended. When the extensor carpi radialis brevis is weakened from overuse, microscopic tears form in the tendon where it attaches to the lateral epicondyle. This leads to inflammation and pain. There is some evidence that the inflammation can extend back along the tendon to the periosteum of the lateral epicondyle.

Athletes are not the only people who get tennis elbow and are actually in the minority — leading some to suggest the condition be referred to as "lateral elbow syndrome". Workers whose activities require repetitive and vigorous use of the forearm muscles, such as common to painters, plumbers, and carpenters, are particularly prone to developing this pathology. Studies show a high incidence also among auto workers, cooks, and butchers. Common signs and symptoms of tennis elbow include pain with wrist extension against resistance, point tenderness or burning on the lateral epicondyle, and weak grip strength. Symptoms are intensified with forearm activity.

Table 26.3 **Posterior compartment of the forearm: Radialis muscles**

Muscle	Origin	Insertion	Innervation	Action
① Brachioradialis	Distal humerus (lateral surface), lateral intermuscular septum	Styloid process of the radius	Radial n. (C5, C6)	Elbow: flexion Forearm: semipronation
② Extensor carpi radialis longus	Lateral supracondylar ridge of distal humerus, lateral intermuscular septum	2nd metacarpal (base)	Radial n. (C6, C7)	Elbow: weak flexion Wrist: extension and abduction
③ Extensor carpi radialis brevis	Lateral epicondyle of humerus	3rd metacarpal (base)	Radial n. (C7, C8)	

Fig. 26.15 **Posterior compartment of the forearm: Radialis muscles**
Right forearm.

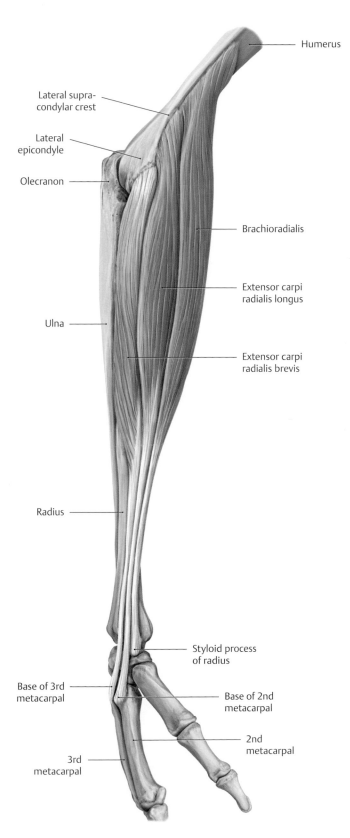

A Lateral (radial) view.

Humerus

Lateral supra-condylar crest

Lateral epicondyle

Olecranon

Brachioradialis

Extensor carpi radialis longus

Ulna

Extensor carpi radialis brevis

Radius

Styloid process of radius

Base of 3rd metacarpal

Base of 2nd metacarpal

3rd metacarpal

2nd metacarpal

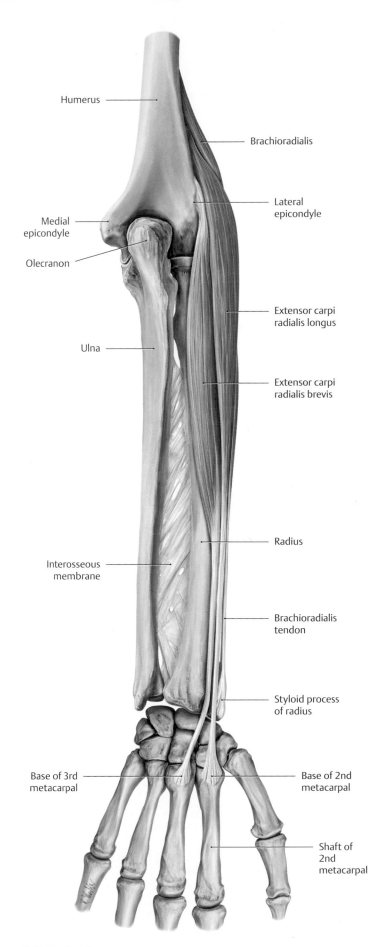

B Posterior view.

Humerus

Brachioradialis

Medial epicondyle

Olecranon

Lateral epicondyle

Extensor carpi radialis longus

Ulna

Extensor carpi radialis brevis

Radius

Interosseous membrane

Brachioradialis tendon

Styloid process of radius

Base of 3rd metacarpal

Base of 2nd metacarpal

Shaft of 2nd metacarpal

Muscle Facts (III)

***Fig. 26.16* Posterior compartment of the forearm**
Right forearm, posterior view.

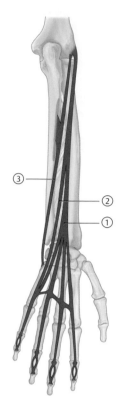

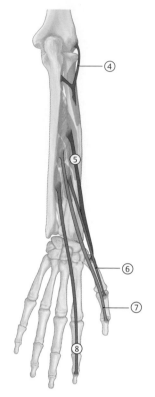

A Superficial muscles.　　　**B** Deep muscles.

Table 26.4	Posterior compartment of the forearm			
Muscle	**Origin**	**Insertion**	**Innervation**	**Action**
Superficial muscles				
① Extensor digitorum	Common head (lateral epicondyle of humerus)	Dorsal digital expansion of 2nd to 5th digits	Radial n. (C7, C8)	Wrist: extension MCP, PIP, and DIP joints of 2nd to 5th digits: extension/abduction of fingers
② Extensor digiti minimi		Dorsal digital expansion of 5th digit		Wrist: extension, ulnar abduction of hand MCP, PIP, and DIP joints of 5th digit: extension and abduction of 5th digit
③ Extensor carpi ulnaris	Common head (lateral epicondyle of humerus) Ulnar head (dorsal surface)	Base of 5th metacarpal		Wrist: extension, adduction (ulnar deviation) of hand
Deep muscles				
④ Supinator	Olecranon, lateral epicondyle of humerus, radial collateral ligament, annular ligament of radius	Radius (between radial tuberosity and insertion of pronator teres)	Radial n. (C6, C7)	Radioulnar joints: supination
⑤ Abductor pollicis longus	Radius and ulna (dorsal surfaces, interosseous membrane)	Base of 1st metacarpal	Radial n. (C7, C8)	Radiocarpal joint: abduction of the hand Carpometacarpal joint of thumb: abduction
⑥ Extensor pollicis brevis	Radius (posterior surface) and interosseous membrane	Base of proximal phalanx of thumb		Radiocarpal joint: abduction (radial deviation) of hand Carpometacarpal and MCP joints of thumb: extension
⑦ Extensor pollicis longus	Ulna (posterior surface) and interosseous membrane	Base of distal phalanx of thumb		Wrist: extension and abduction (radial deviation) of hand Carpometacarpal joint of thumb: adduction MCP and IP joints of thumb: extension
⑧ Extensor indicis	Ulna (posterior surface) and interosseous membrane	Posterior digital extension of 2nd digit		Wrist: extension MCP, PIP, and DIP joints of 2nd digit: extension
DIP, distal interphalangeal; IP, interphalangeal; MCP, metacarpophalangeal; PIP, proximal interphalangeal.				

Fig. 26.17 **Posterior compartment of the forearm: Superficial and deep muscles**
Right forearm, posterior view.

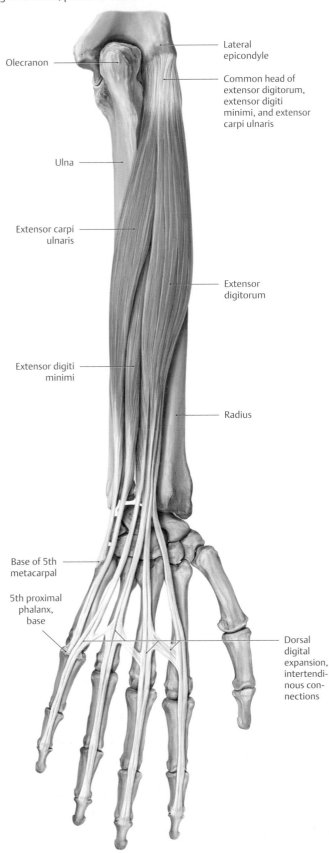

Olecranon

Lateral epicondyle

Common head of extensor digitorum, extensor digiti minimi, and extensor carpi ulnaris

Ulna

Extensor carpi ulnaris

Extensor digitorum

Extensor digiti minimi

Radius

Base of 5th metacarpal

5th proximal phalanx, base

Dorsal digital expansion, intertendinous connections

A Superficial extensors.

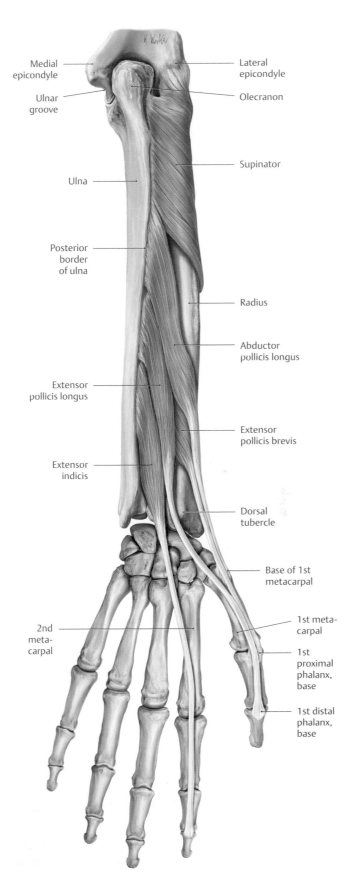

Medial epicondyle

Ulnar groove

Lateral epicondyle

Olecranon

Ulna

Supinator

Posterior border of ulna

Radius

Abductor pollicis longus

Extensor pollicis longus

Extensor pollicis brevis

Extensor indicis

Dorsal tubercle

Base of 1st metacarpal

2nd metacarpal

1st metacarpal

1st proximal phalanx, base

1st distal phalanx, base

B Deep extensors with supinator.

341

27 Wrist & Hand
Bones of the Wrist & Hand

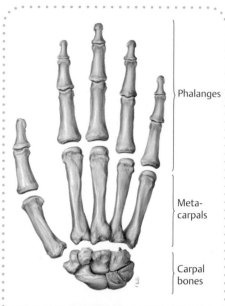

Table 27.1	Bones of the wrist and hand	
Phalanges	1st to 5th proximal phalanges	
	2nd to 5th middle phalanges*	
	1st to 5th distal phalanges	
Metacarpal bones	1st to 5th metacarpals	
Carpal bones	Trapezium	Scaphoid
	Trapezoid	Lunate
	Capitate	Triquetrum
	Hamate	Pisiform

*There are only four middle phalanges (the thumb has only a proximal and a distal phalanx).

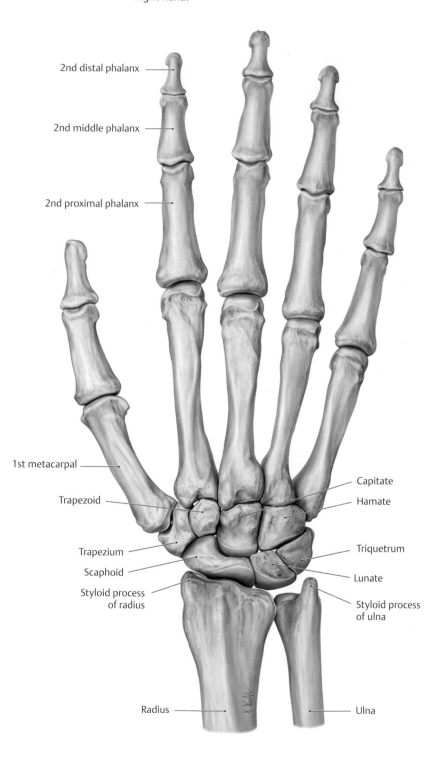

Fig. 27.1 Dorsal view
Right hand.

2nd distal phalanx

2nd middle phalanx

2nd proximal phalanx

1st metacarpal

Trapezoid

Trapezium

Scaphoid

Styloid process of radius

Capitate

Hamate

Triquetrum

Lunate

Styloid process of ulna

Radius

Ulna

Fig. 27.2 Palmar view
Right hand.

Tuberosity of distal phalanx

Head
Shaft — Middle phalanx
Base

Head
Meta-carpal — Shaft
Base

Hook of hamate
Pisiform
Triquetrum
Lunate
Ulna — Styloid process
Head

Sesamoid bones

Trapezoid
Tubercle of trapezium
Capitate
Tubercle of scaphoid
Styloid process of radius

Radius

Fig. 27.3 Radiograph of the wrist
Anteroposterior view of left limb.

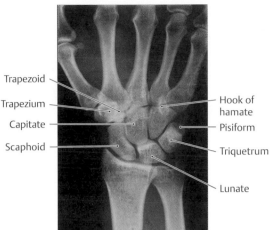

Trapezoid
Trapezium
Capitate
Scaphoid
Hook of hamate
Pisiform
Triquetrum
Lunate

Clinical box 27.1

Scaphoid Fractures
Scaphoid fractures are the most common carpal bone fractures, generally occurring at the narrowed waist between the proximal and distal poles (**A**, right scaphoid red line; **B**, white arrow). Because blood supply to the scaphoid is transmitted via the distal segment, fractures at the waist can compromise the supply to the proximal segment, often resulting in nonunion and avascular necrosis.

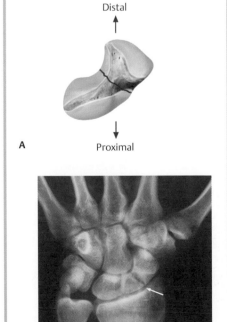

Distal
Proximal
A
B

Carpal Bones

Fig. 27.4 Carpal bones of the right wrist

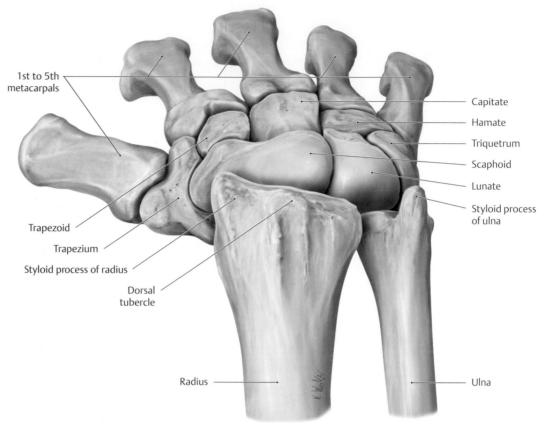

1st to 5th metacarpals

Capitate

Hamate

Triquetrum

Scaphoid

Lunate

Styloid process of ulna

Trapezoid

Trapezium

Styloid process of radius

Dorsal tubercle

Radius

Ulna

A Carpal bones of the right wrist with the wrist in flexion, proximal view.

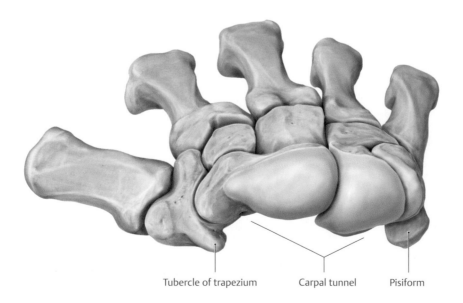

Tubercle of trapezium

Carpal tunnel

Pisiform

B Carpal and metacarpal bones of the right wrist with radius and ulna removed, proximal view.

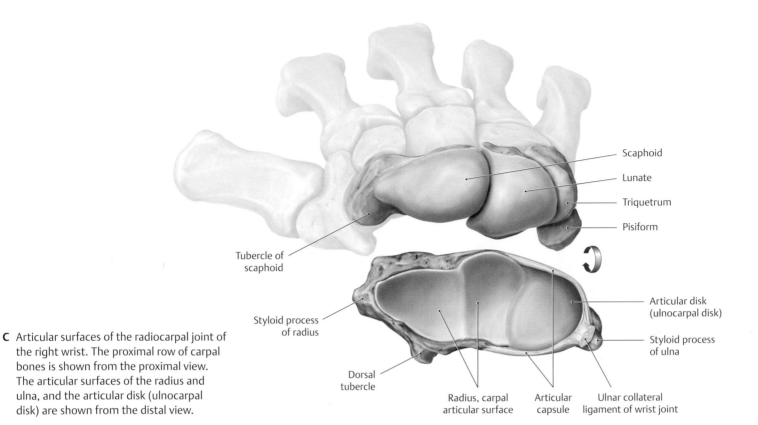

Scaphoid

Lunate

Triquetrum

Pisiform

Tubercle of scaphoid

Styloid process of radius

Articular disk (ulnocarpal disk)

Styloid process of ulna

Dorsal tubercle

Radius, carpal articular surface

Articular capsule

Ulnar collateral ligament of wrist joint

C Articular surfaces of the radiocarpal joint of the right wrist. The proximal row of carpal bones is shown from the proximal view. The articular surfaces of the radius and ulna, and the articular disk (ulnocarpal disk) are shown from the distal view.

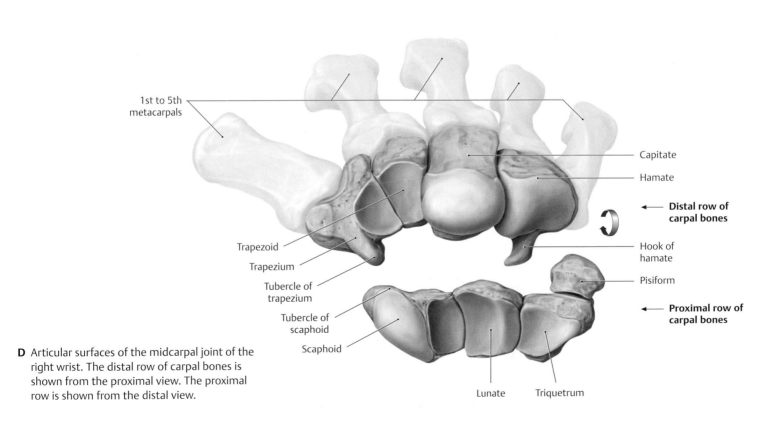

1st to 5th metacarpals

Capitate

Hamate

Distal row of carpal bones

Trapezoid

Trapezium

Hook of hamate

Pisiform

Tubercle of trapezium

Tubercle of scaphoid

Proximal row of carpal bones

Scaphoid

Lunate

Triquetrum

D Articular surfaces of the midcarpal joint of the right wrist. The distal row of carpal bones is shown from the proximal view. The proximal row is shown from the distal view.

Joints of the Wrist & Hand

Fig. 27.5 Joints of the wrist and hand

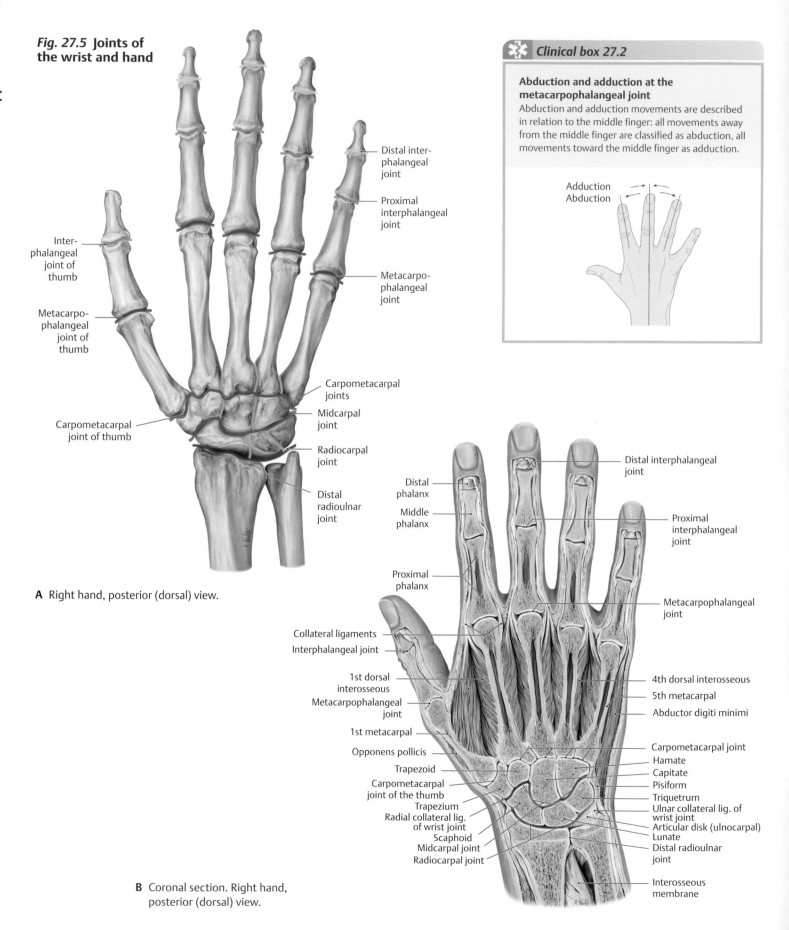

Distal inter-phalangeal joint

Proximal interphalangeal joint

Inter-phalangeal joint of thumb

Metacarpo-phalangeal joint of thumb

Metacarpo-phalangeal joint

Carpometacarpal joints

Midcarpal joint

Carpometacarpal joint of thumb

Radiocarpal joint

Distal radioulnar joint

A Right hand, posterior (dorsal) view.

Distal interphalangeal joint

Proximal interphalangeal joint

Distal phalanx

Middle phalanx

Proximal phalanx

Metacarpophalangeal joint

Collateral ligaments

Interphalangeal joint

1st dorsal interosseous

Metacarpophalangeal joint

1st metacarpal

Opponens pollicis

Trapezoid

Carpometacarpal joint of the thumb

Trapezium

Radial collateral lig. of wrist joint

Scaphoid

Midcarpal joint

Radiocarpal joint

4th dorsal interosseous

5th metacarpal

Abductor digiti minimi

Carpometacarpal joint

Hamate

Capitate

Pisiform

Triquetrum

Ulnar collateral lig. of wrist joint

Articular disk (ulnocarpal)

Lunate

Distal radioulnar joint

Interosseous membrane

B Coronal section. Right hand, posterior (dorsal) view.

Fig. 27.6 Carpometacarpal joint of the thumb

Right hand, radial view. The 1st metacarpal bone has been moved slightly distally to expose the articular surface of the trapezium. Two cardinal axes of motion are shown here: (**a**) abduction/adduction and (**b**) flexion/extension.

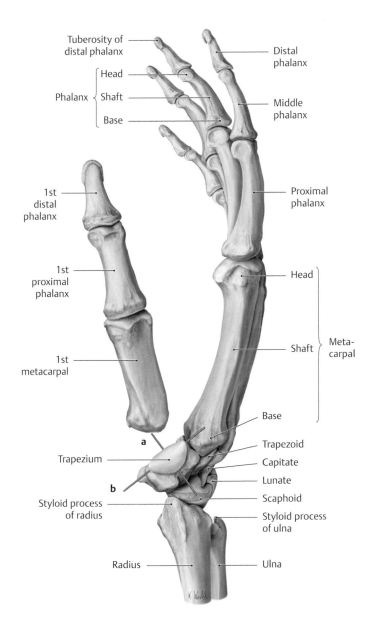

Fig. 27.7 Movements of the carpometacarpal joint of the thumb

Right hand, Palmar view.

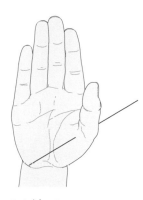

A The neutral (0°) position.

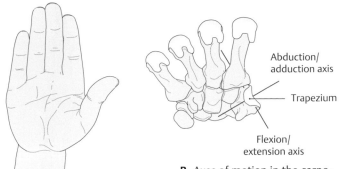

B Axes of motion in the carpometacarpal joint of the thumb.

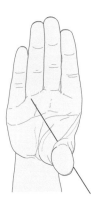

C Adduction.

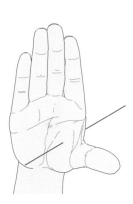

D Abduction.

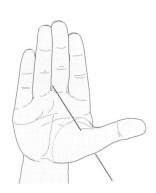

E Flexion.

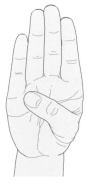

F Extension.

G Opposition.

Ligaments of the Hand

***Fig. 27.8* Ligaments of the hand**
Right hand.

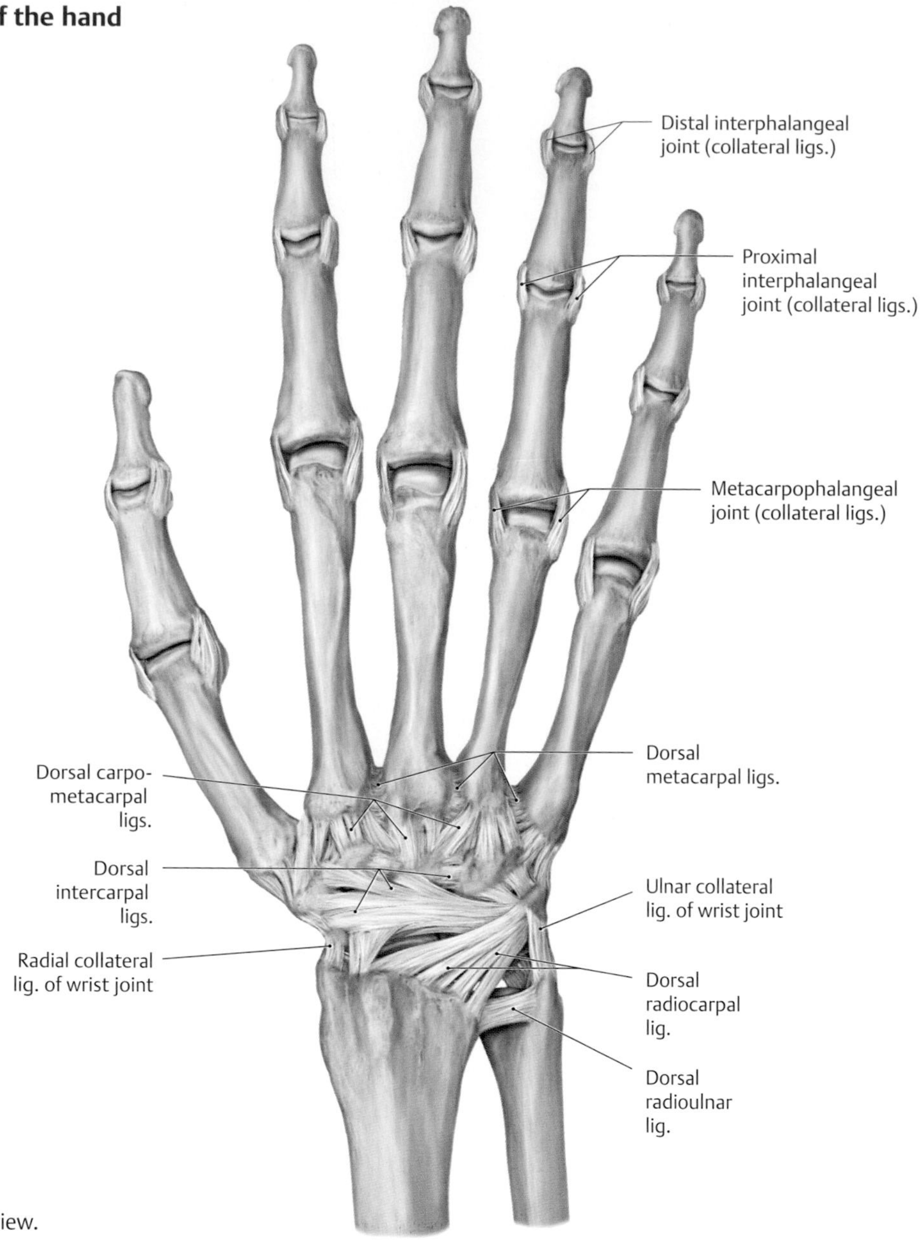

Distal interphalangeal joint (collateral ligs.)

Proximal interphalangeal joint (collateral ligs.)

Metacarpophalangeal joint (collateral ligs.)

Dorsal metacarpal ligs.

Dorsal carpo-metacarpal ligs.

Dorsal intercarpal ligs.

Radial collateral lig. of wrist joint

Ulnar collateral lig. of wrist joint

Dorsal radiocarpal lig.

Dorsal radioulnar lig.

A Posterior (dorsal) view.

✴ *Clinical box 27.3*

Movements at the radiocarpal and midcarpal joints

Palmar flexion and dorsal extension occur around a transverse axis (**A**) that runs through the lunate bone (radiocarpal joint) and capitate bone (midcarpal joint). Radial and ulnar deviation (**B**) occur around a dorsopalmar axis that runs through the capitate bone.

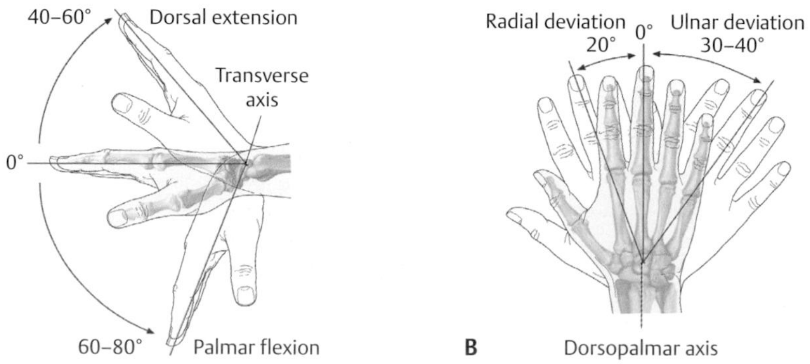

40–60° Dorsal extension

Transverse axis

0°

A 60–80° Palmar flexion

Radial deviation 0° Ulnar deviation
20° 30–40°

B Dorsopalmar axis

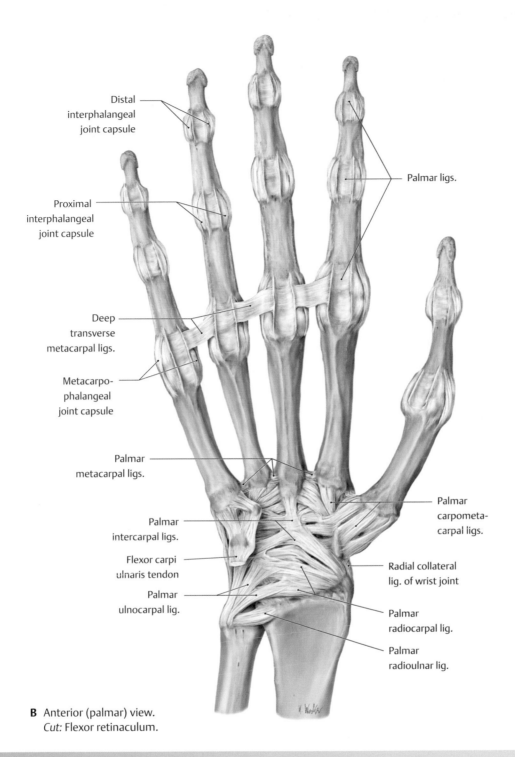

Distal
interphalangeal
joint capsule

Proximal
interphalangeal
joint capsule

Palmar ligs.

Deep
transverse
metacarpal ligs.

Metacarpo-
phalangeal
joint capsule

Palmar
metacarpal ligs.

Palmar carpometa-
carpal ligs.

Palmar
intercarpal ligs.

Flexor carpi
ulnaris tendon

Radial collateral
lig. of wrist joint

Palmar
ulnocarpal lig.

Palmar
radiocarpal lig.

Palmar
radioulnar lig.

B Anterior (palmar) view.
Cut: Flexor retinaculum.

✳ *Clinical box 27.4*

Functional position of the hand

The anatomic position of the hand, in which the palm is flat, the fingers are extended, and the forearm is supinated (palm facing forward), differs from the normal relaxed position of the hand. At rest, the forearm is in mid-supination/pronation (palm facing the body), the wrist is slightly extended, the fingers form an arcade of flexion, and the thumb is in the neutral position. Postoperative immobilization of the hand (by a cast or splint) fixes the fingers in flexion and the wrist in extension to prevent shortening of the ligaments and to maintain the ability of the hand to assume normal resting position.

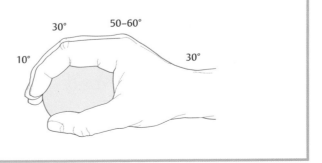

Ligaments & Compartments of the Wrist

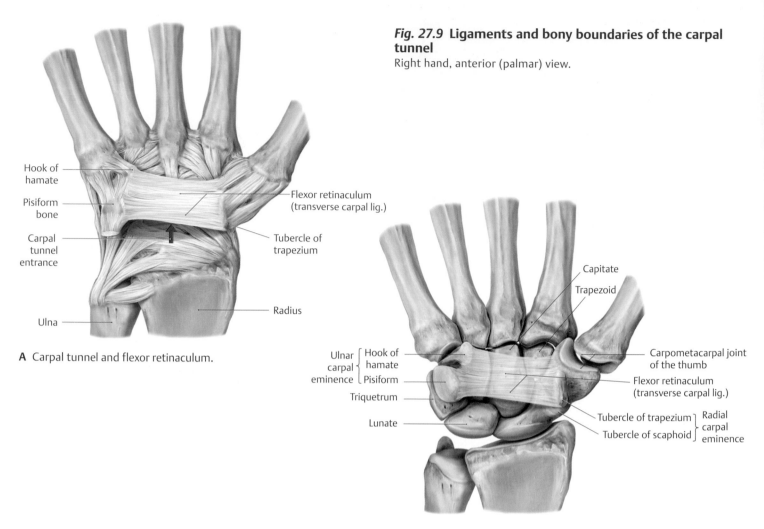

Fig. 27.9 Ligaments and bony boundaries of the carpal tunnel

Right hand, anterior (palmar) view.

A Carpal tunnel and flexor retinaculum.

B Bony boundaries of the carpal tunnel.

Fig. 27.10 Carpal tunnel

Right hand, transverse section. The contents of the carpal and ulnar tunnels are discussed on **p. 391**.

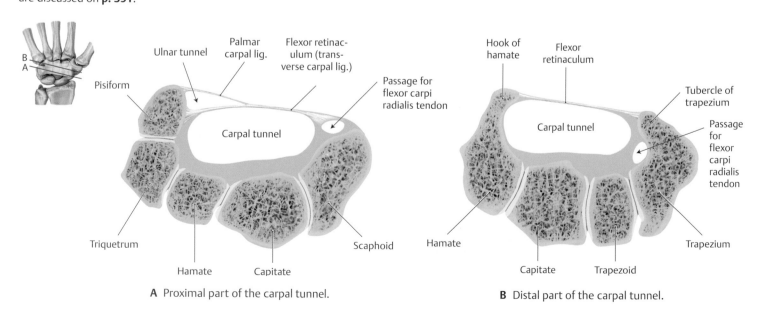

A Proximal part of the carpal tunnel.

B Distal part of the carpal tunnel.

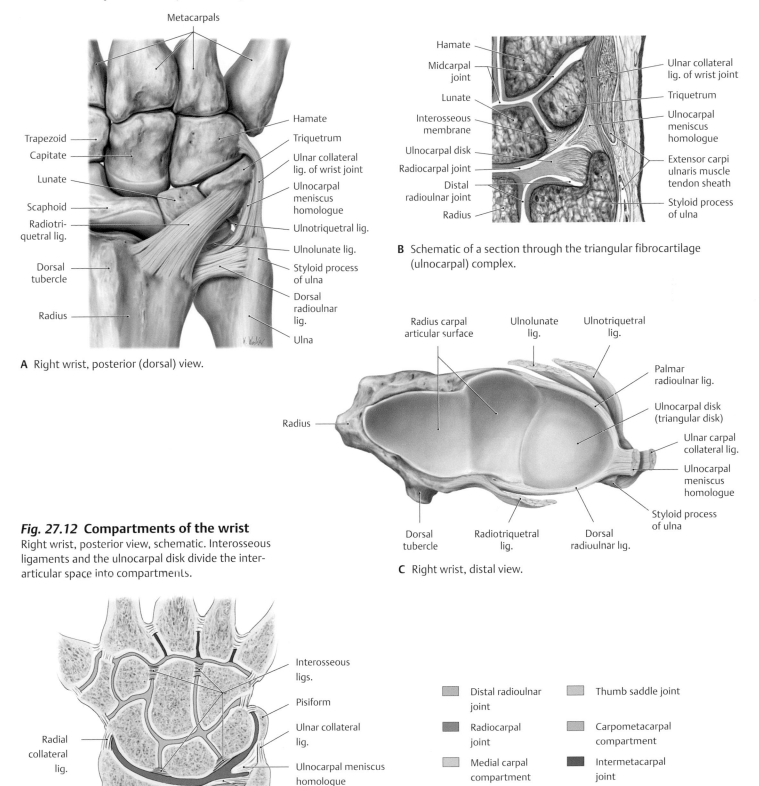

Fig. 27.11 Ulnocarpal complex

Right hand. The ulnocarpal complex (triangular fibrocartilage complex) consists of ligaments and disks that connect the distal ulna, distal radioulnar joint, and the proximal carpal row.

Metacarpals

Trapezoid
Capitate
Lunate
Scaphoid
Radiotriquetral lig.
Dorsal tubercle
Radius

Hamate
Triquetrum
Ulnar collateral lig. of wrist joint
Ulnocarpal meniscus homologue
Ulnotriquetral lig.
Ulnolunate lig.
Styloid process of ulna
Dorsal radioulnar lig.
Ulna

A Right wrist, posterior (dorsal) view.

Hamate
Midcarpal joint
Lunate
Interosseous membrane
Ulnocarpal disk
Radiocarpal joint
Distal radioulnar joint
Radius

Ulnar collateral lig. of wrist joint
Triquetrum
Ulnocarpal meniscus homologue
Extensor carpi ulnaris muscle tendon sheath
Styloid process of ulna

B Schematic of a section through the triangular fibrocartilage (ulnocarpal) complex.

Radius carpal articular surface
Ulnolunate lig.
Ulnotriquetral lig.
Palmar radioulnar lig.
Ulnocarpal disk (triangular disk)
Ulnar carpal collateral lig.
Ulnocarpal meniscus homologue
Styloid process of ulna

Radius

Dorsal tubercle
Radiotriquetral lig.
Dorsal radioulnar lig.

C Right wrist, distal view.

Fig. 27.12 Compartments of the wrist

Right wrist, posterior view, schematic. Interosseous ligaments and the ulnocarpal disk divide the interarticular space into compartments.

Radial collateral lig.

Interosseous ligs.
Pisiform
Ulnar collateral lig.
Ulnocarpal meniscus homologue
Ulnocarpal disk

- Distal radioulnar joint
- Radiocarpal joint
- Medial carpal compartment
- Thumb saddle joint
- Carpometacarpal compartment
- Intermetacarpal joint

Ligaments of the Fingers

Fig. 27.13 Ligaments of the fingers: Lateral view

Right middle finger. Joint capsules, ligaments, and digital tendon sheaths. The outer fibrous layer of the tendon sheaths (stratum fibrosum) is strengthened by the anular and cruciform ligaments, which also bind the sheaths to the palmar surface of the phalanx and prevent palmar deviation of the sheaths during flexion.

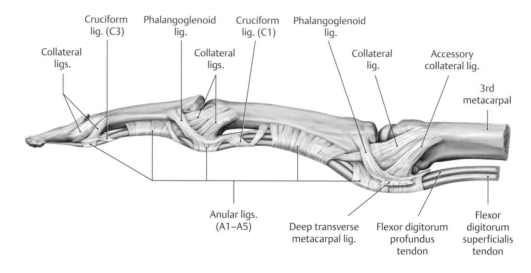

Fig. 27.14 Ligaments during extension and flexion of fingers: Lateral view

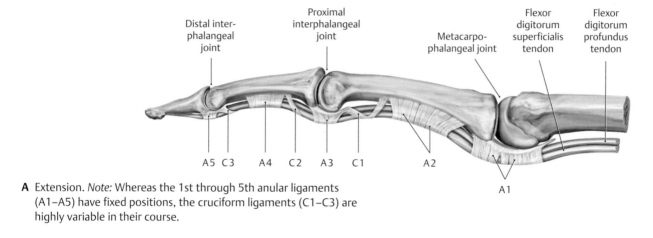

A Extension. *Note:* Whereas the 1st through 5th anular ligaments (A1–A5) have fixed positions, the cruciform ligaments (C1–C3) are highly variable in their course.

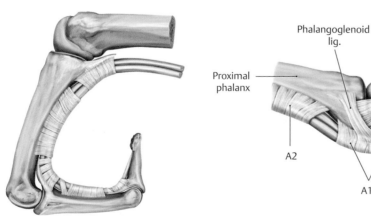

B Flexion.

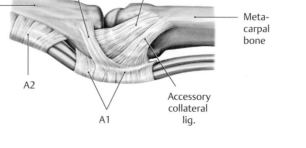

C Extension of the metacarpophalangeal joint. *Note:* The collateral ligament is lax.

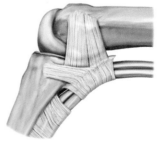

D Flexion of the metacarpophalangeal joint. *Note:* The collateral ligament is taut.

Fig. 27.15 Ligaments of the fingers: Anterior (palmar) view

Right middle finger.

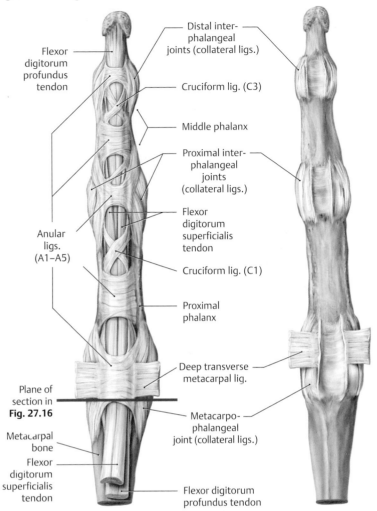

Flexor digitorum profundus tendon

Distal inter-phalangeal joints (collateral ligs.)

Cruciform lig. (C3)

Middle phalanx

Proximal inter-phalangeal joints (collateral ligs.)

Flexor digitorum superficialis tendon

Cruciform lig. (C1)

Anular ligs. (A1–A5)

Proximal phalanx

Deep transverse metacarpal lig.

Plane of section in **Fig. 27.16**

Metacarpo-phalangeal joint (collateral ligs.)

Metacarpal bone

Flexor digitorum superficialis tendon

Flexor digitorum profundus tendon

A Superficial ligaments.

B Deep ligaments with digital tendon sheath removed.

Fig. 27.16 Third metacarpal: Transverse section

Proximal view.

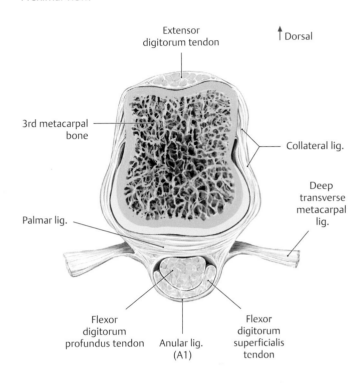

Extensor digitorum tendon

↑ Dorsal

3rd metacarpal bone

Collateral lig.

Deep transverse metacarpal lig.

Palmar lig.

Flexor digitorum profundus tendon

Anular lig. (A1)

Flexor digitorum superficialis tendon

Fig. 27.17 Fingertip: Longitudinal section

The palmar articular surfaces of the phalanges are enlarged proximally at the joints by the palmar ligament. This fibrocartilaginous plate, also known as the volar plate, forms the floor of the digital tendon sheaths.

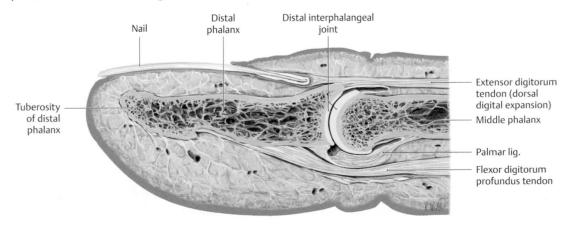

Nail

Distal phalanx

Distal interphalangeal joint

Tuberosity of distal phalanx

Extensor digitorum tendon (dorsal digital expansion)

Middle phalanx

Palmar lig.

Flexor digitorum profundus tendon

Muscles of the Hand: Superficial & Middle Layers

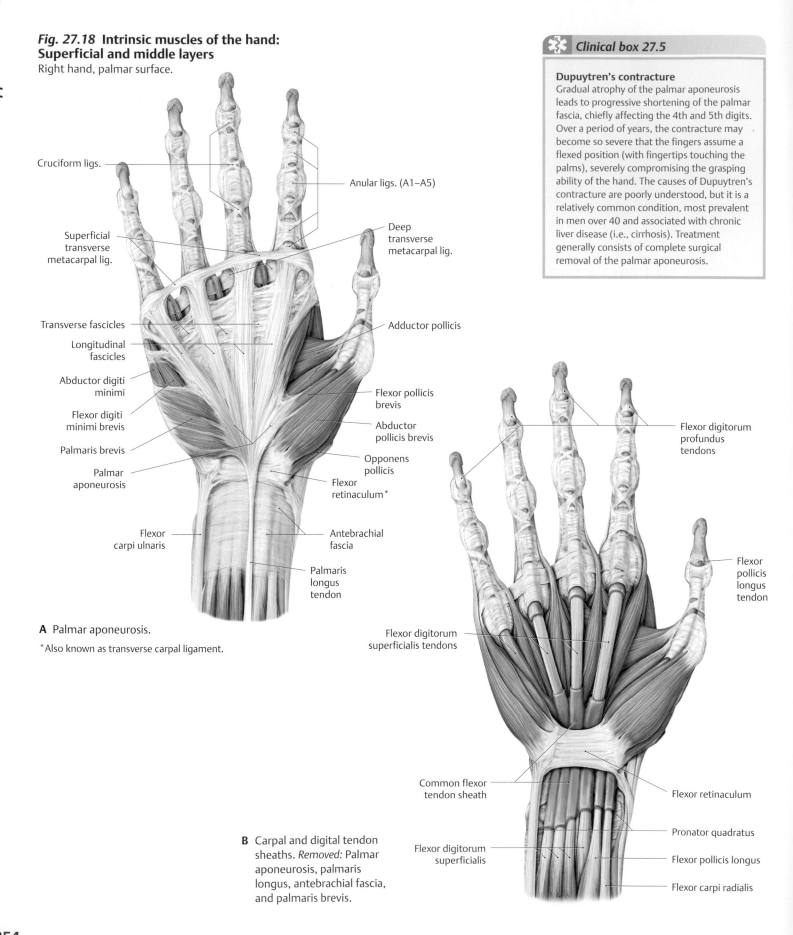

***Fig. 27.18* Intrinsic muscles of the hand: Superficial and middle layers**
Right hand, palmar surface.

Cruciform ligs.

Anular ligs. (A1–A5)

Superficial transverse metacarpal lig.

Deep transverse metacarpal lig.

Transverse fascicles

Adductor pollicis

Longitudinal fascicles

Abductor digiti minimi

Flexor pollicis brevis

Flexor digiti minimi brevis

Abductor pollicis brevis

Palmaris brevis

Opponens pollicis

Palmar aponeurosis

Flexor retinaculum*

Flexor carpi ulnaris

Antebrachial fascia

Palmaris longus tendon

A Palmar aponeurosis.

*Also known as transverse carpal ligament.

Flexor digitorum profundus tendons

Flexor pollicis longus tendon

Flexor digitorum superficialis tendons

Common flexor tendon sheath

Flexor retinaculum

Pronator quadratus

Flexor digitorum superficialis

Flexor pollicis longus

Flexor carpi radialis

B Carpal and digital tendon sheaths. *Removed:* Palmar aponeurosis, palmaris longus, antebrachial fascia, and palmaris brevis.

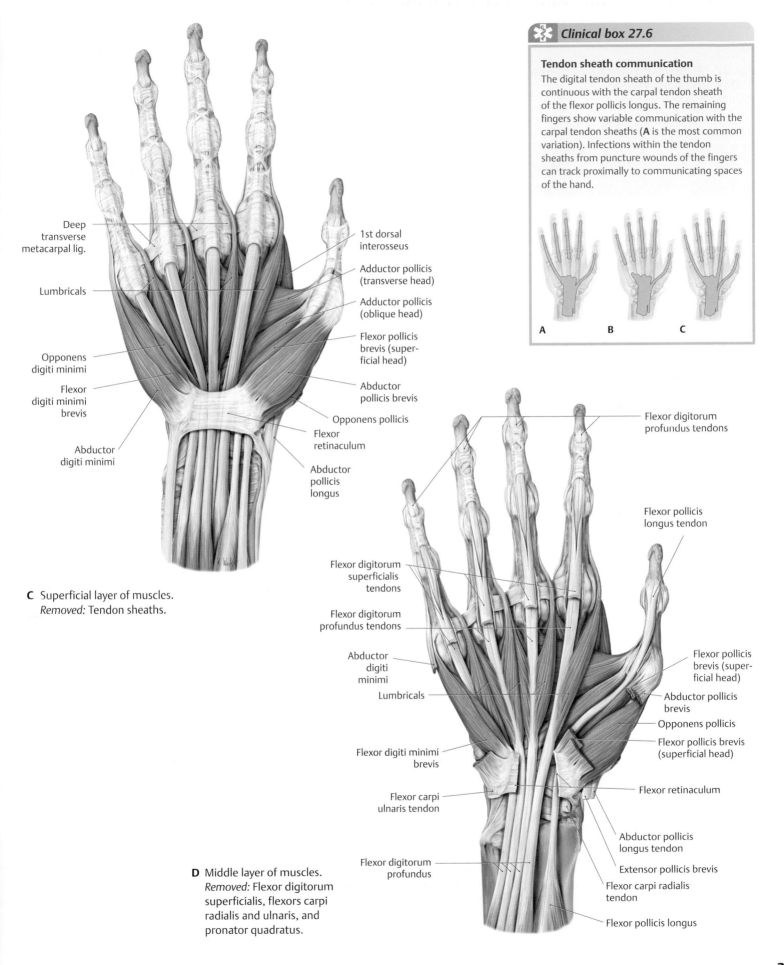

Deep transverse metacarpal lig.

Lumbricals

Opponens digiti minimi

Flexor digiti minimi brevis

Abductor digiti minimi

1st dorsal interosseus

Adductor pollicis (transverse head)

Adductor pollicis (oblique head)

Flexor pollicis brevis (superficial head)

Abductor pollicis brevis

Opponens pollicis

Flexor retinaculum

Abductor pollicis longus

C Superficial layer of muscles.
Removed: Tendon sheaths.

Flexor digitorum profundus tendons

Flexor pollicis longus tendon

Flexor digitorum superficialis tendons

Flexor digitorum profundus tendons

Abductor digiti minimi

Lumbricals

Flexor digiti minimi brevis

Flexor carpi ulnaris tendon

Flexor digitorum profundus

Flexor pollicis brevis (superficial head)

Abductor pollicis brevis

Opponens pollicis

Flexor pollicis brevis (superficial head)

Flexor retinaculum

Abductor pollicis longus tendon

Extensor pollicis brevis

Flexor carpi radialis tendon

Flexor pollicis longus

D Middle layer of muscles.
Removed: Flexor digitorum superficialis, flexors carpi radialis and ulnaris, and pronator quadratus.

Muscles of the Hand: Middle & Deep Layers

Fig. 27.19 **Intrinsic muscles of the hand: Middle and deep layers**

Right hand, palmar surface.

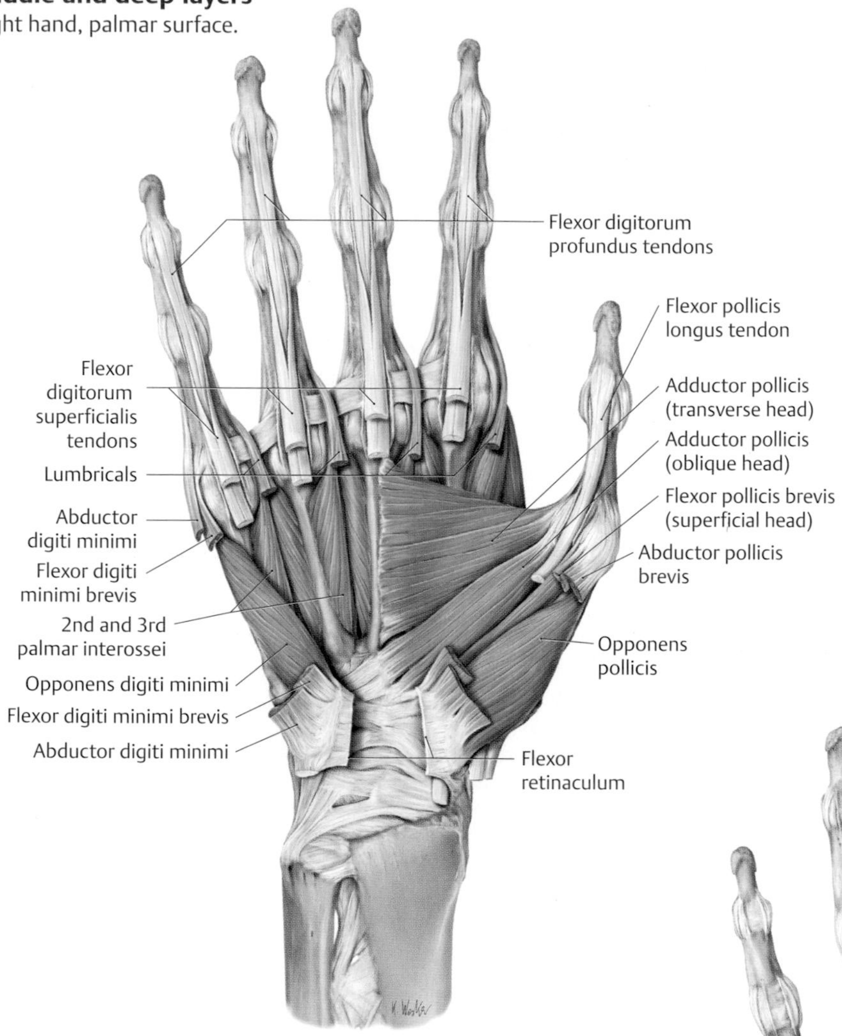

Flexor digitorum profundus tendons

Flexor digitorum superficialis tendons

Lumbricals

Abductor digiti minimi

Flexor digiti minimi brevis

2nd and 3rd palmar interossei

Opponens digiti minimi

Flexor digiti minimi brevis

Abductor digiti minimi

Flexor pollicis longus tendon

Adductor pollicis (transverse head)

Adductor pollicis (oblique head)

Flexor pollicis brevis (superficial head)

Abductor pollicis brevis

Opponens pollicis

Flexor retinaculum

A Middle layer of muscles. *Cut:* Flexor digitorum profundus, lumbricals, flexor pollicis longus, and flexor digiti minimi brevis.

Palmar ligs.

1st through 4th dorsal interossei

Opponens digiti minimi

1st through 3rd palmar interossei

Flexor carpi ulnaris tendon

Adductor pollicis

Flexor pollicis brevis (superficial head)

Flexor pollicis brevis (deep head)

Opponens pollicis

Abductor pollicis longus tendon

Extensor pollicis brevis

Flexor carpi radialis tendon

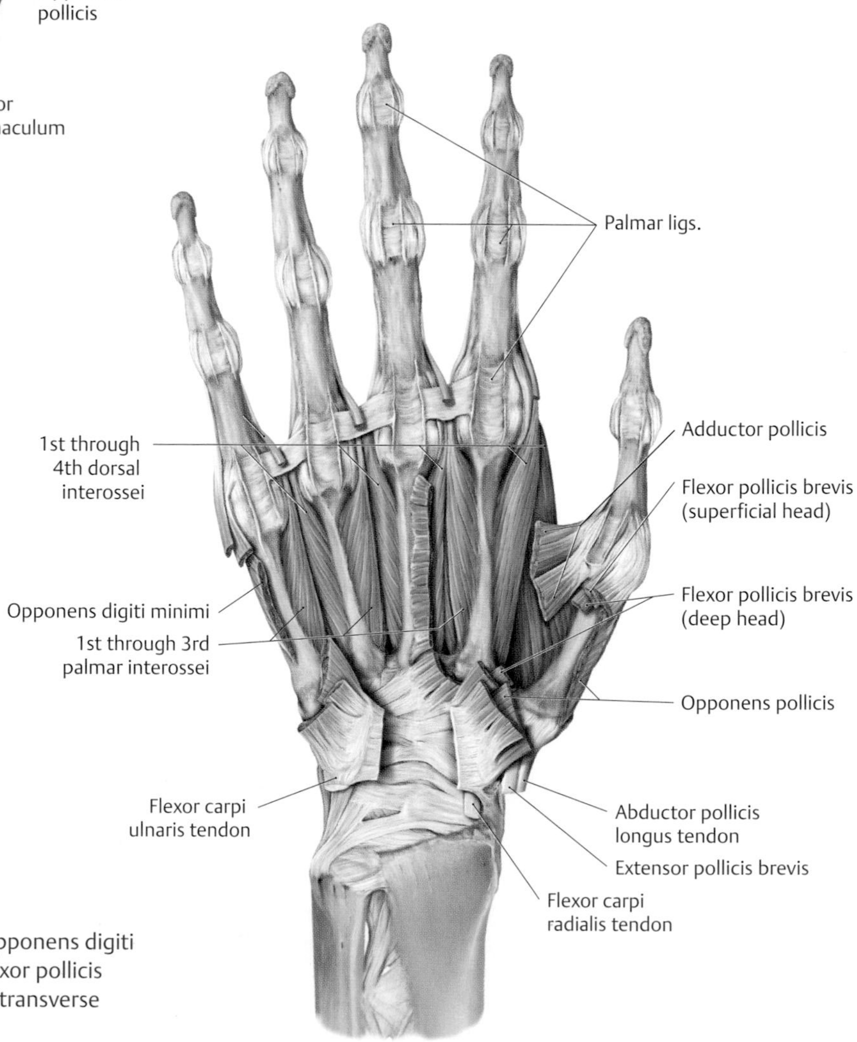

B Deep layer of muscles. *Cut:* Opponens digiti minimi, opponens pollicis, flexor pollicis brevis, and adductor pollicis (transverse and oblique heads).

Fig. 27.20 Origins and insertions of muscles of the hand

Right hand. Muscle origins shown in red, insertions in blue.

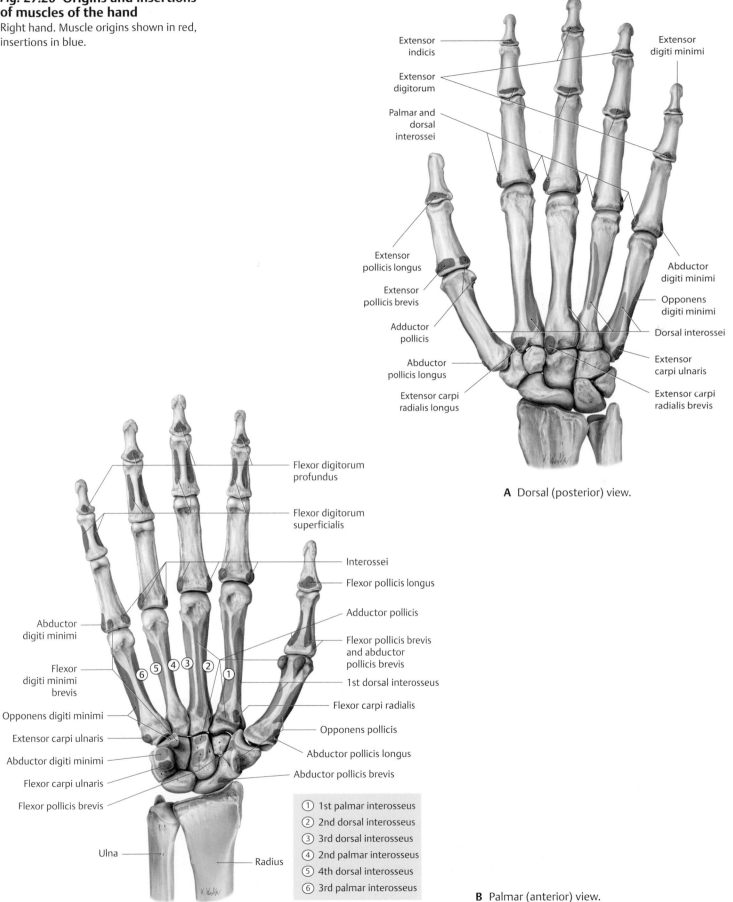

Extensor indicis

Extensor digitorum

Palmar and dorsal interossei

Extensor pollicis longus

Extensor pollicis brevis

Adductor pollicis

Abductor pollicis longus

Extensor carpi radialis longus

Extensor digiti minimi

Abductor digiti minimi

Opponens digiti minimi

Dorsal interossei

Extensor carpi ulnaris

Extensor carpi radialis brevis

A Dorsal (posterior) view.

Flexor digitorum profundus

Flexor digitorum superficialis

Abductor digiti minimi

Flexor digiti minimi brevis

Opponens digiti minimi

Extensor carpi ulnaris

Abductor digiti minimi

Flexor carpi ulnaris

Flexor pollicis brevis

Ulna

Radius

Interossei

Flexor pollicis longus

Adductor pollicis

Flexor pollicis brevis and abductor pollicis brevis

1st dorsal interosseus

Flexor carpi radialis

Opponens pollicis

Abductor pollicis longus

Abductor pollicis brevis

① 1st palmar interosseus
② 2nd dorsal interosseus
③ 3rd dorsal interosseus
④ 2nd palmar interosseus
⑤ 4th dorsal interosseus
⑥ 3rd palmar interosseus

B Palmar (anterior) view.

357

Dorsum of the Hand

Fig. 27.21 Extensor retinaculum and dorsal carpal tendon sheaths

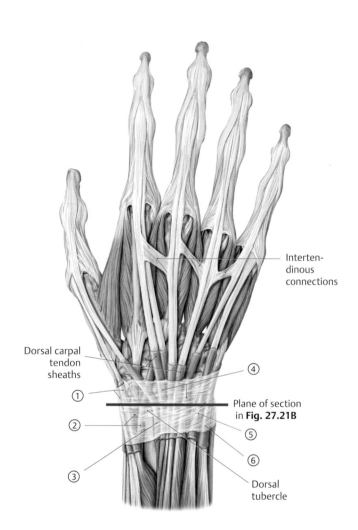

Intertendinous connections

Dorsal carpal tendon sheaths

①

Plane of section in **Fig. 27.21B**

②

⑤

④

⑥

③

Dorsal tubercle

A Right hand, posterior (dorsal) view.

Fig. 27.22 Muscles and tendons of the dorsum
Right hand, posterior (dorsal) view.

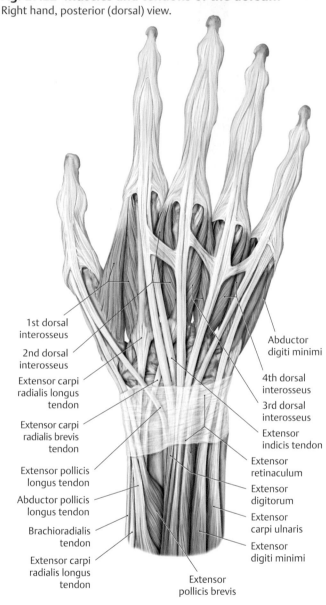

1st dorsal interosseus

2nd dorsal interosseus

Extensor carpi radialis longus tendon

Extensor carpi radialis brevis tendon

Extensor pollicis longus tendon

Abductor pollicis longus tendon

Brachioradialis tendon

Extensor carpi radialis longus tendon

Abductor digiti minimi

4th dorsal interosseus

3rd dorsal interosseus

Extensor indicis tendon

Extensor retinaculum

Extensor digitorum

Extensor carpi ulnaris

Extensor digiti minimi

Extensor pollicis brevis

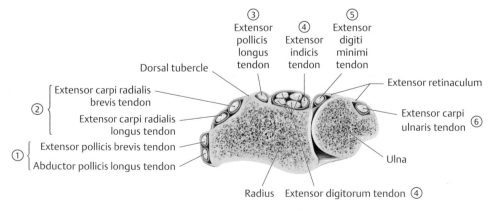

③ Extensor pollicis longus tendon

④ Extensor indicis tendon

⑤ Extensor digiti minimi tendon

Dorsal tubercle

② { Extensor carpi radialis brevis tendon
Extensor carpi radialis longus tendon

① { Extensor pollicis brevis tendon
Abductor pollicis longus tendon

Extensor retinaculum

Extensor carpi ulnaris tendon ⑥

Ulna

Radius   Extensor digitorum tendon ④

B Posterior (dorsal) compartments, proximal view of section in **Fig. 27.21A.**

Table 27.2	Dorsal compartments for extensor tendons
①	Abductor pollicis longus
	Extensor pollicis brevis
②	Extensor carpi radialis longus
	Extensor carpi radialis brevis
③	Extensor pollicis longus
④	Extensor digitorum
	Extensor indicis
⑤	Extensor digiti minimi
⑥	Extensor carpi ulnaris

Fig. 27.23 Dorsal digital expansion

Right hand, middle finger. The dorsal digital expansion permits the long digital flexors and the short muscles of the hand to act on all three finger joints.

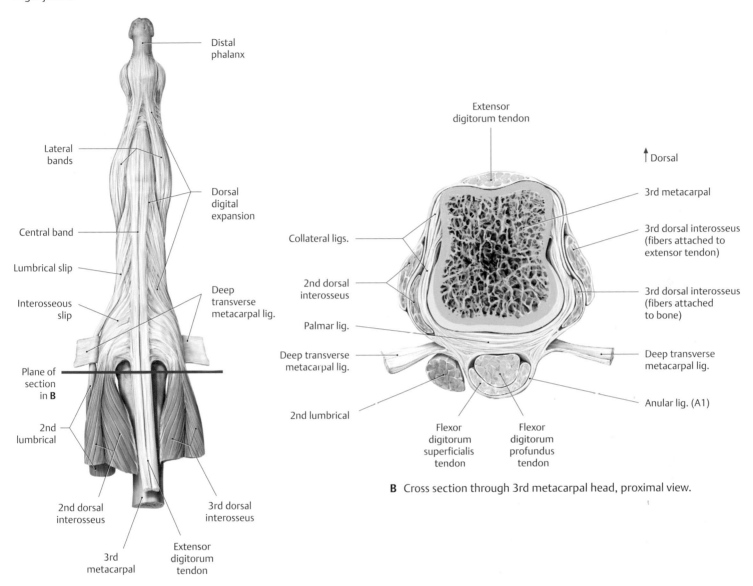

A Posterior view.

B Cross section through 3rd metacarpal head, proximal view.

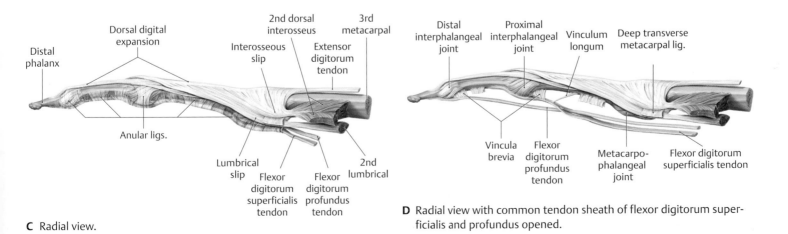

C Radial view.

D Radial view with common tendon sheath of flexor digitorum superficialis and profundus opened.

Muscle Facts (I)

The intrinsic muscles of the hand are divided into three groups: the thenar, hypothenar, and metacarpal muscles (see **p. 362**). The thenar muscles are responsible for movement of the thumb, while the hypothenar muscles move the 5th digit.

Table 27.3	Thenar muscles					
Muscle	**Origin**	**Insertion**		**Innervation**		**Action**
① Adductor pollicis	Transverse head: 3rd metacarpal (palmar surface)	Thumb (base of proximal phalanx) via the ulnar sesamoid	Via the ulnar sesamoid	Ulnar n. (C8, T1)		CMC joint of thumb: adduction MCP joint of thumb: flexion
	Oblique head: capitate bone, 2nd and 3rd metacarpals (bases)					
② Abductor pollicis brevis	Scaphoid bone and trapezium, flexor retinaculum	Thumb (base of proximal phalanx) via the radial sesamoid	Via the radial sesamoid	Median n. (C8, T1)	C8, T1	CMC joint of thumb: abduction
③ Flexor pollicis brevis	Superficial head: flexor retinaculum			Superficial head: median n. (C8, T1)		CMC joint of thumb: flexion
	Deep head: capitate bone, trapezium			Deep head: ulnar n. (C8, T1)		
④ Opponens pollicis	Trapezium	1st metacarpal (radial border)		Median n. (C8, T1)		CMC joint of thumb: opposition

CMC, carpometacarpal; MCP, metacarpophalangeal.

Fig. 27.24 Thenar and hypothenar muscles

Right hand, palmar (anterior) view, schematic.

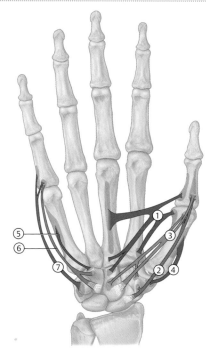

Table 27.4	Hypothenar muscles			
Muscle	**Origin**	**Insertion**	**Innervation**	**Action**
⑤ Opponens digiti minimi	Hook of hamate, flexor retinaculum	5th metacarpal (ulnar border)	Ulnar n. (C8, T1)	Draws metacarpal in palmar direction (opposition)
⑥ Flexor digiti minimi brevis		5th proximal phalanx (base)		MCP joint of little finger: flexion
⑦ Abductor digiti minimi	Pisiform bone	5th proximal phalanx (ulnar base) and dorsal digital expansion of 5th digit		MCP joint of little finger: flexion and abduction of little finger PIP and DIP joints of little finger: extension
Palmaris brevis	Palmar aponeurosis (ulnar border)	Skin of hypothenar eminence		Tightens the palmar aponeurosis (protective function)

DIP, distal interphalangeal; MCP, metacarpophalangeal; PIP, proximal interphalangeal.

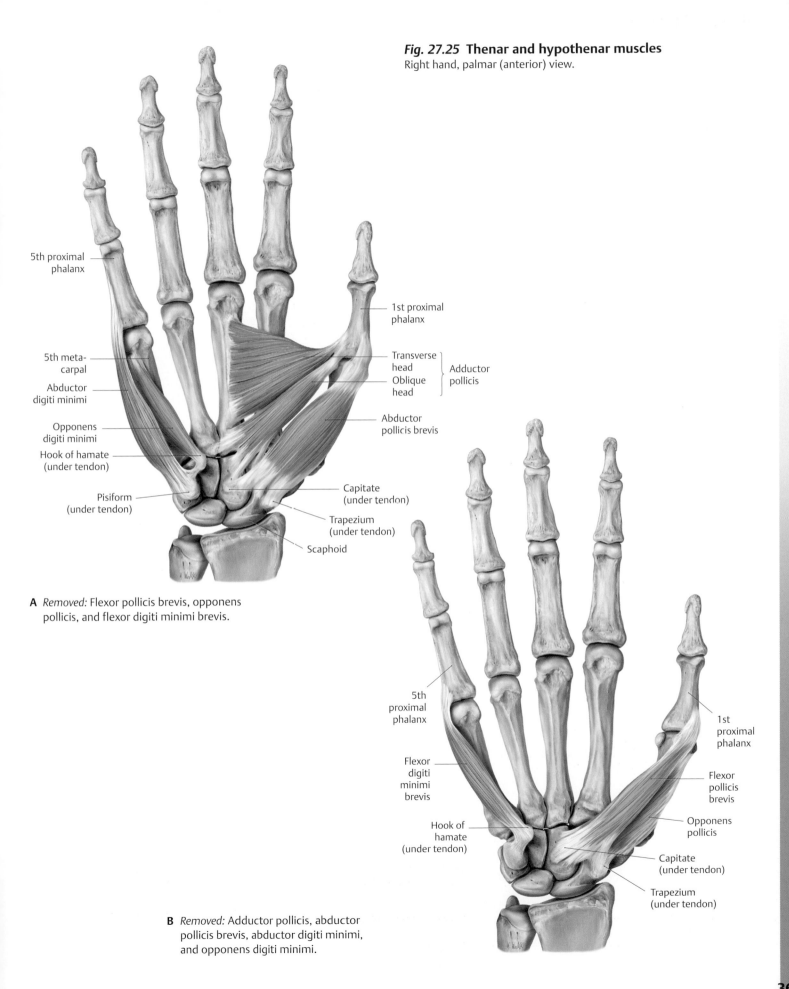

Fig. 27.25 Thenar and hypothenar muscles
Right hand, palmar (anterior) view.

5th proximal phalanx

5th meta-carpal

Abductor digiti minimi

Opponens digiti minimi

Hook of hamate (under tendon)

Pisiform (under tendon)

1st proximal phalanx

Transverse head
Oblique head
} Adductor pollicis

Abductor pollicis brevis

Capitate (under tendon)

Trapezium (under tendon)

Scaphoid

A *Removed:* Flexor pollicis brevis, opponens pollicis, and flexor digiti minimi brevis.

5th proximal phalanx

Flexor digiti minimi brevis

Hook of hamate (under tendon)

1st proximal phalanx

Flexor pollicis brevis

Opponens pollicis

Capitate (under tendon)

Trapezium (under tendon)

B *Removed:* Adductor pollicis, abductor pollicis brevis, abductor digiti minimi, and opponens digiti minimi.

Muscle Facts (II)

The metacarpal muscles of the hand consist of the lumbricals and interossei. They are responsible for the movement of the digits (with the hypothenars, which act on the 5th digit).

Fig. 27.26 **Metacarpal muscles of the hand**
Right hand, palmar view, schematic.

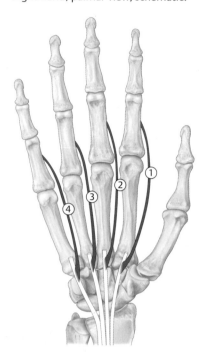

A Lumbricals.

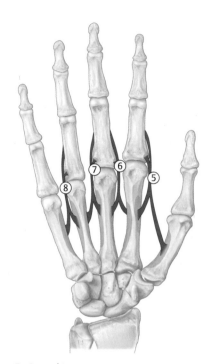

B Dorsal interossei.

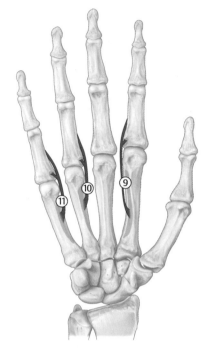

C Palmar interossei.

Table 27.5		Metacarpal muscles			
Muscle group	**Muscle**	**Origin**	**Insertion**	**Innervation**	**Action**
Lumbricals	① 1st	Tendons of flexor digitorum profundus (radial sides)	2nd digit (dde)	Median n. (C8, T1)	2nd to 5th digits: • MCP joints: flexion • Proximal and distal IP joints: extension
	② 2nd		3rd digit (dde)		
	③ 3rd	Tendons of flexor digitorum profundus (bipennate from medial and lateral sides)	4th digit (dde)	Ulnar n. (C8, T1)	
	④ 4th		5th digit (dde)		
Dorsal interossei	⑤ 1st	1st and 2nd metacarpals (adjacent sides, two heads)	2nd digit (dde) 2nd proximal phalanx (radial side)		2nd to 4th digits: • MCP joints: flexion • Proximal and distal IP joints: extension and abduction from 3rd digit
	⑥ 2nd	2nd and 3rd metacarpals (adjacent sides, two heads)	3rd digit (dde) 3rd proximal phalanx (radial side)		
	⑦ 3rd	3rd and 4th metacarpals (adjacent sides, two heads)	3rd digit (dde) 3rd proximal phalanx (ulnar side)		
	⑧ 4th	4th and 5th metacarpals (adjacent sides, two heads)	4th digit (dde) 4th proximal phalanx (ulnar side)		
Palmar interossei	⑨ 1st	2nd metacarpal (ulnar side)	2nd digit (dde) 2nd proximal phalanx (base)		2nd, 4th, and 5th digits: • MCP joints: flexion • Proximal and distal IP joints: extension and adduction toward 3rd digit
	⑩ 2nd	4th metacarpal (radial side)	4th digit (dde) 4th proximal phalanx (base)		
	⑪ 3rd	5th metacarpal (radial side)	5th digit (dde) 5th proximal phalanx (base)		

dde, dorsal digital expansion; IP, interphalangeal; MCP, metacarpophalangeal.

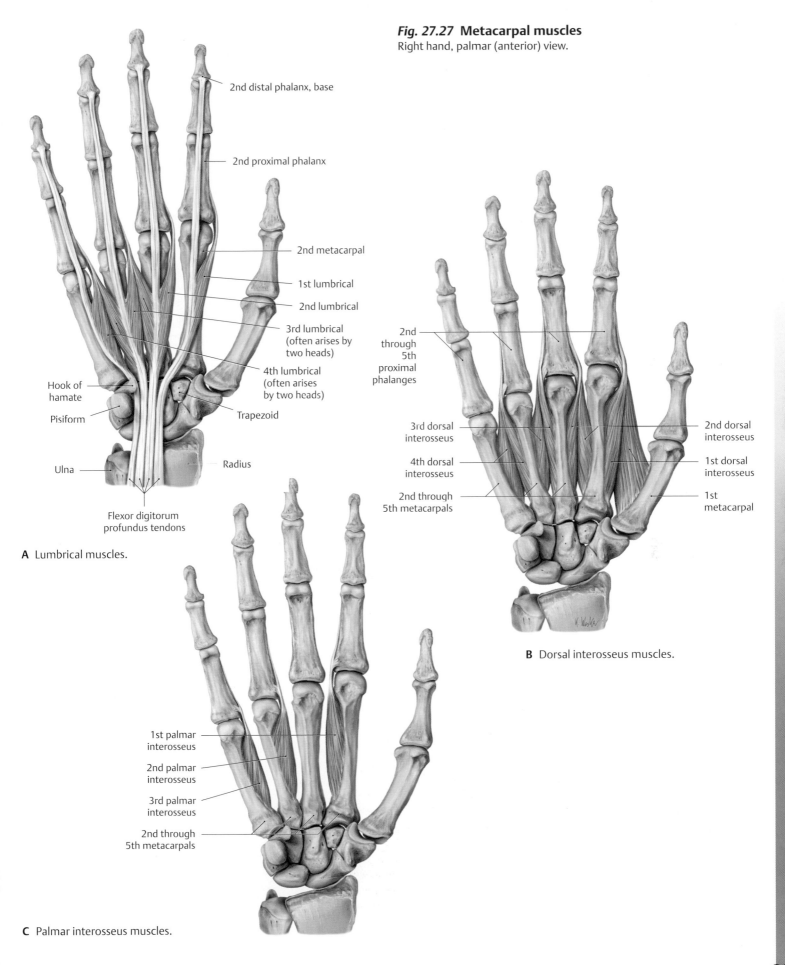

Fig. 27.27 Metacarpal muscles
Right hand, palmar (anterior) view.

2nd distal phalanx, base

2nd proximal phalanx

2nd metacarpal

1st lumbrical

2nd lumbrical

3rd lumbrical
(often arises by
two heads)

4th lumbrical
(often arises
by two heads)

Hook of
hamate

Pisiform

Trapezoid

Ulna

Radius

Flexor digitorum
profundus tendons

A Lumbrical muscles.

2nd
through
5th
proximal
phalanges

3rd dorsal
interosseus

4th dorsal
interosseus

2nd through
5th metacarpals

2nd dorsal
interosseus

1st dorsal
interosseus

1st
metacarpal

B Dorsal interosseus muscles.

1st palmar
interosseus

2nd palmar
interosseus

3rd palmar
interosseus

2nd through
5th metacarpals

C Palmar interosseus muscles.

28 Neurovasculature
Arteries of the Upper Limb

Fig. 28.1 **Arteries of the upper limb**
Right limb with the forearm supinated, anterior view.

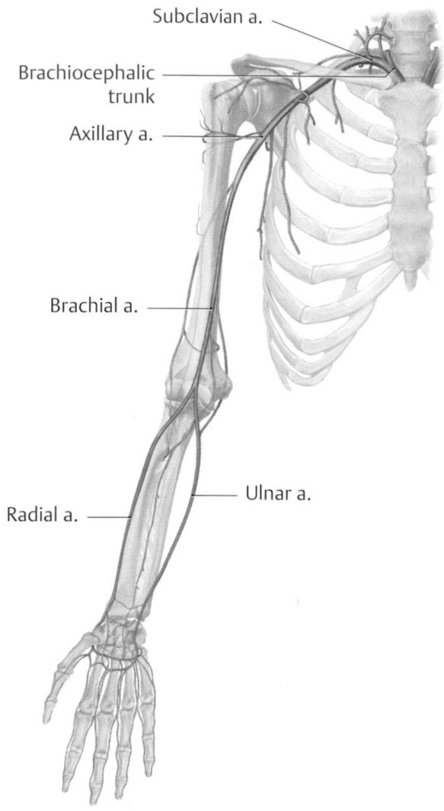

A Main arterial segments.

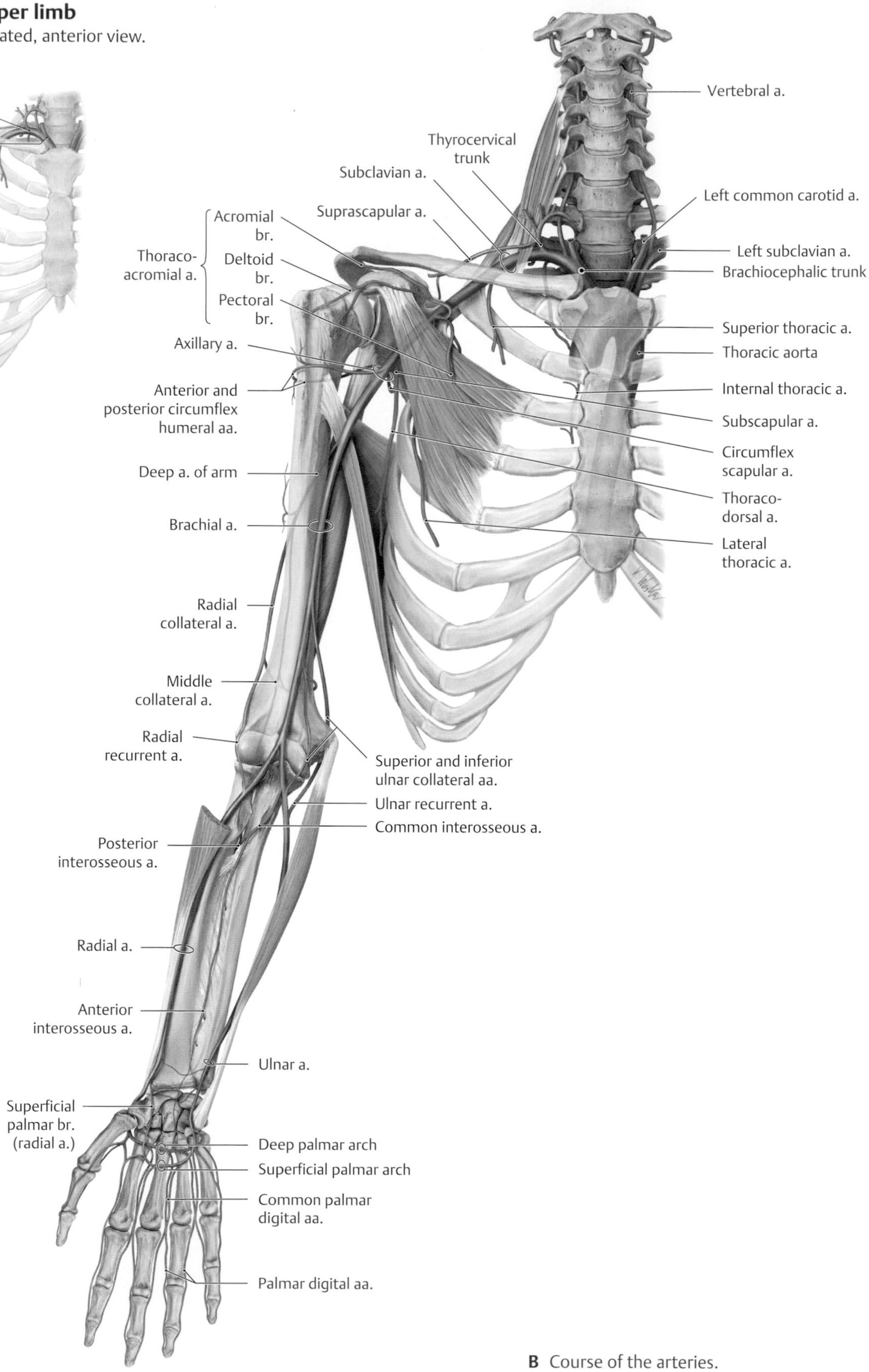

B Course of the arteries.

Fig. 28.2 Branches of the subclavian artery
Right side, anterior view.

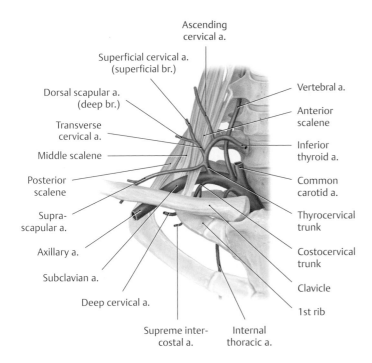

- Ascending cervical a.
- Superficial cervical a. (superficial br.)
- Dorsal scapular a. (deep br.)
- Transverse cervical a.
- Middle scalene
- Posterior scalene
- Supra-scapular a.
- Axillary a.
- Subclavian a.
- Deep cervical a.
- Supreme inter-costal a.
- Internal thoracic a.
- Vertebral a.
- Anterior scalene
- Inferior thyroid a.
- Common carotid a.
- Thyrocervical trunk
- Costocervical trunk
- Clavicle
- 1st rib

Fig. 28.3 Scapular arcade
Right side, posterior view.

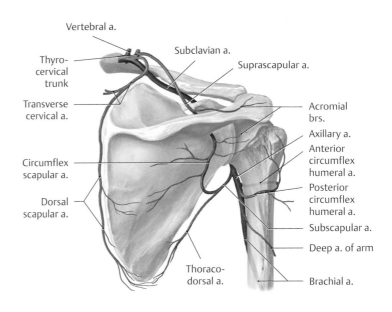

- Vertebral a.
- Thyro-cervical trunk
- Transverse cervical a.
- Circumflex scapular a.
- Dorsal scapular a.
- Thoraco-dorsal a.
- Subclavian a.
- Suprascapular a.
- Acromial brs.
- Axillary a.
- Anterior circumflex humeral a.
- Posterior circumflex humeral a.
- Subscapular a.
- Deep a. of arm
- Brachial a.

Fig. 28.4 Arteries of the forearm and hand
Right limb. The ulnar and radial arteries are interconnected by the superficial and deep palmar arches, the perforating branches, and the dorsal carpal network.

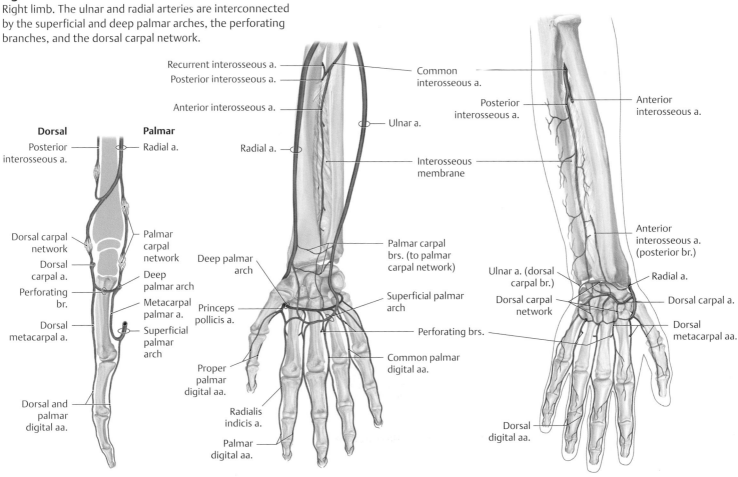

- Recurrent interosseous a.
- Posterior interosseous a.
- Anterior interosseous a.
- Common interosseous a.
- Posterior interosseous a.
- Anterior interosseous a.
- Ulnar a.
- Radial a.
- Interosseous membrane

Dorsal   **Palmar**
- Posterior interosseous a.
- Radial a.
- Dorsal carpal network
- Palmar carpal network
- Dorsal carpal a.
- Deep palmar arch
- Perforating br.
- Metacarpal palmar a.
- Dorsal metacarpal a.
- Superficial palmar arch
- Dorsal and palmar digital aa.

- Deep palmar arch
- Princeps pollicis a.
- Proper palmar digital aa.
- Radialis indicis a.
- Palmar digital aa.
- Palmar carpal brs. (to palmar carpal network)
- Superficial palmar arch
- Perforating brs.
- Common palmar digital aa.

- Posterior interosseous a.
- Anterior interosseous a.
- Anterior interosseous a. (posterior br.)
- Ulnar a. (dorsal carpal br.)
- Dorsal carpal network
- Dorsal digital aa.
- Radial a.
- Dorsal carpal a.
- Dorsal metacarpal aa.

A Right middle finger, lateral view.
B Anterior (palmar) view.
C Posterior (dorsal) view.

Veins & Lymphatics of the Upper Limb

Fig. 28.5 **Veins of the upper limb**
Right limb, anterior view.

Deltopectoral groove

Cephalic v.

Basilic hiatus

Basilic v.

Median cubital v.

Median ante-brachial v.

Cephalic v.

Perforator vv.

Superficial palmar venous arch

Intercapitular vv.

Basilic v.

A Superficial veins.

Axillary v.

Subscapular v.

Basilic v.

Brachial vv.

Anterior inter-osseous vv.

Radial vv.

Ulnar vv.

Deep palmar venous arch

Palmar metacarpal vv.

Palmar digital vv.

B Deep veins.

Fig. 28.6 **Veins of the dorsum**
Right hand, posterior view.

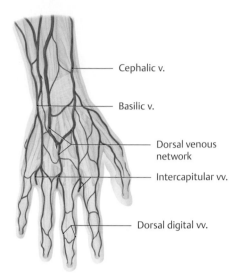

Cephalic v.

Basilic v.

Dorsal venous network

Intercapitular vv.

Dorsal digital vv.

Clinical box 28.1

Venipuncture
The veins of the cubital fossa are frequently used when drawing blood. In preparation, a tourniquet is applied above the cubital fossa. This allows arterial blood to flow, but blocks the return of venous blood. The resulting swelling makes the veins more visible and palpable.

Fig. 28.7 **Cubital fossa**
Right limb, anterior view. The subcutaneous veins of the cubital fossa have a highly variable course.

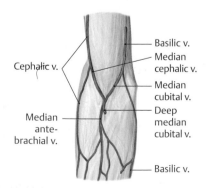

Cephalic v.

Median ante-brachial v.

Basilic v.

Median cephalic v.

Median cubital v.

Deep median cubital v.

Basilic v.

A M-shaped.

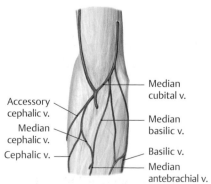

Accessory cephalic v.

Median cephalic v.

Cephalic v.

Median cubital v.

Median basilic v.

Basilic v.

Median antebrachial v.

B Accessory cephalic vein.

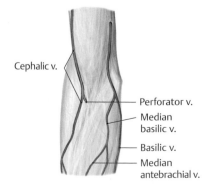

Cephalic v.

Perforator v.

Median basilic v.

Basilic v.

Median antebrachial v.

C Absent median cubital vein.

Lymph from the upper limb and breast drains to the axillary lymph nodes. The superficial lymphatics of the upper limb lie in the subcutaneous tissue, while the deep lymphatics accompany the arteries and deep veins. Numerous anastomoses exist between the two systems.

Fig. 28.8 Lymph vessels of the upper limb
Right limb.

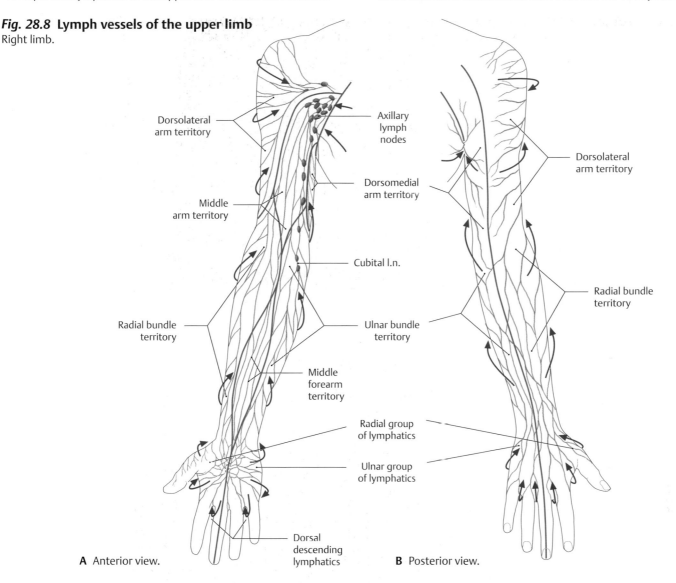

Dorsolateral arm territory

Axillary lymph nodes

Dorsomedial arm territory

Middle arm territory

Cubital l.n.

Radial bundle territory

Ulnar bundle territory

Middle forearm territory

Radial group of lymphatics

Ulnar group of lymphatics

Dorsal descending lymphatics

Dorsolateral arm territory

Radial bundle territory

A Anterior view.

B Posterior view.

Fig. 28.9 Lymphatic drainage of the hand
Right hand, radial view. Most of the hand drains to the axillary nodes via cubital nodes. However, the thumb, index finger, and dorsum of the hand drain directly.

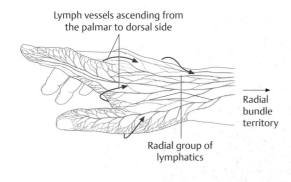

Lymph vessels ascending from the palmar to dorsal side

Radial bundle territory

Radial group of lymphatics

Fig. 28.10 Axillary lymph nodes
Right side, anterior view. For surgical purposes, the axillary lymph nodes are divided into three levels with respect to their relationship with the pectoralis minor: lateral (level I), posterior (level II), or medial (level III). They have major clinical importance in breast cancer (see **p. 76**).

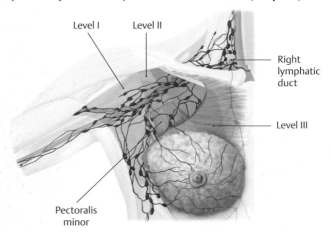

Level I

Level II

Right lymphatic duct

Level III

Pectoralis minor

Nerves of the Upper Limb: Brachial Plexus

Almost all muscles in the upper limb are innervated by the brachial plexus, which arises from spinal cord segments C5 to T1. The anterior rami of the spinal nerves give off direct branches (supraclavicular part of the brachial plexus) and merge to form three trunks, six divisions (three anterior and three posterior), and three cords. The infraclavicular part of the brachial plexus consists of short branches that arise directly from the cords and long (terminal) branches that traverse the limb.

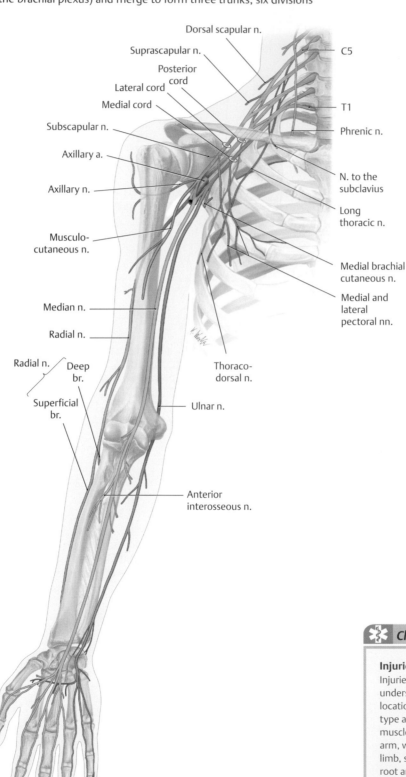

Table 28.1	Nerves of the brachial plexus		
Supraclavicular part			
Direct branches from the anterior rami or plexus trunks			
●	Dorsal scapular n.		C4–C5
	Suprascapular n.		C5, C6
	N. to the subclavius		C5–C6
	Long thoracic n.		C5–C7
Infraclavicular part			
Short and long branches from the plexus cords			
●	**Lateral cord**	Lateral pectoral n.	C5–C7
		Musculocutaneous n.	
●		Median n.	Lateral root	C6–C7
			Medial root	
	Medial cord	Medial pectoral n.	C8–T1
		Medial antebrachial cutaneous n.	
●		Medial brachial cutaneous n.	T1
		Ulnar n.	C7–T1
	Posterior cord	Upper subscapular n.	C5–C6
		Thoracodorsal n.	C6–C8
●		Lower subscapular n.	C5–C6
		Axillary n.	
		Radial n.	C5–T1

Clinical box 28.2

Injuries to nerves of the brachial plexus
Injuries of the brachial plexus can be complicated to diagnose but an understanding of the basic organization of the plexus is essential. The location of the injury can be determined by careful examination of the type and specificity of the deficit. Nerves of the upper plexus innervate muscles of the proximal limb such as those of the shoulder girdle and arm, while nerves of the lower plexus innervate muscles of the distal limb, such as the forearm and hand. Symptoms from injuries at the root and cord levels will demonstrate this anatomical arrangement. Additionally, a proximal injury to a nerve will elicit more broad-ranging symptoms than a distal injury to that nerve.

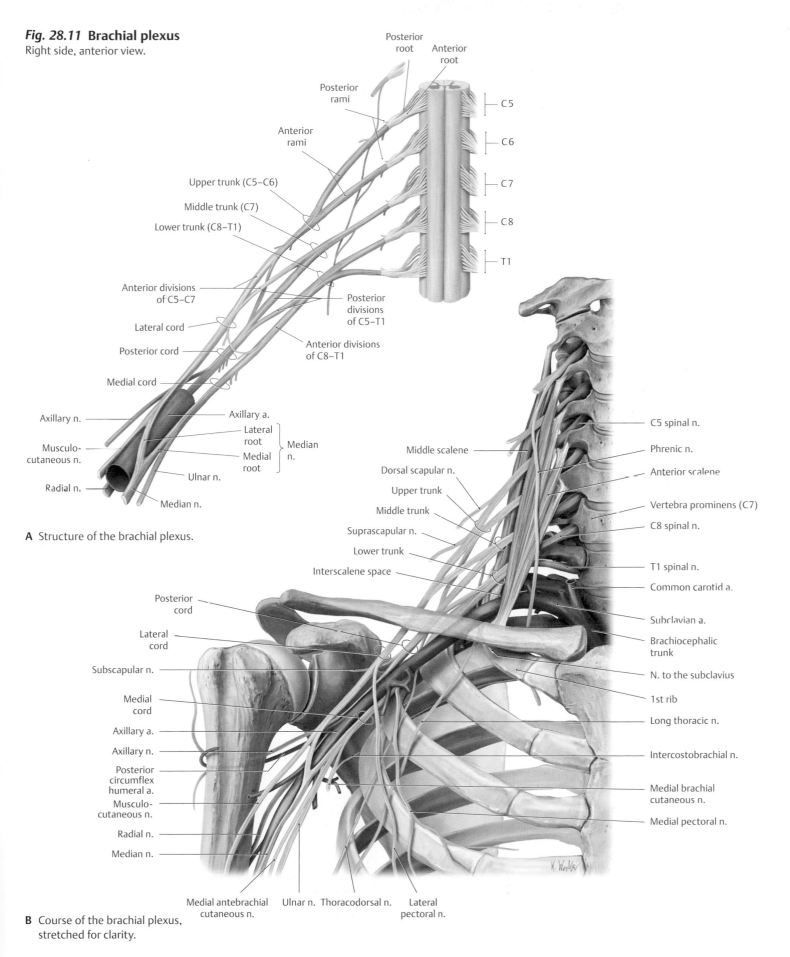

Fig. 28.11 Brachial plexus
Right side, anterior view.

Posterior root

Anterior root

Posterior rami

Anterior rami

C5
C6
C7
C8
T1

Upper trunk (C5–C6)

Middle trunk (C7)

Lower trunk (C8–T1)

Anterior divisions of C5–C7

Posterior divisions of C5–T1

Anterior divisions of C8–T1

Lateral cord

Posterior cord

Medial cord

Axillary n.

Axillary a.

Lateral root

Medial root

} Median n.

Musculo-cutaneous n.

Ulnar n.

Radial n.

Median n.

A Structure of the brachial plexus.

Middle scalene

Dorsal scapular n.

Upper trunk

Middle trunk

Suprascapular n.

Lower trunk

Interscalene space

C5 spinal n.

Phrenic n.

Anterior scalene

Vertebra prominens (C7)

C8 spinal n.

T1 spinal n.

Common carotid a.

Subclavian a.

Brachiocephalic trunk

Posterior cord

Lateral cord

Subscapular n.

Medial cord

Axillary a.

Axillary n.

Posterior circumflex humeral a.

Musculo-cutaneous n.

Radial n.

Median n.

N. to the subclavius

1st rib

Long thoracic n.

Intercostobrachial n.

Medial brachial cutaneous n.

Medial pectoral n.

Medial antebrachial cutaneous n.

Ulnar n.

Thoracodorsal n.

Lateral pectoral n.

B Course of the brachial plexus, stretched for clarity.

Supraclavicular Branches & Posterior Cord

Fig. 28.12 Supraclavicular branches
Right shoulder.

The supraclavicular branches of the brachial plexus arise directly from the plexus roots (anterior rami of the spinal nerves) or from the plexus trunks in the lateral cervical triangle.

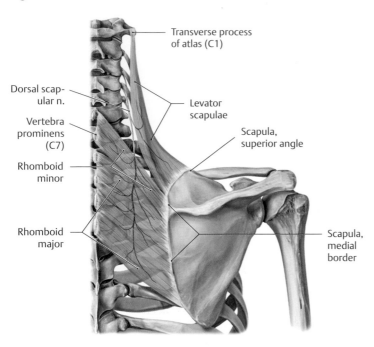

A Dorsal scapular nerve. Posterior view.

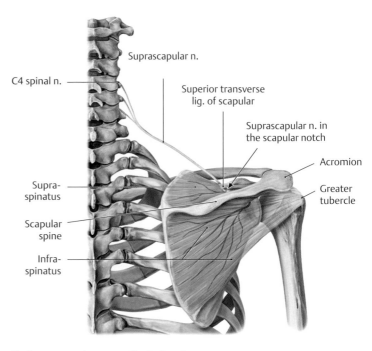

B Suprascapular nerve. Posterior view.

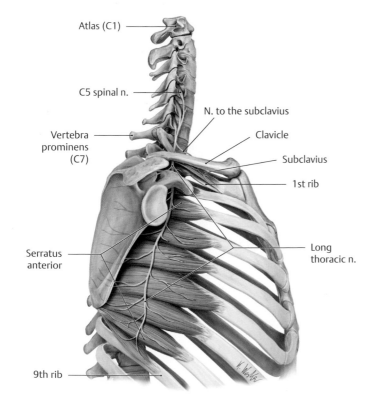

C Long thoracic nerve and nerve to the subclavius. Right lateral view.

Table 28.2	Supraclavicular branches	
Nerve	**Level**	**Innervated muscle**
Dorsal scapular n.	C4–C5	Levator scapulae Rhomboids major and minor
Suprascapular n.	C5, C6	Supraspinatus Infraspinatus
N. to the subclavius	C5–C6	Subclavius
Long thoracic n.	C5–C7	Serratus anterior

Fig. 28.13 Posterior cord: Short branches
Right shoulder.

The posterior cord gives off three short branches (arising at the level of the plexus cords) and two long branches (terminal nerves, see **pp. 372–373**).

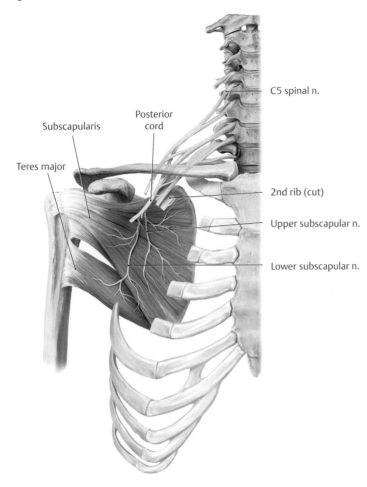

A Subscapular nerves. Anterior view.

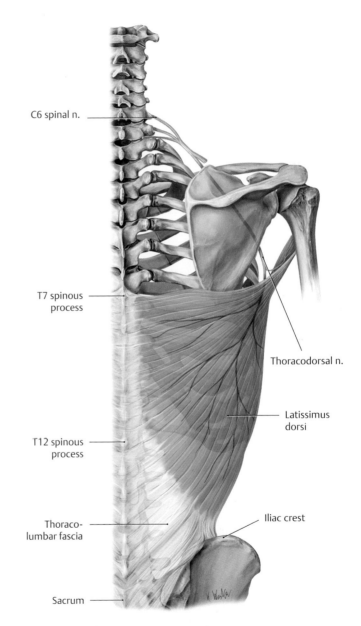

B Thoracodorsal nerve. Posterior view.

Table 28.3	Branches of the posterior cord	
Nerve	**Level**	**Innervated muscle**
Short branches		
Upper subscapular n.	C5–C6	Subscapularis
Lower subscapular n.		Subscapularis Teres major
Thoracodorsal n.	C6–C8	Latissimus dorsi
Long (terminal) branches		
Axillary n.	C5–C6	See **p. 372**
Radial n.	C5–T1	See **p. 373**

Posterior Cord: Axillary & Radial Nerves

Fig. 28.14 Axillary nerve: Cutaneous distribution
Right limb.

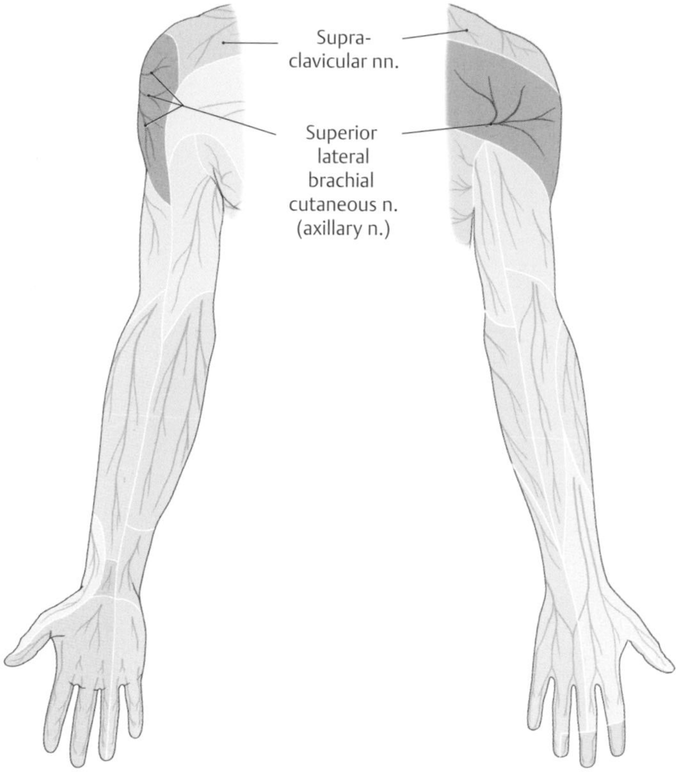

Supra-clavicular nn.

Superior lateral brachial cutaneous n. (axillary n.)

A Anterior view. **B** Posterior view.

The axillary nerve may be damaged in a fracture of the surgical neck of the humerus. This results in limited ability to abduct the arm and may cause a loss of profile of the shoulder.

Fig. 28.15 Axillary nerve
Right side, anterior view, stretched for clarity.

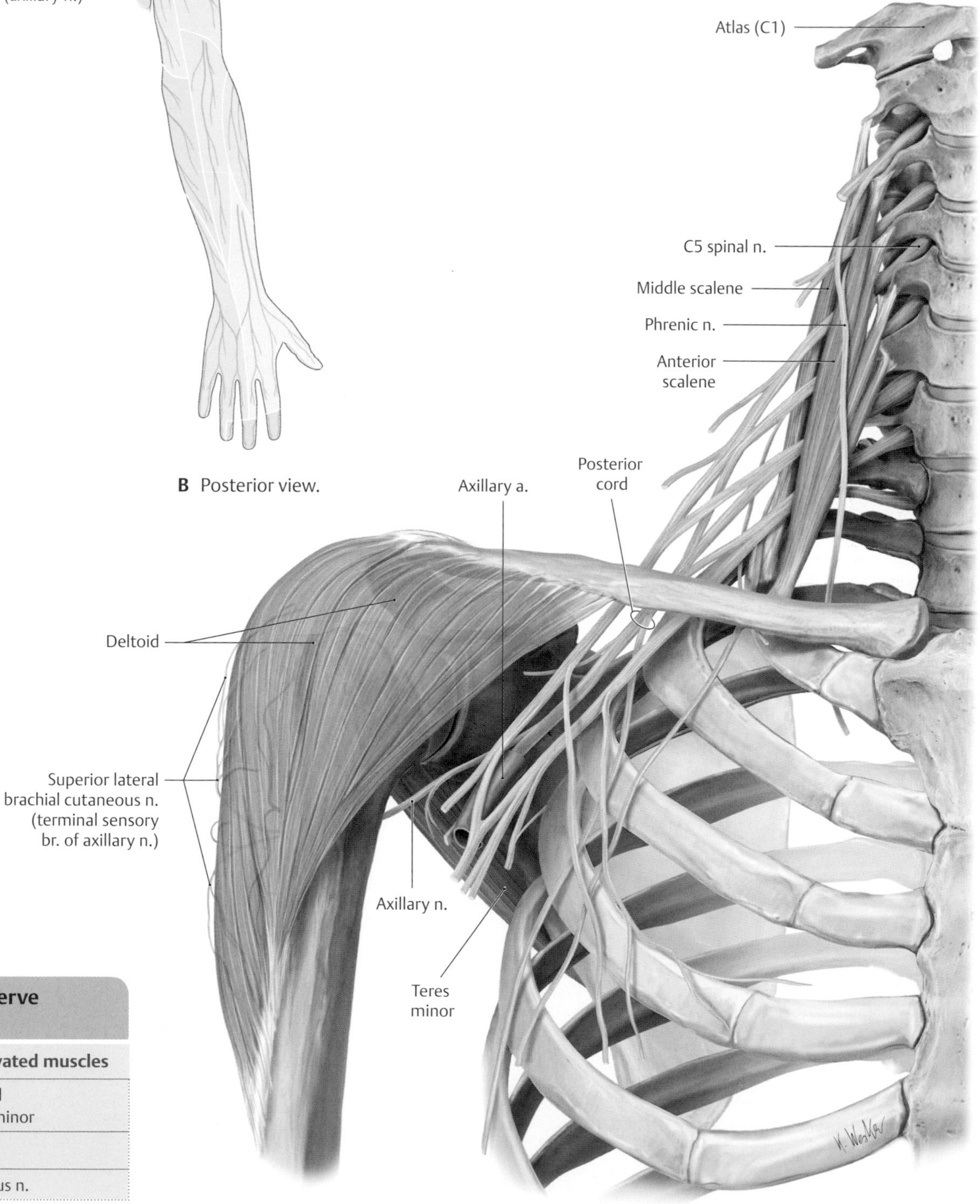

Atlas (C1)

C5 spinal n.

Middle scalene

Phrenic n.

Anterior scalene

Posterior cord

Axillary a.

Deltoid

Superior lateral brachial cutaneous n. (terminal sensory br. of axillary n.)

Axillary n.

Teres minor

Table 28.4	Axillary nerve (C5–C6)
Motor branches	**Innervated muscles**
Muscular brs.	Deltoid Teres minor
Sensory branch	
Superior lateral brachial cutaneous n.	

Fig. 28.16 Radial nerve: Cutaneous distribution

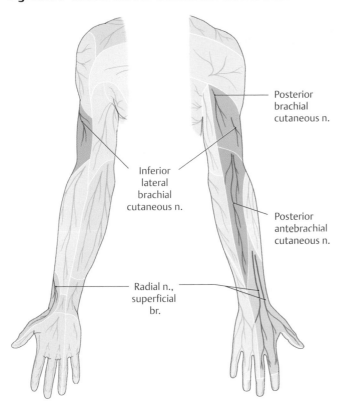

A Anterior view.   **B** Posterior view.

Fig. 28.17 Radial nerve

Right limb, anterior view with forearm pronated.

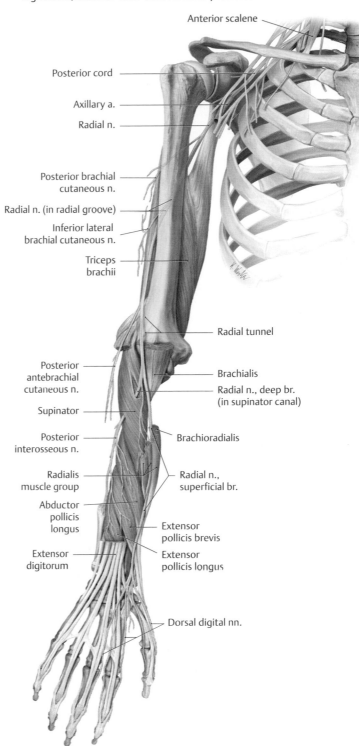

Table 28.5	Radial nerve (C5–T1)
Motor branches	**Innervated muscles**
Muscular brs.	Brachialis (partial)
	Triceps brachii
	Anconeus
	Brachioradialis
	Extensors carpi radialis longus and brevis
Deep br. (terminal br.: posterior interosseous n.)	Supinator
	Extensor digitorum
	Extensor digiti minimi
	Extensor carpi ulnaris
	Extensors pollicis brevis and longus
	Extensor indicis
	Abductor pollicis longus
Sensory branches	
Articular brs. from radial n.: Capsule of the shoulder joint	
Articular brs. from posterior interosseous n.: Joint capsule of the wrist and four radial metacarpophalangeal joints	
Posterior brachial cutaneous n.	
Inferior lateral brachial cutaneous n.	
Posterior antebrachial cutaneous n.	
Superficial brs.	Dorsal digital nn.
	Ulnar communicating br.

✳ Clinical box 28.4

Chronic radial nerve compression in the axilla (e.g., due to extended/improper crutch use) may cause loss of sensation or motor function in the hand, forearm, and posterior arm. More distal injuries (e.g., during anesthesia) affect fewer muscles, potentially resulting in wrist drop with intact triceps brachii function.

Medial & Lateral Cords

The medial and lateral cords give off four short branches. The intercostobrachial nerves are included with the short branches of the brachial plexus, although they are actually the cutaneous branches of the 2nd and 3rd intercostal nerves.

Table 28.6		Branches of the medial and lateral cords	
Nerve	**Level**	**Cord**	**Innervated muscle**
Short branches			
Lateral pectoral n.	C5–C7	Lateral cord	Pectoralis major
Medial pectoral n.	C8–T1	Medial cord	Pectoralis major and minor
Medial brachial cutaneous n.	T1		— (sensory brs., do not innervate any muscles)
Medial antebrachial cutaneous n.	C8–T1		
Intercostobrachial nn.	T2–T3		
Long (terminal) branches			
Musculocutaneous n.	C5–C7	Lateral cord	Coracobrachialis Biceps brachii Brachialis
Median n.	C6–T1	Medial cord	See **p. 376**
Ulnar n.	C7–T1		See **p. 377**

Fig. 28.19 **Short branches of medial and lateral cords: Cutaneous distribution**

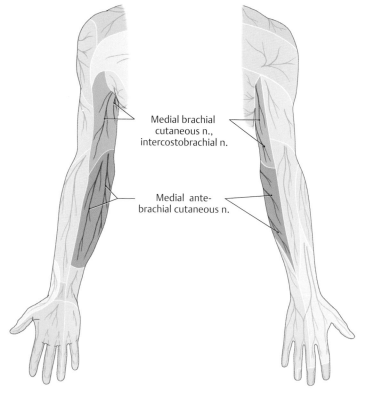

Medial brachial cutaneous n., intercostobrachial n.

Medial antebrachial cutaneous n.

A Anterior view.   **B** Posterior view.

Fig. 28.18 **Medial and lateral cords: Short branches**
Right side, anterior view.

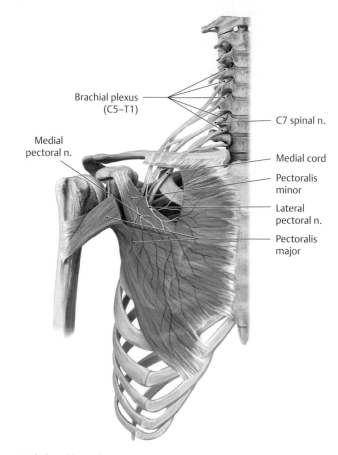

Brachial plexus (C5–T1)

Medial pectoral n.

C7 spinal n.

Medial cord

Pectoralis minor

Lateral pectoral n.

Pectoralis major

A Medial and lateral pectoral nerves.

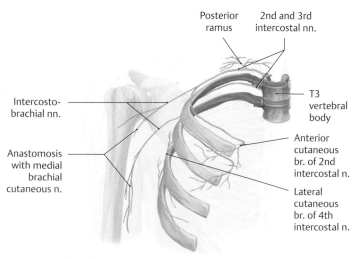

Posterior ramus

2nd and 3rd intercostal nn.

Intercostobrachial nn.

T3 vertebral body

Anterior cutaneous br. of 2nd intercostal n.

Anastomosis with medial brachial cutaneous n.

Lateral cutaneous br. of 4th intercostal n.

B Intercostobrachial nerves.

Fig. 28.20 Musculocutaneous nerve

Right limb, anterior view.

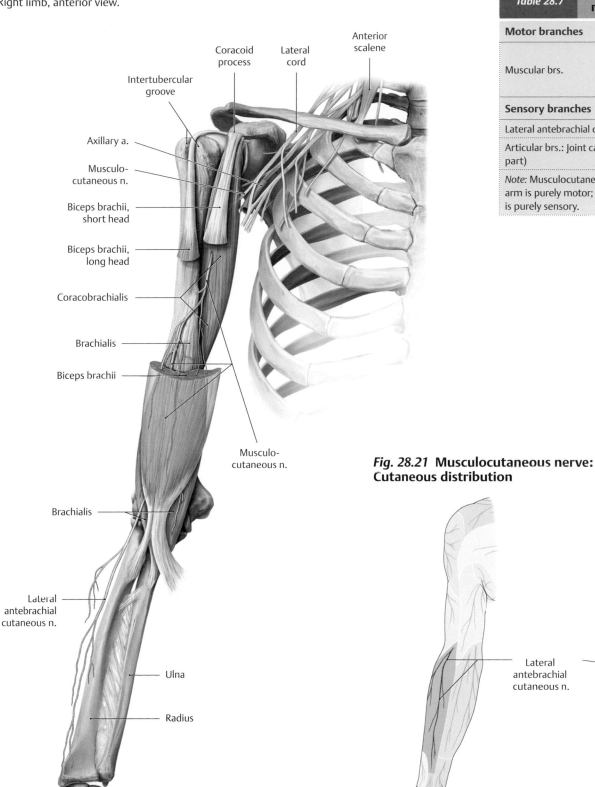

Table 28.7	Musculocutaneous nerve (C5–C7)
Motor branches	**Innervated muscles**
Muscular brs.	Coracobrachialis
	Biceps brachii
	Brachialis
Sensory branches	
Lateral antebrachial cutaneous n.	
Articular brs.: Joint capsule of the elbow (anterior part)	
Note: Musculocutaneous n. innervation of the arm is purely motor; innervation of the forearm is purely sensory.	

Fig. 28.21 Musculocutaneous nerve: Cutaneous distribution

Lateral antebrachial cutaneous n.

A Anterior view.   **B** Posterior view.

Median & Ulnar Nerves

The median nerve is a terminal branch arising from both the medial and the lateral cords. The ulnar nerve arises exclusively from the medial cord.

Fig. 28.22 **Median nerve**
Right limb, anterior view.

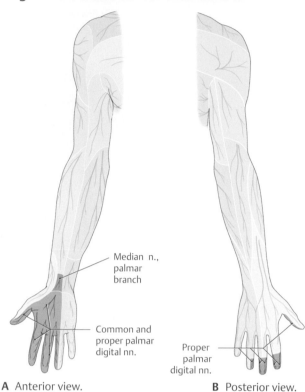

Anterior scalene

Lateral cord

Medial cord

Axillary a.

Median n. { Lateral root / Medial root

Median n.

Articular br.

Medial epicondyle

Pronator teres, humeral head

Flexor carpi radialis

Pronator teres, ulnar head

Palmaris longus

Flexor digitorum superficialis

Anterior interosseous n.

Flexor digitorum profundus

Flexor pollicis longus

Pronator quadratus

Recurrent br.

Median n., palmar br.

Flexor retinaculum

Common palmar digital nn.

1st and 2nd lumbricals

Proper palmar digital nn.

Fig. 28.23 **Median nerve: Cutaneous distribution**

Median n., palmar branch

Common and proper palmar digital nn.

Proper palmar digital nn.

A Anterior view.

B Posterior view.

Table 28.8	Median nerve (C6–T1)	
Motor branches	**Innervated muscles**	
Direct muscular brs.	Pronator teres	
	Flexor carpi radialis	
	Palmaris longus	
	Flexor digitorum superficialis	
Muscular brs. from anterior interosseous n.	Pronator quadratus	
	Flexor pollicis longus	
	Flexor digitorum profundus (radial half)	
Recurrent br.	Abductor pollicis brevis	
	Flexor pollicis brevis (superficial head)	
	Opponens pollicis	
Muscular brs. from common palmar digital nn.	1st and 2nd lumbricals	
Sensory branches		
Articular brs.: Capsules of the elbow and wrist joints		
Palmar br. of median n. (thenar eminence)		
Communicating br. to ulnar n.		
Common palmar digital nn.		
Proper palmar digital nn.		

✚ *Clinical box 28.5*

Median nerve injury caused by fracture/dislocation of the elbow joint may result in compromised grasping ability and sensory loss in the fingertips (see **Fig. 28.23** for territories). See also carpal tunnel syndrome (**p. 391**).

Fig. 28.24 Ulnar nerve: Cutaneous distribution

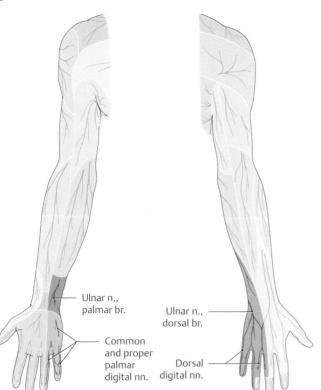

A Anterior view.

B Posterior view.

Ulnar n., palmar br.

Common and proper palmar digital nn.

Ulnar n., dorsal br.

Dorsal digital nn.

Fig. 28.25 Ulnar nerve
Right limb, anterior view.

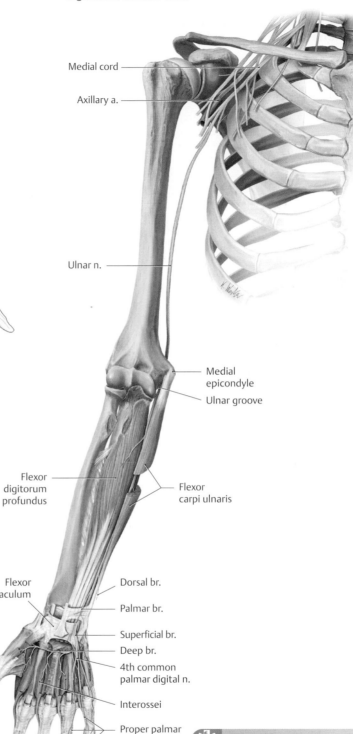

Medial cord

Axillary a.

Ulnar n.

Medial epicondyle

Ulnar groove

Flexor digitorum profundus

Flexor carpi ulnaris

Flexor retinaculum

Dorsal br.

Palmar br.

Superficial br.

Deep br.

4th common palmar digital n.

Interossei

Proper palmar digital nn.

Table 28.9	Ulnar nerve (C7–T1)
Motor branches	**Innervated muscles**
Direct muscular brs.	Flexor carpi ulnaris
	Flexor digitorum profundus (ulnar half)
Muscular br. from superior ulnar n.	Palmaris brevis
Muscular brs. from deep ulnar n.	Abductor digiti minimi
	Flexor digiti minimi brevis
	Opponens digiti minimi
	3rd and 4th lumbricals
	Palmar and dorsal interosseous muscles
	Adductor pollicis
	Flexor pollicis brevis (deep head)
Sensory branches	
Articular brs.: Capsules of the elbow, carpal, and metacarpophalangeal joints	
Dorsal br. (terminal brs.: dorsal digital nn.)	
Palmar br.	
Proper palmar digital n. (from superficial br.)	
Common palmar digital n. (from superficial br.; terminal brs.: proper palmar digital nn.)	

✳ Clinical box 28.6

Ulnar nerve palsy is the most common peripheral nerve damage. The ulnar nerve is most vulnerable to trauma or chronic compression in the elbow joint and ulnar tunnel (see **p. 391**). Nerve damage causes "clawing" of the hand and atrophy of the interossei. Sensory losses are often limited to the 5th digit.

Superficial Veins & Nerves of the Upper Limb

Fig. 28.26 **Superficial cutaneous veins and nerves of the upper limb**

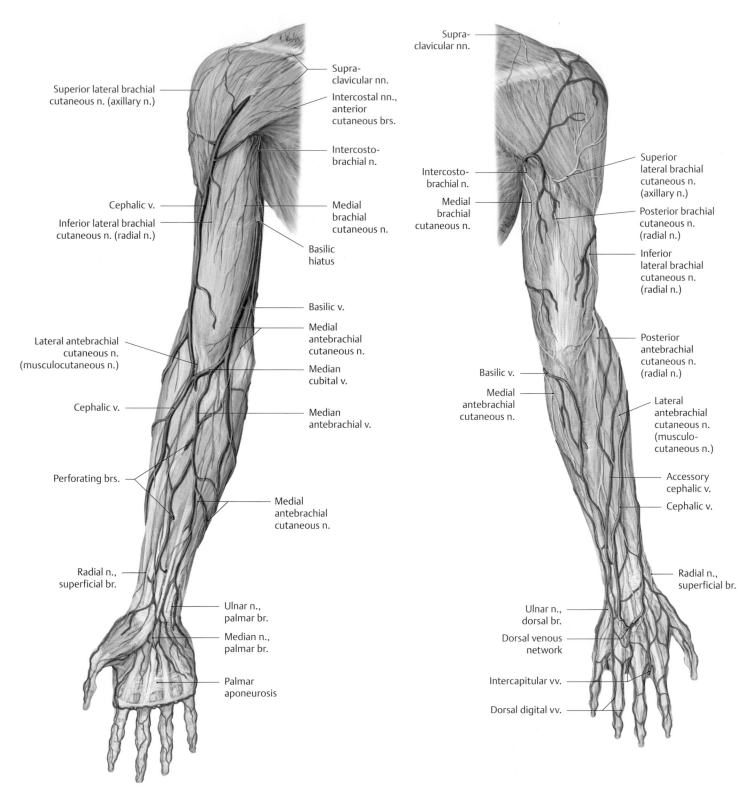

Superior lateral brachial cutaneous n. (axillary n.)

Supra-clavicular nn.

Intercostal nn., anterior cutaneous brs.

Intercosto-brachial n.

Cephalic v.

Inferior lateral brachial cutaneous n. (radial n.)

Medial brachial cutaneous n.

Basilic hiatus

Basilic v.

Medial antebrachial cutaneous n.

Median cubital v.

Median antebrachial v.

Lateral antebrachial cutaneous n. (musculocutaneous n.)

Cephalic v.

Perforating brs.

Medial antebrachial cutaneous n.

Radial n., superficial br.

Ulnar n., palmar br.

Median n., palmar br.

Palmar aponeurosis

Supra-clavicular nn.

Intercosto-brachial n.

Medial brachial cutaneous n.

Superior lateral brachial cutaneous n. (axillary n.)

Posterior brachial cutaneous n. (radial n.)

Inferior lateral brachial cutaneous n. (radial n.)

Posterior antebrachial cutaneous n. (radial n.)

Basilic v.

Medial antebrachial cutaneous n.

Lateral antebrachial cutaneous n. (musculo-cutaneous n.)

Accessory cephalic v.

Cephalic v.

Radial n., superficial br.

Ulnar n., dorsal br.

Dorsal venous network

Intercapitular vv.

Dorsal digital vv.

A Anterior view. See **pp. 392–393** for nerves of the palm.

B Posterior view. See **pp. 394–395** for nerves of the dorsum.

Fig. 28.27 Cutaneous innervation of the upper limb

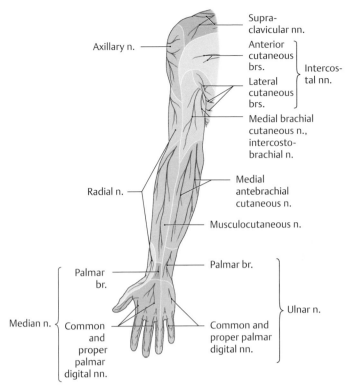

Supra-clavicular nn.

Axillary n.

Anterior cutaneous brs.

Lateral cutaneous brs.

} Intercostal nn.

Medial brachial cutaneous n., intercosto-brachial n.

Radial n.

Medial antebrachial cutaneous n.

Musculocutaneous n.

Palmar br.

Palmar br.

Median n. {

Palmar br.

Common and proper palmar digital nn.

Common and proper palmar digital nn.

} Ulnar n.

A Anterior view.

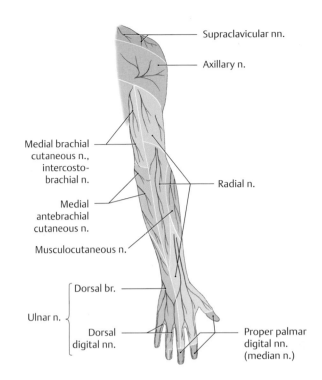

Supraclavicular nn.

Axillary n.

Medial brachial cutaneous n., intercosto-brachial n.

Radial n.

Medial antebrachial cutaneous n.

Musculocutaneous n.

Ulnar n. {

Dorsal br.

Dorsal digital nn.

Proper palmar digital nn. (median n.)

B Posterior view.

Fig. 28.28 Dermatomes of the upper limb

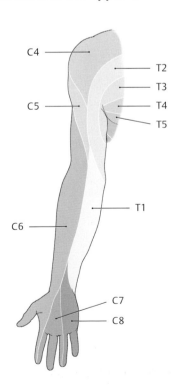

C4

T2

T3

C5

T4

T5

C6

T1

C7

C8

A Anterior view.

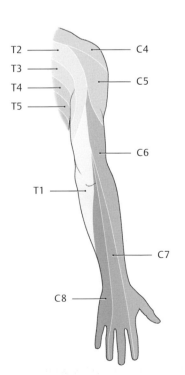

T2

T3

T4

T5

C4

C5

C6

T1

C7

C8

B Posterior view.

Posterior Shoulder & Arm

Fig. 28.29 **Posterior shoulder**
Right shoulder, posterior view. *Raised:* Trapezius (transverse part).
Windowed: Supraspinatus. *Revealed:* Suprascapular region.

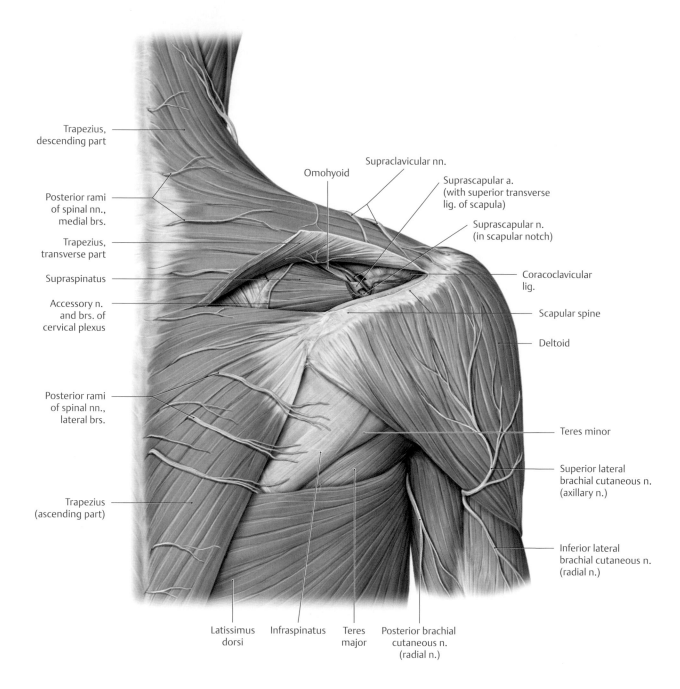

Trapezius, descending part

Posterior rami of spinal nn., medial brs.

Trapezius, transverse part

Supraspinatus

Accessory n. and brs. of cervical plexus

Posterior rami of spinal nn., lateral brs.

Trapezius (ascending part)

Omohyoid

Supraclavicular nn.

Suprascapular a. (with superior transverse lig. of scapula)

Suprascapular n. (in scapular notch)

Coracoclavicular lig.

Scapular spine

Deltoid

Teres minor

Superior lateral brachial cutaneous n. (axillary n.)

Inferior lateral brachial cutaneous n. (radial n.)

Latissimus dorsi

Infraspinatus

Teres major

Posterior brachial cutaneous n. (radial n.)

Table 28.10	Neurovascular tracts of the scapula	

Passageway		Boundaries	Transmitted structures
①	Scapular notch	Superior transverse lig. of scapula, scapula	Suprascapular a., v. and n.
②	Medial border	Scapula	Dorsal scapular a., v. and n.
③	Triangular space	Teres major and minor, triceps brachii	Circumflex scapular a. and v.
④	Triceps hiatus	Triceps brachii, humerus, teres major	Deep a. and v. of arm and radial n.
⑤	Quadrangular space	Teres major and minor, triceps brachii, humerus	Posterior circumflex humeral a. and v. and axillary n.

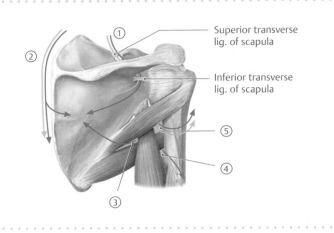

Fig. 28.30 Triangular and quadrangular spaces

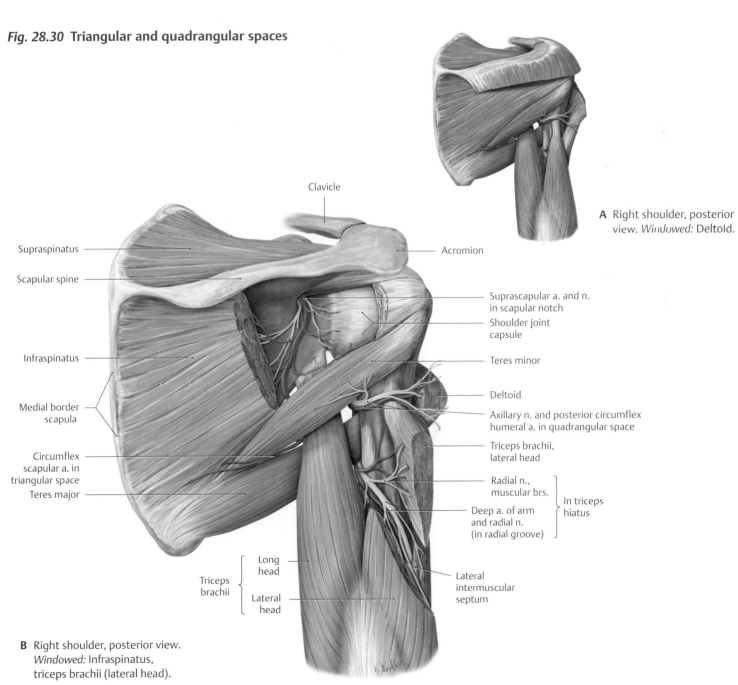

A Right shoulder, posterior view. *Windowed:* Deltoid.

B Right shoulder, posterior view. *Windowed:* Infraspinatus, triceps brachii (lateral head).

Anterior Shoulder

Fig. 28.31 Anterior shoulder: Superficial dissection
Right shoulder.

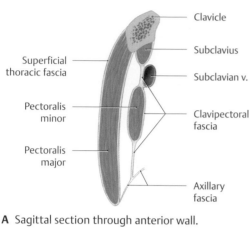

- Clavicle
- Subclavius
- Subclavian v.
- Clavipectoral fascia
- Superficial thoracic fascia
- Pectoralis minor
- Pectoralis major
- Axillary fascia

A Sagittal section through anterior wall.

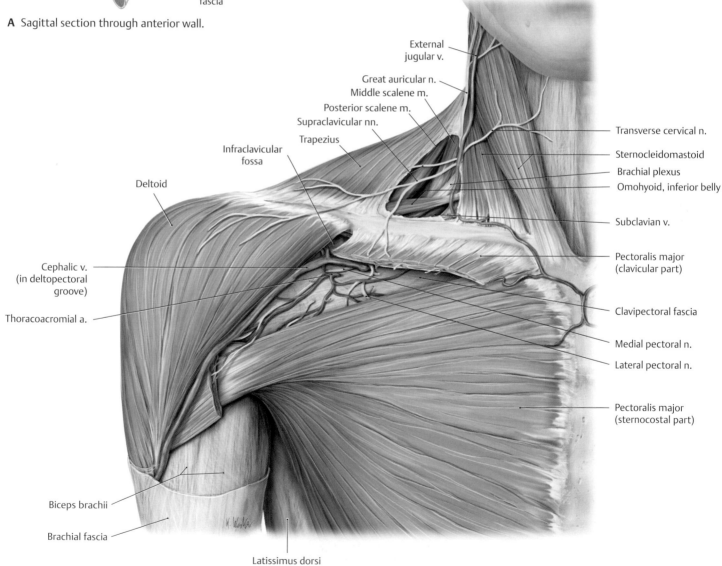

- External jugular v.
- Great auricular n.
- Middle scalene m.
- Posterior scalene m.
- Supraclavicular nn.
- Trapezius
- Infraclavicular fossa
- Deltoid
- Cephalic v. (in deltopectoral groove)
- Thoracoacromial a.
- Biceps brachii
- Brachial fascia
- Latissimus dorsi
- Transverse cervical n.
- Sternocleidomastoid
- Brachial plexus
- Omohyoid, inferior belly
- Subclavian v.
- Pectoralis major (clavicular part)
- Clavipectoral fascia
- Medial pectoral n.
- Lateral pectoral n.
- Pectoralis major (sternocostal part)

B Anterior view. *Removed:* Platysma, muscle fasciae, superficial layer of cervical fascia, and pectoralis major (clavicular part). *Revealed:* Clavipectoral triangle.

Fig. 28.32 **Shoulder: Transverse section**

Right shoulder, inferior view.

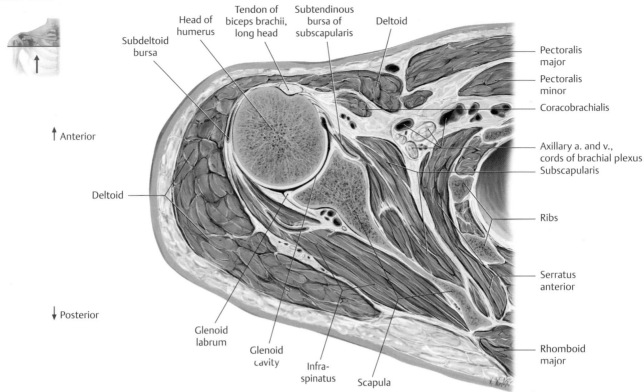

Fig. 28.33 **Anterior shoulder: Deep dissection**

Right limb, anterior view. *Removed:* Sternocleidomastoid, omohyoid, and pectoralis major. This dissection reveals the neurovascular contents of the lateral cervical triangle (see **pp. 538–539**) and axilla (see **pp. 384–385**).

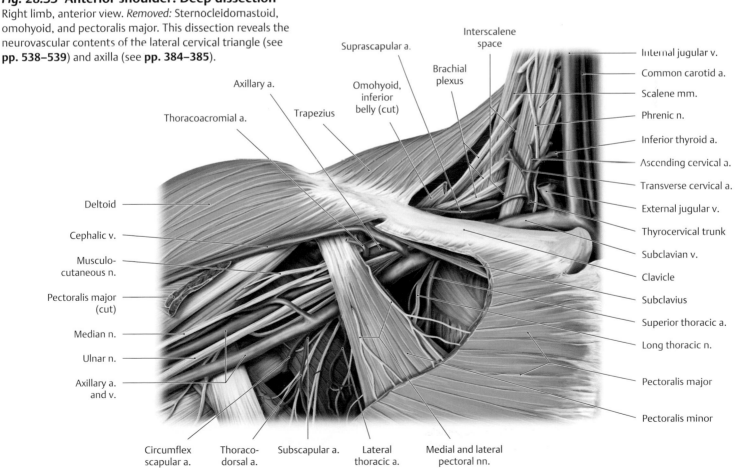

Fig. 28.34 **Axilla: Dissection**
Right shoulder, anterior view.

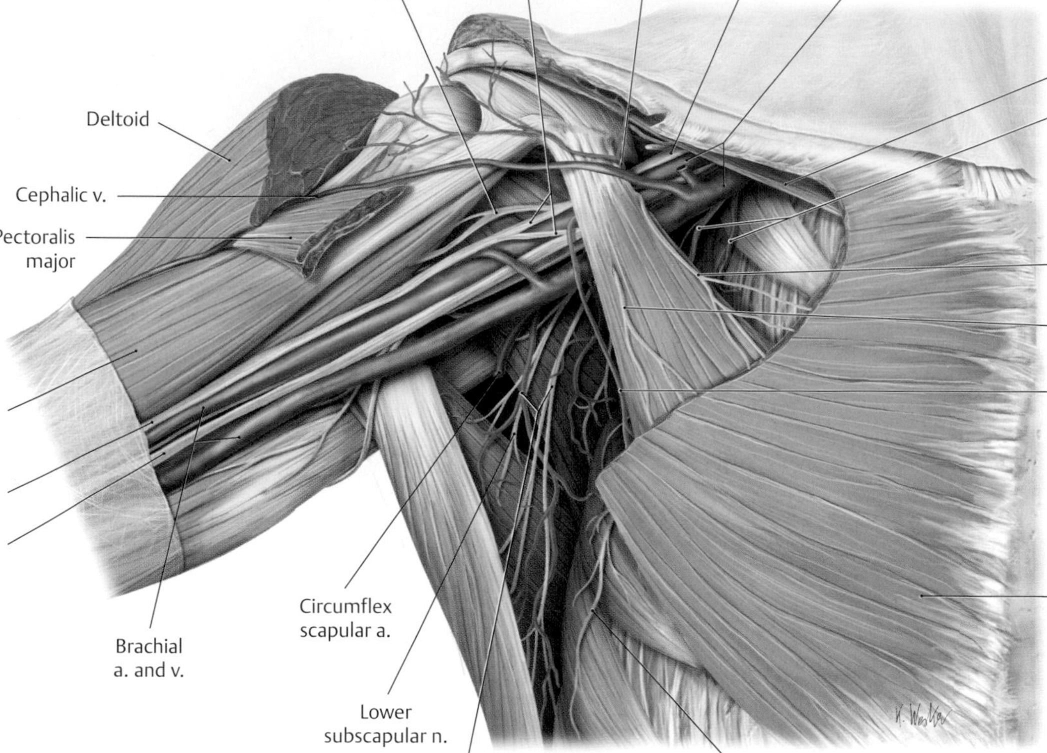

A *Removed:* Pectoralis major and clavipectoral fascia.

Table 28.11	Walls of the axilla
Anterior wall	Pectoralis major Pectoralis minor Clavipectoral fascia
Lateral wall	Intertubercular groove of humerus
Posterior wall	Subscapularis Teres major Latissimus dorsi
Medial wall	Lateral thoracic wall Serratus anterior

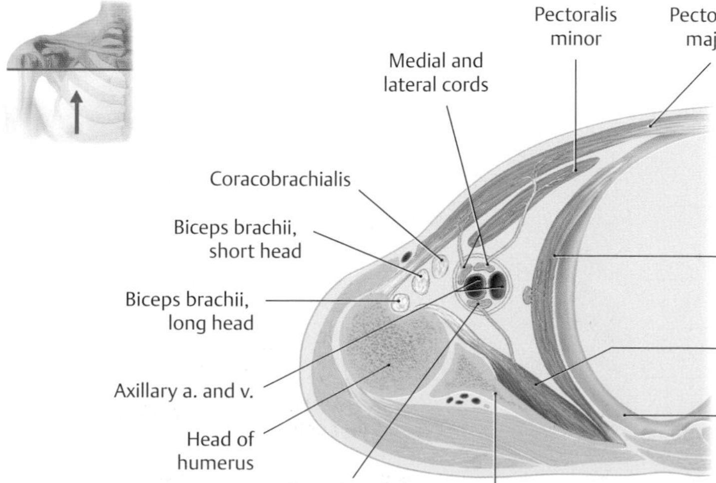

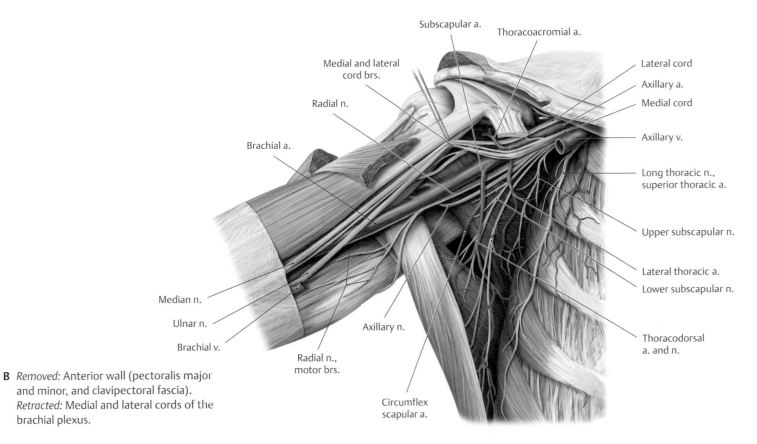

Subscapular a.

Thoracoacromial a.

Medial and lateral cord brs.

Radial n.

Brachial a.

Median n.

Ulnar n.

Brachial v.

Radial n., motor brs.

Axillary n.

Circumflex scapular a.

Lateral cord

Axillary a.

Medial cord

Axillary v.

Long thoracic n., superior thoracic a.

Upper subscapular n.

Lateral thoracic a.

Lower subscapular n.

Thoracodorsal a. and n.

B *Removed:* Anterior wall (pectoralis major and minor, and clavipectoral fascia). *Retracted:* Medial and lateral cords of the brachial plexus.

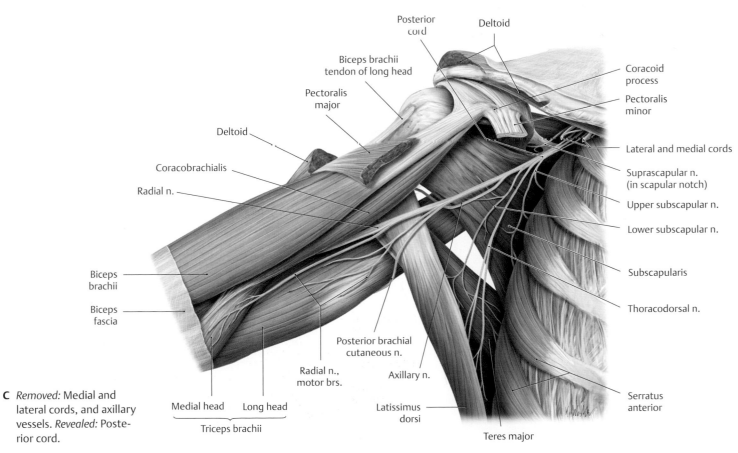

Posterior cord

Deltoid

Biceps brachii tendon of long head

Pectoralis major

Deltoid

Coracobrachialis

Radial n.

Biceps brachii

Biceps fascia

Medial head   Long head

Triceps brachii

Posterior brachial cutaneous n.

Radial n., motor brs.

Axillary n.

Latissimus dorsi

Teres major

Coracoid process

Pectoralis minor

Lateral and medial cords

Suprascapular n. (in scapular notch)

Upper subscapular n.

Lower subscapular n.

Subscapularis

Thoracodorsal n.

Serratus anterior

C *Removed:* Medial and lateral cords, and axillary vessels. *Revealed:* Posterior cord.

Fig. 28.35 Brachial region

Right arm, anterior view. *Removed:* Deltoid, pectoralis major and minor. *Revealed:* Medial bicipital groove.

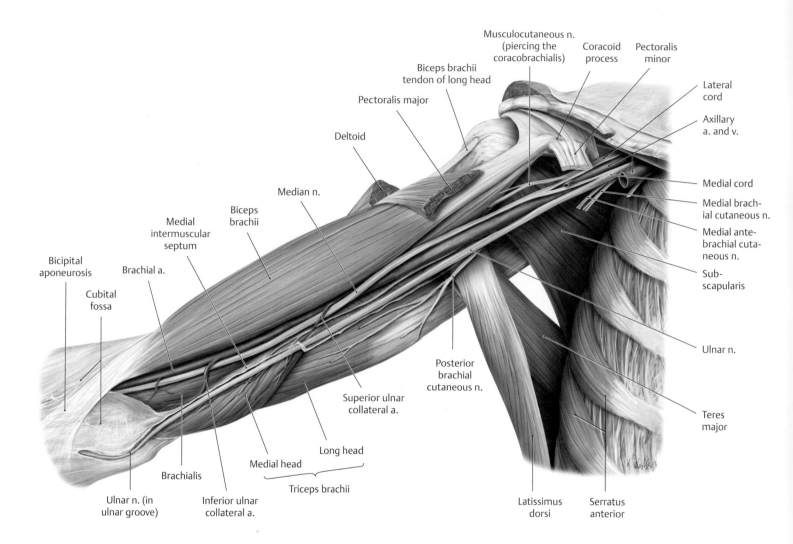

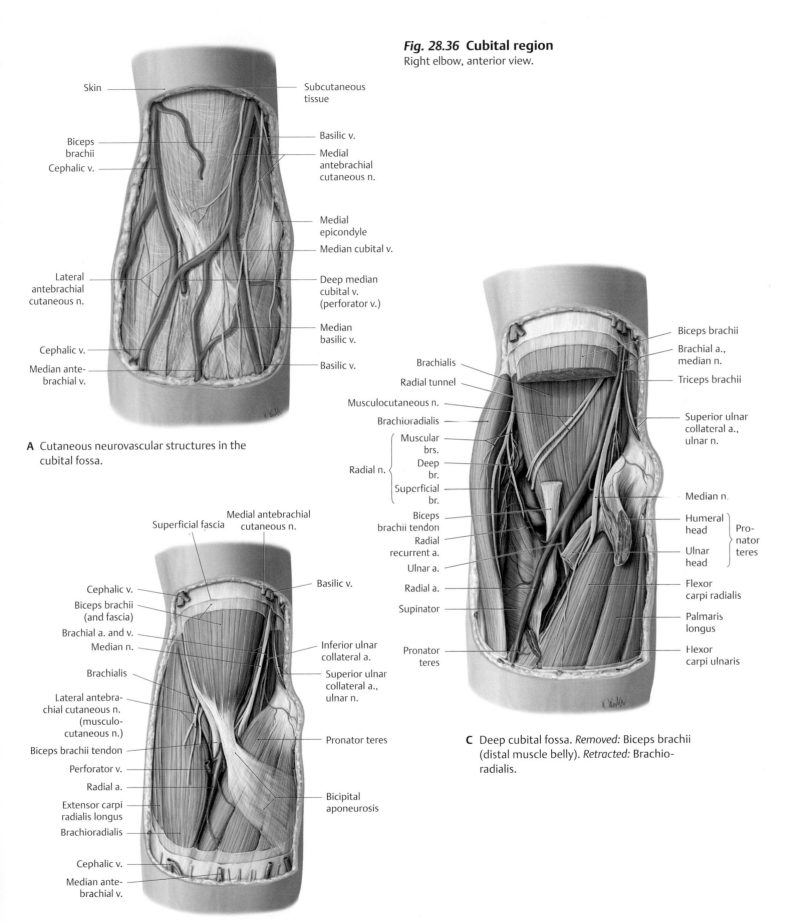

Fig. 28.36 **Cubital region**
Right elbow, anterior view.

Skin

Subcutaneous tissue

Biceps brachii

Cephalic v.

Basilic v.

Medial antebrachial cutaneous n.

Medial epicondyle

Median cubital v.

Lateral antebrachial cutaneous n.

Deep median cubital v. (perforator v.)

Median basilic v.

Cephalic v.

Basilic v.

Median antebrachial v.

A Cutaneous neurovascular structures in the cubital fossa.

Superficial fascia

Medial antebrachial cutaneous n.

Cephalic v.

Basilic v.

Biceps brachii (and fascia)

Brachial a. and v.

Median n.

Brachialis

Inferior ulnar collateral a.

Superior ulnar collateral a., ulnar n.

Lateral antebrachial cutaneous n. (musculocutaneous n.)

Biceps brachii tendon

Perforator v.

Radial a.

Pronator teres

Extensor carpi radialis longus

Brachioradialis

Cephalic v.

Bicipital aponeurosis

Median antebrachial v.

B Superficial cubital fossa. *Removed:* Fasciae and epifascial neurovascular structures.

Brachialis

Radial tunnel

Musculocutaneous n.

Brachioradialis

Radial n. {
Muscular brs.
Deep br.
Superficial br.
}

Biceps brachii tendon

Radial recurrent a.

Ulnar a.

Radial a.

Supinator

Pronator teres

Biceps brachii

Brachial a., median n.

Triceps brachii

Superior ulnar collateral a., ulnar n.

Median n.

Humeral head } Pronator teres
Ulnar head

Flexor carpi radialis

Palmaris longus

Flexor carpi ulnaris

C Deep cubital fossa. *Removed:* Biceps brachii (distal muscle belly). *Retracted:* Brachioradialis.

387

Anterior & Posterior Forearm

Fig. 28.37 Anterior forearm
Right forearm, anterior view.

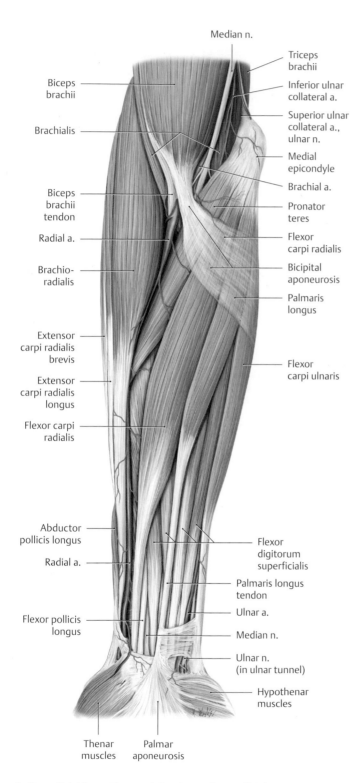

Median n.
Triceps brachii
Biceps brachii
Inferior ulnar collateral a.
Brachialis
Superior ulnar collateral a., ulnar n.
Medial epicondyle
Biceps brachii tendon
Brachial a.
Pronator teres
Radial a.
Flexor carpi radialis
Brachio-radialis
Bicipital aponeurosis
Palmaris longus
Extensor carpi radialis brevis
Extensor carpi radialis longus
Flexor carpi ulnaris
Flexor carpi radialis
Abductor pollicis longus
Flexor digitorum superficialis
Radial a.
Palmaris longus tendon
Ulnar a.
Flexor pollicis longus
Median n.
Ulnar n. (in ulnar tunnel)
Hypothenar muscles
Thenar muscles
Palmar aponeurosis

A Superficial layer. *Removed:* Fasciae and superficial neurovasculature.

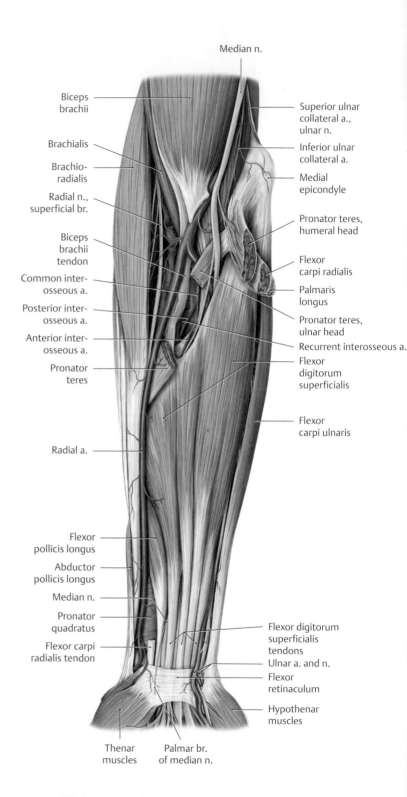

Median n.
Biceps brachii
Superior ulnar collateral a., ulnar n.
Brachialis
Inferior ulnar collateral a.
Brachio-radialis
Medial epicondyle
Radial n., superficial br.
Pronator teres, humeral head
Biceps brachii tendon
Flexor carpi radialis
Common inter-osseous a.
Palmaris longus
Posterior inter-osseous a.
Pronator teres, ulnar head
Anterior inter-osseous a.
Recurrent interosseous a.
Pronator teres
Flexor digitorum superficialis
Radial a.
Flexor carpi ulnaris
Flexor pollicis longus
Abductor pollicis longus
Median n.
Pronator quadratus
Flexor digitorum superficialis tendons
Flexor carpi radialis tendon
Ulnar a. and n.
Flexor retinaculum
Hypothenar muscles
Thenar muscles
Palmar br. of median n.

B Middle layer. *Partially removed:* Superficial flexors (pronator teres, flexor digitorum superficialis, palmaris longus, and flexor carpi radialis).

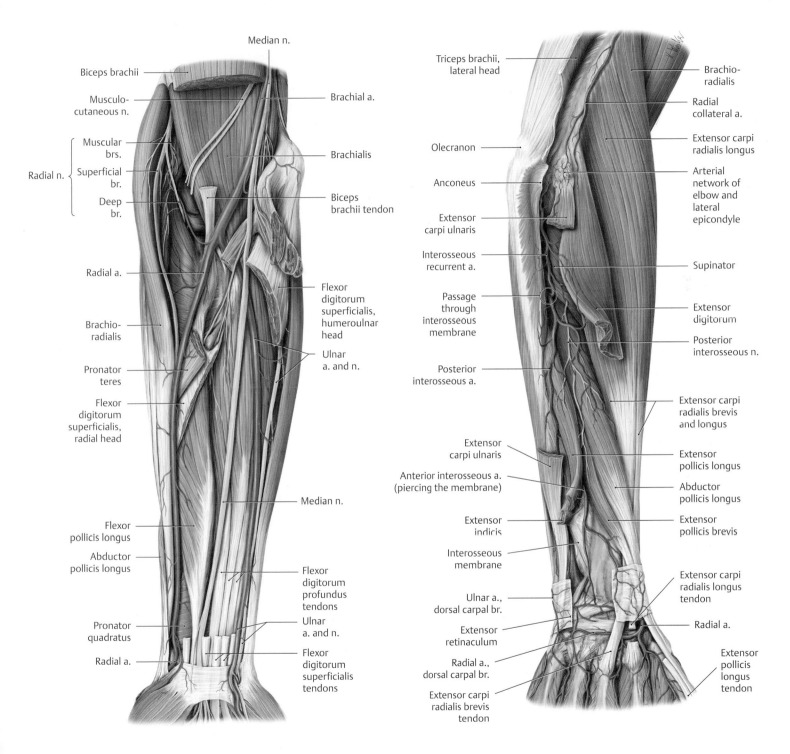

Fig. 28.38 Posterior forearm

Right forearm, anterior view during pronation. *Reflected:* Anconeus and triceps brachii. *Removed:* Extensor carpi ulnaris and extensor digitorum.

Left diagram labels:

Biceps brachii

Musculo-cutaneous n.

Radial n. {
  Muscular brs.
  Superficial br.
  Deep br.
}

Median n.

Brachial a.

Brachialis

Biceps brachii tendon

Radial a.

Brachio-radialis

Pronator teres

Flexor digitorum superficialis, radial head

Flexor digitorum superficialis, humeroulnar head

Ulnar a. and n.

Median n.

Flexor pollicis longus

Abductor pollicis longus

Pronator quadratus

Radial a.

Flexor digitorum profundus tendons

Ulnar a. and n.

Flexor digitorum superficialis tendons

Right diagram labels:

Triceps brachii, lateral head

Olecranon

Anconeus

Extensor carpi ulnaris

Interosseous recurrent a.

Passage through interosseous membrane

Posterior interosseous a.

Extensor carpi ulnaris

Anterior interosseous a. (piercing the membrane)

Extensor indicis

Interosseous membrane

Ulnar a., dorsal carpal br.

Extensor retinaculum

Radial a., dorsal carpal br.

Extensor carpi radialis brevis tendon

Brachio-radialis

Radial collateral a.

Extensor carpi radialis longus

Arterial network of elbow and lateral epicondyle

Supinator

Extensor digitorum

Posterior interosseous n.

Extensor carpi radialis brevis and longus

Extensor pollicis longus

Abductor pollicis longus

Extensor pollicis brevis

Extensor carpi radialis longus tendon

Radial a.

Extensor pollicis longus tendon

C Deep layer. *Removed:* Deep flexors.

***Fig. 28.39* Anterior carpal region**
Right hand, anterior (palmar) view.

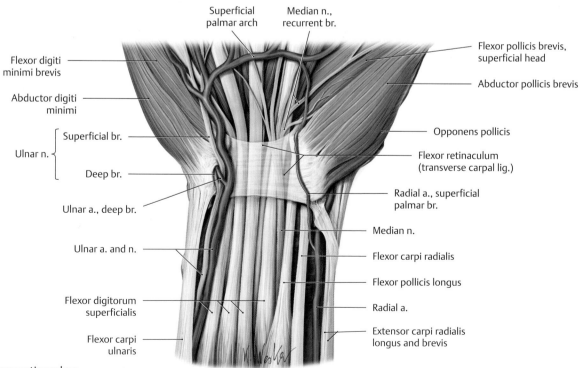

Superficial palmar arch

Median n., recurrent br.

Flexor digiti minimi brevis

Abductor digiti minimi

Palmaris brevis

Palmar aponeurosis (cut)

Pisiform

Ulnar tunnel

Palmar carpal lig.

Ulnar a. and n.

Flexor carpi ulnaris

Palmaris longus tendon

Flexor pollicis brevis, superficial head

Abductor pollicis brevis

Opponens pollicis

Flexor retinaculum (transverse carpal lig.)

Radial a., superficial palmar br.

Median n.

Pronator quadratus

Flexor carpi radialis

Flexor pollicis longus

Radial a.

Flexor digitorum superficialis

A Ulnar tunnel and deep palm.

Superficial palmar arch

Median n., recurrent br.

Flexor digiti minimi brevis

Abductor digiti minimi

Ulnar n.
 Superficial br.
 Deep br.

Ulnar a., deep br.

Ulnar a. and n.

Flexor digitorum superficialis

Flexor carpi ulnaris

Flexor pollicis brevis, superficial head

Abductor pollicis brevis

Opponens pollicis

Flexor retinaculum (transverse carpal lig.)

Radial a., superficial palmar br.

Median n.

Flexor carpi radialis

Flexor pollicis longus

Radial a.

Extensor carpi radialis longus and brevis

B Carpal tunnel with flexor retinaculum transparent. *Removed:* palmaris brevis, palmaris longus, palmar aponeurosis, and palmar carpal ligament.

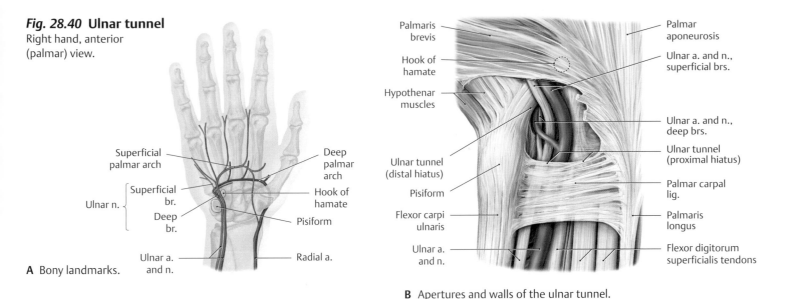

Fig. 28.40 Ulnar tunnel
Right hand, anterior (palmar) view.

Superficial palmar arch

Deep palmar arch

Ulnar n. {
 Superficial br.
 Deep br.
}

Hook of hamate

Pisiform

Ulnar a. and n.

Radial a.

A Bony landmarks.

Palmaris brevis

Hook of hamate

Hypothenar muscles

Ulnar tunnel (distal hiatus)

Pisiform

Flexor carpi ulnaris

Ulnar a. and n.

Palmar aponeurosis

Ulnar a. and n., superficial brs.

Ulnar a. and n., deep brs.

Ulnar tunnel (proximal hiatus)

Palmar carpal lig.

Palmaris longus

Flexor digitorum superficialis tendons

B Apertures and walls of the ulnar tunnel.

Fig. 28.41 Carpal tunnel: Cross section

Right hand, proximal view. The tight fit of sensitive neurovascular structures with closely apposed, frequently moving tendons in the carpal tunnel often causes problems (carpal tunnel syndrome) when any of the structures swell or degenerate.

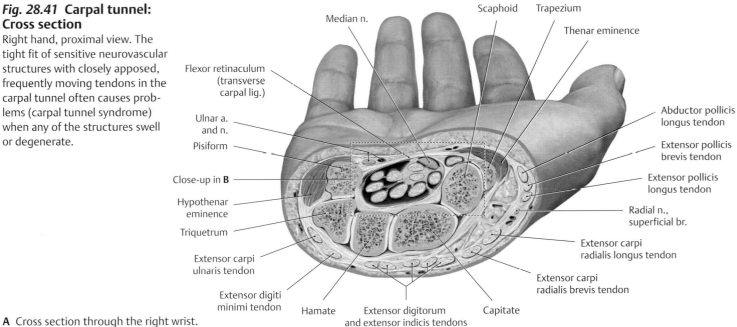

Median n.

Scaphoid

Trapezium

Thenar eminence

Flexor retinaculum (transverse carpal lig.)

Ulnar a. and n.

Pisiform

Close-up in **B**

Hypothenar eminence

Triquetrum

Extensor carpi ulnaris tendon

Extensor digiti minimi tendon

Hamate

Extensor digitorum and extensor indicis tendons

Capitate

Abductor pollicis longus tendon

Extensor pollicis brevis tendon

Extensor pollicis longus tendon

Radial n., superficial br.

Extensor carpi radialis longus tendon

Extensor carpi radialis brevis tendon

A Cross section through the right wrist.

Flexor retinaculum (transverse carpal lig.)

Flexor digitorum superficialis tendons

Superficial palmar a. and v.

Palmar carpal lig.

Ulnar a. and n.

Pisiform

Synovial cavity

Triquetrum

Hamate

Flexor digitorum profundus tendons

Flexor carpi radialis tendon

Median n.

Flexor pollicis longus tendon

Scaphoid

Capitate

B Structures in the ulnar tunnel (green) and carpal tunnel (blue).

Palm of the Hand

Fig. 28.42 Superficial neurovascular structures of the palm

Right hand, anterior view.

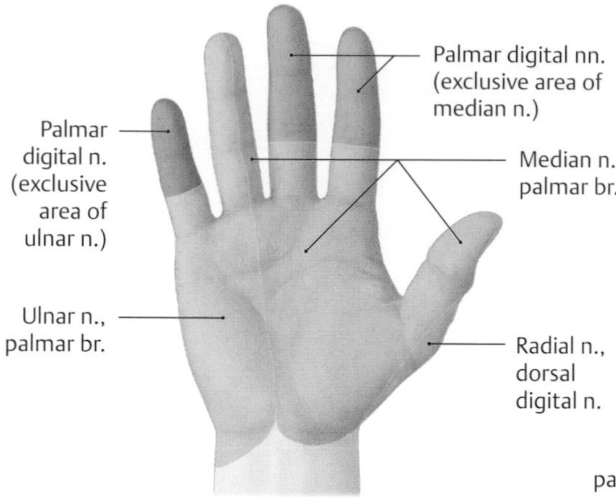

Palmar digital nn. (exclusive area of median n.)

Palmar digital n. (exclusive area of ulnar n.)

Median n., palmar br.

Ulnar n., palmar br.

Radial n., dorsal digital n.

A Sensory territories. Extensive overlap exists between adjacent areas. *Exclusive* nerve territories indicated with darker shading.

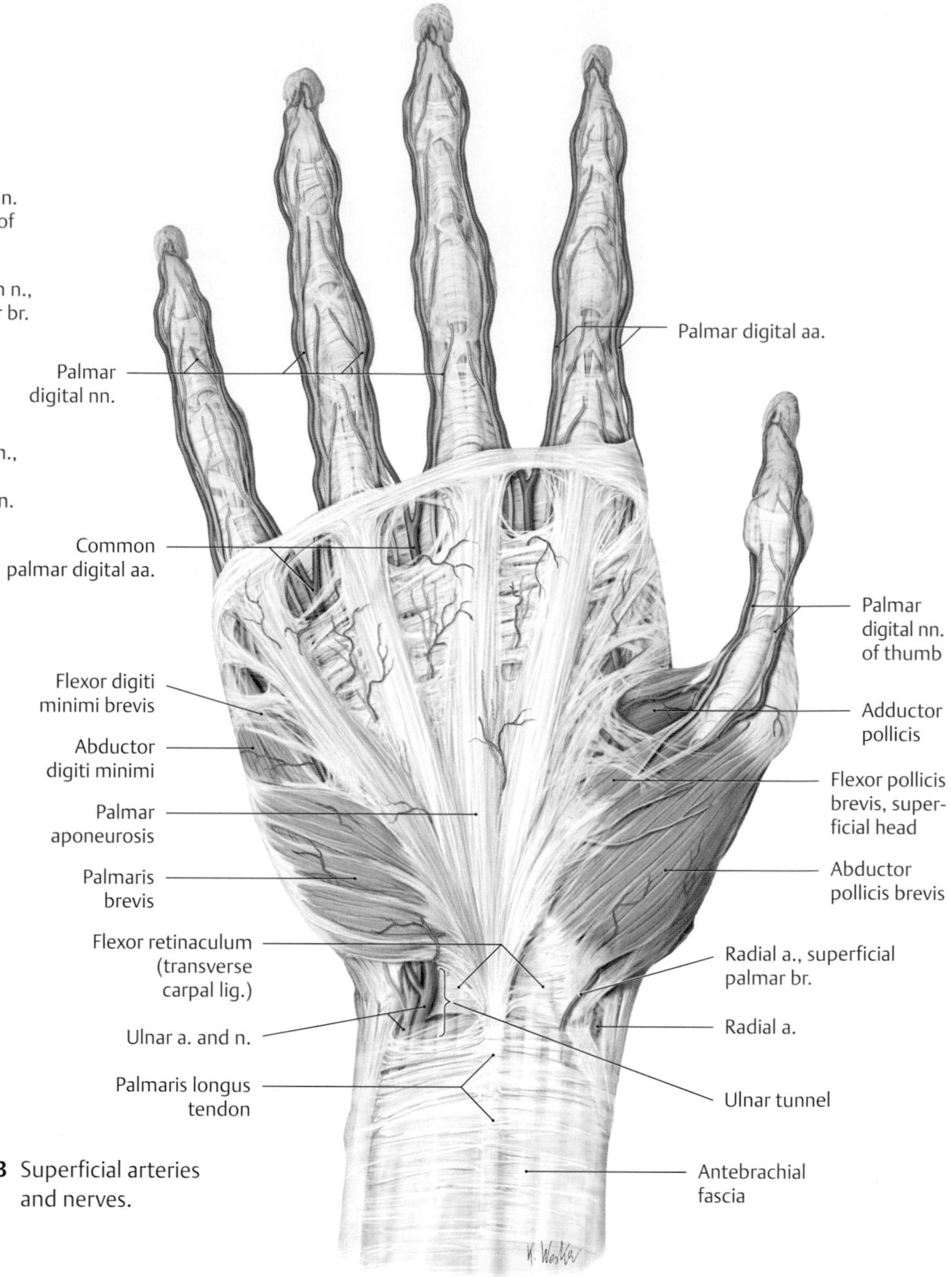

Palmar digital nn.

Palmar digital aa.

Common palmar digital aa.

Palmar digital nn. of thumb

Flexor digiti minimi brevis

Adductor pollicis

Abductor digiti minimi

Flexor pollicis brevis, superficial head

Palmar aponeurosis

Palmaris brevis

Abductor pollicis brevis

Flexor retinaculum (transverse carpal lig.)

Radial a., superficial palmar br.

Ulnar a. and n.

Radial a.

Palmaris longus tendon

Ulnar tunnel

Antebrachial fascia

B Superficial arteries and nerves.

Fig. 28.43 Neurovasculature of the finger

Right middle finger, lateral view.

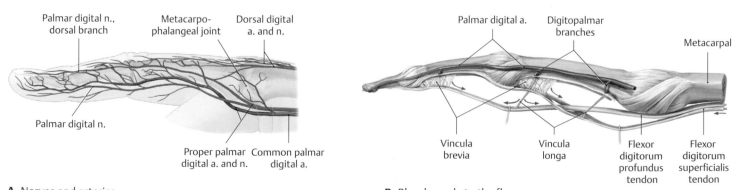

Palmar digital n., dorsal branch

Metacarpophalangeal joint

Dorsal digital a. and n.

Palmar digital n.

Proper palmar digital a. and n.

Common palmar digital a.

Palmar digital a.

Digitopalmar branches

Metacarpal

Vincula brevia

Vincula longa

Flexor digitorum profundus tendon

Flexor digitorum superficialis tendon

A Nerves and arteries.

B Blood supply to the flexor tendons in the tendon sheath.

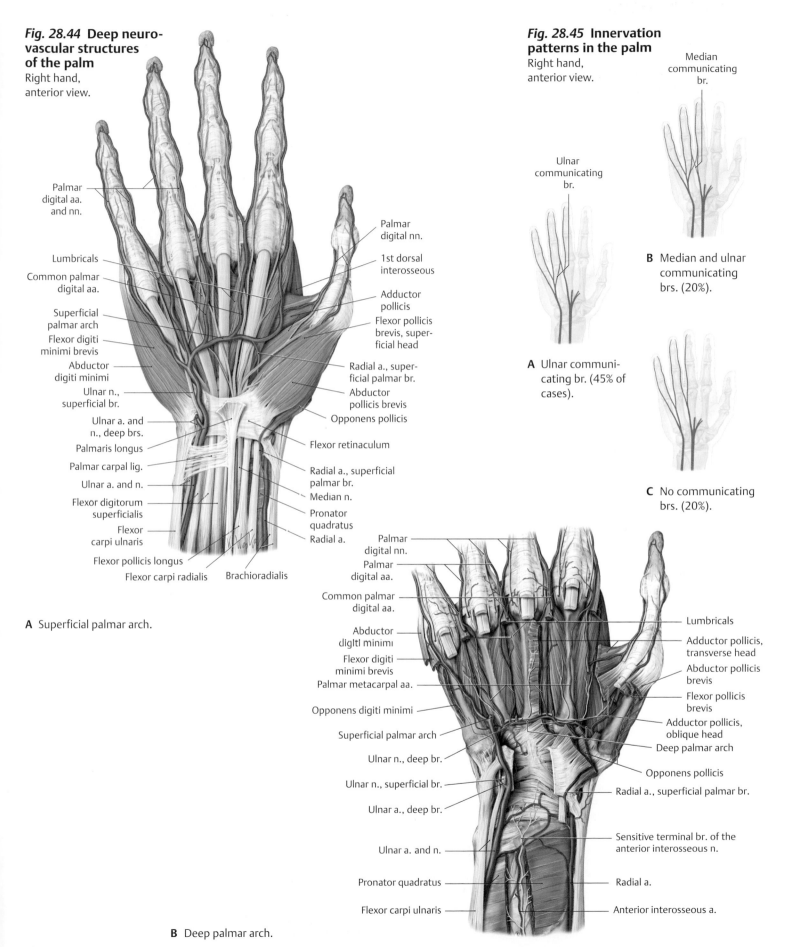

Fig. 28.44 Deep neuro-vascular structures of the palm
Right hand, anterior view.

Palmar digital aa. and nn.

Lumbricals

Common palmar digital aa.

Superficial palmar arch

Flexor digiti minimi brevis

Abductor digiti minimi

Ulnar n., superficial br.

Ulnar a. and n., deep brs.

Palmaris longus

Palmar carpal lig.

Ulnar a. and n.

Flexor digitorum superficialis

Flexor carpi ulnaris

Flexor pollicis longus

Flexor carpi radialis

Brachioradialis

Palmar digital nn.

1st dorsal interosseous

Adductor pollicis

Flexor pollicis brevis, superficial head

Radial a., superficial palmar br.

Abductor pollicis brevis

Opponens pollicis

Flexor retinaculum

Radial a., superficial palmar br.

Median n.

Pronator quadratus

Radial a.

A Superficial palmar arch.

Fig. 28.45 Innervation patterns in the palm
Right hand, anterior view.

Median communicating br.

Ulnar communicating br.

B Median and ulnar communicating brs. (20%).

A Ulnar communicating br. (45% of cases).

C No communicating brs. (20%).

Palmar digital nn.

Palmar digital aa.

Common palmar digital aa.

Abductor digiti minimi

Flexor digiti minimi brevis

Palmar metacarpal aa.

Opponens digiti minimi

Superficial palmar arch

Ulnar n., deep br.

Ulnar n., superficial br.

Ulnar a., deep br.

Ulnar a. and n.

Pronator quadratus

Flexor carpi ulnaris

Lumbricals

Adductor pollicis, transverse head

Abductor pollicis brevis

Flexor pollicis brevis

Adductor pollicis, oblique head

Deep palmar arch

Opponens pollicis

Radial a., superficial palmar br.

Sensitive terminal br. of the anterior interosseous n.

Radial a.

Anterior interosseous a.

B Deep palmar arch.

Dorsum of the Hand

Fig. 28.46 Cutaneous innervation of the dorsum of the hand
Right hand, posterior view.

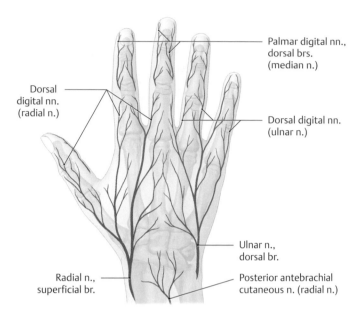

A Nerves of the dorsum.

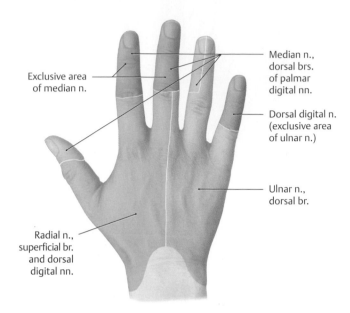

B Sensory territories. Extensive overlap exists between adjacent areas. *Exclusive* nerve territories indicated with darker shading.

Fig. 28.47 Anatomic snuffbox
Right hand, radial view. The three-sided "anatomic snuffbox" (shaded green) is bounded by the tendons of insertion of the abductor pollicis longus and extensors pollicis brevis and longus.

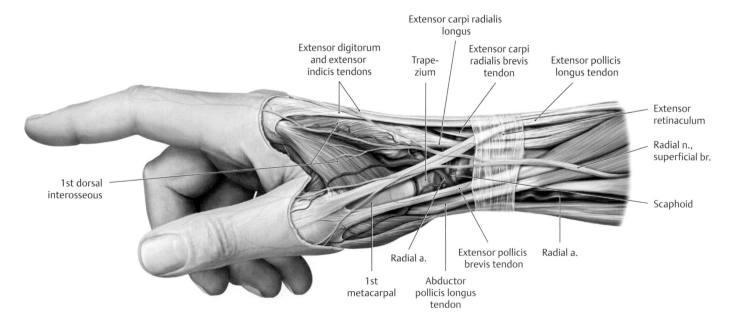

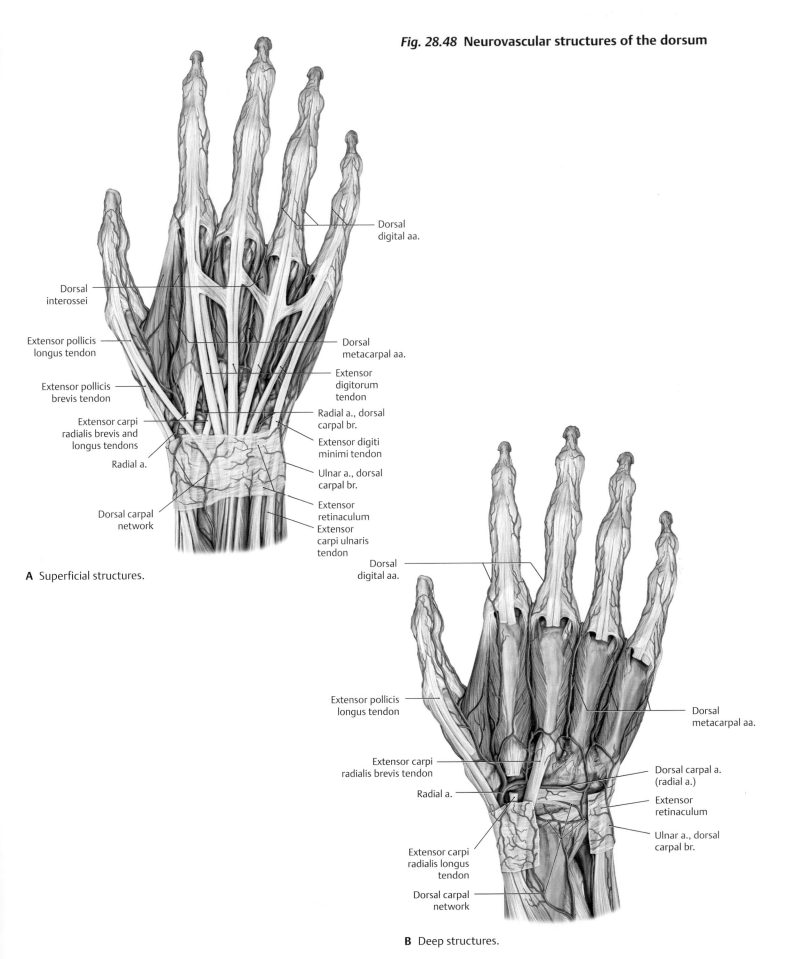

Fig. 28.48 Neurovascular structures of the dorsum

A Superficial structures.

Dorsal digital aa.

Dorsal interossei

Extensor pollicis longus tendon

Extensor pollicis brevis tendon

Extensor carpi radialis brevis and longus tendons

Radial a.

Dorsal carpal network

Dorsal metacarpal aa.

Extensor digitorum tendon

Radial a., dorsal carpal br.

Extensor digiti minimi tendon

Ulnar a., dorsal carpal br.

Extensor retinaculum

Extensor carpi ulnaris tendon

B Deep structures.

Dorsal digital aa.

Extensor pollicis longus tendon

Extensor carpi radialis brevis tendon

Radial a.

Extensor carpi radialis longus tendon

Dorsal carpal network

Dorsal metacarpal aa.

Dorsal carpal a. (radial a.)

Extensor retinaculum

Ulnar a., dorsal carpal br.

29 Sectional & Radiographic Anatomy

Sectional Anatomy of the Upper Limb

Fig. 29.1 **Windowed dissection of the arm and forearm**

Right limb, anterior view.

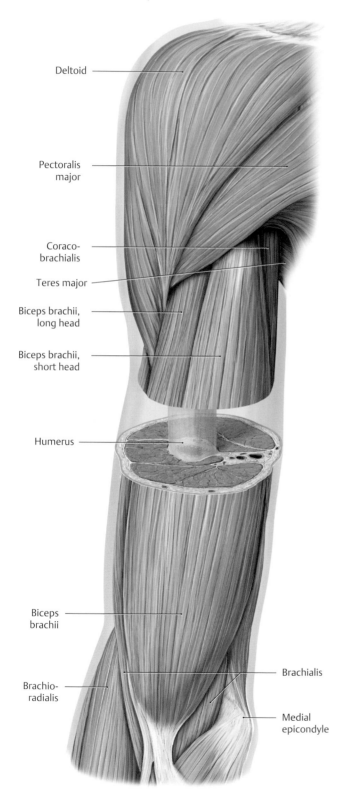

A Dissection of the arm.

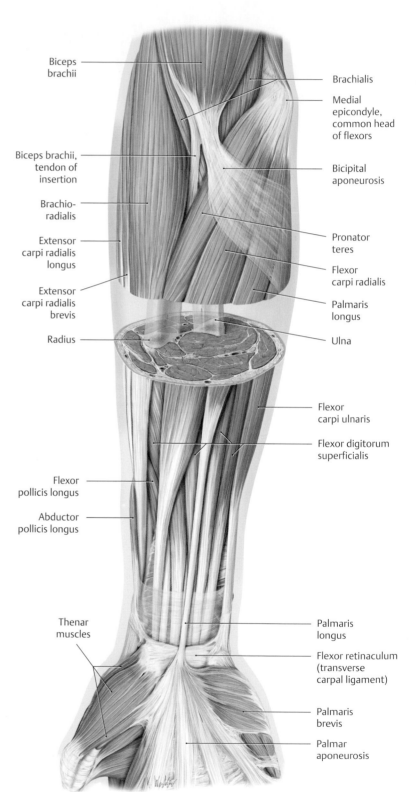

B Right forearm

Fig. 29.2 **Cross-section through the arm and forearm**

Right limb, proximal view.

Posterior

Anterior

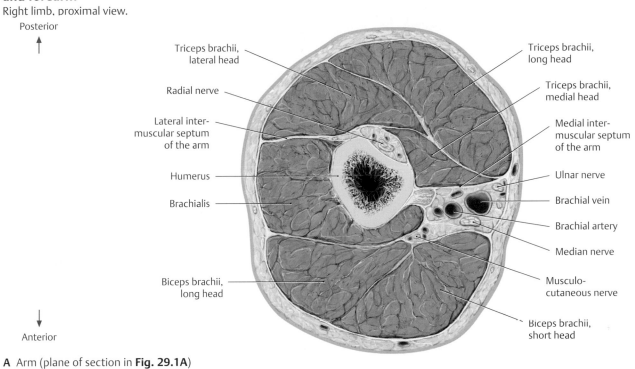

Triceps brachii, lateral head

Radial nerve

Lateral inter-muscular septum of the arm

Humerus

Brachialis

Biceps brachii, long head

Triceps brachii, long head

Triceps brachii, medial head

Medial inter-muscular septum of the arm

Ulnar nerve

Brachial vein

Brachial artery

Median nerve

Musculo-cutaneous nerve

Biceps brachii, short head

A Arm (plane of section in **Fig. 29.1A**)

Posterior (dorsal)

Anterior (palmar)

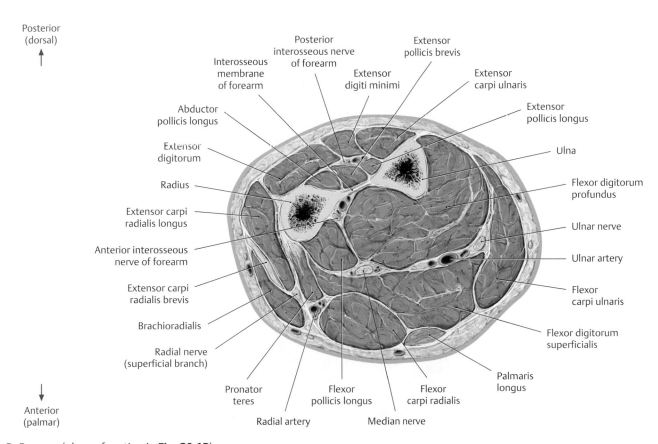

Interosseous membrane of forearm

Posterior interosseous nerve of forearm

Extensor pollicis brevis

Extensor digiti minimi

Extensor carpi ulnaris

Abductor pollicis longus

Extensor pollicis longus

Extensor digitorum

Ulna

Radius

Flexor digitorum profundus

Extensor carpi radialis longus

Ulnar nerve

Anterior interosseous nerve of forearm

Ulnar artery

Extensor carpi radialis brevis

Flexor carpi ulnaris

Brachioradialis

Flexor digitorum superficialis

Radial nerve (superficial branch)

Pronator teres

Flexor pollicis longus

Flexor carpi radialis

Palmaris longus

Radial artery

Median nerve

B Forearm (plane of section in **Fig. 29.1B**)

Radiographic Anatomy of the Upper Limb (I)

Fig. 29.3 MRI of the arm
Transverse section, distal (inferior) view.

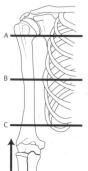

A Proximal arm. (Reproduced from Moeller TB, Reif E. Pocket Atlas of Sectional Anatomy, Vol 2, 4th ed. New York, NY: Thieme; 2014.)

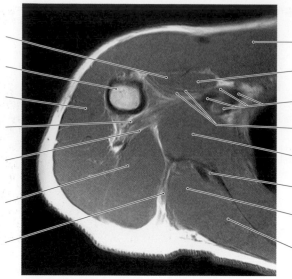

- Biceps brachii (short head, tendon)
- Humerus
- Deltoid
- Axillary n.
- Posterior humeral circumflex a. and v.
- Triceps brachii (long head)
- Circumflex scapular a. and v.
- Pectoralis major
- Coracobrachialis
- Axillary a. and v., brachial plexus
- Anterior humeral circumflex a. and v.
- Subscapularis
- Scapula
- Teres minor
- Infraspinatus

B Mid-arm. (Reproduced from Moeller TB, Reif E. Atlas of Sectional Anatomy: The Musculoskeletal System. New York, NY: Thieme; 2009.)

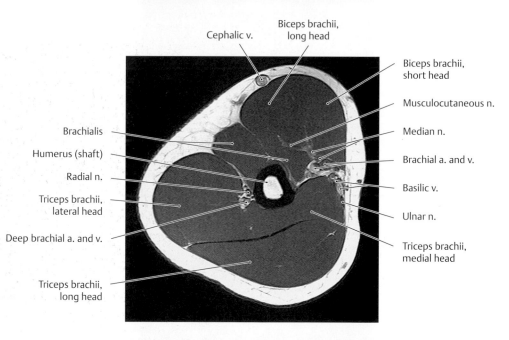

- Cephalic v.
- Biceps brachii, long head
- Brachialis
- Humerus (shaft)
- Radial n.
- Triceps brachii, lateral head
- Deep brachial a. and v.
- Triceps brachii, long head
- Biceps brachii, short head
- Musculocutaneous n.
- Median n.
- Brachial a. and v.
- Basilic v.
- Ulnar n.
- Triceps brachii, medial head

C Distal arm. (Reproduced from Moeller TB, Reif E. Pocket Atlas of Sectional Anatomy, Vol 2, 4th ed. New York, NY: Thieme; 2014.)

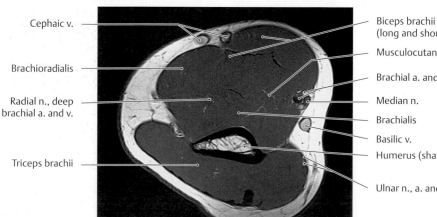

- Cephaic v.
- Brachioradialis
- Radial n., deep brachial a. and v.
- Triceps brachii
- Biceps brachii (long and short heads)
- Musculocutaneous n.
- Brachial a. and v.
- Median n.
- Brachialis
- Basilic v.
- Humerus (shaft)
- Ulnar n., a. and v.

Fig. 29.4 MRI of the forearm

Transverse section, distal view.

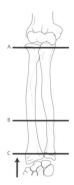

A Proximal forearm. (Reproduced from Moeller TB, Reif E. Pocket Atlas of Sectional Anatomy, Vol 2, 4th ed. New York, NY: Thieme; 2014.)

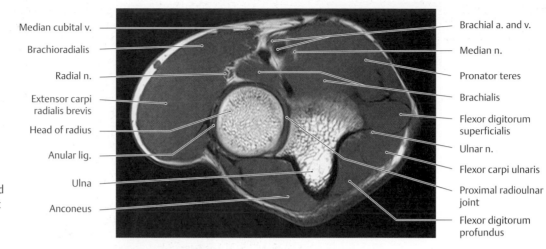

Median cubital v. — Brachioradialis — Radial n. — Extensor carpi radialis brevis — Head of radius — Anular lig. — Ulna — Anconeus

Brachial a. and v. — Median n. — Pronator teres — Brachialis — Flexor digitorum superficialis — Ulnar n. — Flexor carpi ulnaris — Proximal radioulnar joint — Flexor digitorum profundus

B Mid-forearm. (Reproduced from Moeller TB, Reif E. Atlas of Sectional Anatomy: The Musculoskeletal System. New York, NY: Thieme; 2009.)

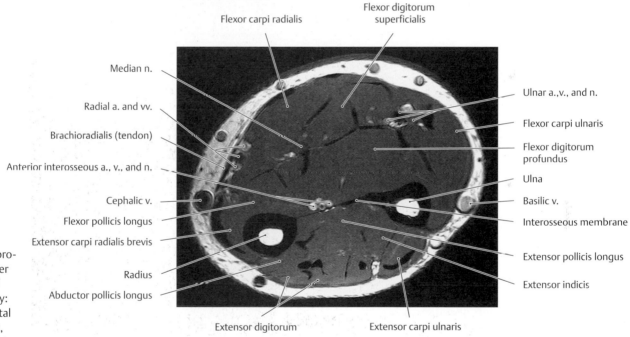

Flexor carpi radialis — Flexor digitorum superficialis

Median n. — Radial a. and vv. — Brachioradialis (tendon) — Anterior interosseous a., v., and n. — Cephalic v. — Flexor pollicis longus — Extensor carpi radialis brevis — Radius — Abductor pollicis longus

Ulnar a., v., and n. — Flexor carpi ulnaris — Flexor digitorum profundus — Ulna — Basilic v. — Interosseous membrane — Extensor pollicis longus — Extensor indicis

Extensor digitorum — Extensor carpi ulnaris

C Distal forearm. (Reproduced from Moeller TB, Reif E. Pocket Atlas of Sectional Anatomy, Vol 2, 4th ed. New York, NY: Thieme; 2014.)

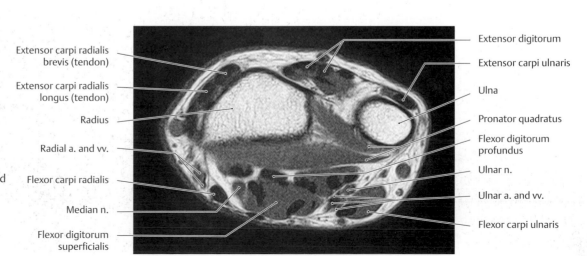

Extensor carpi radialis brevis (tendon) — Extensor carpi radialis longus (tendon) — Radius — Radial a. and vv. — Flexor carpi radialis — Median n. — Flexor digitorum superficialis

Extensor digitorum — Extensor carpi ulnaris — Ulna — Pronator quadratus — Flexor digitorum profundus — Ulnar n. — Ulnar a. and vv. — Flexor carpi ulnaris

Radiographic Anatomy of the Upper Limb (II)

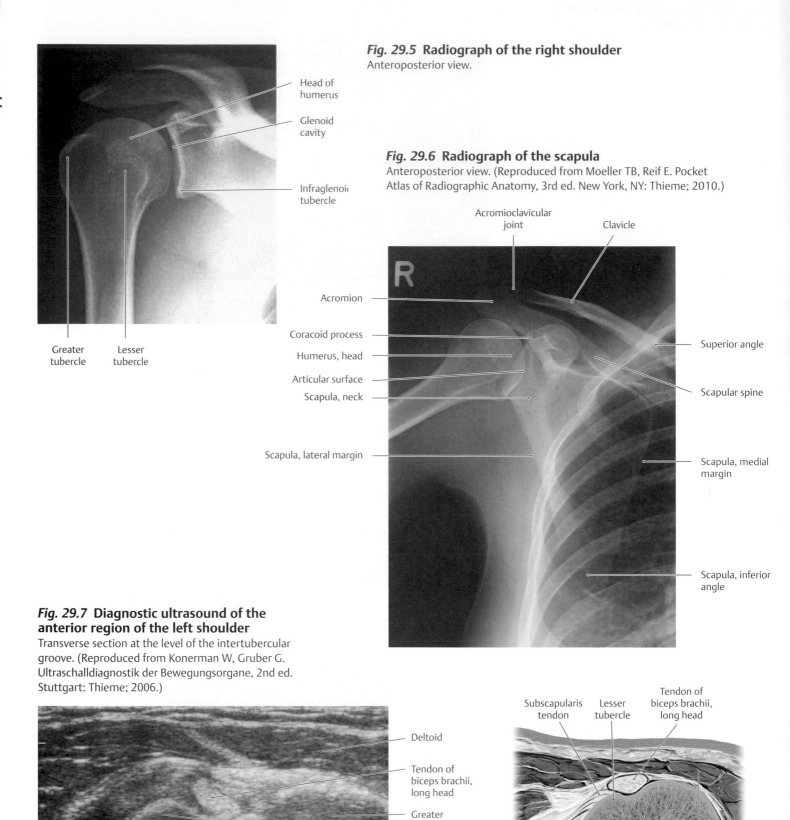

Fig. 29.5 Radiograph of the right shoulder
Anteroposterior view.

Head of humerus

Glenoid cavity

Infraglenoid tubercle

Greater tubercle   Lesser tubercle

Fig. 29.6 Radiograph of the scapula
Anteroposterior view. (Reproduced from Moeller TB, Reif E. Pocket Atlas of Radiographic Anatomy, 3rd ed. New York, NY: Thieme; 2010.)

Acromioclavicular joint

Clavicle

Acromion

Coracoid process

Humerus, head

Articular surface

Scapula, neck

Scapula, lateral margin

Superior angle

Scapular spine

Scapula, medial margin

Scapula, inferior angle

Fig. 29.7 Diagnostic ultrasound of the anterior region of the left shoulder
Transverse section at the level of the intertubercular groove. (Reproduced from Konerman W, Gruber G. Ultraschalldiagnostik der Bewegungsorgane, 2nd ed. Stuttgart: Thieme; 2006.)

Deltoid

Tendon of biceps brachii, long head

Greater tubercle

Lesser tubercle

Subscapularis tendon   Lesser tubercle

Tendon of biceps brachii, long head

Greater tubercle   Deltoid

A Sonogram.

B Schematic of the transverse section.

Fig. 29.8 MRI of the right shoulder joint in three planes

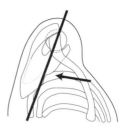

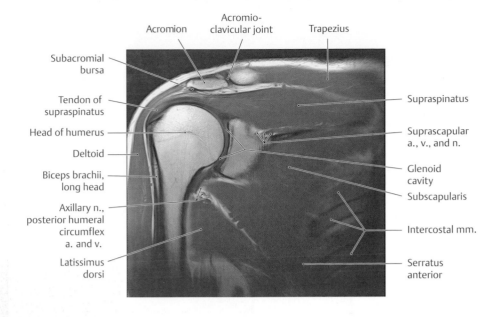

Acromion
Acromio-clavicular joint
Trapezius
Subacromial bursa
Tendon of supraspinatus
Head of humerus
Deltoid
Biceps brachii, long head
Axillary n., posterior humeral circumflex a. and v.
Latissimus dorsi
Supraspinatus
Suprascapular a., v., and n.
Glenoid cavity
Subscapularis
Intercostal mm.
Serratus anterior

A Coronal section, anterior view.

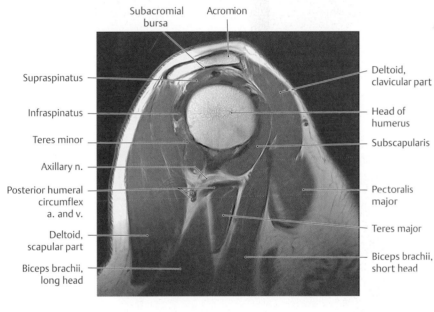

Subacromial bursa
Acromion
Supraspinatus
Infraspinatus
Teres minor
Axillary n.
Posterior humeral circumflex a. and v.
Deltoid, scapular part
Biceps brachii, long head
Deltoid, clavicular part
Head of humerus
Subscapularis
Pectoralis major
Teres major
Biceps brachii, short head

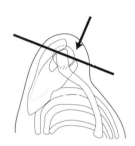

B Sagittal section, lateral view.

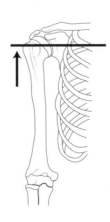

C Transverse section, inferior view.

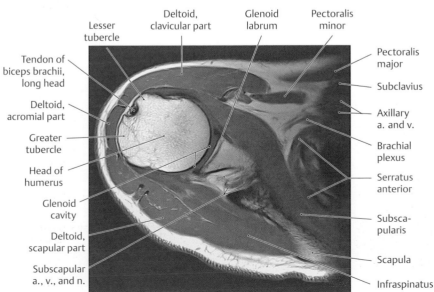

Lesser tubercle
Deltoid, clavicular part
Glenoid labrum
Pectoralis minor
Tendon of biceps brachii, long head
Deltoid, acromial part
Greater tubercle
Head of humerus
Glenoid cavity
Deltoid, scapular part
Subscapular a., v., and n.
Pectoralis major
Subclavius
Axillary a. and v.
Brachial plexus
Serratus anterior
Subscapularis
Scapula
Infraspinatus

Radiographic Anatomy of the Upper Limb (III)

Fig. 29.9 Radiograph of the elbow

Anteroposterior view. (Reproduced from Moeller TB, Reif E. Pocket Atlas of Radiographic Anatomy, 3rd ed. New York, NY: Thieme; 2010.)

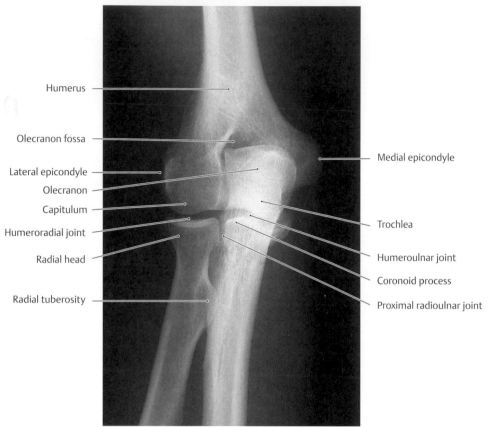

Fig. 29.10 Radiograph of the elbow

Lateral view. (Reproduced from Moeller TB, Reif E. Pocket Atlas of Radiographic Anatomy, 3rd ed. New York, NY: Thieme; 2010.)

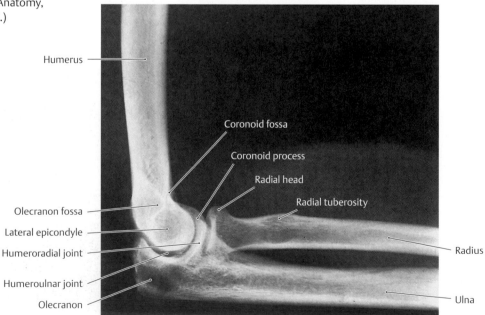

Fig. 29.11 MRI of the elbow
(Reproduced from Moeller TB, Reif E. Atlas of Sectional Anatomy: The Musculoskeletal System. New York, NY: Thieme; 2009.)

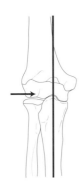

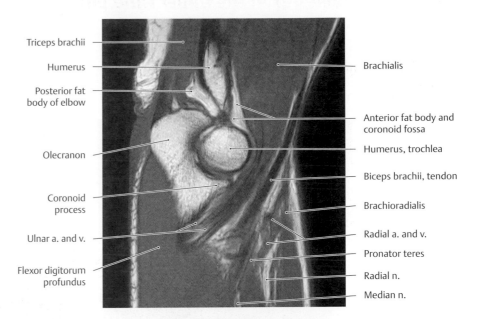

Triceps brachii

Humerus

Posterior fat body of elbow

Olecranon

Coronoid process

Ulnar a. and v.

Flexor digitorum profundus

Brachialis

Anterior fat body and coronoid fossa

Humerus, trochlea

Biceps brachii, tendon

Brachioradialis

Radial a. and v.

Pronator teres

Radial n.

Median n.

A Sagittal section through the humeroulnar joint.

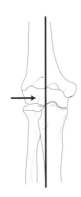

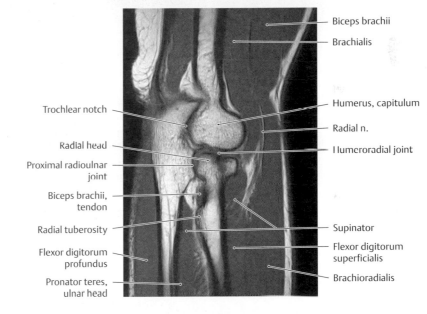

Trochlear notch

Radial head

Proximal radioulnar joint

Biceps brachii, tendon

Radial tuberosity

Flexor digitorum profundus

Pronator teres, ulnar head

Biceps brachii

Brachialis

Humerus, capitulum

Radial n.

Humeroradial joint

Supinator

Flexor digitorum superficialis

Brachioradialis

B Sagittal section through the humeroulnar and humeroradial joints.

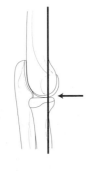

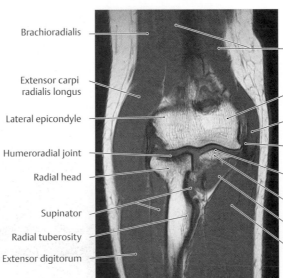

Brachioradialis

Extensor carpi radialis longus

Lateral epicondyle

Humeroradial joint

Radial head

Supinator

Radial tuberosity

Extensor digitorum

Brachialis

Medial epicondyle

Pronator teres

Medial collateral lig.

Humeroulnar joint

Ulna, coronoid process

Brachialis

Flexor carpi radialis

C Coronal section through the humeroulnar and humeroradial joints.

Radiographic Anatomy of the Upper Limb (IV)

Fig. 29.12 **Radiograph of the hand**
(Reproduced from Moeller TB, Reif E. Pocket Atlas of Radiographic Anatomy, 3rd ed. New York, NY: Thieme; 2010.)

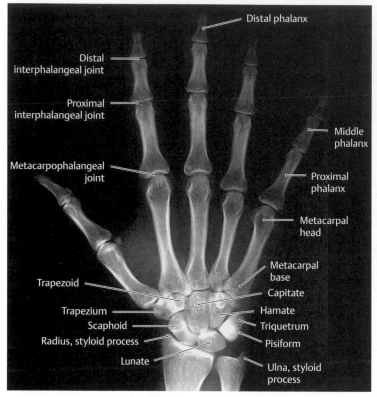

A Anteroposterior view.

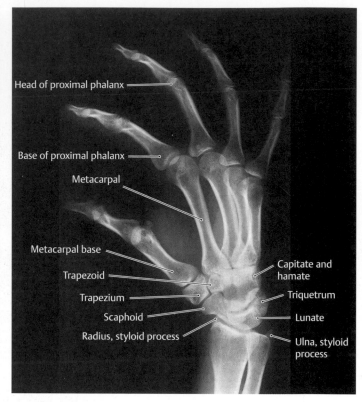

B Oblique view.

Fig. 29.13 **MRI of the right wrist**
Transverse section, distal view. (Reproduced from Moeller TB, Reif E. Atlas of Sectional Anatomy: The Musculoskeletal System. New York, NY: Thieme; 2009.)

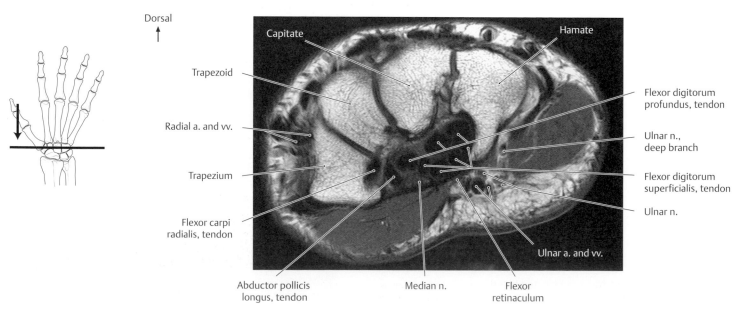

Fig. 29.14 MRI of the hand

(Reproduced from Moeller TB, Reif E. Atlas of Sectional Anatomy: The Musculoskeletal System. New York, NY: Thieme; 2009.)

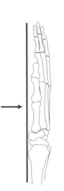

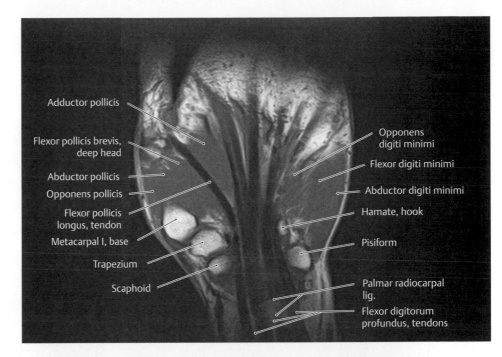

Adductor pollicis

Flexor pollicis brevis, deep head

Abductor pollicis

Opponens pollicis

Flexor pollicis longus, tendon

Metacarpal I, base

Trapezium

Scaphoid

Opponens digiti minimi

Flexor digiti minimi

Abductor digiti minimi

Hamate, hook

Pisiform

Palmar radiocarpal lig.

Flexor digitorum profundus, tendons

A Coronal section through the carpal tunnel.

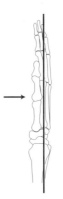

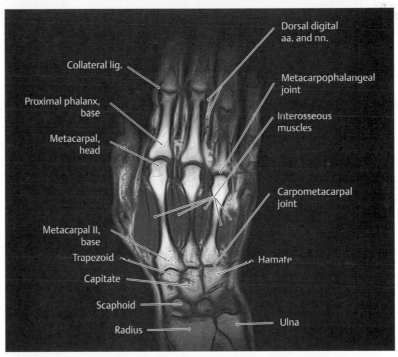

Dorsal digital aa. and nn.

Collateral lig.

Proximal phalanx, base

Metacarpal, head

Metacarpophalangeal joint

Interosseous muscles

Carpometacarpal joint

Metacarpal II, base

Trapezoid

Capitate

Scaphoid

Radius

Hamate

Ulna

B Coronal section through the palm.

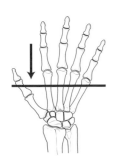

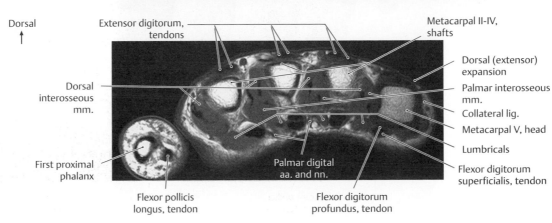

Dorsal

Extensor digitorum, tendons

Metacarpal II-IV, shafts

Dorsal interosseous mm.

Dorsal (extensor) expansion

Palmar interosseous mm.

Collateral lig.

Metacarpal V, head

Lumbricals

Flexor digitorum superficialis, tendon

First proximal phalanx

Palmar digital aa. and nn.

Flexor digitorum profundus, tendon

Flexor pollicis longus, tendon

C Transverse section through the palm, distal view.

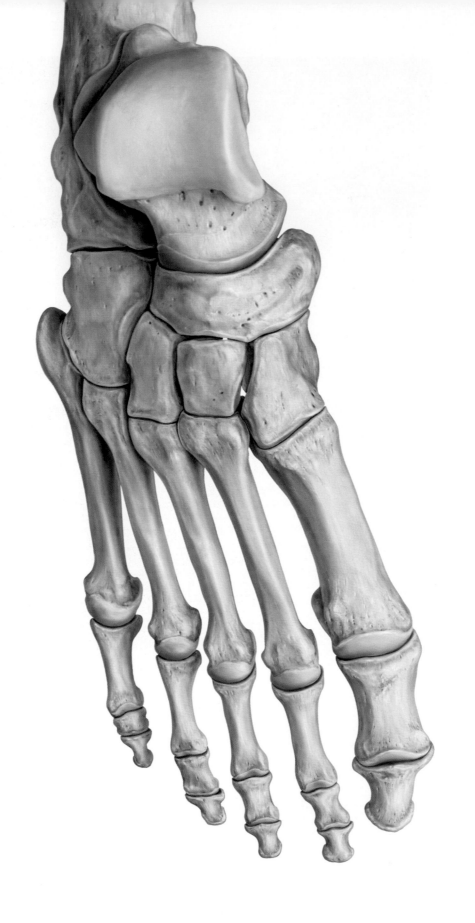

Lower Limb

30 Surface Anatomy

Surface Anatomy

Fig. 30.1 Palpable bony prominences of the lower limb
Right limb.

Fig. 30.2 Regions of the lower limb
Right leg.

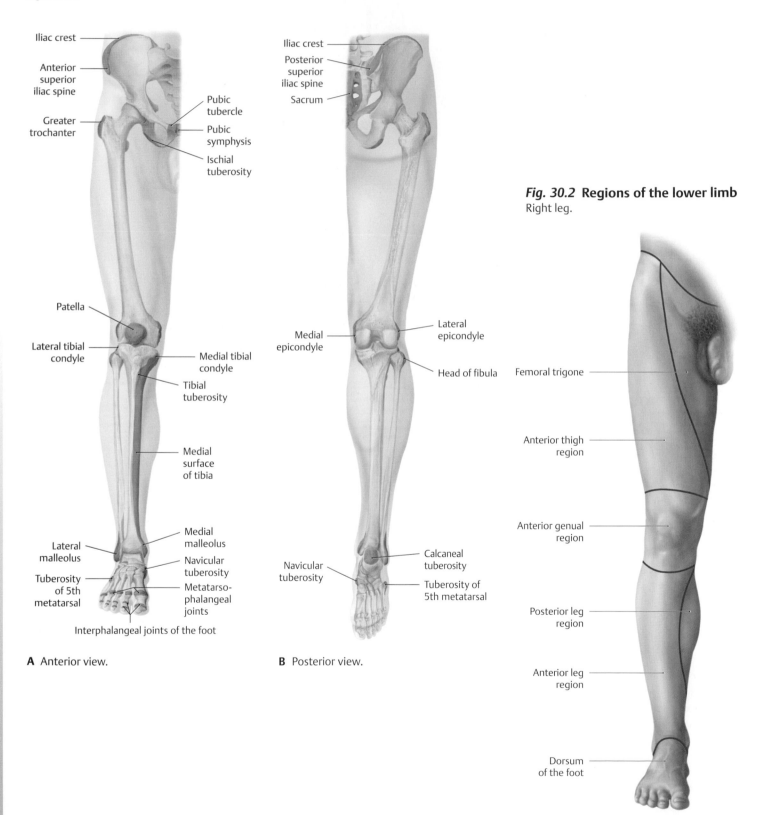

Iliac crest

Anterior superior iliac spine

Greater trochanter

Pubic tubercle

Pubic symphysis

Ischial tuberosity

Iliac crest

Posterior superior iliac spine

Sacrum

Patella

Lateral tibial condyle

Medial tibial condyle

Tibial tuberosity

Medial surface of tibia

Medial epicondyle

Lateral epicondyle

Head of fibula

Femoral trigone

Anterior thigh region

Anterior genual region

Lateral malleolus

Medial malleolus

Navicular tuberosity

Tuberosity of 5th metatarsal

Metatarso-phalangeal joints

Navicular tuberosity

Calcaneal tuberosity

Tuberosity of 5th metatarsal

Posterior leg region

Anterior leg region

Interphalangeal joints of the foot

A Anterior view.

B Posterior view.

Dorsum of the foot

A Anterior view.

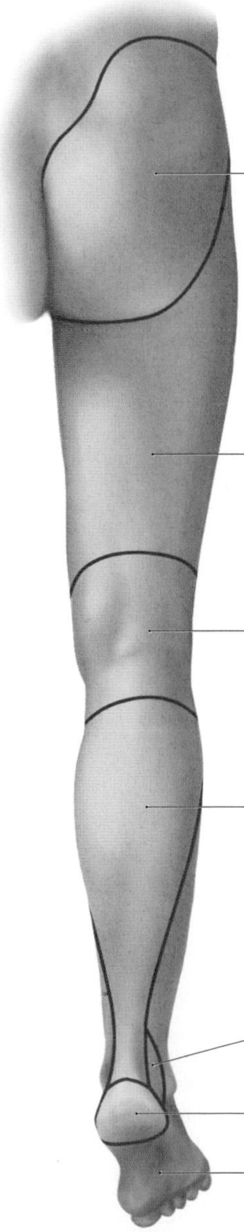
Gluteal region
Posterior thigh region
Popliteal region
Posterior leg region
Lateral retro-malleolar region
Calcaneal region
Sole of the foot

B Posterior view.

Fig. 30.3 **Palpable musculature of the lower limb**

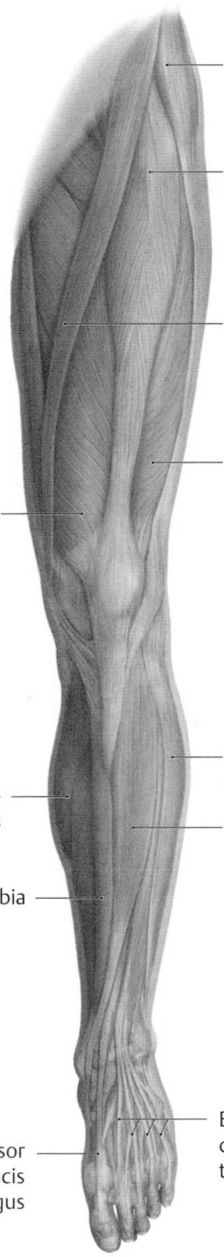
Tensor fascia lata
Rectus femoris
Sartorius
Vastus lateralis
Vastus medialis
Fibularis longus
Gastroc-nemius
Tibialis anterior
Tibia
Extensor digitorum tendons
Extensor hallucis longus

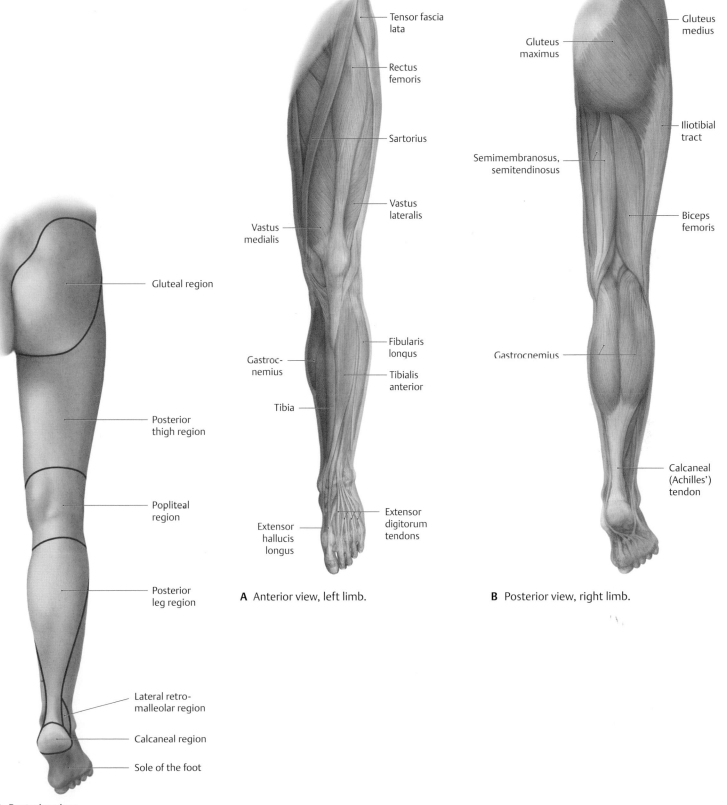

A Anterior view, left limb.

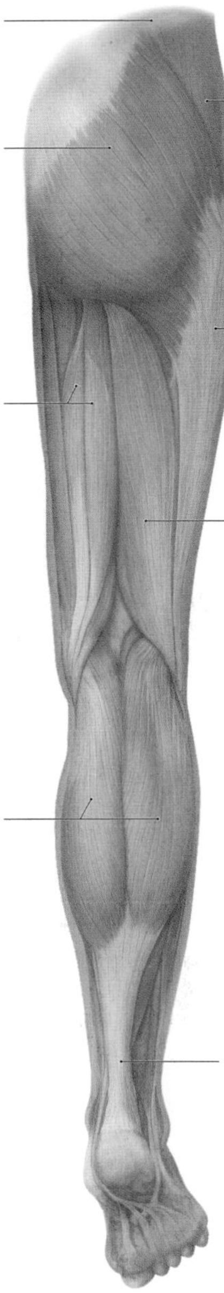
Iliac crest
Gluteus medius
Gluteus maximus
Iliotibial tract
Semimembranosus, semitendinosus
Biceps femoris
Gastrocnemius
Calcaneal (Achilles') tendon

B Posterior view, right limb.

31 Hip & Thigh
Bones of the Lower Limb

The skeleton of the lower limb consists of a coxal (hip) bone and a free limb. The paired coxal bones attach to the trunk at the sacroiliac joint to form the pelvic girdle (see **p. 230**), and the free limb, divided into a thigh, leg, and foot, attaches to the pelvic girdle at the hip joint. Stability of the pelvic girdle is important in the distribution of weight from the upper body to the lower limbs.

***Fig. 31.1* Bones of the lower limb**

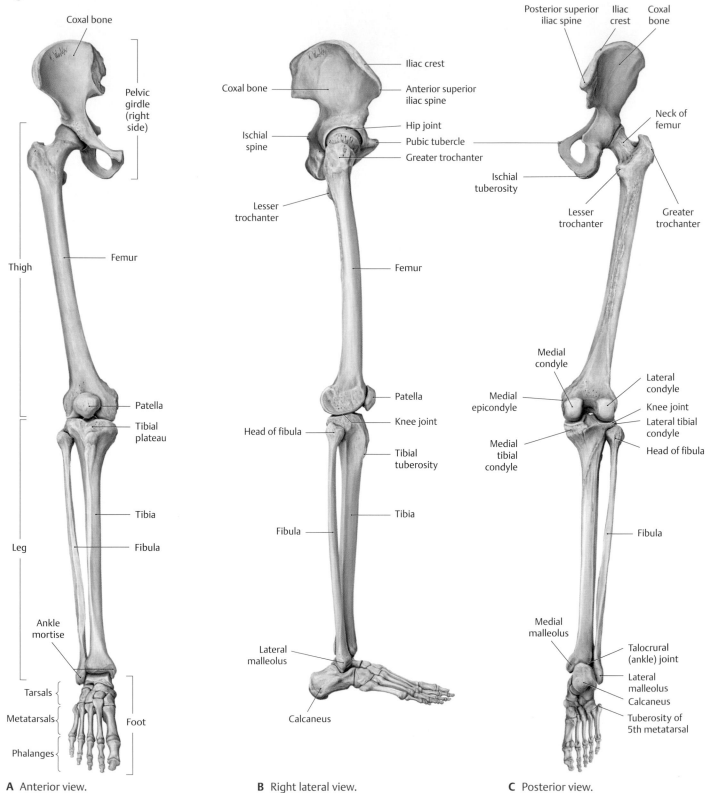

A Anterior view.　　　**B** Right lateral view.　　　**C** Posterior view.

Fig. 31.2 **Line of gravity**

Right lateral view. The line of gravity runs vertically from the whole-body center of gravity to the ground with characteristic points of intersection.

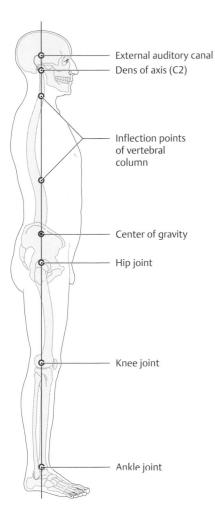

External auditory canal
Dens of axis (C2)

Inflection points of vertebral column

Center of gravity

Hip joint

Knee joint

Ankle joint

Fig. 31.3 **The coxal bones and their relation to the vertebral column.**

The paired coxal bones and sacrum form the pelvic girdle (see **p. 230**).

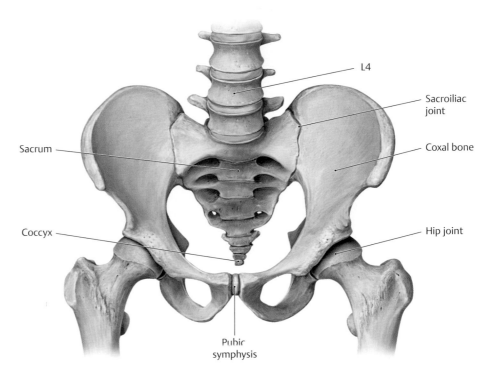

L4

Sacroiliac joint

Coxal bone

Sacrum

Coccyx

Hip joint

Pubic symphysis

A Anterior view.

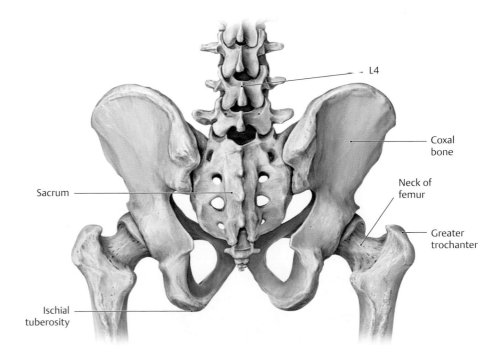

L4

Coxal bone

Neck of femur

Sacrum

Greater trochanter

Ischial tuberosity

B Posterior view.

411

Femur

Fig. 31.4 **Femur**
Right femur. The femur articulates proximally with the acetabulum of the pelvis at the hip joint and distally with the tibia at the knee joint.

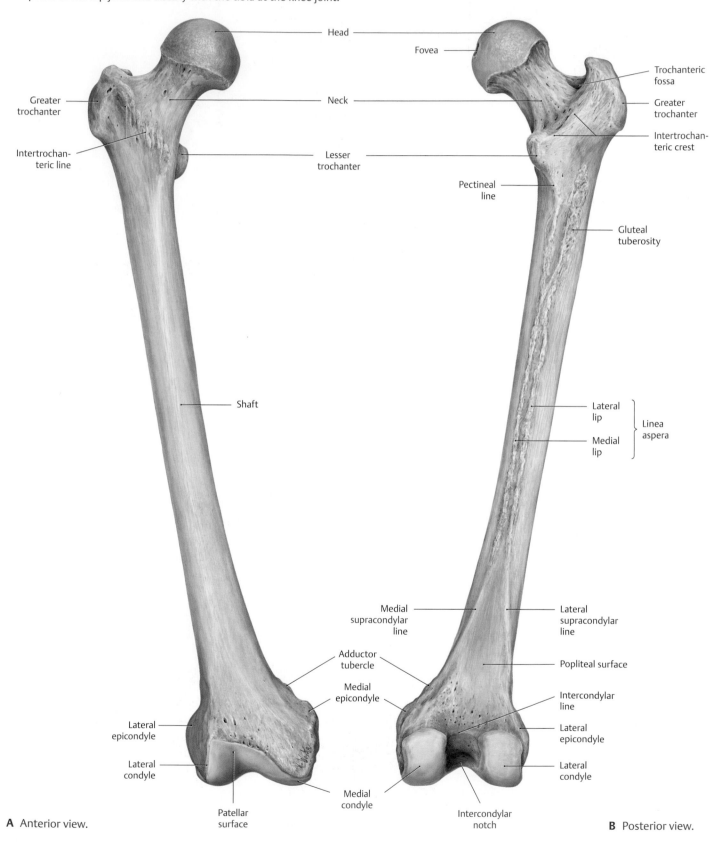

A Anterior view.

B Posterior view.

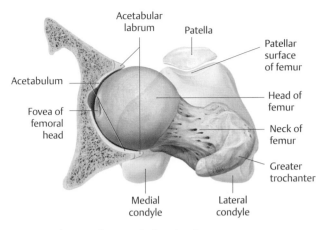

C Proximal view. The acetabulum has been sectioned in the horizontal plane.

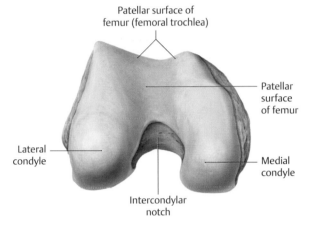

D Distal view.

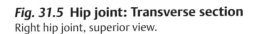

Fig. 31.5 Hip joint: Transverse section
Right hip joint, superior view.

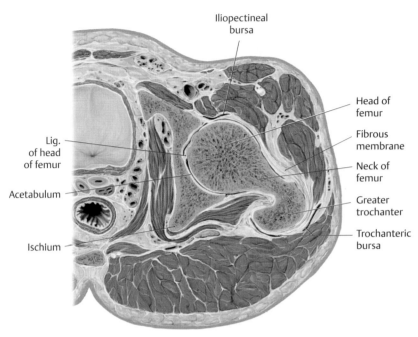

Clinical box 31.1

Rotation of the femoral head

The acetabular rim is oriented anteroinferiorly relative to the sagittal plane. At birth, the aperture angle measures approximately 7 degrees but increases to 17 degrees by adulthood (**A**). This angle affects the stability and "seating" of the femoral head in the hip joint. When the femoral head is centered in the acetabulum, the distal femur and thus the knee joint, point slightly inward. Note how external (**B**) and internal (**C**) rotation of the femoral head affect the orientation of the knee joint.

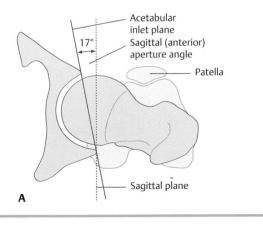

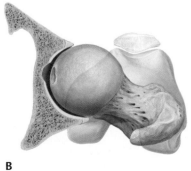

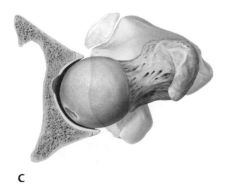

Hip Joint: Overview

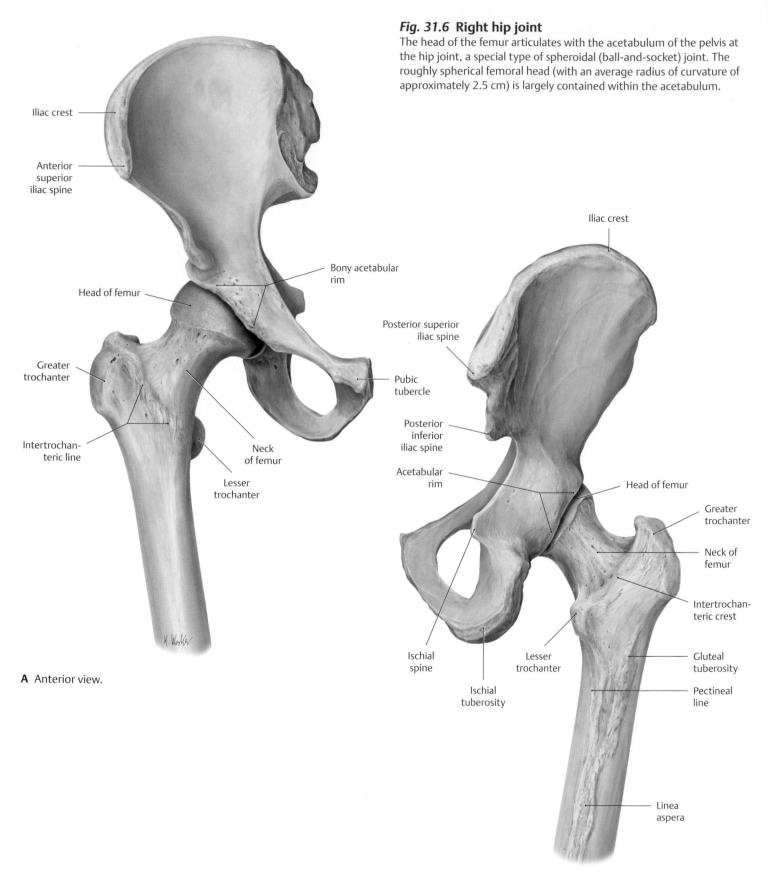

Fig. 31.6 Right hip joint
The head of the femur articulates with the acetabulum of the pelvis at the hip joint, a special type of spheroidal (ball-and-socket) joint. The roughly spherical femoral head (with an average radius of curvature of approximately 2.5 cm) is largely contained within the acetabulum.

A Anterior view.

B Posterior view.

Fig. 31.7 **Hip joint: Coronal section**
Right hip joint, anterior view.

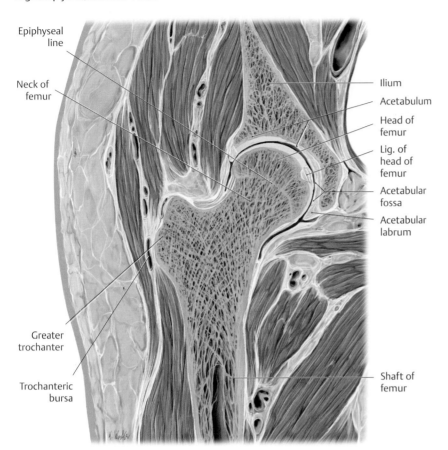

Epiphyseal line
Neck of femur
Ilium
Acetabulum
Head of femur
Lig. of head of femur
Acetabular fossa
Acetabular labrum
Greater trochanter
Trochanteric bursa
Shaft of femur

Clinical box 31.2

Fractures of the femur
Femoral fractures caused by falls in patients with osteoporosis are most frequently located in the neck of the femur. Femoral shaft fractures are less frequent and are usually caused by strong trauma (e.g., a car accident).

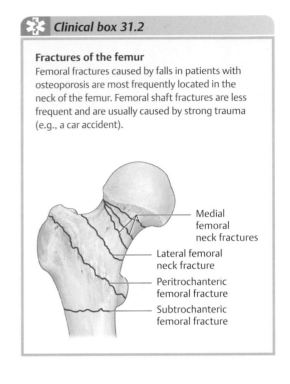

Medial femoral neck fractures
Lateral femoral neck fracture
Peritrochanteric femoral fracture
Subtrochanteric femoral fracture

Clinical box 31.3

Diagnosing hip dysplasia and dislocation
Ultrasonography, the most important imaging method for screening the infant hip, is used to identify morphological changes such as hip dysplasia and dislocation. Clinically, hip dislocation presents with instability and limited abduction of the hip joint, and leg shortening with asymmetry of the gluteal folds.

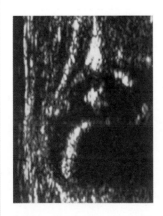
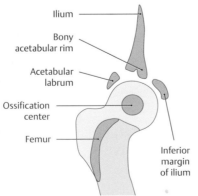

Ilium
Bony acetabular rim
Acetabular labrum
Ossification center
Femur
Inferior margin of ilium

A Normal hip joint in a 5-month-old.

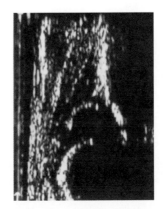
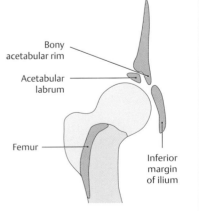

Bony acetabular rim
Acetabular labrum
Femur
Inferior margin of ilium

B Hip dislocation and dysplasia in a 3-month-old.

Hip Joint: Ligaments & Capsule

The hip joint has three major ligaments: iliofemoral, pubofemoral, and ischiofemoral. The iliofemoral, the strongest of these, provides an important constraint for the hip joint: it prevents the pelvis from tilting posteriorly in the upright stance, without the need for muscular effort.

It also limits adduction of the extended limb and stabilizes the pelvis on the stance side during gait. A fourth ligament, the zona orbicularis (anular ligament) is not visible externally and encircles the femoral neck like a buttonhole.

Fig. 31.8 Ligaments of the hip joint
Right hip joint.

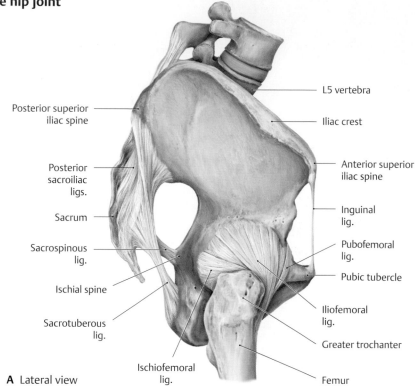

Posterior superior iliac spine
Posterior sacroiliac ligs.
Sacrum
Sacrospinous lig.
Ischial spine
Sacrotuberous lig.
Ischiofemoral lig.

L5 vertebra
Iliac crest
Anterior superior iliac spine
Inguinal lig.
Pubofemoral lig.
Pubic tubercle
Iliofemoral lig.
Greater trochanter
Femur

A Lateral view

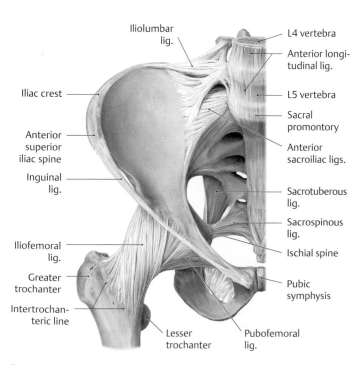

Iliolumbar lig.
Iliac crest
Anterior superior iliac spine
Inguinal lig.
Iliofemoral lig.
Greater trochanter
Intertrochanteric line
Lesser trochanter

L4 vertebra
Anterior longitudinal lig.
L5 vertebra
Sacral promontory
Anterior sacroiliac ligs.
Sacrotuberous lig.
Sacrospinous lig.
Ischial spine
Pubic symphysis
Pubofemoral lig.

B Anterior view

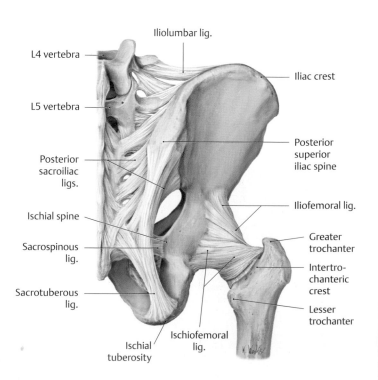

Iliolumbar lig.
L4 vertebra
L5 vertebra
Posterior sacroiliac ligs.
Ischial spine
Sacrospinous lig.
Sacrotuberous lig.
Ischial tuberosity
Ischiofemoral lig.

Iliac crest
Posterior superior iliac spine
Iliofemoral lig.
Greater trochanter
Intertrochanteric crest
Lesser trochanter

C Posterior view

Fig. 31.9 Weakness in the joint capsule

Right hip joint. Weak spots in the joint capsule (color-shaded areas) are located between the joint ligaments. External trauma may cause the femoral head to dislocate from the acetabulum at these sites.

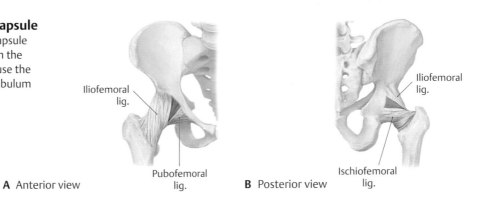

A Anterior view

B Posterior view

Fig 31.10 Synovial membrane of the joint capsule

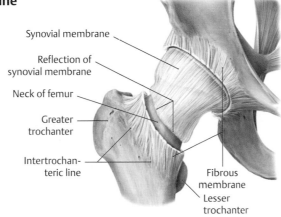

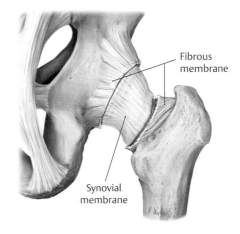

A Anterior view

B Posterior view

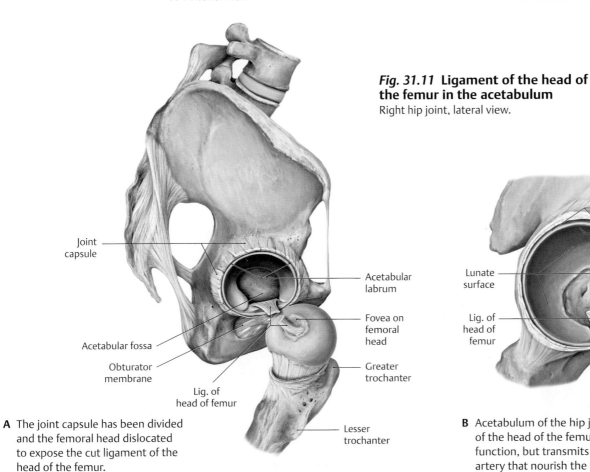

A The joint capsule has been divided and the femoral head dislocated to expose the cut ligament of the head of the femur.

Fig. 31.11 Ligament of the head of the femur in the acetabulum

Right hip joint, lateral view.

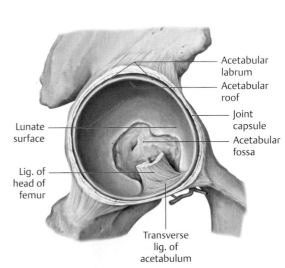

B Acetabulum of the hip joint. *Note:* The ligament of the head of the femur (cut) has no mechanical function, but transmits branches from the obturator artery that nourish the femoral head (see **p. 473**).

Anterior Muscles of the Hip, Thigh & Gluteal Region (I)

Fig. 31.12 Anterior muscles of the hip and thigh (I)
Right limb. Muscle origins are shown in red, insertions in blue.

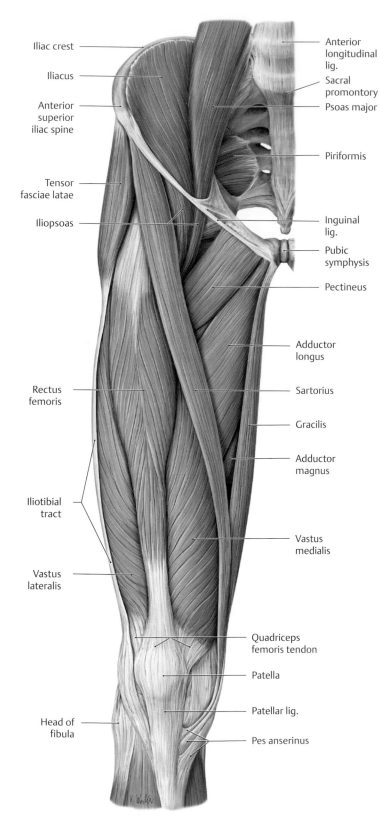

Iliac crest
Iliacus
Anterior superior iliac spine
Tensor fasciae latae
Iliopsoas
Rectus femoris
Iliotibial tract
Vastus lateralis
Head of fibula

Anterior longitudinal lig.
Sacral promontory
Psoas major
Piriformis
Inguinal lig.
Pubic symphysis
Pectineus
Adductor longus
Sartorius
Gracilis
Adductor magnus
Vastus medialis
Quadriceps femoris tendon
Patella
Patellar lig.
Pes anserinus

A *Removed:* Fascia lata of thigh (to the lateral iliotibial tract).

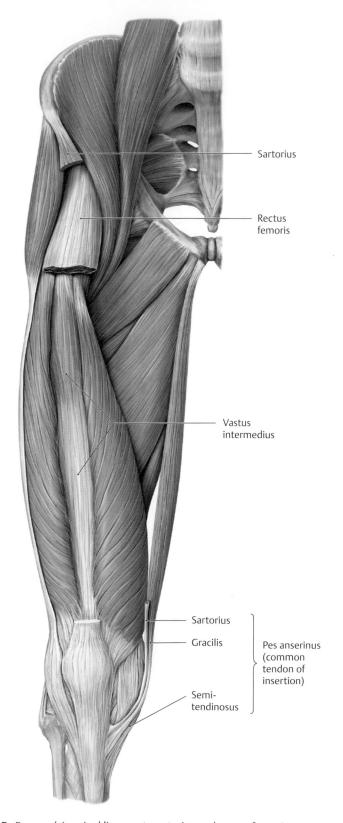

Sartorius
Rectus femoris
Vastus intermedius
Sartorius
Gracilis
Pes anserinus (common tendon of insertion)
Semi-tendinosus

B *Removed:* Inguinal ligament, sartorius and rectus femoris.

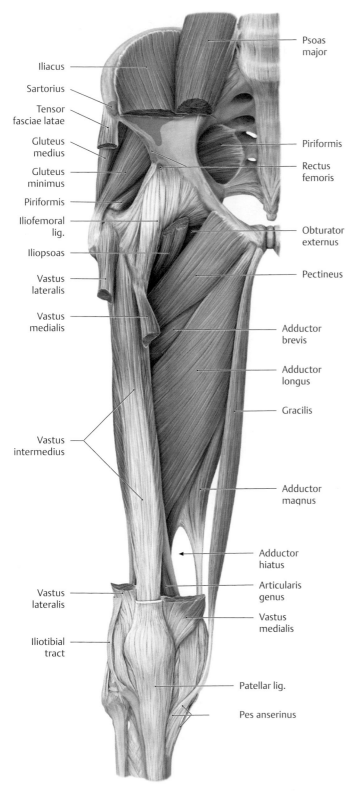

Iliacus

Sartorius

Tensor fasciae latae

Gluteus medius

Gluteus minimus

Piriformis

Iliofemoral lig.

Iliopsoas

Vastus lateralis

Vastus medialis

Vastus intermedius

Vastus lateralis

Iliotibial tract

Psoas major

Piriformis

Rectus femoris

Obturator externus

Pectineus

Adductor brevis

Adductor longus

Gracilis

Adductor magnus

Adductor hiatus

Articularis genus

Vastus medialis

Patellar lig.

Pes anserinus

C *Removed:* Rectus femoris (completely), vastus lateralis, vastus medialis, iliopsoas, and tensor fasciae latae.

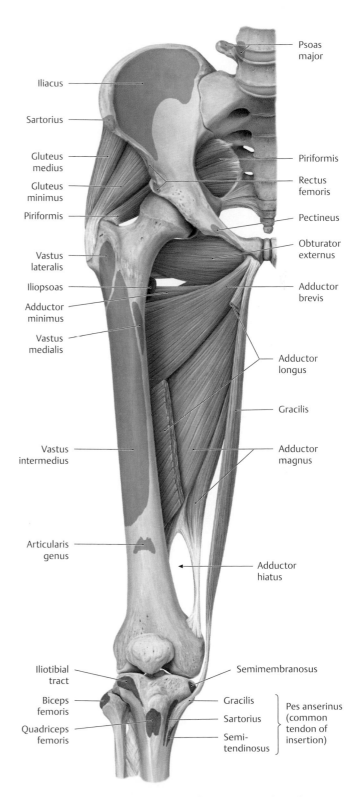

Iliacus

Sartorius

Gluteus medius

Gluteus minimus

Piriformis

Vastus lateralis

Iliopsoas

Adductor minimus

Vastus medialis

Vastus intermedius

Articularis genus

Iliotibial tract

Biceps femoris

Quadriceps femoris

Psoas major

Piriformis

Rectus femoris

Pectineus

Obturator externus

Adductor brevis

Adductor longus

Gracilis

Adductor magnus

Adductor hiatus

Semimembranosus

Gracilis

Sartorius

Semi-tendinosus

Pes anserinus (common tendon of insertion)

D *Removed:* Quadriceps femoris (rectus femoris, vastus lateralis, vastus medialis, vastus intermedius), iliopsoas, tensor fasciae latae, pectineus, and midportion of adductor longus.

419

Anterior Muscles of the Hip, Thigh & Gluteal Region (II)

***Fig. 31.13* Anterior muscles of the hip and thigh (II)**
Right limb. Muscle origins are shown in red, insertions in blue.

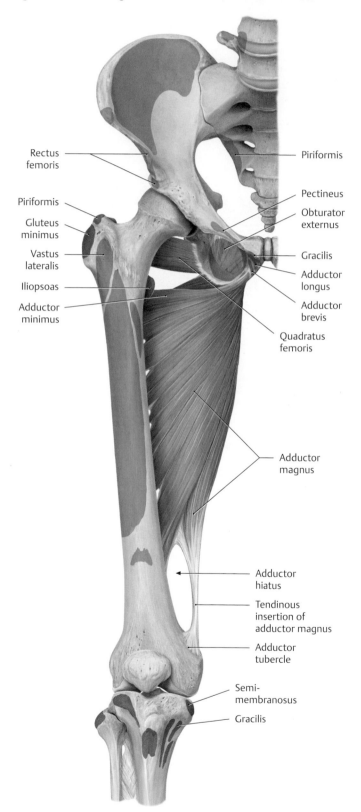

Rectus femoris
Piriformis
Gluteus minimus
Vastus lateralis
Iliopsoas
Adductor minimus

Piriformis
Pectineus
Obturator externus
Gracilis
Adductor longus
Adductor brevis
Quadratus femoris

Adductor magnus

Adductor hiatus
Tendinous insertion of adductor magnus
Adductor tubercle

Semi-membranosus
Gracilis

A *Removed:* Gluteus medius and minimus, piriformis, obturator externus, adductor brevis and longus, and gracilis.

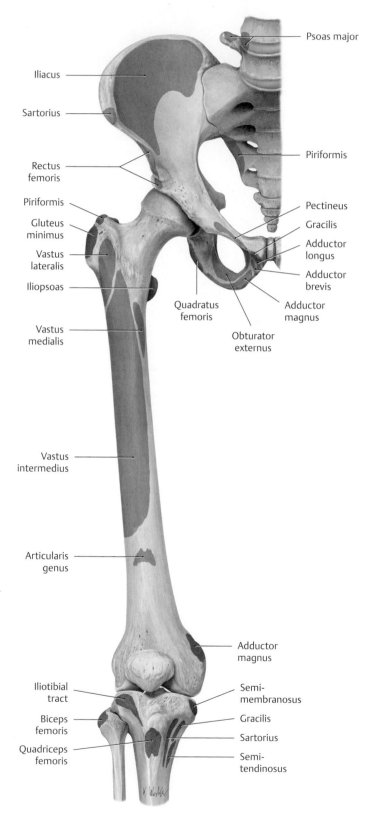

Iliacus
Sartorius

Rectus femoris
Piriformis
Gluteus minimus
Vastus lateralis
Iliopsoas
Quadratus femoris

Vastus medialis

Psoas major

Piriformis
Pectineus
Gracilis
Adductor longus
Adductor brevis
Adductor magnus
Obturator externus

Vastus intermedius

Articularis genus

Adductor magnus

Iliotibial tract
Biceps femoris
Quadriceps femoris

Semi-membranosus
Gracilis
Sartorius
Semi-tendinosus

B *Removed:* All muscles.

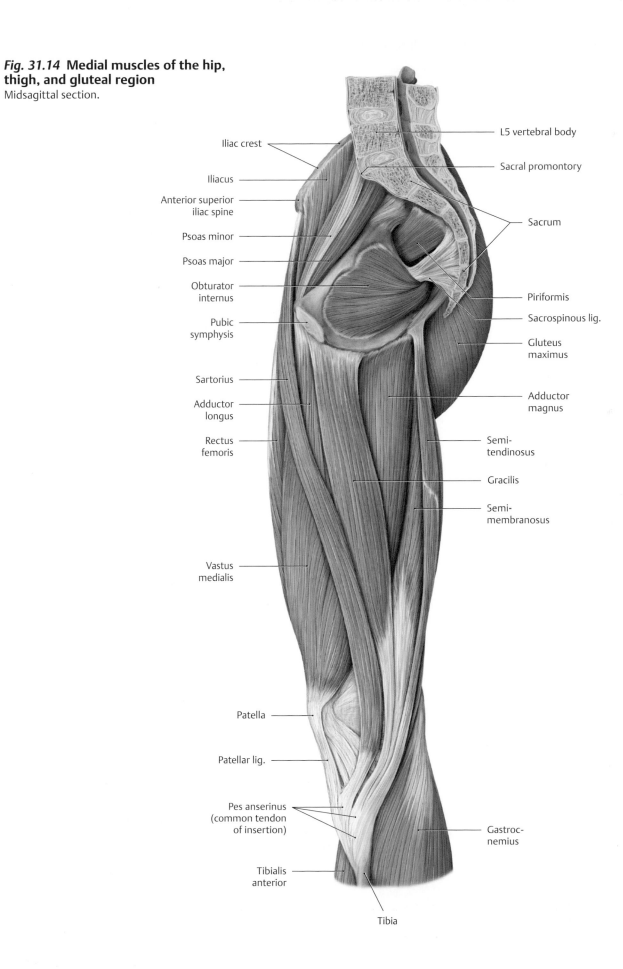

Fig. 31.14 **Medial muscles of the hip, thigh, and gluteal region**
Midsagittal section.

Iliac crest

Iliacus

Anterior superior iliac spine

Psoas minor

Psoas major

Obturator internus

Pubic symphysis

Sartorius

Adductor longus

Rectus femoris

Vastus medialis

Patella

Patellar lig.

Pes anserinus (common tendon of insertion)

Tibialis anterior

Tibia

L5 vertebral body

Sacral promontory

Sacrum

Piriformis

Sacrospinous lig.

Gluteus maximus

Adductor magnus

Semi-tendinosus

Gracilis

Semi-membranosus

Gastrocnemius

Posterior Muscles of the Hip, Thigh & Gluteal Region (I)

Fig. 31.15 Posterior muscles of the hip, thigh, and gluteal region (I)
Right limb. Muscle origins are shown in red, insertions in blue.

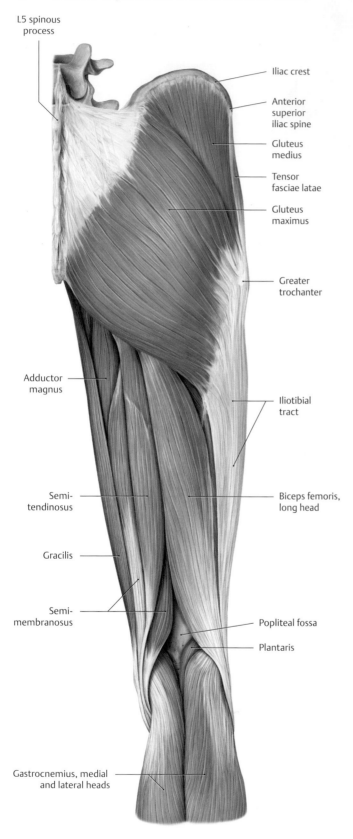

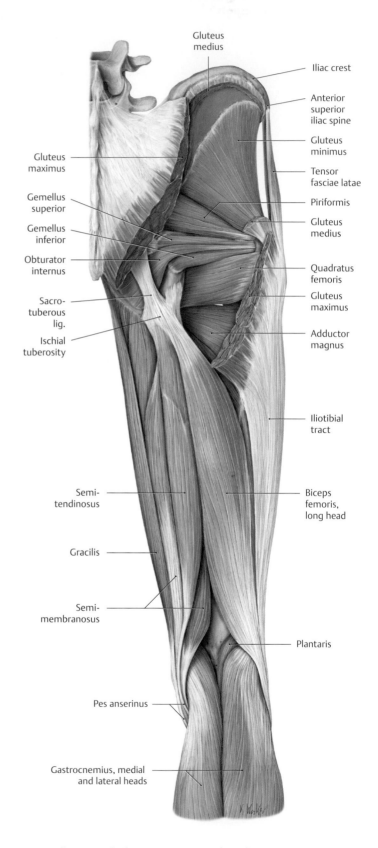

A *Removed:* Fascia lata (to iliotibial tract).

B *Partially removed:* Gluteus maximus and medius.

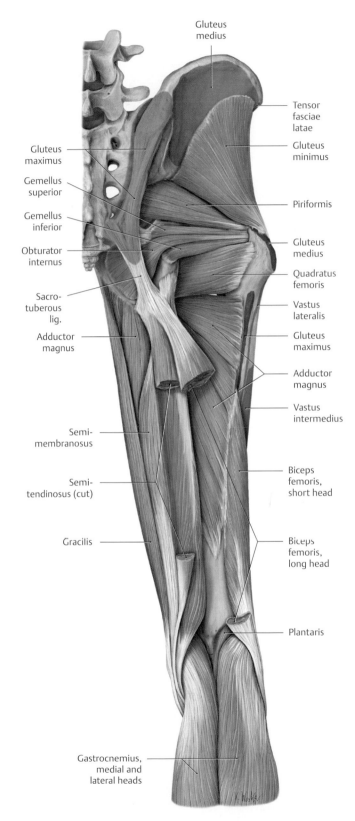

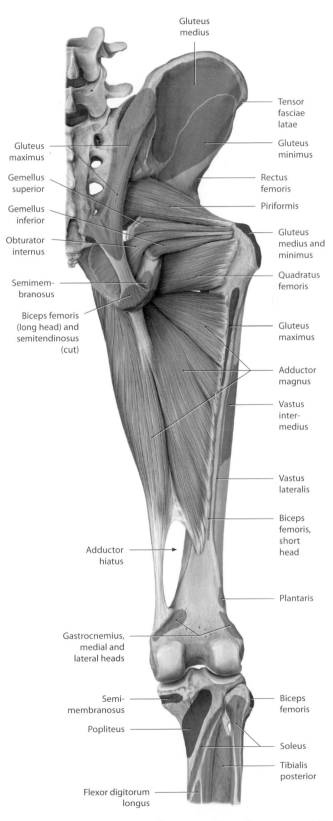

Gluteus medius

Gluteus maximus

Gemellus superior

Gemellus inferior

Obturator internus

Sacro-tuberous lig.

Adductor magnus

Semi-membranosus

Semi-tendinosus (cut)

Gracilis

Gastrocnemius, medial and lateral heads

Tensor fasciae latae

Gluteus minimus

Piriformis

Gluteus medius

Quadratus femoris

Vastus lateralis

Gluteus maximus

Adductor magnus

Vastus intermedius

Biceps femoris, short head

Biceps femoris, long head

Plantaris

Gluteus medius

Gluteus maximus

Gemellus superior

Gemellus inferior

Obturator internus

Semimem-branosus

Biceps femoris (long head) and semitendinosus (cut)

Adductor hiatus

Gastrocnemius, medial and lateral heads

Semi-membranosus

Popliteus

Flexor digitorum longus

Tensor fasciae latae

Gluteus minimus

Rectus femoris

Piriformis

Gluteus medius and minimus

Quadratus femoris

Gluteus maximus

Adductor magnus

Vastus inter-medius

Vastus lateralis

Biceps femoris, short head

Plantaris

Biceps femoris

Soleus

Tibialis posterior

C *Removed:* Semitendinosus and biceps femoris (partially); gluteus maximus and medius (completely).

D *Removed:* Hamstrings (semitendinosus, semimembranosus, and biceps femoris), gluteus minimus, gastrocnemius, and muscles of the leg.

Posterior Muscles of the Hip, Thigh & Gluteal Region (II)

Fig. 31.16 Posterior muscles of the hip, thigh, and gluteal region (II)

Right limb. Muscle origins are shown in red, insertions in blue.

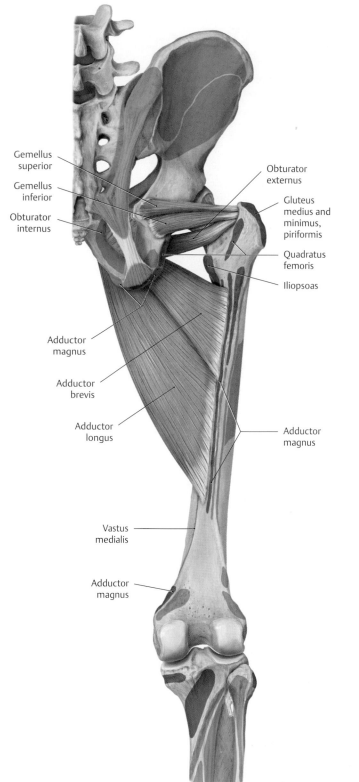

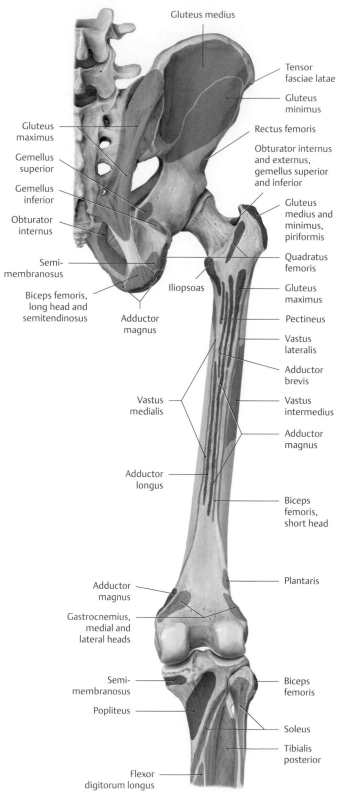

A *Removed:* Piriformis, obturator internus, quadratus femoris, and adductor magnus.

B *Removed:* All muscles.

Fig. 31.17 Lateral muscles of the hip, thigh, and gluteal region
Note: The iliotibial tract (the thickened band of fascia lata) functions as a tension band
to reduce the bending loads on the proximal femur.

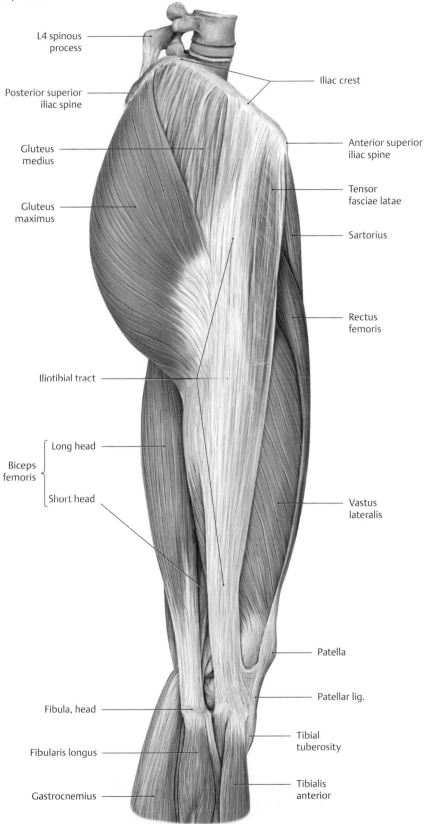

L4 spinous process

Iliac crest

Posterior superior iliac spine

Gluteus medius

Anterior superior iliac spine

Gluteus maximus

Tensor fasciae latae

Sartorius

Rectus femoris

Iliotibial tract

Long head

Biceps femoris

Short head

Vastus lateralis

Patella

Patellar lig.

Fibula, head

Fibularis longus

Tibial tuberosity

Gastrocnemius

Tibialis anterior

Muscle Facts (I)

Table 31.1		Iliopsoas muscle			
Muscles		**Origin**	**Insertion**	**Innervation**	**Action**
③ Iliopsoas	① Psoas major*	*Superficial:* T12–L4 and associated intervertebral disks (lateral surfaces) *Deep:* L1–L5 vertebrae (costal processes)	Femur (lesser trochanter)	Lumbar plexus L1, L2(L3)	• Hip joint: flexion and external rotation • Lumbar spine: *unilateral* contraction (with the femur fixed) flexes the trunk laterally to the same side; *bilateral* contraction raises the trunk from the supine position
	② Iliacus	Iliac fossa		Femoral n. (L2–L3)	

* The psoas minor, present in approximately 50% of the population, is often found on the superficial surface of the psoas major (see **Fig. 31.19**). It is not a muscle of the lower limb. It originates, inserts, and exerts its action on the abdomen (see **Table 13.1, p. 148**).

Fig. 31.18 Muscles of the hip
Right side, schematic.

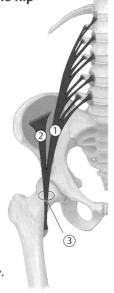

A Iliopsoas muscle, anterior view.

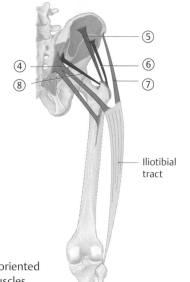

Iliotibial tract

B Vertically oriented gluteal muscles, posterior view.

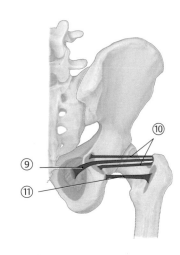

C Horizontally oriented gluteal muscles, posterior view.

Table 31.2	Gluteal muscles			
Muscle	**Origin**	**Insertion**	**Innervation**	**Action**
④ Gluteus maximus	Sacrum (dorsal surface, lateral part), ilium (gluteal surface, posterior part), thoracolumbar fascia, sacrotuberous lig.	• Upper fibers: iliotibial tract • Lower fibers: gluteal tuberosity	Inferior gluteal n. (L5–S2)	• Entire muscle: extends and externally rotates the hip in sagittal and coronal planes • Upper fibers: abduction • Lower fibers: adduction
⑤ Gluteus medius	Ilium (gluteal surface below the iliac crest between the anterior and posterior gluteal line)	Greater trochanter of the femur (lateral surface)	Superior gluteal n. (L4–S1)	• Entire muscle: abducts the hip, stabilizes the pelvis in the coronal plane • Anterior part: flexion and internal rotation • Posterior part: extension and external rotation
⑥ Gluteus minimus	Ilium (gluteal surface below the origin of gluteus medius)	Greater trochanter of the femur (anterolateral surface)		
⑦ Tensor fasciae latae	Anterior superior iliac spine	Iliotibial tract		• Tenses the fascia lata • Hip joint: abduction, flexion, and internal rotation
⑧ Piriformis	Pelvic surface of the sacrum	Apex of the greater trochanter of the femur	Sacral plexus (S1, S2)	• External rotation, abduction, and extension of the hip joint • Stabilizes the hip joint
⑨ Obturator internus	Inner surface of the obturator membrane and its bony boundaries	Medial surface of the greater trochanter		External rotation and extension of the hip joint (also active in abduction, depending on the joint's position)
⑩ Gemelli	• Gemellus superior: ischial spine • Gemellus inferior: ischial tuberosity	Jointly with obturator internus tendon (medial surface, greater trochanter)	Sacral plexus (L5, S1)	
⑪ Quadratus femoris	Lateral border of the ischial tuberosity	Intertrochanteric crest of the femur		External rotation of the hip joint

Fig. 31.19 Psoas and iliacus muscles

Right side, anterior view.

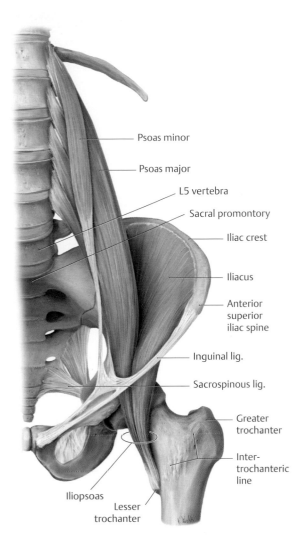

- Psoas minor
- Psoas major
- L5 vertebra
- Sacral promontory
- Iliac crest
- Iliacus
- Anterior superior iliac spine
- Inguinal lig.
- Sacrospinous lig.
- Greater trochanter
- Inter-trochanteric line
- Iliopsoas
- Lesser trochanter

Fig. 31.20 Superficial muscles of the gluteal region

Right side, posterior view.

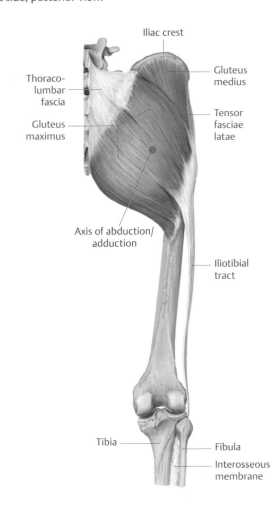

- Iliac crest
- Thoraco-lumbar fascia
- Gluteus medius
- Gluteus maximus
- Tensor fasciae latae
- Axis of abduction/adduction
- Iliotibial tract
- Tibia
- Fibula
- Interosseous membrane

Fig. 31.21 Deep muscles of the gluteal region

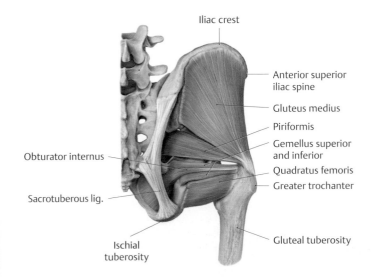

- Iliac crest
- Anterior superior iliac spine
- Gluteus medius
- Piriformis
- Gemellus superior and inferior
- Quadratus femoris
- Greater trochanter
- Obturator internus
- Sacrotuberous lig.
- Ischial tuberosity
- Gluteal tuberosity

A Deep layer with gluteus maximus removed.

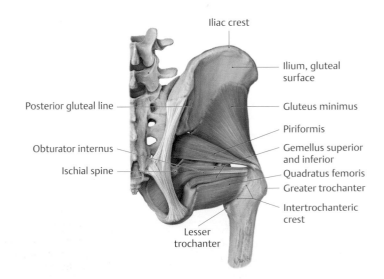

- Iliac crest
- Ilium, gluteal surface
- Posterior gluteal line
- Gluteus minimus
- Piriformis
- Obturator internus
- Gemellus superior and inferior
- Ischial spine
- Quadratus femoris
- Greater trochanter
- Intertrochanteric crest
- Lesser trochanter

B Deep layer with gluteus maximus and gluteus medius removed.

Muscle Facts (II)

Functionally, the medial thigh muscles are considered the adductors of the hip.

Fig. 31.22 **Medial thigh muscles: Superficial layer**
Right side, anterior view.

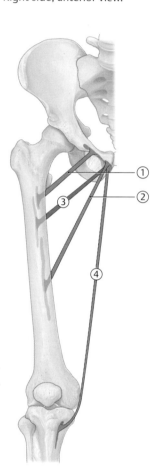

A Schematic.

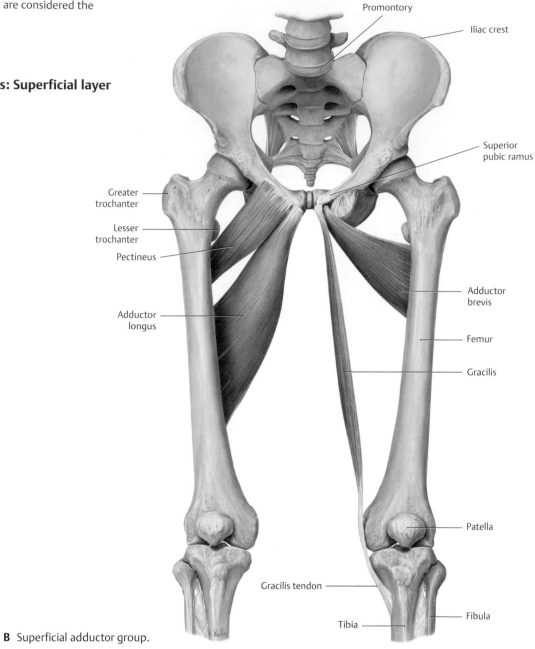

B Superficial adductor group.

Table 31.3	**Medial thigh muscles: Superficial layer**			
Muscle	**Origin**	**Insertion**	**Innervation**	**Action**
① Pectineus	Pecten pubis	Femur (pectineal line and the proximal linea aspera)	Femoral n., obturator n. (L2, L3)	• Hip joint: adduction, external rotation, and slight flexion • Stabilizes the pelvis in the coronal and sagittal planes
② Adductor longus	Superior pubic ramus and anterior side of the pubic symphysis	Femur (linea aspera, medial lip in the middle third of the femur)	Obturator n. (L2–L4)	• Hip joint: adduction and flexion (up to 70 degrees); extension (past 80 degrees of flexion) • Stabilizes the pelvis in the coronal and sagittal planes
③ Adductor brevis	Inferior pubic ramus			
④ Gracilis	Inferior pubic ramus below the pubic symphysis	Tibia (medial border of the tuberosity, along with the tendons of sartorius and semitendinosus)	Obturator n. (L2, L3)	• Hip joint: adduction and flexion • Knee joint: flexion and internal rotation

Fig. 31.23 Medial thigh muscles: Deep layer

Right side, anterior view.

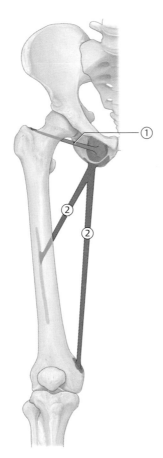

A Schematic.

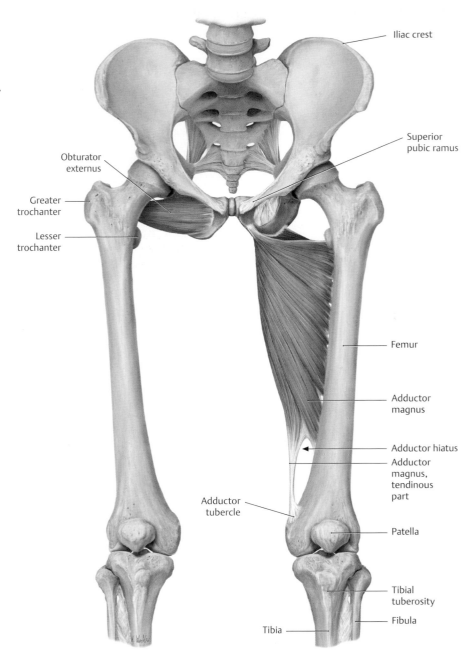

B Deep adductor group.

Table 31.4	Medial thigh muscles: Deep layer			
Muscle	**Origin**	**Insertion**	**Innervation**	**Action**
① Obturator externus	Outer surface of the obturator membrane and its bony boundaries	Trochanteric fossa of the femur	Obturator n. (L3, L4)	• Hip joint: adduction and external rotation • Stabilizes the pelvis in the sagittal plane
② Adductor magnus	Inferior pubic ramus, ischial ramus, and ischial tuberosity	• Deep part ("fleshy insertion"): medial lip of the linea aspera	• Deep part: obturator n. (L2–L4)	• Hip joint: adduction, extension, and slight flexion (the tendinous insertion is also active in internal rotation) • Stabilizes the pelvis in the coronal and sagittal planes
		• Superficial part ("tendinous insertion"): adductor tubercle of the femur	• Superficial part: tibial n. (L4)	

Muscle Facts (III)

The anterior and posterior muscles of the thigh can be classified as extensors and flexors, respectively, with regard to the knee joint.

Fig. 31.24 Anterior thigh muscles

Right side, anterior view.

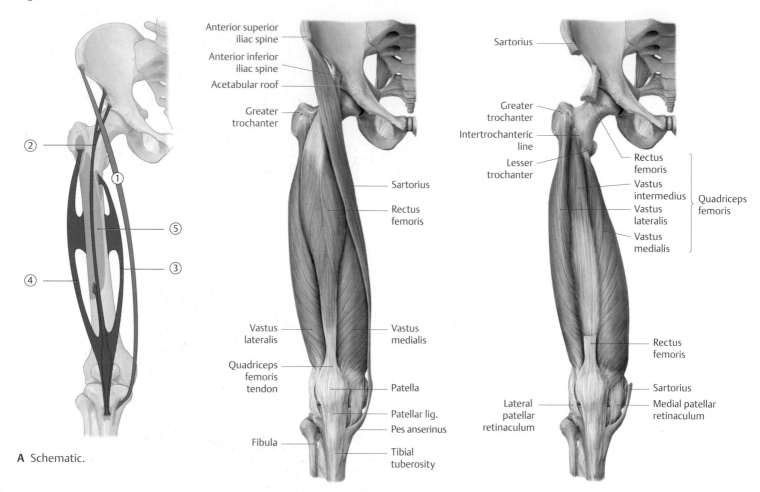

A Schematic.

B Superficial group.

C Deep group. *Removed:* Sartorius and rectus femoris.

Table 31.5		Anterior thigh muscles			
Muscle		**Origin**	**Insertion**	**Innervation**	**Action**
① Sartorius		Anterior superior iliac spine	Medial to the tibial tuberosity (together with gracilis and semitendinosus)	Femoral n. (L2, L3)	• Hip joint: flexion, abduction, and external rotation • Knee joint: flexion and internal rotation
Quadriceps femoris*	② Rectus femoris	Anterior inferior iliac spine, acetabular roof of hip joint	Tibial tuberosity (via patellar lig.)	Femoral n. (L2–L4)	• Hip joint: flexion • Knee joint: extension
	③ Vastus medialis	Linea aspera (medial lip), intertrochanteric line (distal part)	Tibial tuberosity via patellar lig.; patella and tibial tuberosity via respective medial and lateral patellar retinacula		Knee joint: extension
	④ Vastus lateralis	Linea aspera (lateral lip), greater trochanter (lateral surface)			
	⑤ Vastus intermedius	Femoral shaft (anterior side)	Tibial tuberosity (via patellar lig.)		
	Articularis genus (distal fibers of vastus intermedius)	Anterior side of femoral shaft at level of the suprapatellar recess	Suprapatellar recess of knee joint capsule		Knee joint: extension; retracts the suprapatellar bursa to prevent entrapment of capsule
*The entire muscle inserts on the tibial tuberosity via the patellar lig.					

Fig. 31.25 Posterior thigh muscles

Right side, posterior view.

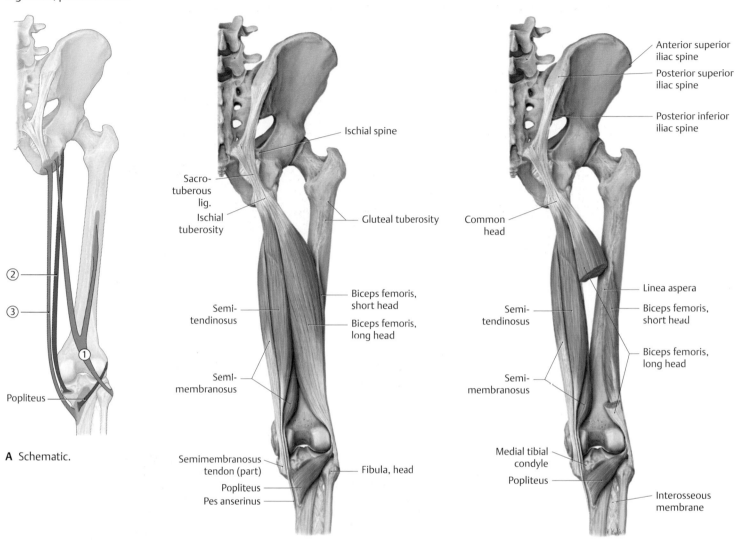

A Schematic.

B Superficial group.

C Deep group. *Removed:* Biceps femoris (long head) and semitendinosus.

Table 31.6	**Posterior thigh muscles**			
Muscle	**Origin**	**Insertion**	**Innervation**	**Action**
① Biceps femoris	Long head: ischial tuberosity, sacrotuberous lig. (common head with semitendinosus)	Head of fibula	Tibial n. (L5–S2)	• Hip joint (long head): extends the hip, stabilizes the pelvis in the sagittal plane • Knee joint: flexion and external rotation
	Short head: lateral lip of the linea aspera in the middle third of the femur		Common fibular n. (L5–S2)	Knee joint: flexion and external rotation
② Semimembranosus	Ischial tuberosity	Medial tibial condyle, oblique popliteal lig., popliteus fascia	Tibial n. (L5–S2)	• Hip joint: extends the hip, stabilizes the pelvis in the sagittal plane • Knee joint: flexion and internal rotation
③ Semitendinosus	Ischial tuberosity and sacrotuberous lig. (common head with long head of biceps femoris)	Medial to the tibial tuberosity in the pes anserinus (along with the tendons of gracilis and sartorius)		
See **p. 451** for the popliteus.				

32 Knee & Leg
Tibia & Fibula

The tibia and fibula articulate at two joints, allowing limited motion (rotation). The crural interosseous membrane is a sheet of tough connective tissue that serves as an origin for several muscles in the leg. It also acts with the tibiofibular syndesmosis to stabilize the ankle joint.

***Fig. 32.1* Tibia and fibula**
Right leg.

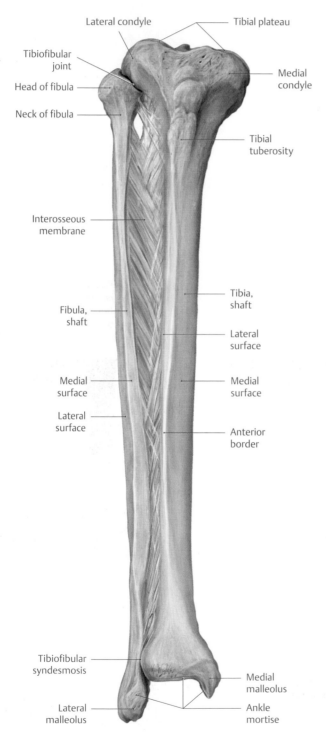

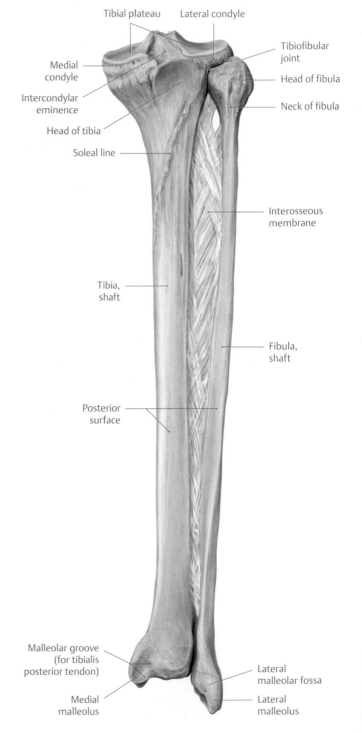

A Anterior view.

B Posterior view.

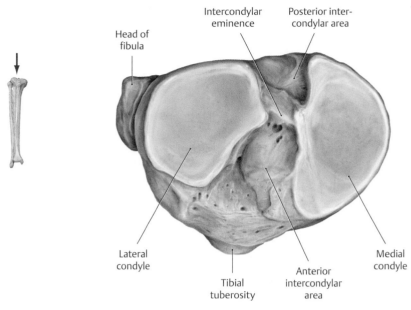

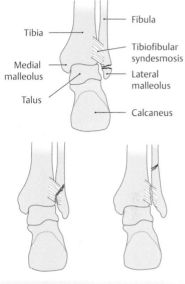

Clinical box 32.1

Fibular fracture

When diagnosing a fibular fracture, it is important to determine whether the tibiofibular syndesmosis (see **p. 432**) is disrupted. Fibular fractures may occur distal to, level with, or proximal to the tibiofibular syndesmosis; the latter two frequently involve tearing of the syndesmosis.

C Proximal view.

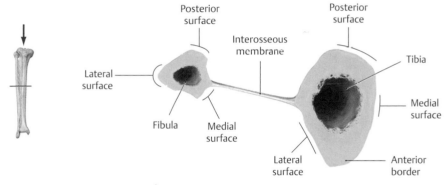

D Transverse section, proximal view.

In this fracture located proximal to the syndesmosis (*arrow*), the syndesmosis is torn, as indicated by the widened medial joint space of the upper ankle joint (see **pp. 456–457**).

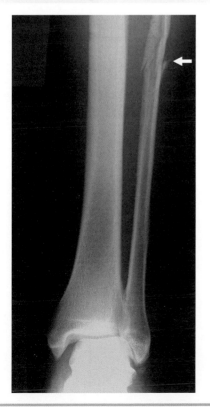

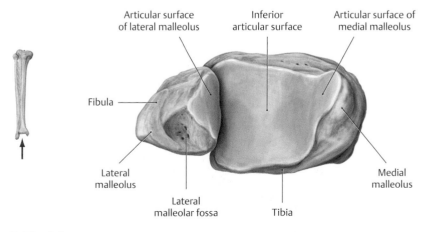

E Distal view.

Knee Joint: Overview

In the knee joint, the femur articulates with the tibia and patella. Both joints are contained within a common capsule and have communicating articular cavities. *Note:* The fibula is not included in the knee joint (contrast to the humerus in the elbow; see **p. 326**). Instead, it forms a separate rigid articulation with the tibia.

Fig. 32.2 **Right knee joint**

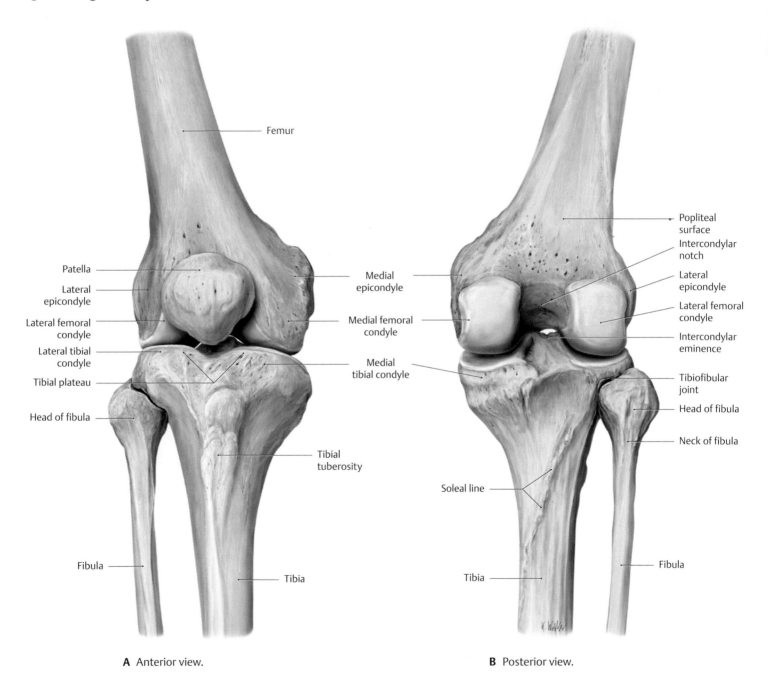

A Anterior view.

B Posterior view.

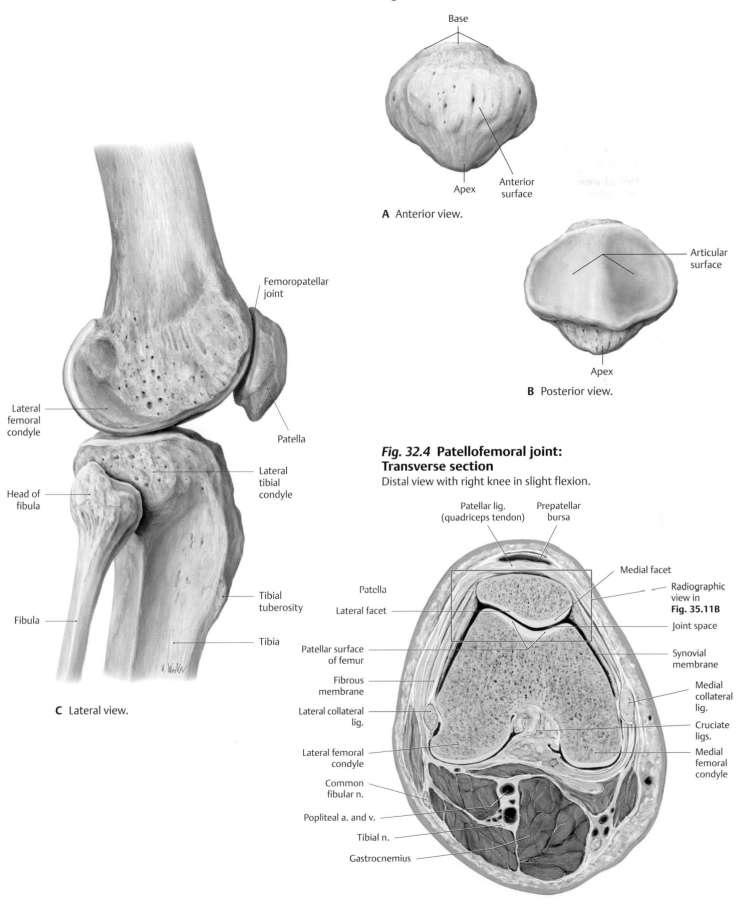

Fig. 32.3 Patella

Base

Apex — Anterior surface

A Anterior view.

Articular surface

Apex

B Posterior view.

Femoropatellar joint

Lateral femoral condyle

Patella

Head of fibula

Lateral tibial condyle

Fibula

Tibial tuberosity

Tibia

C Lateral view.

Fig. 32.4 Patellofemoral joint: Transverse section
Distal view with right knee in slight flexion.

Patellar lig. (quadriceps tendon) Prepatellar bursa

Patella

Lateral facet

Medial facet

Radiographic view in **Fig. 35.11B**

Joint space

Patellar surface of femur

Fibrous membrane

Lateral collateral lig.

Lateral femoral condyle

Common fibular n.

Popliteal a. and v.

Tibial n.

Gastrocnemius

Synovial membrane

Medial collateral lig.

Cruciate ligs.

Medial femoral condyle

Knee Joint: Capsule, Ligaments & Bursae

Table 32.1	Ligaments of the knee joint	
Extrinsic ligaments		
Anterior side	Patellar lig.	
	Medial longitudinal patellar retinaculum	
	Lateral longitudinal patellar retinaculum	
	Medial transverse patellar retinaculum	
	Lateral transverse patellar retinaculum	
Medial and lateral sides	Medial (tibial) collateral lig.	
	Lateral (fibular) collateral lig.	
Posterior side	Oblique popliteal lig.	
	Arcuate popliteal lig.	
Intrinsic ligaments		
Anterior cruciate lig.		
Posterior cruciate lig.		
Transverse lig. of knee		
Posterior meniscofemoral lig.		

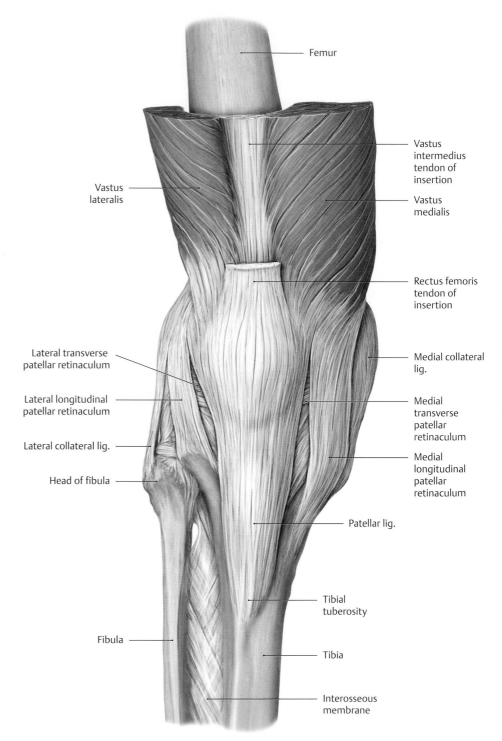

***Fig. 32.5* Ligaments of the knee joint**
Anterior view of right knee.

- Femur
- Vastus intermedius tendon of insertion
- Vastus lateralis
- Vastus medialis
- Rectus femoris tendon of insertion
- Lateral transverse patellar retinaculum
- Medial collateral lig.
- Lateral longitudinal patellar retinaculum
- Medial transverse patellar retinaculum
- Lateral collateral lig.
- Medial longitudinal patellar retinaculum
- Head of fibula
- Patellar lig.
- Tibial tuberosity
- Fibula
- Tibia
- Interosseous membrane

Fig. 32.6 Capsule, ligaments, and periarticular bursae

Posterior view of right knee. The joint cavity communicates with peri-articular bursae at the subpopliteal recess, semimembranosus bursa, and medial subtendinous bursa of the gastrocnemius.

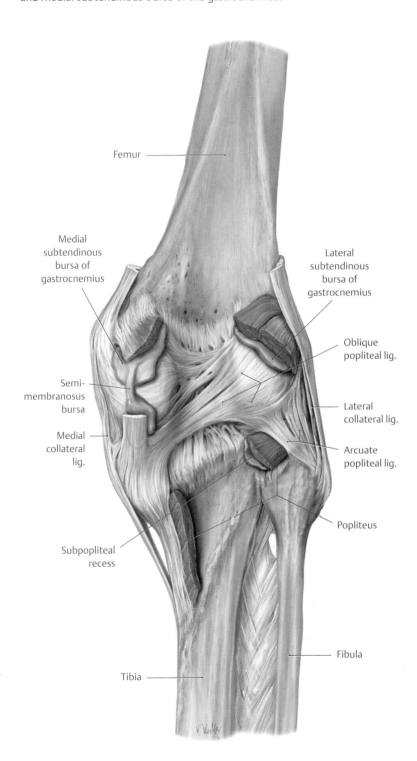

Femur

Medial subtendinous bursa of gastrocnemius

Lateral subtendinous bursa of gastrocnemius

Semi-membranosus bursa

Oblique popliteal lig.

Medial collateral lig.

Lateral collateral lig.

Arcuate popliteal lig.

Subpopliteal recess

Popliteus

Fibula

Tibia

 Clinical box 32.2

Gastrocnemio-semimembranosus bursa (Baker's cyst)

Painful swelling behind the knee may be caused by a cystic outpouching of the joint capsule (synovial popliteal cyst). This frequently results from an increase in intra-articular pressure (e.g., in rheumatoid arthritis).

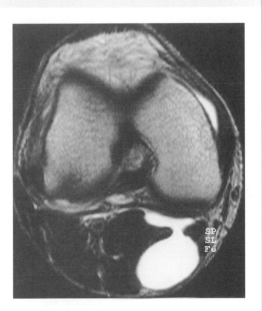

Axial MRI of a Baker's cyst in the right popliteal fossa, inferior view. Baker's cysts often occur in the medial part of the popliteal fossa between the semimem-branosus tendon and the medial head of the gas-trocnemius at the level of the posteromedial femoral condyle.

Knee Joint: Ligaments & Menisci

Fig. 32.7 Collateral and patellar ligaments of the knee joint
Right knee joint. Each knee joint has medial and lateral collateral ligaments. The medial collateral ligament is attached to both the capsule
and the medial meniscus, whereas the lateral collateral ligament has no
direct contact with either the capsule or the lateral meniscus. Both
collateral ligaments are taut when the knee is in extension and stabilize
the joint in the coronal plane.

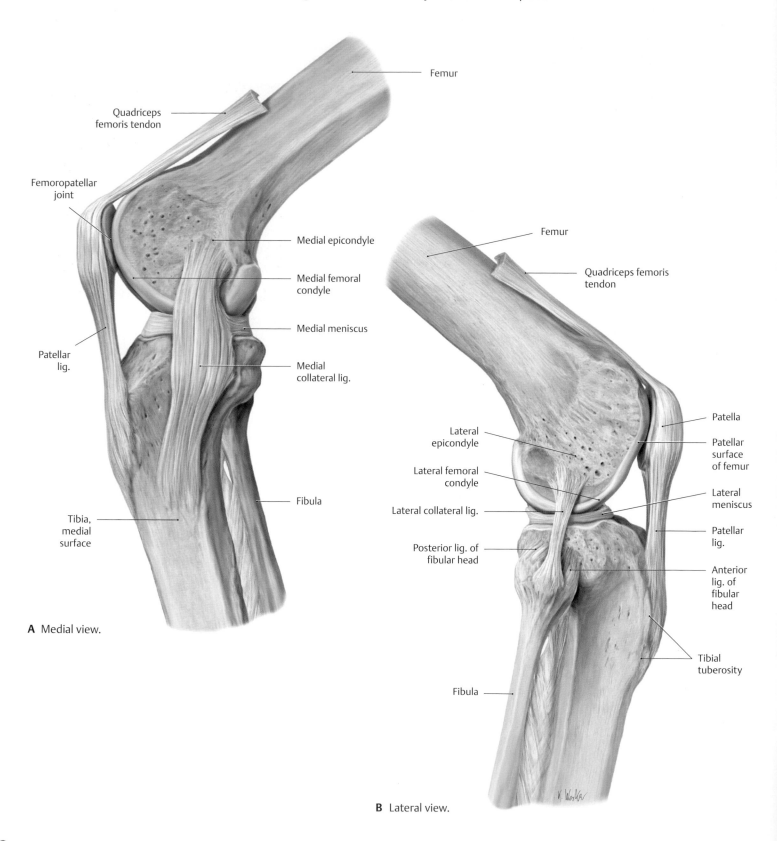

A Medial view.

B Lateral view.

Fig. 32.8 Menisci in the knee joint

Right tibial plateau, proximal view.

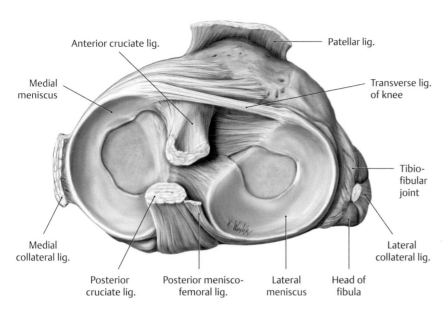

A Right tibial plateau with cruciate, patellar, and collateral ligaments divided.

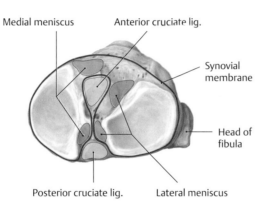

B Attachment sites of menisci and cruciate ligaments. Red line indicates the tibial attachment of the synovial membrane that covers the cruciate ligaments. The cruciate ligaments lie in the subsynovial connective tissue.

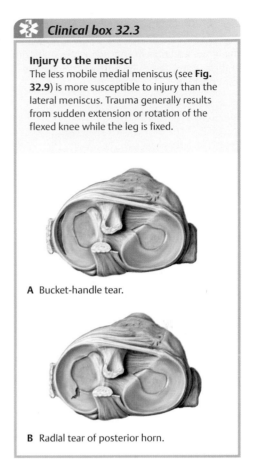

Clinical box 32.3

Injury to the menisci

The less mobile medial meniscus (see **Fig. 32.9**) is more susceptible to injury than the lateral meniscus. Trauma generally results from sudden extension or rotation of the flexed knee while the leg is fixed.

A Bucket-handle tear.

B Radial tear of posterior horn.

Fig. 32.9 Movements of the menisci

Right knee joint. The medial meniscus, which is anchored more securely than the lateral meniscus, undergoes less displacement during knee flexion.

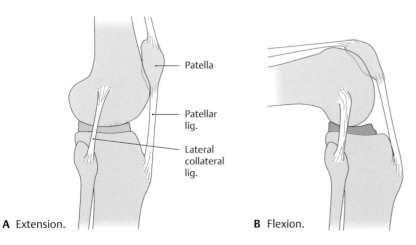

A Extension.

B Flexion.

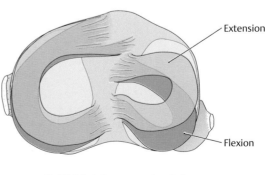

C Tibial plateau, proximal view.

Cruciate Ligaments

Fig. 32.10 **Cruciate and collateral ligaments**

Right knee joint. The cruciate ligaments keep the articular surfaces of the femur and tibia in contact, while stabilizing the knee joint primarily in the sagittal plane. Portions of the cruciate ligaments are taut in every joint position.

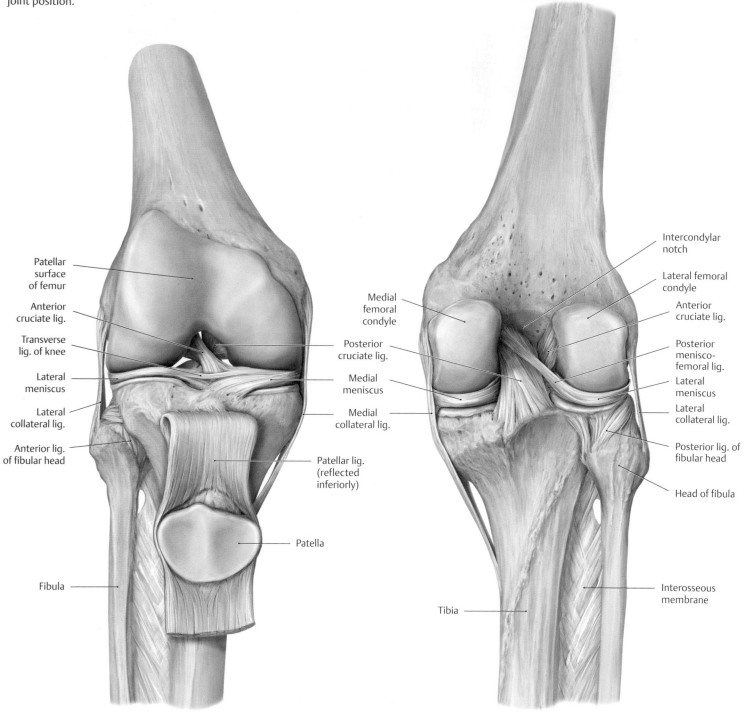

Patellar surface of femur

Anterior cruciate lig.

Transverse lig. of knee

Lateral meniscus

Lateral collateral lig.

Anterior lig. of fibular head

Fibula

Posterior cruciate lig.

Medial meniscus

Medial collateral lig.

Patellar lig. (reflected inferiorly)

Patella

Intercondylar notch

Lateral femoral condyle

Anterior cruciate lig.

Posterior menisco-femoral lig.

Lateral meniscus

Lateral collateral lig.

Posterior lig. of fibular head

Head of fibula

Interosseous membrane

Medial femoral condyle

Tibia

A Anterior view.

B Posterior view.

Fig. 32.11 Right knee joint in flexion

Anterior view with joint capsule and patella removed.

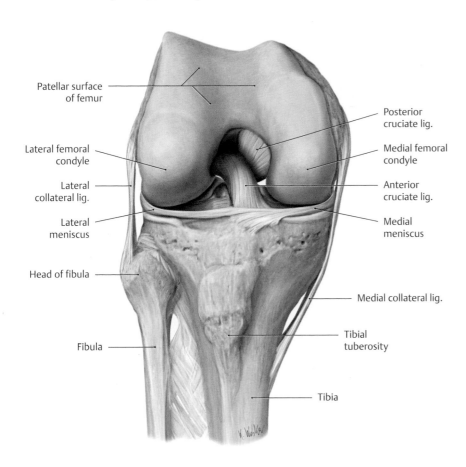

Patellar surface
of femur

Lateral femoral
condyle

Lateral
collateral lig.

Lateral
meniscus

Head of fibula

Fibula

Posterior
cruciate lig.

Medial femoral
condyle

Anterior
cruciate lig.

Medial
meniscus

Medial collateral lig.

Tibial
tuberosity

Tibia

Rupture of cruciate ligaments

Cruciate ligament rupture destabilizes the knee joint, allowing the tibia to move forward (anterior "drawer sign") or backward (posterior "drawer sign") relative to the femur. *Anterior* cruciate ligament ruptures are approximately 10 times more common than posterior ligament ruptures. The most common mechanism of injury is an internal rotation trauma with the leg fixed. A lateral blow to the fully extended knee with the foot planted tends to cause concomitant rupture of the anterior cruciate and medial collateral ligaments, as well as tearing of the attached medial meniscus.

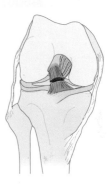

A Right knee in flexion, rupture of anterior cruciate ligament, anterior view.

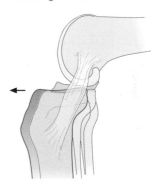

B Right knee in flexion, anterior "drawer sign," medial view. During examination of the flexed knee, the tibia can be pulled forward.

Fig. 32.12 Cruciate and collateral ligaments in flexion and extension

Right knee, anterior view. Taut ligament fibers shown in red. While most parts of the collateral ligaments are taut only in extension (**A**), the cruciate ligaments, or portions of them, are taut in flexion, extension and internal rotation (**B,C**). The cruciate ligaments thus help stabilize the knee in any joint position.

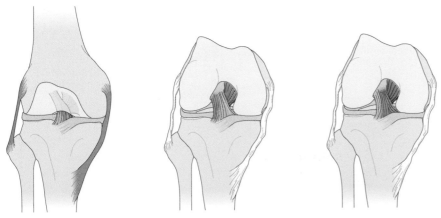

A Extension. **B** Flexion. **C** Flexion and internal rotation.

Knee Joint Cavity

Fig. 32.13 **Opened joint capsule**
Right knee, anterior view with patella reflected downward.

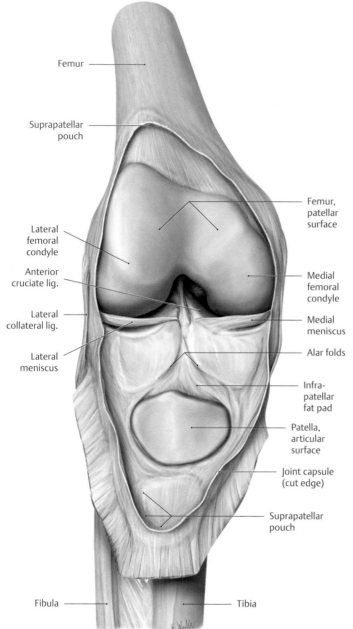

Femur

Suprapatellar pouch

Femur, patellar surface

Lateral femoral condyle

Anterior cruciate lig.

Lateral collateral lig.

Lateral meniscus

Medial femoral condyle

Medial meniscus

Alar folds

Infra-patellar fat pad

Patella, articular surface

Joint capsule (cut edge)

Suprapatellar pouch

Fibula

Tibia

Fig. 32.14 **Joint cavity**
Right knee, lateral view. The joint cavity was demonstrated by injecting liquid plastic into the knee joint and later removing the capsule.

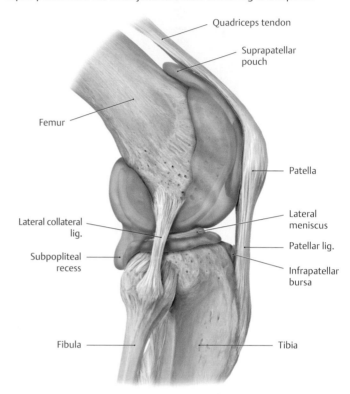

Quadriceps tendon

Suprapatellar pouch

Femur

Patella

Lateral collateral lig.

Lateral meniscus

Subpopliteal recess

Patellar lig.

Infrapatellar bursa

Fibula

Tibia

Fig 32.15 **Relations of structures to the joint capsule and articular cavity**
Right knee joint, proximal view.
Several joint structures provide strength or stability to the knee from outside of, or within, the joint space.

- Extracapsular structures (lateral collateral ligament) remain outside of the joint capsule.
- Intracapsular structures (medial collateral and cruciate ligaments) lie within the joint capsule but run in the subsynovial tissue outside the synovial membrane and are therefore also extra-articular.
- Intra-articular structures (menici) lie within the articular cavity, enclosed by the synovial membrane, and are bathed in synovial fluid.

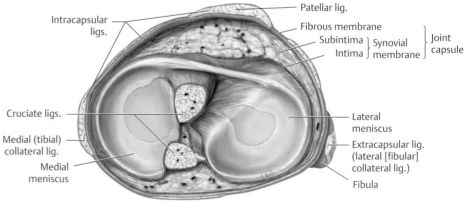

Intracapsular ligs.

Patellar lig.

Fibrous membrane

Subintima ⎱ Synovial
Intima ⎰ membrane

Joint capsule

Cruciate ligs.

Medial (tibial) collateral lig.

Medial meniscus

Lateral meniscus

Extracapsular lig. (lateral [fibular] collateral lig.)

Fibula

Fig. 32.16 Right knee joint: Midsagittal section
Lateral view.

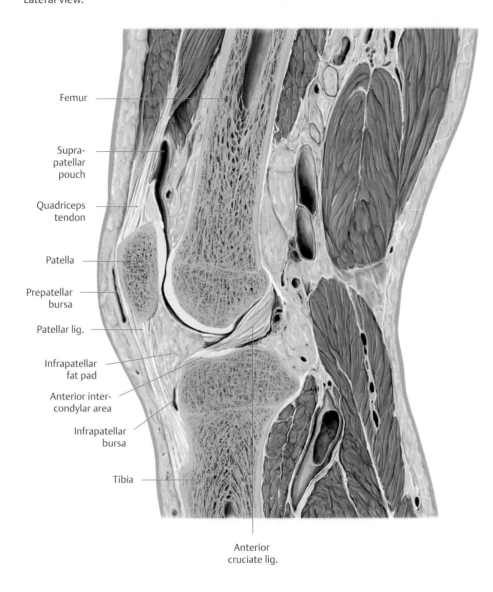

Femur
Supra-patellar pouch
Quadriceps tendon
Patella
Prepatellar bursa
Patellar lig.
Infrapatellar fat pad
Anterior inter-condylar area
Infrapatellar bursa
Tibia
Anterior cruciate lig.

Fig. 32.17 Suprapatellar pouch during flexion
Right knee joint, medial view.

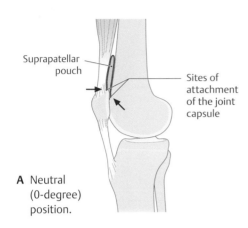

Suprapatellar pouch
Sites of attachment of the joint capsule

A Neutral (0-degree) position.

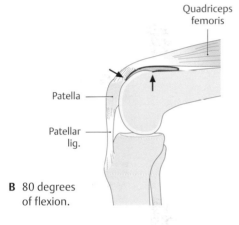

Quadriceps femoris
Patella
Patellar lig.

B 80 degrees of flexion.

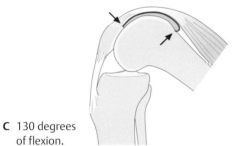

C 130 degrees of flexion.

Clinical box 32.5

The ballottable patella sign of knee effusion

Intra-articular effusion due to inflammatory changes or injury can be differentiated from swelling of the joint capsule by pushing down on the patella of the extended knee. If there is excessive fluid in the joint, the patella will rebound when released, signifying a positive test.

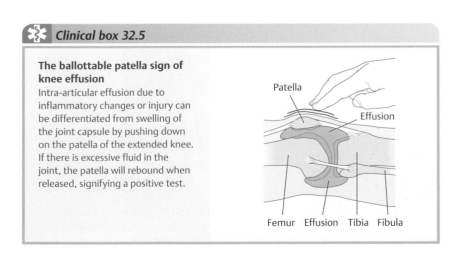

Patella
Effusion
Femur   Effusion   Tibia   Fibula

Muscles of the Leg: Anterior & Lateral Compartments

***Fig. 32.18* Muscles of the anterior compartment of the leg**
Right leg. Muscle origins shown in red, insertions in blue.

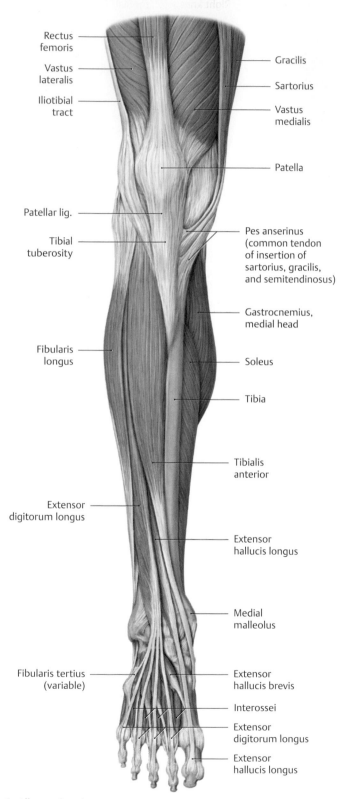

A All muscles shown.

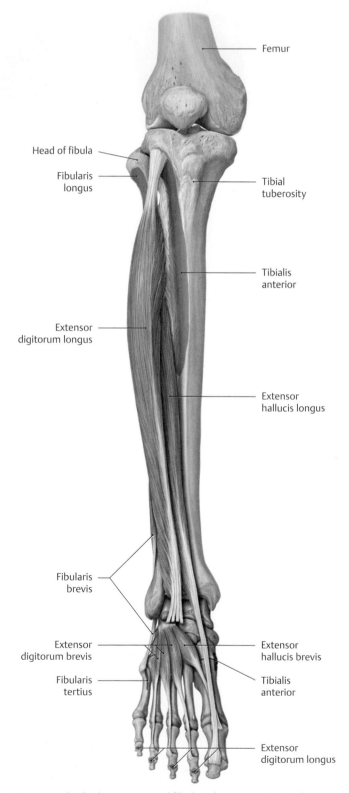

B *Removed:* Tibialis anterior and fibularis longus; extensor digitorum longus tendons (distal portions). *Note:* The fibularis tertius is a division of the extensor digitorum longus.

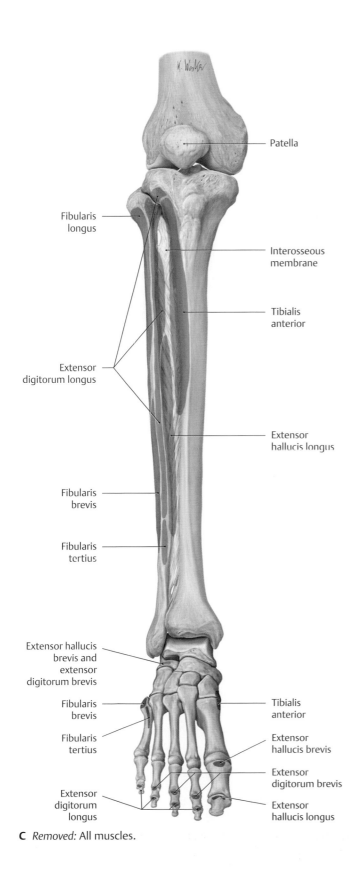

Patella

Fibularis longus

Interosseous membrane

Tibialis anterior

Extensor digitorum longus

Extensor hallucis longus

Fibularis brevis

Fibularis tertius

Extensor hallucis brevis and extensor digitorum brevis

Fibularis brevis

Tibialis anterior

Fibularis tertius

Extensor hallucis brevis

Extensor digitorum brevis

Extensor digitorum longus

Extensor hallucis longus

C *Removed:* All muscles.

Fig. 32.19 Muscles of the lateral compartment of the leg
Right leg. The triceps surae is comprised of the soleus and two heads of the gastrocnemius.

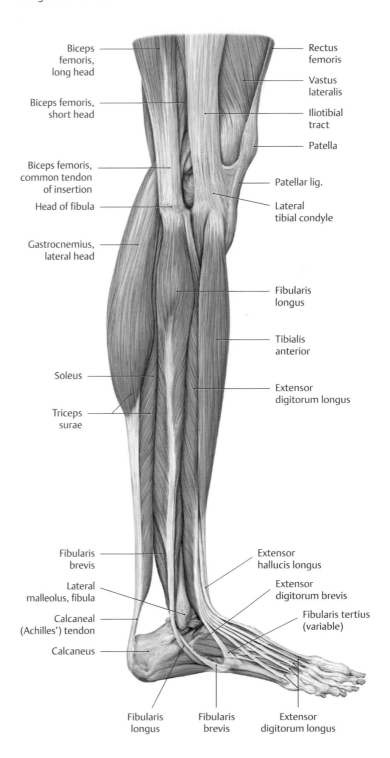

Biceps femoris, long head

Biceps femoris, short head

Biceps femoris, common tendon of insertion

Head of fibula

Gastrocnemius, lateral head

Soleus

Triceps surae

Fibularis brevis

Lateral malleolus, fibula

Calcaneal (Achilles') tendon

Calcaneus

Fibularis longus

Fibularis brevis

Extensor digitorum longus

Rectus femoris

Vastus lateralis

Iliotibial tract

Patella

Patellar lig.

Lateral tibial condyle

Fibularis longus

Tibialis anterior

Extensor digitorum longus

Extensor hallucis longus

Extensor digitorum brevis

Fibularis tertius (variable)

445

Muscles of the Leg: Posterior Compartment

***Fig. 32.20* Muscles of the posterior compartment of the leg**
Right leg. Muscle origins shown in red, insertions in blue.

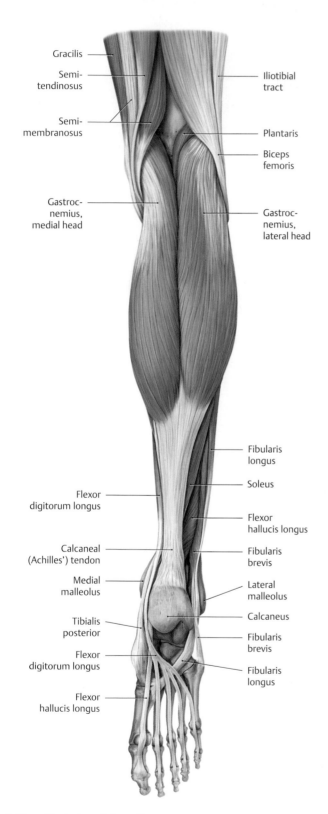

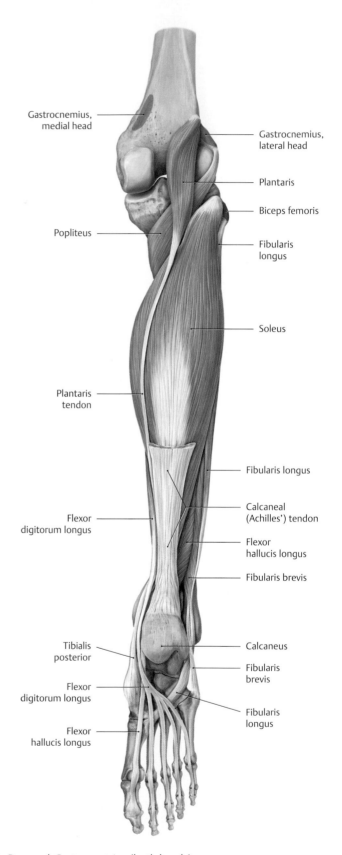

A *Note:* The bulge of the calf is produced mainly by the triceps surae (soleus and the two heads of the gastrocnemius).

B *Removed:* Gastrocnemius (both heads).

446

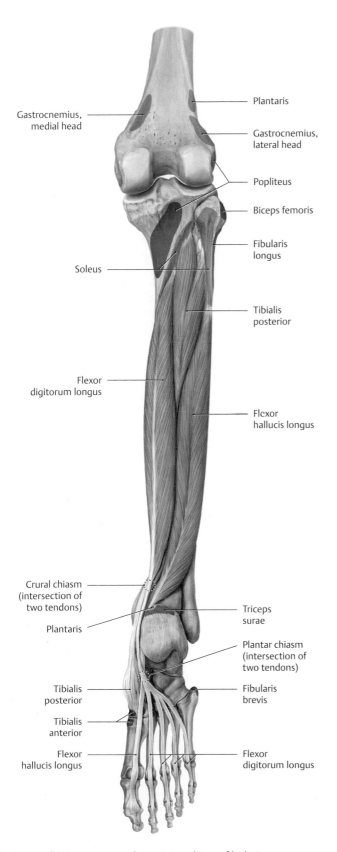

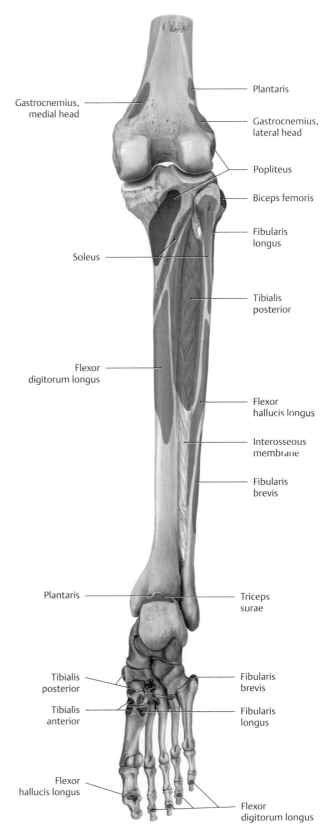

Gastrocnemius, medial head

Plantaris

Gastrocnemius, lateral head

Popliteus

Biceps femoris

Fibularis longus

Soleus

Tibialis posterior

Flexor digitorum longus

Flexor hallucis longus

Crural chiasm (intersection of two tendons)

Plantaris

Triceps surae

Plantar chiasm (intersection of two tendons)

Tibialis posterior

Fibularis brevis

Tibialis anterior

Flexor hallucis longus

Flexor digitorum longus

Gastrocnemius, medial head

Plantaris

Gastrocnemius, lateral head

Popliteus

Biceps femoris

Fibularis longus

Soleus

Tibialis posterior

Flexor digitorum longus

Flexor hallucis longus

Interosseous membrane

Fibularis brevis

Plantaris

Triceps surae

Tibialis posterior

Fibularis brevis

Tibialis anterior

Fibularis longus

Flexor hallucis longus

Flexor digitorum longus

C *Removed:* Triceps surae, plantaris, popliteus, fibularis longus, and fibularis brevis muscles.

D *Removed:* All muscles.

447

Muscle Facts (I)

The muscles of the leg control the flexion/extension and inversion/ eversion of the foot, which provide stability to the lower limb during movements at the knee and hip joint.

Fig. 32.21 **Muscles of the lateral compartment of the leg**
Right leg and foot.

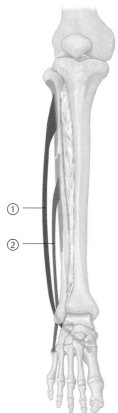

A Fibularis muscles, anterior view, schematic.

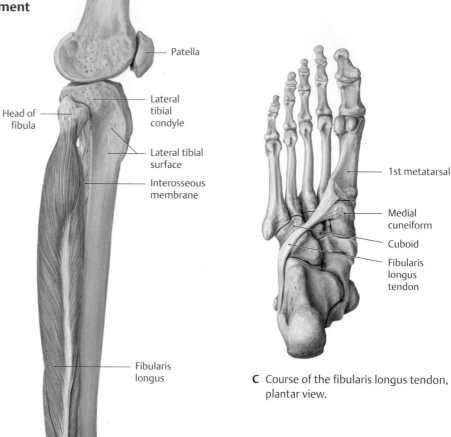

B Lateral compartment, right lateral view.

C Course of the fibularis longus tendon, plantar view.

Table 32.2	Lateral compartment			
Muscle	**Origin**	**Insertion**	**Innervation**	**Action**
① Fibularis longus	Fibula (head and proximal two thirds of the lateral surface, arising partly from the intermuscular septa)	Medial cuneiform (plantar side), 1st metatarsal (base)	Superficial fibular n. (L5, S1)	• Talocrural joint: plantar flexion • Subtalar joint: eversion (pronation) • Supports the transverse arch of the foot
② Fibularis brevis	Fibula (distal half of the lateral surface), intermuscular septa	5th metatarsal (tuberosity at the base, with an occasional division to the dorsal aponeurosis of the 5th toe)		• Talocrural joint: plantar flexion • Subtalar joint: eversion (pronation)

Fig. 32.22 Muscles of the anterior compartment of the leg

Right leg, anterior view.

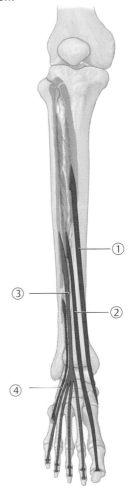

A Schematic.

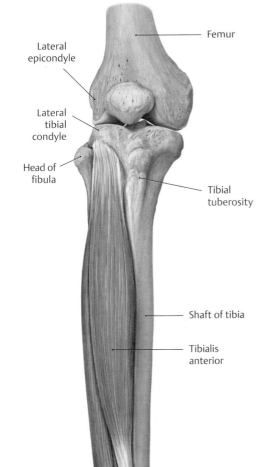

B Anterior compartment.

Table 32.3	Anterior compartment			
Muscle	**Origin**	**Insertion**	**Innervation**	**Action**
① Tibialis anterior	Tibia (upper two thirds of the lateral surface), interosseous membrane, and superficial crural fascia (highest part)	Medial cuneiform (medial and plantar surface), first metatarsal (medial base)	Deep fibular n. (L4, L5)	• Talocrural joint: dorsiflexion • Subtalar joint: inversion (supination)
② Extensor hallucis longus	Fibula (middle third of the medial surface), interosseous membrane	1st toe (at the dorsal aponeurosis at the base of its distal phalanx)	Deep fibular n. (L4, L5)	• Talocrural joint: dorsiflexion • Subtalar joint: active in both eversion and inversion (pronation/supination), depending on the initial position of the foot • Extends the MTP and IP joints of the big toe
③ Extensor digitorum longus	Fibula (head and medial surface), tibia (lateral condyle), and interosseous membrane	2nd to 5th toes (at the dorsal aponeuroses at the bases of the distal phalanges)	Deep fibular n. (L4, L5)	• Talocrural joint: dorsiflexion • Subtalar joint: eversion (pronation) • Extends the MTP and IP joints of the 2nd to 5th toes
④ Fibularis tertius	Distal fibula (anterior border)	5th metatarsal (base)	Deep fibular n. (L4, L5)	• Talocrural joint: dorsiflexion • Subtalar joint: eversion (pronation)

IP, interphalangeal; MTP, metatarsophalangeal.

Muscle Facts (II)

The muscles of the posterior compartment are divided into two groups: the superficial and deep flexors. These groups are separated by the transverse intermuscular septum.

Fig. 32.23 **Muscles of the posterior compartment of the leg: Superficial flexors**
Right leg, posterior view.

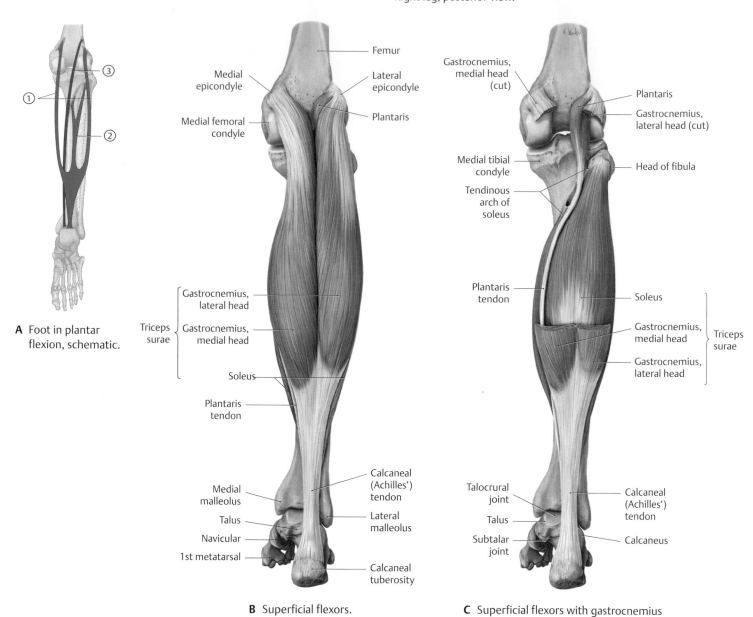

A Foot in plantar flexion, schematic.

B Superficial flexors.

C Superficial flexors with gastrocnemius removed (portions of medial and lateral heads).

Table 32.4		Superficial flexors of the posterior compartment			
Muscle		**Origin**	**Insertion**	**Innervation**	**Action**
Triceps surae	① Gastrocnemius	Femur (medial head: superior posterior part of the medial femoral condyle. lateral head: lateral surface of lateral femoral condyle)	Calcaneal tuberosity via the calcaneal (Achilles') tendon	Tibial n. (S1, S2)	• Talocrural joint: plantar flexion when knee is extended (gastrocnemius) • Knee joint: flexion (gastrocnemius) • Talocrural joint: plantar flexion (soleus)
	② Soleus	Fibula (head and neck, posterior surface), tibia (soleal line via a tendinous arch)			
③ Plantaris		Femur (lateral epicondyle, proximal to lateral head of gastrocnemius)	Calcaneal tuberosity		Negligible; may act with gastrocnemius in plantar flexion

Fig. 32.24 Posterior compartment of the leg: Deep flexors

Right leg with foot in plantar flexion, posterior view.

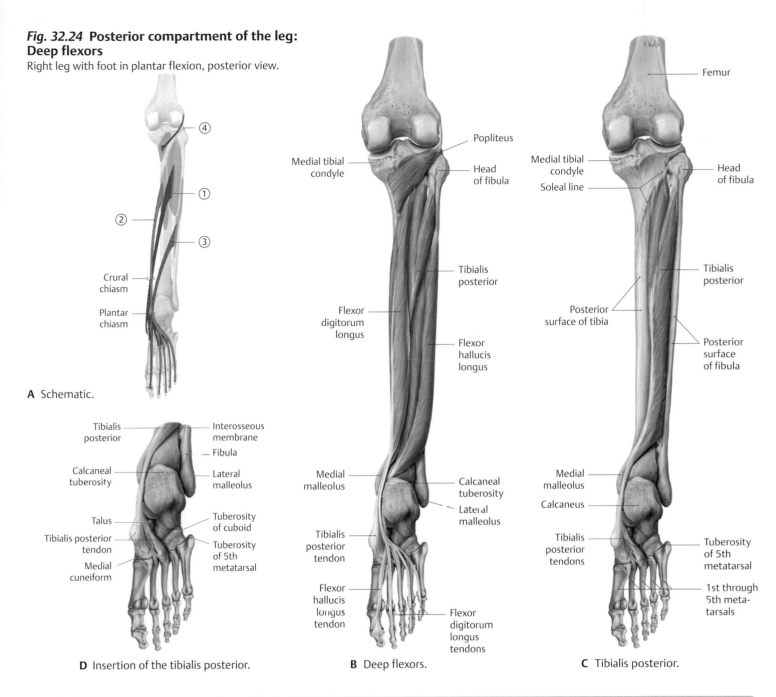

A Schematic.

D Insertion of the tibialis posterior.

B Deep flexors.

C Tibialis posterior.

Table 32.5	Deep flexors of the posterior compartment			
Muscle	**Origin**	**Insertion**	**Innervation**	**Action**
① Tibialis posterior	Interosseous membrane, adjacent borders of tibia and fibula	Navicular tuberosity; cuneiforms (medial, intermediate, and lateral); 2nd to 4th metatarsals (bases)	Tibial n. (L4, L5)	• Talocrural joint: plantar flexion • Subtalar joint: inversion (supination) • Supports the longitudinal and transverse arches
② Flexor digitorum longus	Tibia (middle third of posterior surface)	2nd to 5th distal phalanges (bases)	Tibial n. (L5–S2)	• Talocrural joint: plantar flexion • Subtalar joint: inversion (supination) • MTP and IP joints of the 2nd to 5th toes: plantar flexion
③ Flexor hallucis longus	Fibula (distal two thirds of posterior surface), adjacent interosseous membrane	1st distal phalanx (base)		• Talocrural joint: plantar flexion • Subtalar joint: inversion (supination) • MTP and IP joints of the 1st toe: plantar flexion • Supports the medial longitudinal arch
④ Popliteus	Lateral femoral condyle, posterior horn of the lateral meniscus	Posterior tibial surface (above the origin at the soleus)	Tibial n. (L4–S1)	Knee joint: flexes and unlocks the knee by externally rotating the femur on the fixed tibia
IP, interphalangeal; MTP, metatarsophalangeal.				

33 Ankle & Foot
Bones of the Foot

Fig. 33.1 Subdivisions of the pedal skeleton

Right foot, dorsal view. Descriptive anatomy divides the skeletal elements of the foot into the tarsus, metatarsus, and forefoot (ante-tarsus). Functional and clinical criteria divide the pedal skeleton into hindfoot, midfoot, and forefoot.

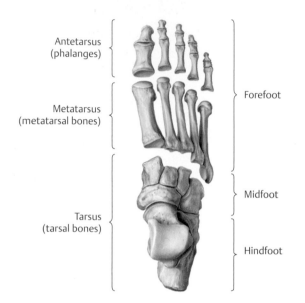

Fig. 33.2 Bones of the foot

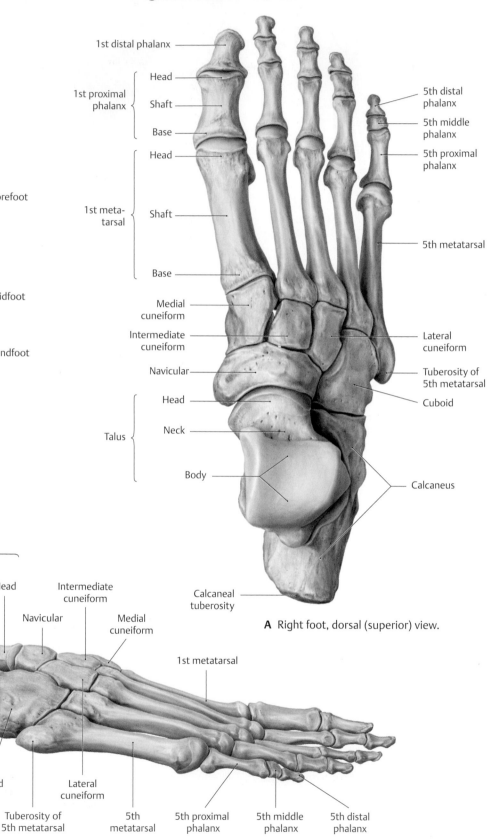

A Right foot, dorsal (superior) view.

B Right foot, lateral view.

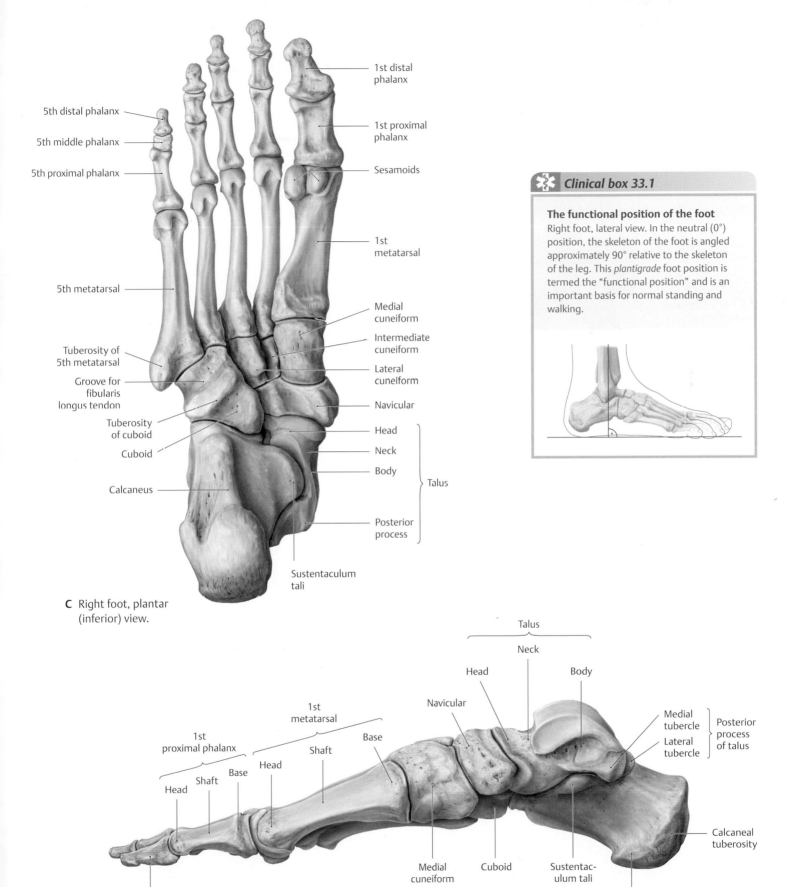

5th distal phalanx

5th middle phalanx

5th proximal phalanx

5th metatarsal

Tuberosity of
5th metatarsal

Groove for
fibularis
longus tendon

Tuberosity
of cuboid

Cuboid

Calcaneus

1st distal
phalanx

1st proximal
phalanx

Sesamoids

1st
metatarsal

Medial
cuneiform

Intermediate
cuneiform

Lateral
cuneiform

Navicular

Head

Neck   } Talus

Body

Posterior
process

Sustentaculum
tali

C Right foot, plantar
(inferior) view.

Clinical box 33.1

The functional position of the foot
Right foot, lateral view. In the neutral (0°)
position, the skeleton of the foot is angled
approximately 90° relative to the skeleton
of the leg. This *plantigrade* foot position is
termed the "functional position" and is an
important basis for normal standing and
walking.

Talus

Neck

Head   Body

Navicular

Medial
tubercle   } Posterior
                process
Lateral   of talus
tubercle

1st
metatarsal

1st
proximal phalanx

Base

Shaft

Base

Head

Shaft

Calcaneal
tuberosity

Head

Medial
cuneiform

Cuboid

Sustentac-
ulum tali

1st distal phalanx

Medial process of
calcaneal tuberosity

D Right foot, medial view.

Joints of the Foot (I)

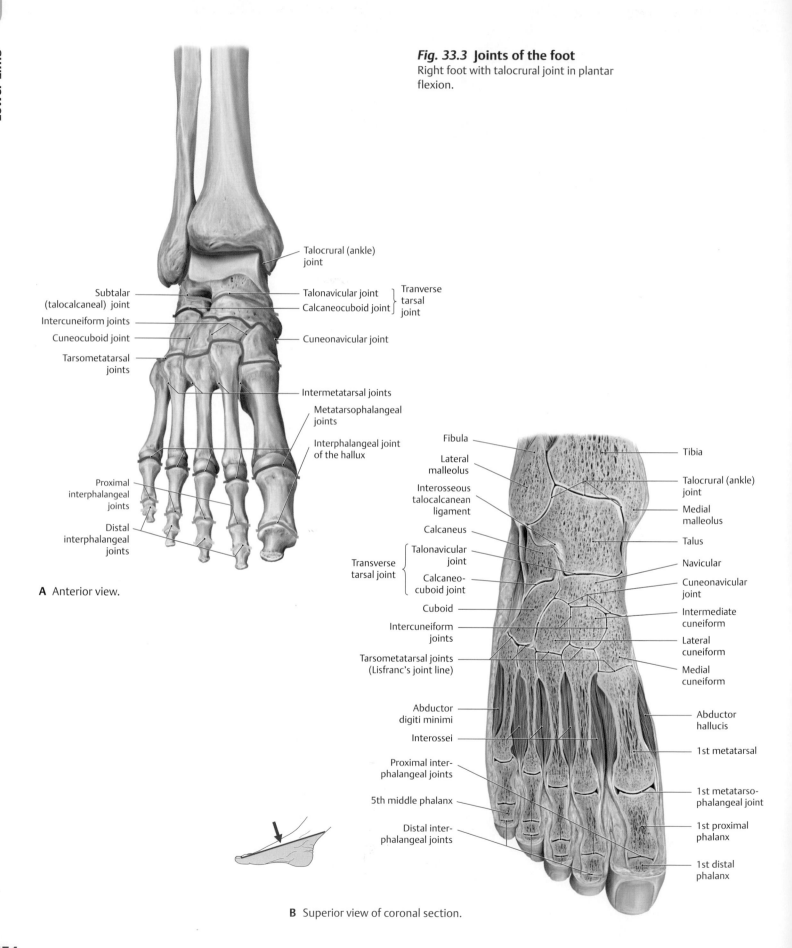

Fig. 33.3 **Joints of the foot**
Right foot with talocrural joint in plantar flexion.

Talocrural (ankle) joint

Subtalar (talocalcaneal) joint
Talonavicular joint ⎱ Tranverse tarsal joint
Calcaneocuboid joint ⎰

Intercuneiform joints

Cuneocuboid joint — Cuneonavicular joint

Tarsometatarsal joints

Intermetatarsal joints

Metatarsophalangeal joints

Interphalangeal joint of the hallux

Proximal interphalangeal joints

Distal interphalangeal joints

A Anterior view.

Fibula — Tibia

Lateral malleolus — Talocrural (ankle) joint

Interosseous talocalcanean ligament — Medial malleolus

Calcaneus — Talus

Talonavicular joint ⎱ Transverse tarsal joint
Calcaneo-cuboid joint ⎰ — Navicular

Cuboid — Cuneonavicular joint

Intercuneiform joints — Intermediate cuneiform

Tarsometatarsal joints (Lisfranc's joint line) — Lateral cuneiform

Abductor digiti minimi — Medial cuneiform

Interossei — Abductor hallucis

Proximal interphalangeal joints — 1st metatarsal

5th middle phalanx — 1st metatarsophalangeal joint

Distal interphalangeal joints — 1st proximal phalanx

— 1st distal phalanx

B Superior view of coronal section.

Fig. 33.4 Proximal articular surfaces
Right foot, proximal view.

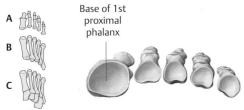

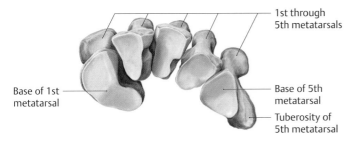

Base of 1st proximal phalanx

A Metatarsophalangeal joints.

1st through 5th metatarsals

Base of 1st metatarsal

Base of 5th metatarsal

Tuberosity of 5th metatarsal

B Tarsometatarsal joints.

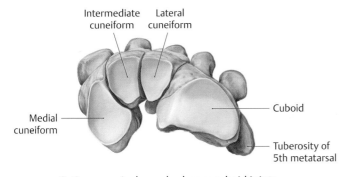

Intermediate cuneiform

Lateral cuneiform

Medial cuneiform

Cuboid

Tuberosity of 5th metatarsal

C Cuneonavicular and calcaneocuboid joints.

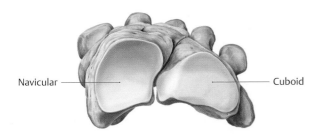

Navicular

Cuboid

D Talonavicular and calcaneocuboid joints.

Fig. 33.5 Distal articular surfaces
Right foot, distal view.

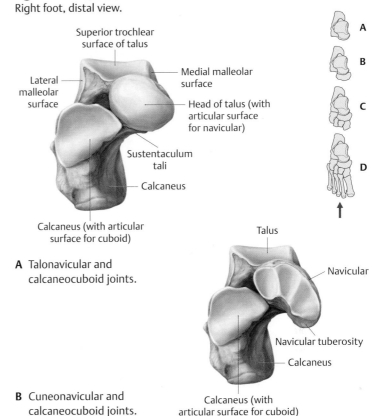

Superior trochlear surface of talus

Lateral malleolar surface

Medial malleolar surface

Head of talus (with articular surface for navicular)

Sustentaculum tali

Calcaneus

Calcaneus (with articular surface for cuboid)

A Talonavicular and calcaneocuboid joints.

Talus

Navicular

Navicular tuberosity

Calcaneus

Calcaneus (with articular surface for cuboid)

B Cuneonavicular and calcaneocuboid joints.

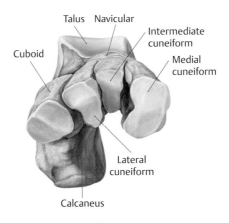

Talus   Navicular

Cuboid

Intermediate cuneiform

Medial cuneiform

Lateral cuneiform

Calcaneus

C Tarsometatarsal joints.

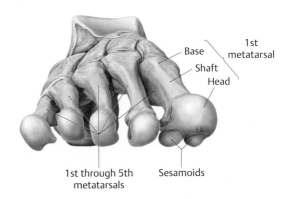

Base

Shaft

Head

1st metatarsal

1st through 5th metatarsals

Sesamoids

D Metatarsophalangeal joints.

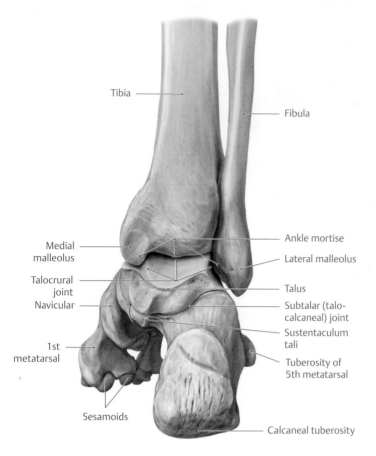

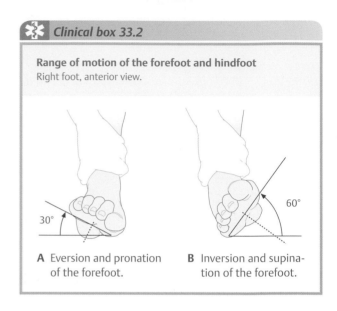

Fig. 33.6 Talocrural and subtalar joints

Right foot. The talocrural (ankle) joint is formed by the distal ends of the tibia and fibula (ankle mortise) articulating with the trochlea of the talus. The subtalar joint consists of an anterior and a posterior compartment (the talocalcaneal and talocalcaneonavicular joints, respectively) divided by the interosseous talocalcaneal ligament (see **p. 458**).

A Posterior view with foot in neutral (0-degree) position.

Clinical box 33.2

Range of motion of the forefoot and hindfoot
Right foot, anterior view.

A Eversion and pronation of the forefoot.

B Inversion and supination of the forefoot.

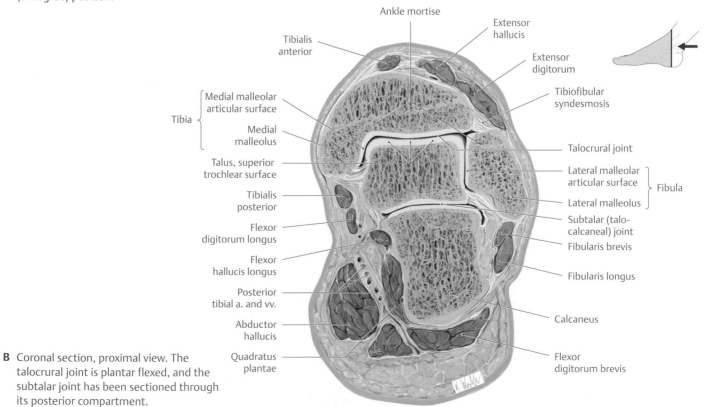

B Coronal section, proximal view. The talocrural joint is plantar flexed, and the subtalar joint has been sectioned through its posterior compartment.

Fig. 33.7 Talocrural and subtalar joints: Sagittal section

Right foot, medial view.

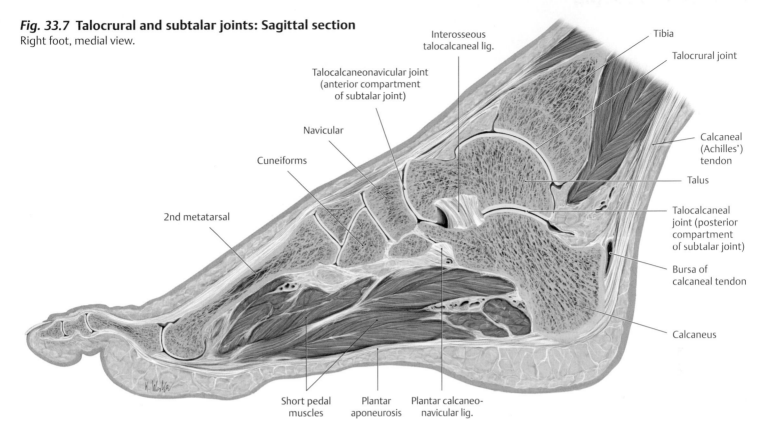

Fig. 33.8 Talocrural joint

Right foot. The talocrural (ankle) joint is tighter and more stable with the foot in dorsiflexion, when the wider, anterior part of the trochlea (of the talus) is wedged within the ankle mortise. Accordingly the joint is looser and less stable in plantar flexion.

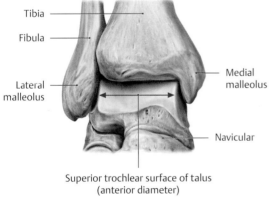

A Anterior view.

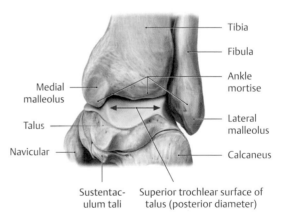

B Posterior view.

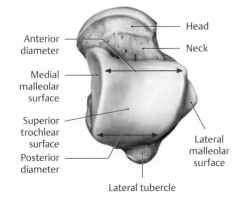

C Proximal (superior) view of talus.

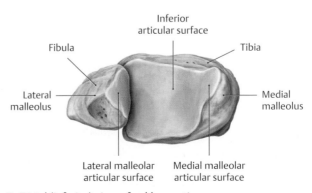

D Distal (inferior) view of ankle mortise.

Joints of the Foot (III)

Fig. 33.9 **Subtalar joint and ligaments**

Right foot with opened subtalar joint. The subtalar joint consists of two distinct articulations separated by the interosseous talocalcaneal liga-ment: the posterior compartment (talocalcaneal joint) and the anterior compartment (talocalcaneonavicular joint).

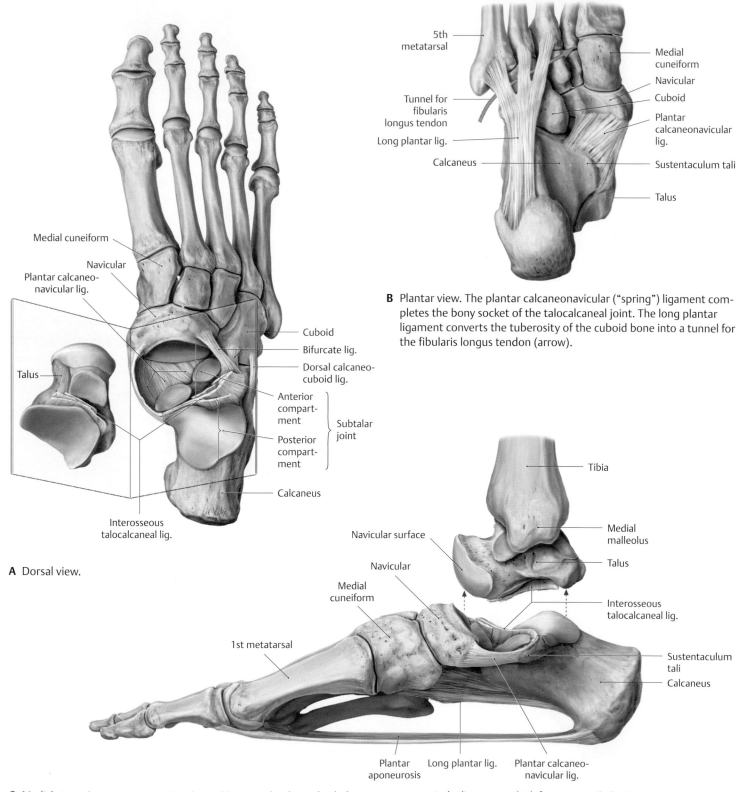

A Dorsal view.

B Plantar view. The plantar calcaneonavicular ("spring") ligament com-pletes the bony socket of the talocalcaneal joint. The long plantar ligament converts the tuberosity of the cuboid bone into a tunnel for the fibularis longus tendon (arrow).

C Medial view. The interosseous talocalcaneal ligament has been divided and the talus displaced upward. Note the course of the plantar calca-neonavicular ligament, which functions with the long plantar ligament and plantar aponeurosis to support the longitudinal arch of the foot.

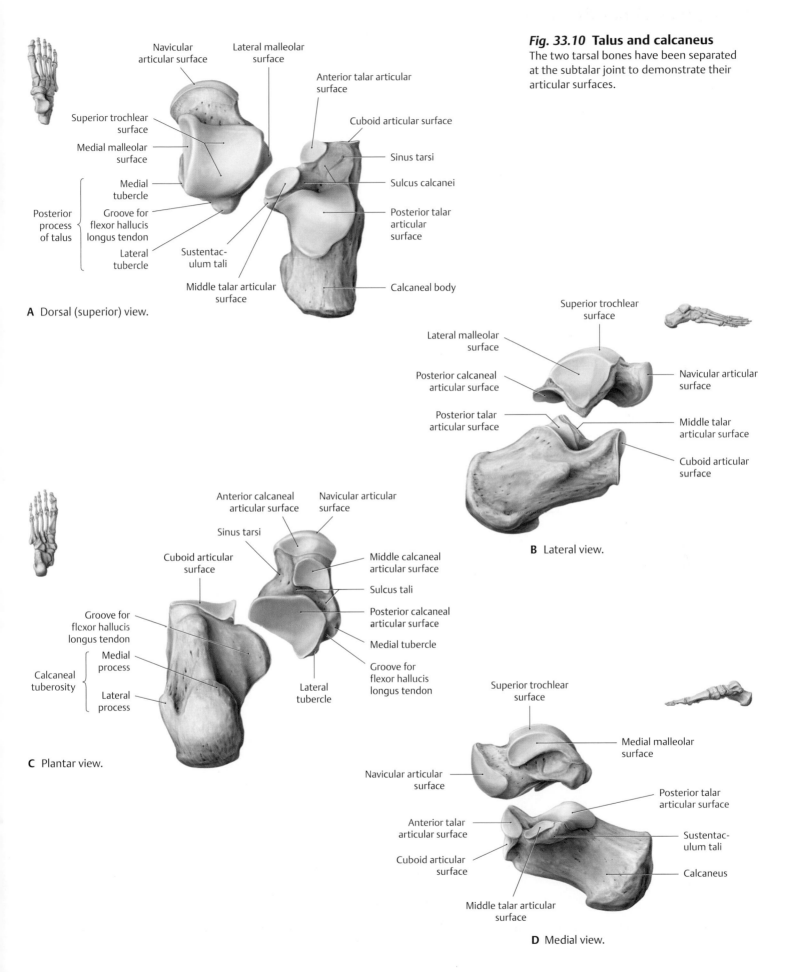

Fig. 33.10 Talus and calcaneus
The two tarsal bones have been separated at the subtalar joint to demonstrate their articular surfaces.

A Dorsal (superior) view.

Navicular articular surface

Lateral malleolar surface

Superior trochlear surface

Medial malleolar surface

Medial tubercle

Posterior process of talus

Groove for flexor hallucis longus tendon

Lateral tubercle

Sustentaculum tali

Middle talar articular surface

Anterior talar articular surface

Cuboid articular surface

Sinus tarsi

Sulcus calcanei

Posterior talar articular surface

Calcaneal body

B Lateral view.

Superior trochlear surface

Lateral malleolar surface

Posterior calcaneal articular surface

Posterior talar articular surface

Navicular articular surface

Middle talar articular surface

Cuboid articular surface

C Plantar view.

Anterior calcaneal articular surface

Navicular articular surface

Sinus tarsi

Cuboid articular surface

Groove for flexor hallucis longus tendon

Medial process

Calcaneal tuberosity

Lateral process

Middle calcaneal articular surface

Sulcus tali

Posterior calcaneal articular surface

Medial tubercle

Groove for flexor hallucis longus tendon

Lateral tubercle

D Medial view.

Superior trochlear surface

Medial malleolar surface

Navicular articular surface

Anterior talar articular surface

Cuboid articular surface

Middle talar articular surface

Posterior talar articular surface

Sustentaculum tali

Calcaneus

Ligaments of the Ankle & Foot

The ligaments of the foot are classified as belonging to the talocrural joint, subtalar joint, metatarsus, forefoot, or sole of the foot. The medial and lateral collateral ligaments, along with the syndesmotic ligaments, are of major importance in the stabilization of the subtalar joint.

Fig. 33.11 Ligaments of the ankle and foot

Right foot. See p. 458 for inferior view.

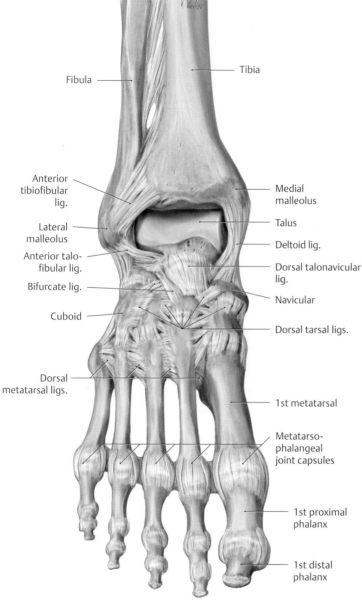

A Anterior view with talocrural joint in plantar flexion.

Table 33.1	Ligaments of the talocrural joint		
Lateral ligs.*	Anterior talofibular lig.		
	Posterior talofibular lig.		
	Calcaneofibular lig.		
Medial ligs.*	Deltoid lig.	Anterior tibiotalar part	
		Posterior tibiotalar part	
		Tibionavicular part	
		Tibiocalcaneal part	
Syndesmotic ligs. of the ankle mortise	Anterior tibiofibular lig.		
	Posterior tibiofibular lig.		

*The medial and lateral ligs. are also known as the medial and lateral collateral ligs.

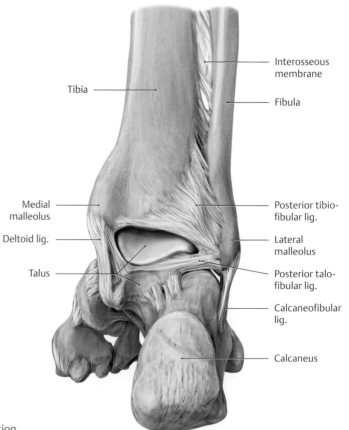

B Posterior view in plantigrade foot position.

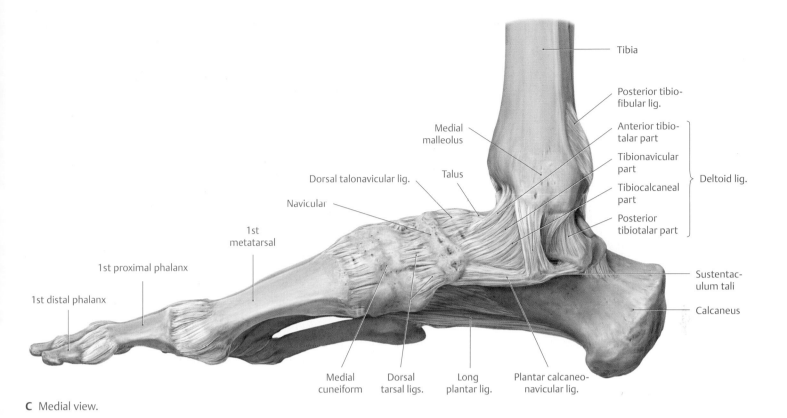

Tibia

Posterior tibio-
fibular lig.

Medial
malleolus

Anterior tibio-
talar part

Dorsal talonavicular lig.

Talus

Tibionavicular
part

Navicular

Tibiocalcaneal
part

Deltoid lig.

1st
metatarsal

Posterior
tibiotalar part

1st proximal phalanx

Sustentac-
ulum tali

1st distal phalanx

Calcaneus

Medial
cuneiform

Dorsal
tarsal ligs.

Long
plantar lig.

Plantar calcaneo-
navicular lig.

C Medial view.

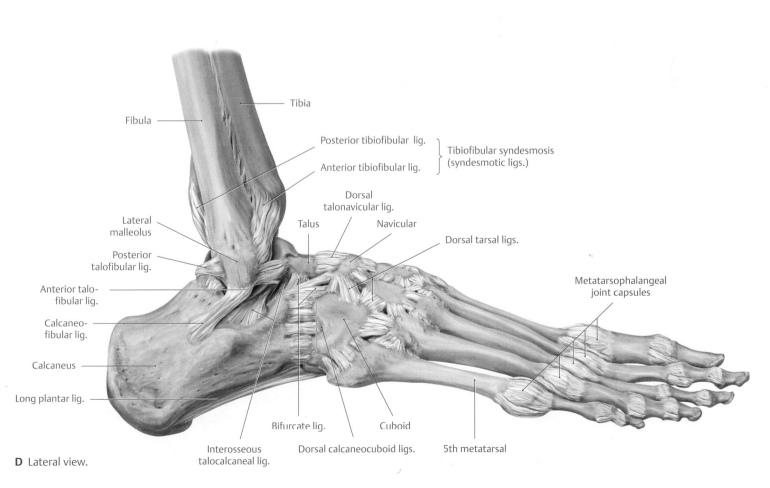

Tibia

Fibula

Posterior tibiofibular lig.

Tibiofibular syndesmosis
(syndesmotic ligs.)

Anterior tibiofibular lig.

Dorsal
talonavicular lig.

Lateral
malleolus

Talus

Navicular

Dorsal tarsal ligs.

Posterior
talofibular lig.

Metatarsophalangeal
joint capsules

Anterior talo-
fibular lig.

Calcaneo-
fibular lig.

Calcaneus

Long plantar lig.

Bifurcate lig.

Cuboid

Interosseous
talocalcaneal lig.

Dorsal calcaneocuboid ligs.

5th metatarsal

D Lateral view.

Plantar Vault & Arches of the Foot

Fig. 33.12 **The plantar vault**

Right foot. The forces of the foot are distributed among two lateral (fibular) and three medial (tibial) rays. The arrangement of these rays creates a longitudinal and a transverse arch in the sole of the foot, helping the foot adapt to uneven terrain and absorb vertical loads.

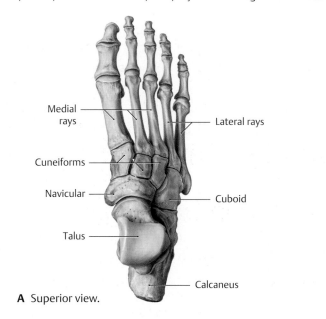

A Superior view.

Medial rays · Lateral rays · Cuneiforms · Navicular · Cuboid · Talus · Calcaneus

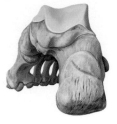
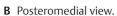

B Posteromedial view.

C Superior view. The area outlined in red by interconnecting the bony points of support for the plantar vault forms a triangle. By contrast, the area of ground contact defined by the plantar soft tissues (the footprint or podogram) is considerably larger.

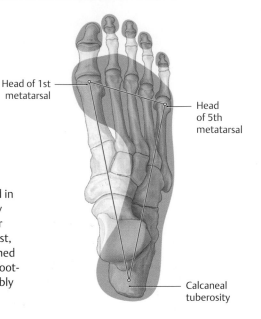

Head of 1st metatarsal · Head of 5th metatarsal · Calcaneal tuberosity

Fig. 33.13 **Stabilizers of the transverse arch**

Right foot. The transverse pedal arch is supported by both active and passive stabilizing structures (muscles and ligaments, respectively).

Note: The arch of the forefoot has only passive stabilizers, whereas the arches of the metatarsus and tarsus have only active stabilizers.

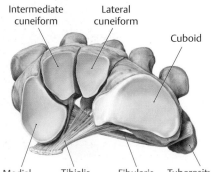

A Plantar view.

Deep transverse metatarsal lig. · Plantar ligs. · Cuboid · Fibularis longus · Calcaneus · Proximal phalanx of great toe · Metatarso-phalangeal joint of great toe · Adductor hallucis, transverse head · 1st metatarsal · Adductor hallucis, oblique head · Medial cuneiform · Tibialis posterior · Medial malleolus · Sustentaculum tali · Talus

B Anterior arch (forefoot), proximal view.

Plantar ligs. · Base of 1st proximal phalanx · Deep transverse metatarsal lig.

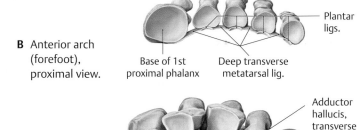

C Metatarsal arch, proximal view.

Adductor hallucis, transverse head · Base of 5th metatarsal · Base of 1st metatarsal · Adductor hallucis, oblique head

D Tarsal region, proximal view.

Intermediate cuneiform · Lateral cuneiform · Cuboid · Medial cuneiform · Tibialis posterior · Fibularis longus · Tuberosity of 5th metatarsal

Fig. 33.14 Stabilizers of the longitudinal arch
Right foot, medial view.

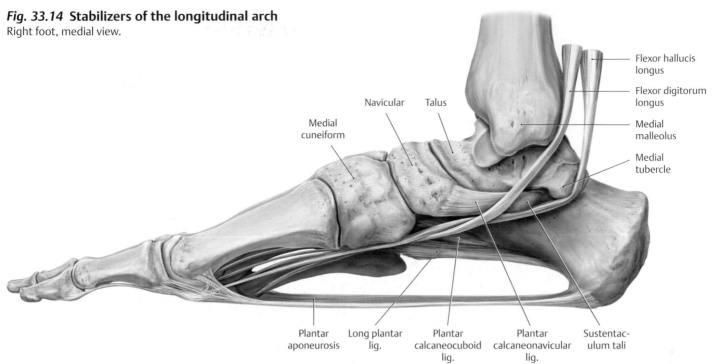

Medial cuneiform · Navicular · Talus · Flexor hallucis longus · Flexor digitorum longus · Medial malleolus · Medial tubercle

Plantar aponeurosis · Long plantar lig. · Plantar calcaneocuboid lig. · Plantar calcaneonavicular lig. · Sustentaculum tali

A Passive stabilizers of the longitudinal arch. The main passive stabilizers of the longitudinal arch are the plantar aponeurosis (strongest component), the long plantar ligament, and the plantar calcaneonavicular ligament (weakest component).

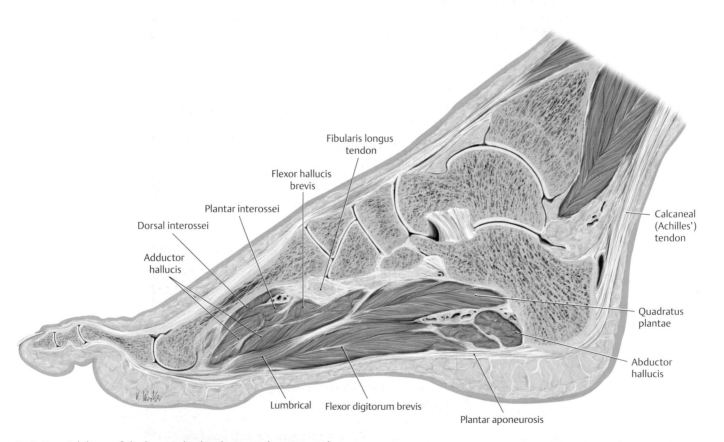

Fibularis longus tendon · Flexor hallucis brevis · Plantar interossei · Dorsal interossei · Adductor hallucis · Calcaneal (Achilles') tendon · Quadratus plantae · Abductor hallucis

Lumbrical · Flexor digitorum brevis · Plantar aponeurosis

B Active stabilizers of the longitudinal arch. Sagittal section at the level of the second ray. The major active stabilizers of the foot are the abductor hallucis, flexor hallucis brevis, flexor digitorum brevis, quadratus plantae, and abductor digiti minimi.

Muscles of the Sole of the Foot

Fig. 33.15 Plantar aponeurosis

Right foot, plantar view. The plantar aponeurosis is a tough aponeurotic sheet, thickest at the center, that blends with the dorsal fascia (not shown) at the borders of the foot.

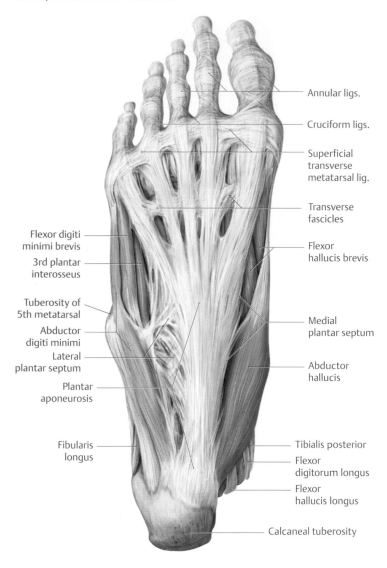

Annular ligs.

Cruciform ligs.

Superficial transverse metatarsal lig.

Transverse fascicles

Flexor hallucis brevis

Medial plantar septum

Abductor hallucis

Tibialis posterior

Flexor digitorum longus

Flexor hallucis longus

Calcaneal tuberosity

Flexor digiti minimi brevis

3rd plantar interosseus

Tuberosity of 5th metatarsal

Abductor digiti minimi

Lateral plantar septum

Plantar aponeurosis

Fibularis longus

Fig. 33.16 Intrinsic muscles of the sole of the foot

Right foot, plantar view.

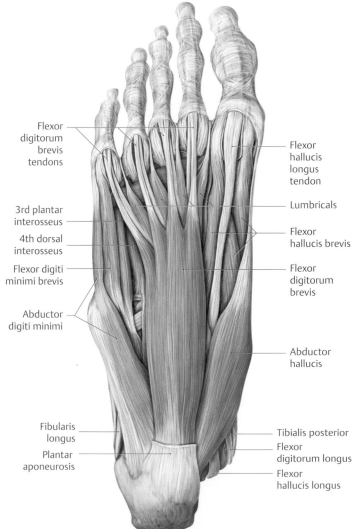

Flexor digitorum brevis tendons

3rd plantar interosseus

4th dorsal interosseus

Flexor digiti minimi brevis

Abductor digiti minimi

Fibularis longus

Plantar aponeurosis

Flexor hallucis longus tendon

Lumbricals

Flexor hallucis brevis

Flexor digitorum brevis

Abductor hallucis

Tibialis posterior

Flexor digitorum longus

Flexor hallucis longus

A Superficial (first) layer. *Removed:* Plantar aponeurosis, including the superficial transverse metacarpal ligament.

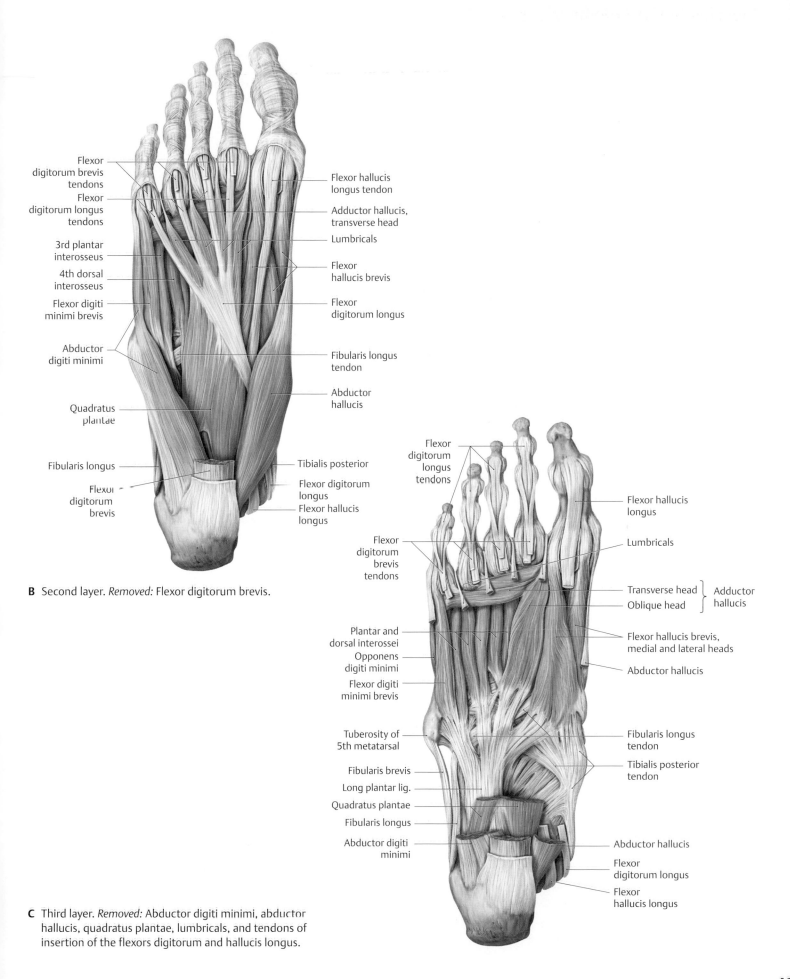

Flexor
digitorum brevis
tendons

Flexor
digitorum longus
tendons

3rd plantar
interosseus

4th dorsal
interosseus

Flexor digiti
minimi brevis

Abductor
digiti minimi

Quadratus
plantae

Fibularis longus

Flexor
digitorum
brevis

Flexor hallucis
longus tendon

Adductor hallucis,
transverse head

Lumbricals

Flexor
hallucis brevis

Flexor
digitorum longus

Fibularis longus
tendon

Abductor
hallucis

Tibialis posterior

Flexor digitorum
longus

Flexor hallucis
longus

B Second layer. *Removed:* Flexor digitorum brevis.

Flexor
digitorum
longus
tendons

Flexor
digitorum
brevis
tendons

Plantar and
dorsal interossei

Opponens
digiti minimi

Flexor digiti
minimi brevis

Tuberosity of
5th metatarsal

Fibularis brevis

Long plantar lig.

Quadratus plantae

Fibularis longus

Abductor digiti
minimi

Flexor hallucis
longus

Lumbricals

Transverse head } Adductor
Oblique head   } hallucis

Flexor hallucis brevis,
medial and lateral heads

Abductor hallucis

Fibularis longus
tendon

Tibialis posterior
tendon

Abductor hallucis

Flexor
digitorum longus

Flexor
hallucis longus

C Third layer. *Removed:* Abductor digiti minimi, abductor
hallucis, quadratus plantae, lumbricals, and tendons of
insertion of the flexors digitorum and hallucis longus.

Muscles & Tendon Sheaths of the Foot

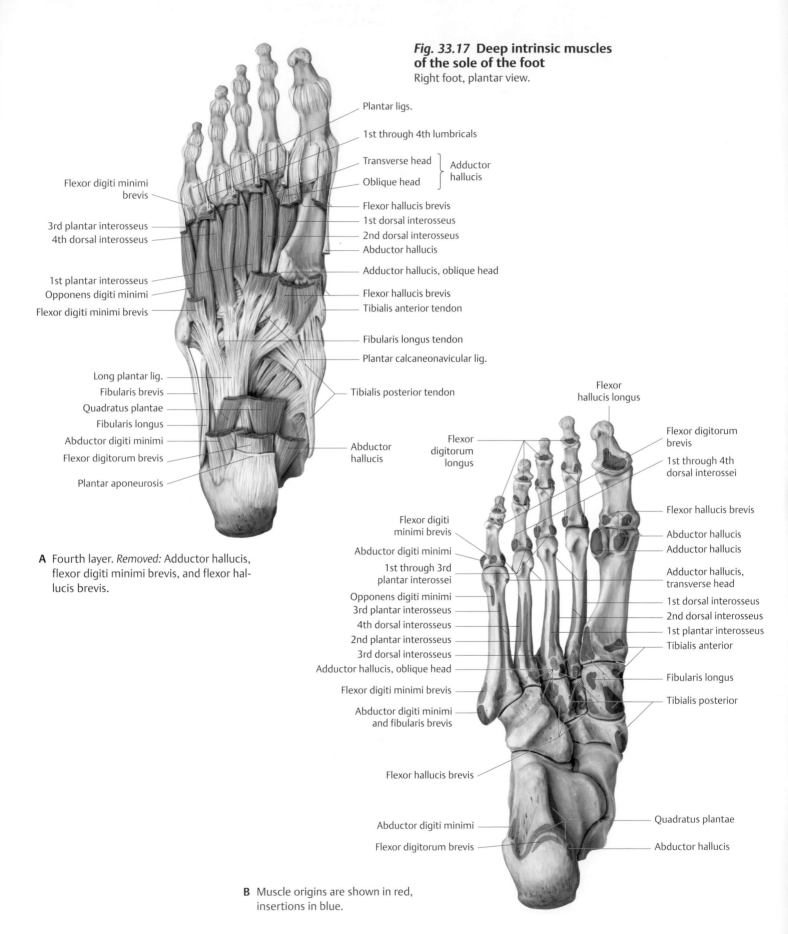

Fig. 33.17 Deep intrinsic muscles of the sole of the foot
Right foot, plantar view.

Plantar ligs.

1st through 4th lumbricals

Transverse head ⎤ Adductor
Oblique head ⎦ hallucis

Flexor digiti minimi brevis

Flexor hallucis brevis
1st dorsal interosseus
2nd dorsal interosseus
Abductor hallucis

3rd plantar interosseus
4th dorsal interosseus

Adductor hallucis, oblique head

1st plantar interosseus
Opponens digiti minimi

Flexor hallucis brevis
Tibialis anterior tendon

Flexor digiti minimi brevis

Fibularis longus tendon

Plantar calcaneonavicular lig.

Long plantar lig.
Fibularis brevis
Quadratus plantae
Fibularis longus
Abductor digiti minimi
Flexor digitorum brevis

Tibialis posterior tendon

Abductor hallucis

Plantar aponeurosis

A Fourth layer. *Removed:* Adductor hallucis, flexor digiti minimi brevis, and flexor hallucis brevis.

Flexor hallucis longus

Flexor digitorum longus

Flexor digitorum brevis
1st through 4th dorsal interossei

Flexor digiti minimi brevis

Flexor hallucis brevis
Abductor hallucis
Adductor hallucis

Abductor digiti minimi

1st through 3rd plantar interossei

Adductor hallucis, transverse head

Opponens digiti minimi
3rd plantar interosseus
4th dorsal interosseus
2nd plantar interosseus
3rd dorsal interosseus

1st dorsal interosseus
2nd dorsal interosseus
1st plantar interosseus
Tibialis anterior

Adductor hallucis, oblique head

Flexor digiti minimi brevis

Fibularis longus

Abductor digiti minimi and fibularis brevis

Tibialis posterior

Flexor hallucis brevis

Abductor digiti minimi

Quadratus plantae

Flexor digitorum brevis

Abductor hallucis

B Muscle origins are shown in red, insertions in blue.

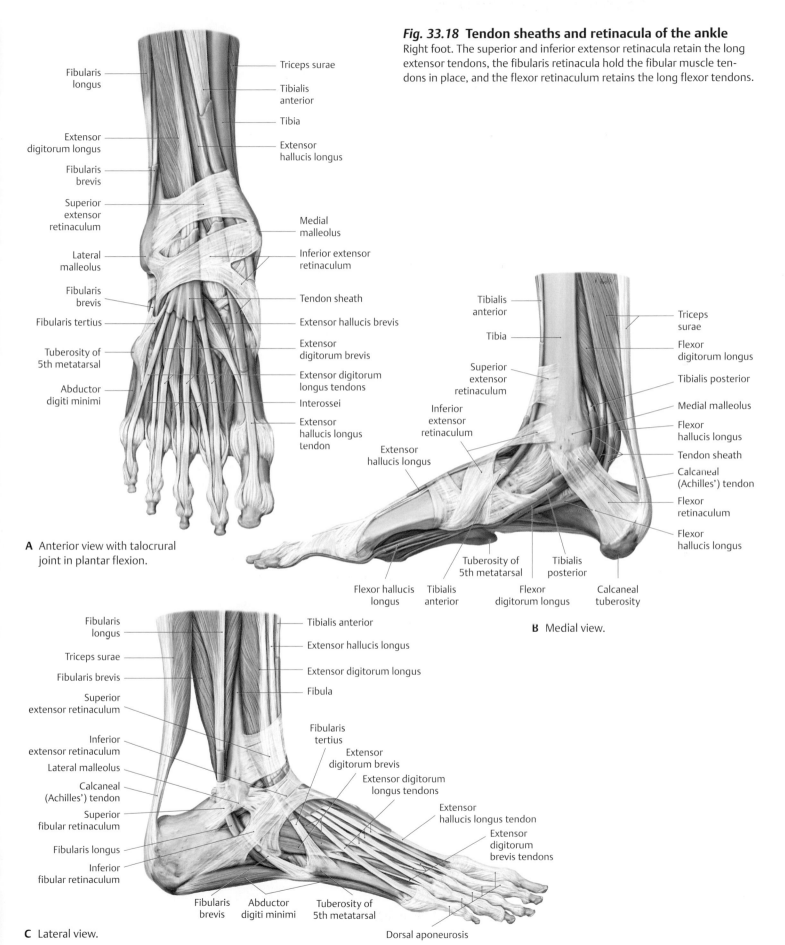

Fig. 33.18 Tendon sheaths and retinacula of the ankle
Right foot. The superior and inferior extensor retinacula retain the long extensor tendons, the fibularis retinacula hold the fibular muscle tendons in place, and the flexor retinaculum retains the long flexor tendons.

A Anterior view with talocrural joint in plantar flexion.

Fibularis longus
Triceps surae
Tibialis anterior
Tibia
Extensor digitorum longus
Extensor hallucis longus
Fibularis brevis
Superior extensor retinaculum
Medial malleolus
Lateral malleolus
Inferior extensor retinaculum
Fibularis brevis
Tendon sheath
Fibularis tertius
Extensor hallucis brevis
Tuberosity of 5th metatarsal
Extensor digitorum brevis
Abductor digiti minimi
Extensor digitorum longus tendons
Interossei
Extensor hallucis longus tendon

B Medial view.

Tibialis anterior
Tibia
Triceps surae
Flexor digitorum longus
Superior extensor retinaculum
Tibialis posterior
Inferior extensor retinaculum
Medial malleolus
Extensor hallucis longus
Flexor hallucis longus
Tendon sheath
Calcaneal (Achilles') tendon
Flexor retinaculum
Flexor hallucis longus
Flexor hallucis longus
Tibialis anterior
Tuberosity of 5th metatarsal
Tibialis posterior
Flexor digitorum longus
Calcaneal tuberosity

C Lateral view.

Fibularis longus
Tibialis anterior
Extensor hallucis longus
Triceps surae
Extensor digitorum longus
Fibularis brevis
Fibula
Superior extensor retinaculum
Inferior extensor retinaculum
Fibularis tertius
Lateral malleolus
Extensor digitorum brevis
Calcaneal (Achilles') tendon
Extensor digitorum longus tendons
Superior fibular retinaculum
Extensor hallucis longus tendon
Fibularis longus
Extensor digitorum brevis tendons
Inferior fibular retinaculum
Fibularis brevis
Abductor digiti minimi
Tuberosity of 5th metatarsal
Dorsal aponeurosis

Muscle Facts (I)

The dorsal surface (dorsum) of the foot contains only two muscles, the extensor digitorum brevis and the extensor hallucis brevis. The sole of the foot, however, is composed of four complex layers that maintain the arches of the foot.

Fig. 33.19 Intrinsic muscles of the dorsum of the foot
Right foot, dorsal view.

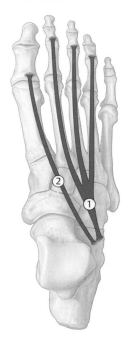

A Schematic.

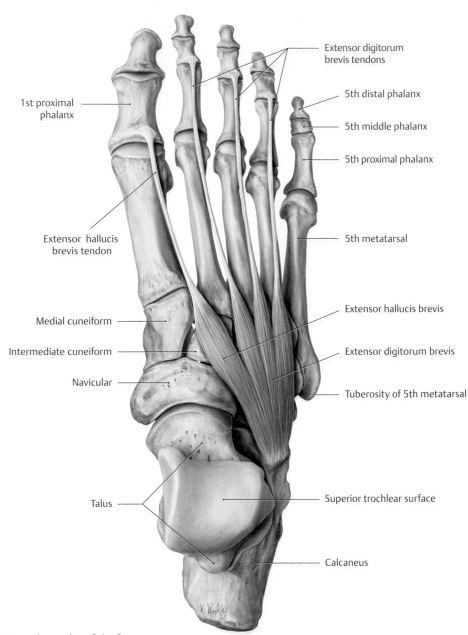

B Dorsal muscles of the foot.

Table 33.2	Intrinsic muscles of the dorsum of the foot			
Muscle	**Origin**	**Insertion**	**Innervation**	**Action**
① Extensor digitorum brevis	Calcaneus (dorsal surface)	2nd to 4th toes (at dorsal aponeuroses and bases of the middle phalanges)	Deep fibular n. (L5, S1)	Extension of the MTP and PIP joints of the 2nd to 4th toes
② Extensor hallucis brevis		1st toe (at dorsal aponeurosis and proximal phalanx)		Extension of the MTP joints of the 1st toe

MTP, metatarsophalangeal; PIP, proximal interphalangeal.

Fig. 33.20 Superficial intrinsic muscles of the sole of the foot

Right foot, plantar view.

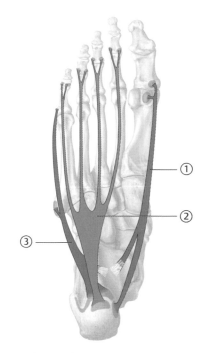

A First layer, schematic.

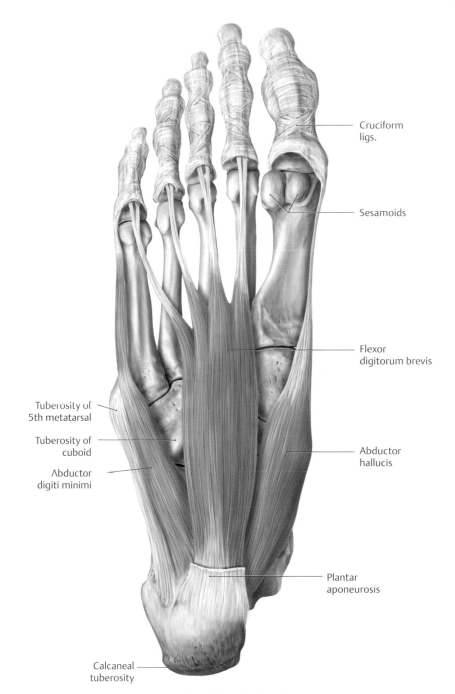

Cruciform ligs.

Sesamoids

Flexor digitorum brevis

Tuberosity of 5th metatarsal

Tuberosity of cuboid

Abductor hallucis

Abductor digiti minimi

Plantar aponeurosis

Calcaneal tuberosity

B Intrinsic muscles of the sole, first layer.

Table 33.3	Superficial intrinsic muscles of the sole of the foot			
Muscle	**Origin**	**Insertion**	**Innervation**	**Action**
① Abductor hallucis	Calcaneal tuberosity (medial process); flexor retinaculum, plantar aponeurosis	1st toe (base of proximal phalanx via the medial sesamoid)	Medial plantar n. (S1, S2)	• 1st MTP joint: flexion and abduction of the 1st toe • Supports the longitudinal arch
② Flexor digitorum brevis	Calcaneal tuberosity (medial tubercle), plantar aponeurosis	2nd to 5th toes (sides of middle phalanges)		• Flexes the MTP and PIP joints of the 2nd to 5th toes • Supports the longitudinal arch
③ Abductor digiti minimi		5th toe (base of proximal phalanx), 5th metatarsal (at tuberosity)	Lateral plantar n. (S1–S3)	• Flexes the MTP joint of the 5th toe • Abducts the 5th toe • Supports the longitudinal arch

MTP, metatarsophalangeal; PIP, proximal interphalangeal.

34 Neurovasculature
Arteries of the Lower Limb

Fig. 34.1 **Arteries of the lower limb and the sole of the foot**

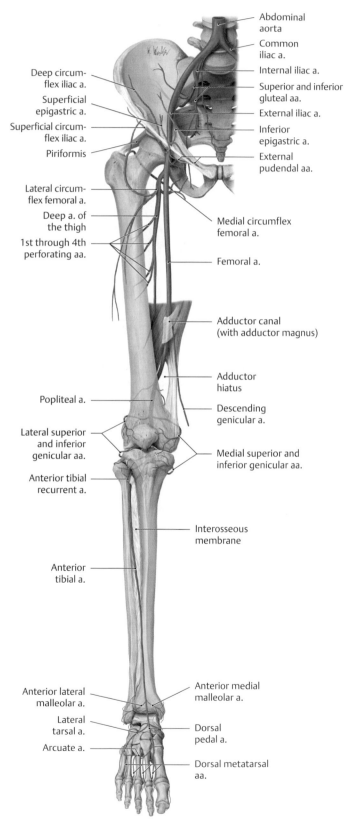

- Abdominal aorta
- Common iliac a.
- Deep circumflex iliac a.
- Internal iliac a.
- Superior and inferior gluteal aa.
- Superficial epigastric a.
- External iliac a.
- Superficial circumflex iliac a.
- Inferior epigastric a.
- Piriformis
- External pudendal aa.
- Lateral circumflex femoral a.
- Medial circumflex femoral a.
- Deep a. of the thigh
- 1st through 4th perforating aa.
- Femoral a.
- Adductor canal (with adductor magnus)
- Adductor hiatus
- Popliteal a.
- Descending genicular a.
- Lateral superior and inferior genicular aa.
- Medial superior and inferior genicular aa.
- Anterior tibial recurrent a.
- Interosseous membrane
- Anterior tibial a.
- Anterior lateral malleolar a.
- Anterior medial malleolar a.
- Lateral tarsal a.
- Dorsal pedal a.
- Arcuate a.
- Dorsal metatarsal aa.

A Right leg, anterior view.

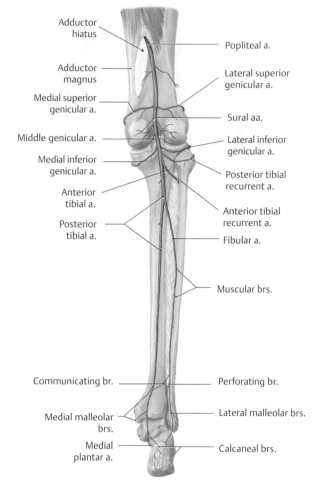

- Adductor hiatus
- Popliteal a.
- Adductor magnus
- Lateral superior genicular a.
- Medial superior genicular a.
- Sural aa.
- Middle genicular a.
- Lateral inferior genicular a.
- Medial inferior genicular a.
- Posterior tibial recurrent a.
- Anterior tibial a.
- Anterior tibial recurrent a.
- Posterior tibial a.
- Fibular a.
- Muscular brs.
- Communicating br.
- Perforating br.
- Medial malleolar brs.
- Lateral malleolar brs.
- Medial plantar a.
- Calcaneal brs.

B Right leg, posterior view.

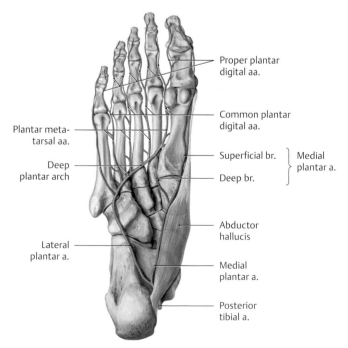

- Proper plantar digital aa.
- Common plantar digital aa.
- Plantar metatarsal aa.
- Superficial br. } Medial plantar a.
- Deep plantar arch
- Deep br.
- Abductor hallucis
- Lateral plantar a.
- Medial plantar a.
- Posterior tibial a.

C Sole of right foot, plantar view.

Fig. 34.2 Segments of the femoral artery

The blood supply to the lower limbs originates from the femoral artery. Color is used to identify the named distal segments of this vessel.

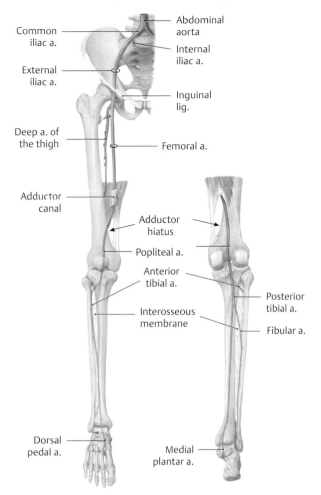

Fig. 34.3 Deep artery of the thigh

Right leg. The artery passes posteriorly through the adductor muscles of the medial thigh to supply the muscles of the posterior compartment via three to five perforating branches. Ligation of the femoral artery proximal to the origin of the deep artery of the thigh (*left*) is well tolerated owing to the collateral blood supply (*arrows*) from branches of the internal iliac artery that anastomose with the perforating branches.

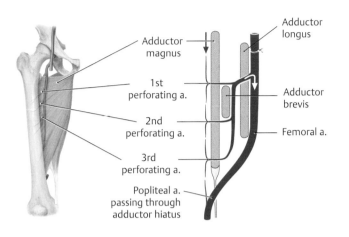

> ### Clinical box 34.1
>
> **Femoral head necrosis**
> Dislocation or fracture of the femoral head (e.g., in patients with osteoporosis) may tear the femoral neck vessels, resulting in femoral head necrosis.

Fig. 34.4 Arteries of the femoral head

Anterior view.

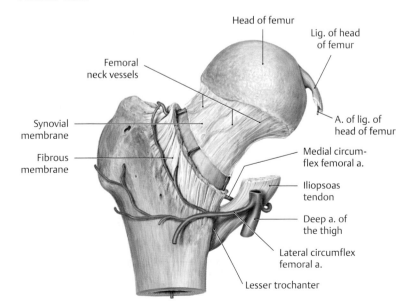

A Right femur.

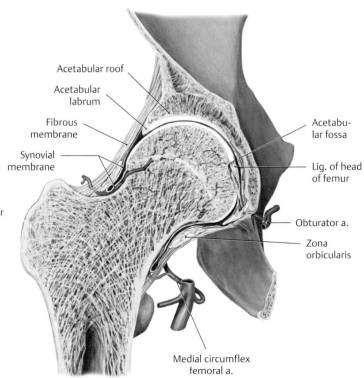

B Right femur, coronal section.

Lumbosacral Plexus

The lumbosacral plexus supplies sensory and motor innervation to the lower limb. It is formed by the anterior (ventral) rami of the lumbar and sacral spinal nerves, with contributions from the subcostal nerve (T12) and coccygeal nerve (Co1). The lumbar plexus mainly supplies the anterior and medial parts of the thigh with a small contribution to the medial leg. The sacral plexus supplies the posterior thigh and most of the leg and foot.

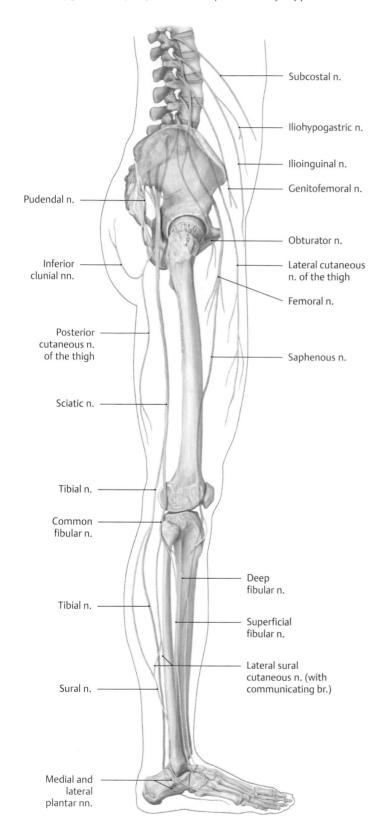

Subcostal n.

Iliohypogastric n.

Ilioinguinal n.

Genitofemoral n.

Pudendal n.

Obturator n.

Inferior clunial nn.

Lateral cutaneous n. of the thigh

Femoral n.

Posterior cutaneous n. of the thigh

Saphenous n.

Sciatic n.

Tibial n.

Common fibular n.

Deep fibular n.

Tibial n.

Superficial fibular n.

Lateral sural cutaneous n. (with communicating br.)

Sural n.

Medial and lateral plantar nn.

Table 34.1	Nerves of the lumbosacral plexus		
Lumbar plexus			
Iliohypogastric n.	L1		
Ilioinguinal n.	L1		
Genitofemoral n.	L1–L2		p. 479
Lateral cutaneous n. of the thigh	L2–L3		
Obturator n.	L2–L4		p. 480
Femoral n.			p. 481
Sacral plexus			
Superior gluteal n.	L4–S1		p. 483
Inferior gluteal n.	L5–S2		
Posterior cutaneous n. of the thigh	S1–S3		p. 482
Sciatic n.	Common fibular n.	L4–S2	p. 484
	Tibial n.	L4–S3	p. 485
Pudendal n.	S2–S4		pp. 284–285

✳ Clinical box 34.2

Injuries to nerves of the lumbar and sacral plexuses

Similar to nerve injuries of the upper limb, injuries involving nerves of the lumbosacral plexus are best understood though an appreciation of the plexus organization. The lumbar plexus arises from higher levels (L1–L4) of the spinal cord and supplies muscles of the abdominal wall and anterior and medial thigh. The sacral plexus arises from lower levels (L4–S4) of the spinal cord and supplies the perineum and, via the large sciatic nerve, the posterior thigh, entire leg and most of the foot. Nerves of the lumbar and sacral plexuses are less likely to be injured at the root level than those of the brachial plexus, although exceptions to this are the obturator and femoral nerves that may be compromised by herniation of intervertebral disks at L4 or L5 as they pass through the intervertebral foramina. Peripheral nerve injuries, such as that of the common fibular nerve, can occur in places where the nerve is superficial and passes close to a bony prominence.

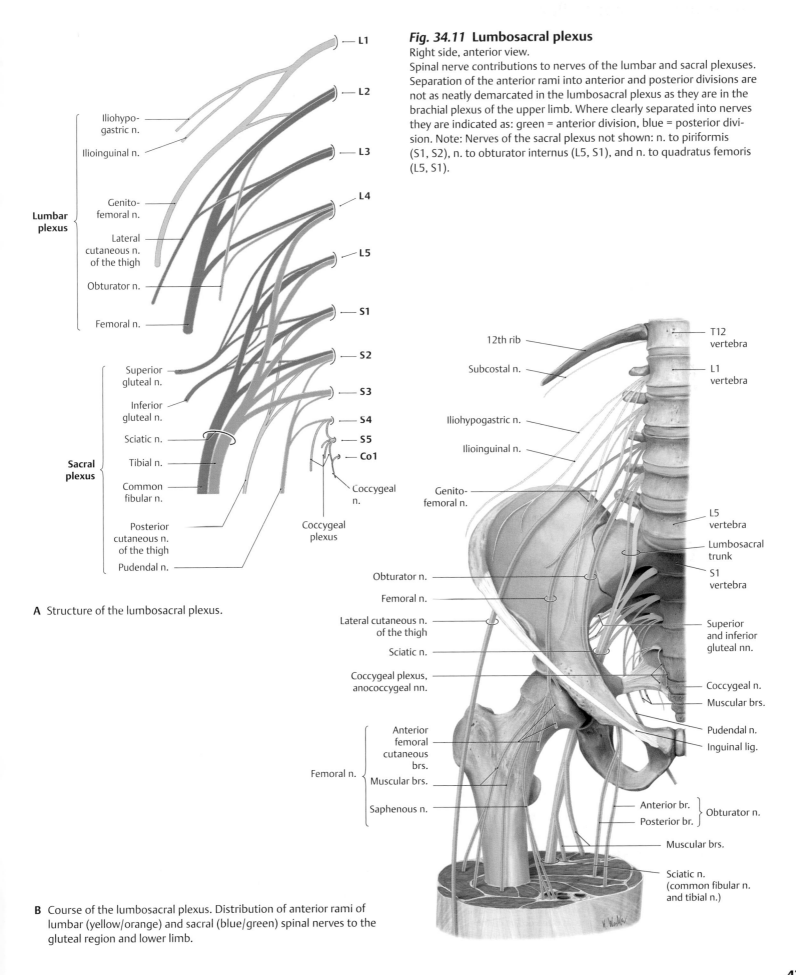

Fig. 34.11 Lumbosacral plexus

Right side, anterior view.
Spinal nerve contributions to nerves of the lumbar and sacral plexuses. Separation of the anterior rami into anterior and posterior divisions are not as neatly demarcated in the lumbosacral plexus as they are in the brachial plexus of the upper limb. Where clearly separated into nerves they are indicated as: green = anterior division, blue = posterior division. Note: Nerves of the sacral plexus not shown: n. to piriformis (S1, S2), n. to obturator internus (L5, S1), and n. to quadratus femoris (L5, S1).

Lumbar plexus

Iliohypo-gastric n.
Ilioinguinal n.
Genito-femoral n.
Lateral cutaneous n. of the thigh
Obturator n.
Femoral n.

L1
L2
L3
L4
L5
S1
S2
S3
S4
S5
Co1

Sacral plexus

Superior gluteal n.
Inferior gluteal n.
Sciatic n.
Tibial n.
Common fibular n.
Posterior cutaneous n. of the thigh
Pudendal n.

Coccygeal n.
Coccygeal plexus

A Structure of the lumbosacral plexus.

12th rib
Subcostal n.
Iliohypogastric n.
Ilioinguinal n.
Genito-femoral n.
Obturator n.
Femoral n.
Lateral cutaneous n. of the thigh
Sciatic n.
Coccygeal plexus, anococcygeal nn.

Anterior femoral cutaneous brs.
Femoral n. { Muscular brs.
Saphenous n.

T12 vertebra
L1 vertebra
L5 vertebra
Lumbosacral trunk
S1 vertebra
Superior and inferior gluteal nn.
Coccygeal n.
Muscular brs.
Pudendal n.
Inguinal lig.
Anterior br. } Obturator n.
Posterior br. }
Muscular brs.
Sciatic n. (common fibular n. and tibial n.)

B Course of the lumbosacral plexus. Distribution of anterior rami of lumbar (yellow/orange) and sacral (blue/green) spinal nerves to the gluteal region and lower limb.

Nerves of the Lumbar Plexus: Obturator & Femoral Nerves

Fig. 34.14 **Obturator nerve: Cutaneous distribution**
Right leg, medial view.

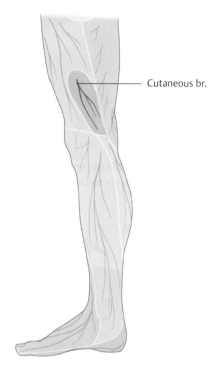

Cutaneous br.

Fig. 34.15 **Obturator nerve**
Right side, anterior view.

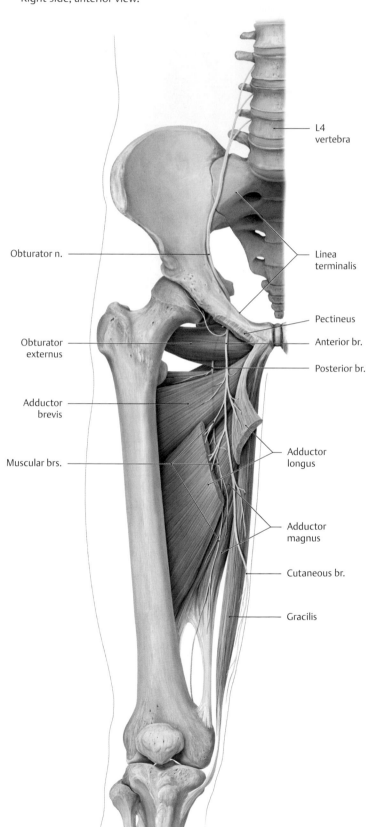

L4 vertebra

Obturator n.

Linea terminalis

Pectineus

Obturator externus

Anterior br.

Posterior br.

Adductor brevis

Muscular brs.

Adductor longus

Adductor magnus

Cutaneous br.

Gracilis

Table 34.3	**Obturator nerve (L2–L4)**
Motor branches	**Innervated muscles**
Direct br.	Obturator externus
Anterior br.	Adductor longus
	Adductor brevis
	Gracilis
	Pectineus
Posterior br.	Adductor magnus
Sensory branches	
Cutaneous br.	

Fig. 34.16 Femoral nerve
Right side, anterior view.

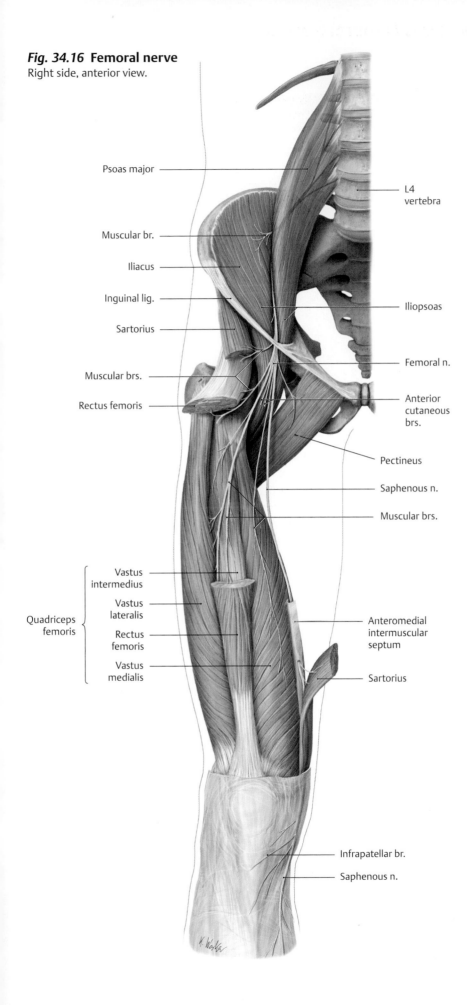

Psoas major

Muscular br.

Iliacus

Inguinal lig.

Sartorius

Muscular brs.

Rectus femoris

Quadriceps
femoris

Vastus
intermedius

Vastus
lateralis

Rectus
femoris

Vastus
medialis

L4
vertebra

Iliopsoas

Femoral n.

Anterior
cutaneous
brs.

Pectineus

Saphenous n.

Muscular brs.

Anteromedial
intermuscular
septum

Sartorius

Infrapatellar br.

Saphenous n.

Fig. 34.17 Femoral nerve: Cutaneous distribution
Right limb, anterior view.

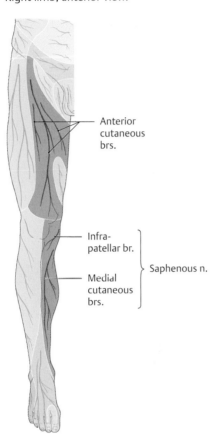

Anterior
cutaneous
brs.

Infra-
patellar br.

Medial
cutaneous
brs.

Saphenous n.

Table 34.4	Femoral nerve (L2–L4)
Motor branches	**Innervated muscles**
Muscular brs.	Iliopsoas
	Pectineus
	Sartorius
	Quadriceps femoris
Sensory branches	
Anterior cutaneous br.	
Saphenous n.	

Nerves of the Sacral Plexus

Table 34.5		Nerves of the sacral plexus		
Nerve		**Level**	**Innervated muscle**	**Cutaneous branches**	

Nerve		Level	Innervated muscle	Cutaneous branches	
Superior gluteal n.		L4–S1	Gluteus medius Gluteus minimus Tensor fasciae latae	—	
Inferior gluteal n.		L5–S2	Gluteus maximus	—	
Posterior cutaneous n. of the thigh		S1–S3	—	Posterior cutaneous n. of the thigh	Inferior clunial nn.
					Perineal brs.
Direct branches	N. of piriformis	S1–S2	Piriformis	—	
	N. of obturator internus	L5–S1	Obturator internus Gemelli	—	
	N. of quadratus femoris		Quadratus femoris	—	
Sciatic n.	Common fibular n.	L4–S2	See **p. 484**		
	Tibial n.	L4–S3	See **p. 485**		
Pudenal n.		S2–S4	See **pp. 284–285**		

Fig. 34.18 **Cutaneous innervation of the gluteal region**
Right limb, posterior view.

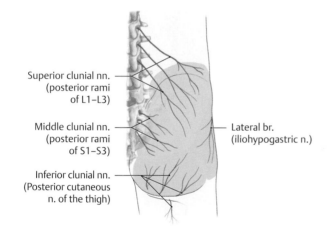

Superior clunial nn.
(posterior rami
of L1–L3)

Middle clunial nn.
(posterior rami
of S1–S3)

Lateral br.
(iliohypogastric n.)

Inferior clunial nn.
(Posterior cutaneous
n. of the thigh)

Fig. 34.19 **Posterior cutaneous nerve of the thigh: Cutaneous distribution**
Right limb, posterior view.

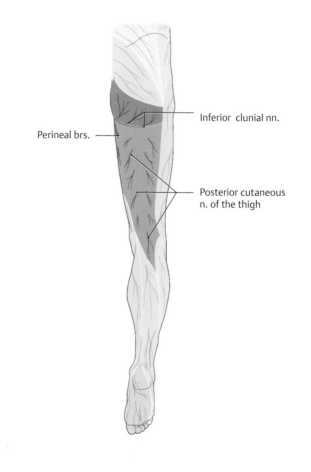

Inferior clunial nn.

Perineal brs.

Posterior cutaneous
n. of the thigh

Fig. 34.20 **Emerging spinal nerve**
Horizontal section, superior view.

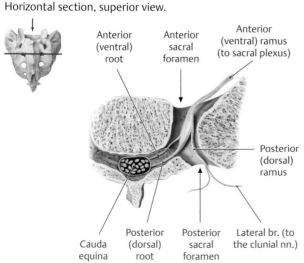

Anterior
(ventral)
root

Anterior
sacral
foramen

Anterior
(ventral) ramus
(to sacral plexus)

Posterior
(dorsal)
ramus

Cauda
equina

Posterior
(dorsal)
root

Posterior
sacral
foramen

Lateral br. (to
the clunial nn.)

Fig. 34.21 **Nerves of the sacral plexus**
Right limb.

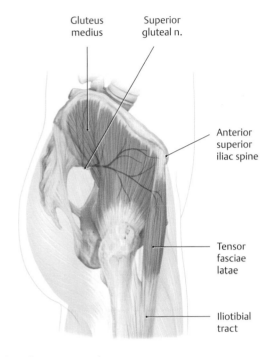

A Superior gluteal nerve. Lateral view.

Gluteus medius

Superior gluteal n.

Anterior superior iliac spine

Tensor fasciae latae

Iliotibial tract

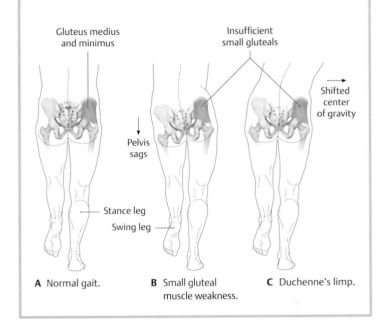
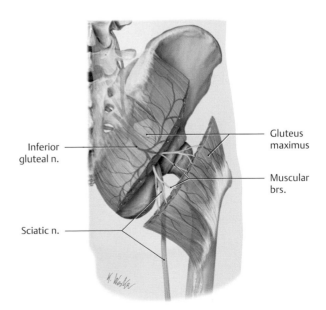

Inferior gluteal n.

Gluteus maximus

Muscular brs.

Sciatic n.

B Inferior gluteal nerve. Posterior view.

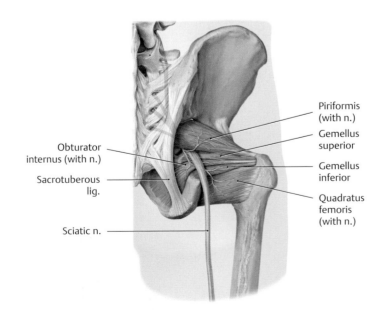

Obturator internus (with n.)

Sacrotuberous lig.

Sciatic n.

Piriformis (with n.)

Gemellus superior

Gemellus inferior

Quadratus femoris (with n.)

C Direct branches. Posterior view.

Nerves of the Sacral Plexus: Sciatic Nerve

The sciatic nerve gives off several direct muscular branches before dividing into the tibial and common fibular nerves proximal to the popliteal fossa.

Fig. 34.22 **Common fibular nerve: Cutaneous distribution**

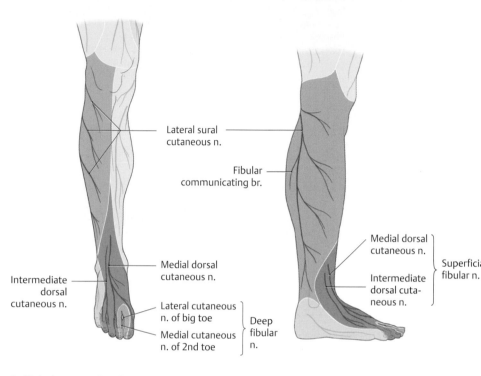

A Right leg, anterior view.   **B** Right leg, lateral view.

Fig. 34.23 **Common fibular nerve**
Right limb, lateral view.

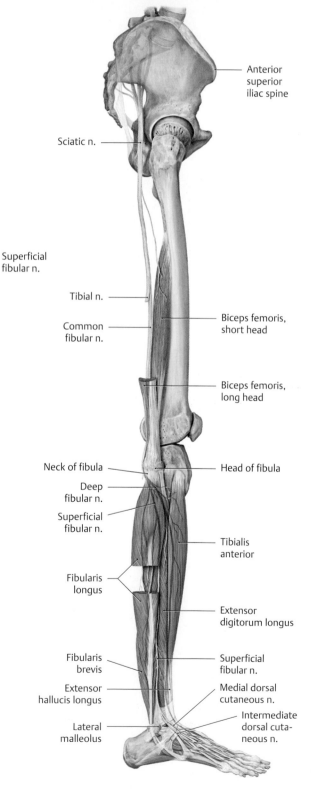

Table 34.6	Common fibular nerve (L4–S2)	
Nerve	**Innervated muscles**	**Sensory branches**
Direct branches from sciatic n.	Bicep femoris (short head)	—
Superficial fibular n.	Fibularis brevis and longus	Medial dorsal cutaneous n. Intermediate dorsal cutaneous n.
Deep fibular n.	Tibialis anterior Extensors digitorum brevis and longus Extensors hallucis brevis and longus Fibularis tertius	Lateral cutaneous n. of big toe Medial cutaneous n. of 2nd toe

Fig. 34.24 Tibial nerve
Right limb.

Fig. 34.25 Tibial nerve: Cutaneous distribution
Right lower limb, posterior view.

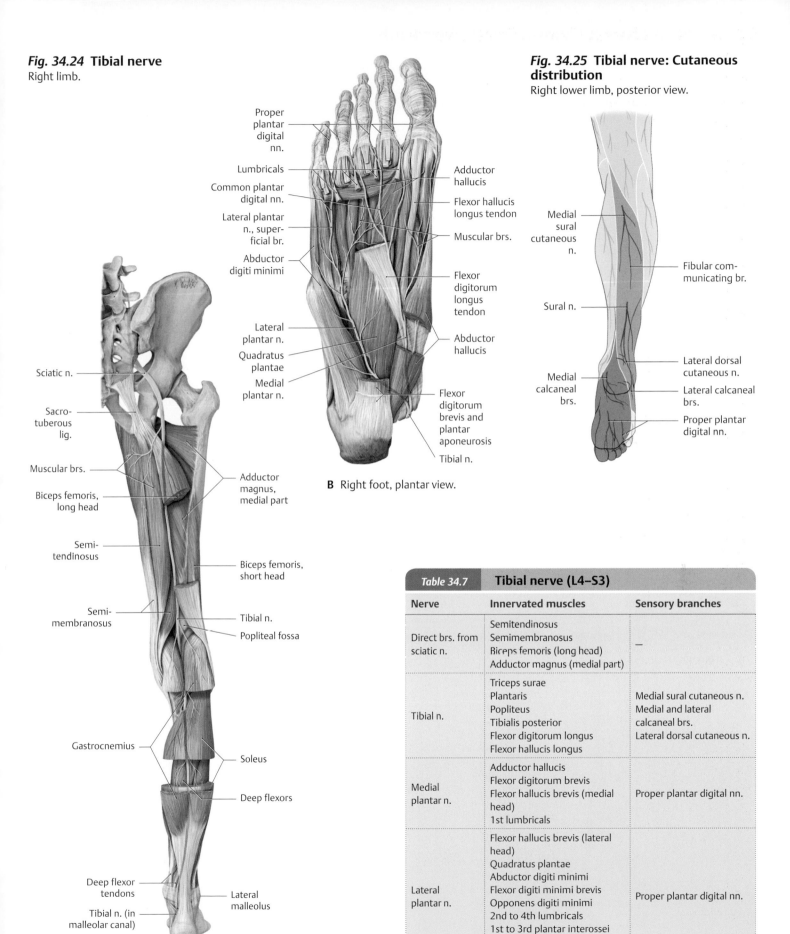

Proper plantar digital nn.

Lumbricals

Common plantar digital nn.

Lateral plantar n., superficial br.

Abductor digiti minimi

Lateral plantar n.

Quadratus plantae

Medial plantar n.

Adductor hallucis

Flexor hallucis longus tendon

Muscular brs.

Flexor digitorum longus tendon

Abductor hallucis

Flexor digitorum brevis and plantar aponeurosis

Tibial n.

B Right foot, plantar view.

Medial sural cutaneous n.

Sural n.

Medial calcaneal brs.

Fibular communicating br.

Lateral dorsal cutaneous n.

Lateral calcaneal brs.

Proper plantar digital nn.

Sciatic n.

Sacro-tuberous lig.

Muscular brs.

Biceps femoris, long head

Semi-tendinosus

Semi-membranosus

Gastrocnemius

Deep flexor tendons

Tibial n. (in malleolar canal)

Adductor magnus, medial part

Biceps femoris, short head

Tibial n.

Popliteal fossa

Soleus

Deep flexors

Lateral malleolus

A Posterior view.

Table 34.7	Tibial nerve (L4–S3)		
Nerve	**Innervated muscles**	**Sensory branches**
Direct brs. from sciatic n.	Semitendinosus Semimembranosus Biceps femoris (long head) Adductor magnus (medial part)	—
Tibial n.	Triceps surae Plantaris Popliteus Tibialis posterior Flexor digitorum longus Flexor hallucis longus	Medial sural cutaneous n. Medial and lateral calcaneal brs. Lateral dorsal cutaneous n.
Medial plantar n.	Adductor hallucis Flexor digitorum brevis Flexor hallucis brevis (medial head) 1st lumbricals	Proper plantar digital nn.
Lateral plantar n.	Flexor hallucis brevis (lateral head) Quadratus plantae Abductor digiti minimi Flexor digiti minimi brevis Opponens digiti minimi 2nd to 4th lumbricals 1st to 3rd plantar interossei 1st to 4th dorsal interossei Adductor hallucis	Proper plantar digital nn.

Superficial Nerves & Veins of the Lower Limb

Fig. 34.26 Superficial cutaneous veins and nerves of right lower limb

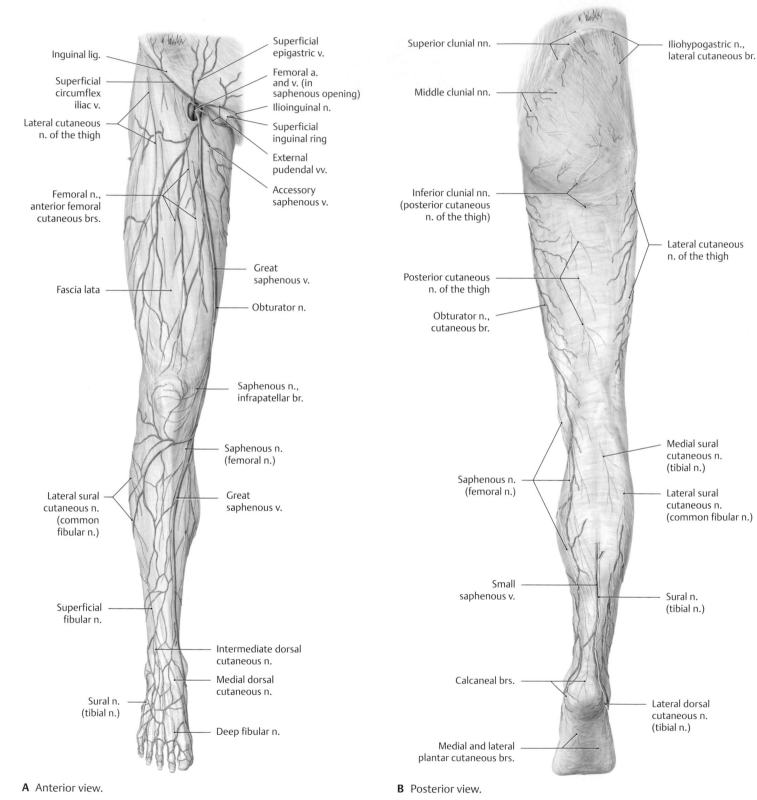

Inguinal lig.

Superficial circumflex iliac v.

Lateral cutaneous n. of the thigh

Femoral n., anterior femoral cutaneous brs.

Fascia lata

Lateral sural cutaneous n. (common fibular n.)

Superficial fibular n.

Sural n. (tibial n.)

Superficial epigastric v.

Femoral a. and v. (in saphenous opening)

Ilioinguinal n.

Superficial inguinal ring

External pudendal vv.

Accessory saphenous v.

Great saphenous v.

Obturator n.

Saphenous n., infrapatellar br.

Saphenous n. (femoral n.)

Great saphenous v.

Intermediate dorsal cutaneous n.

Medial dorsal cutaneous n.

Deep fibular n.

A Anterior view.

Superior clunial nn.

Middle clunial nn.

Inferior clunial nn. (posterior cutaneous n. of the thigh)

Posterior cutaneous n. of the thigh

Obturator n., cutaneous br.

Saphenous n. (femoral n.)

Small saphenous v.

Calcaneal brs.

Medial and lateral plantar cutaneous brs.

Iliohypogastric n., lateral cutaneous br.

Lateral cutaneous n. of the thigh

Medial sural cutaneous n. (tibial n.)

Lateral sural cutaneous n. (common fibular n.)

Sural n. (tibial n.)

Lateral dorsal cutaneous n. (tibial n.)

B Posterior view.

Fig. 34.27 Cutaneous innervation of the lower limb

Right lower limb.

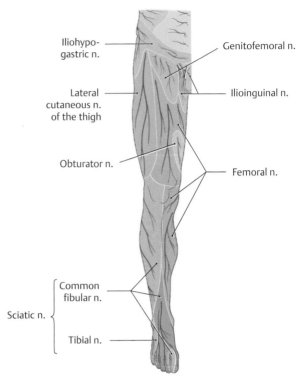

A Anterior view.

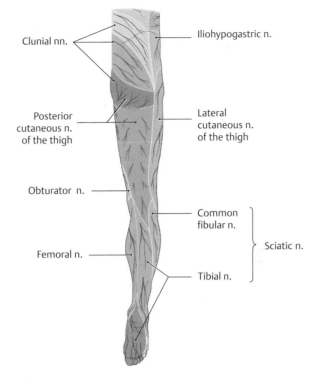

B Posterior view.

Fig. 34.28 Dermatomes of the lower limb

Right lower limb.

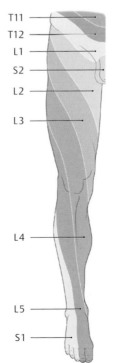

A Anterior view.

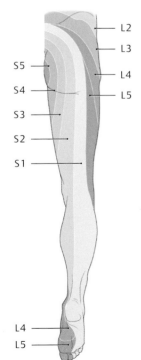

B Posterior view.

Topography of the Inguinal Region

Fig. 34.29 Superficial veins and lymph nodes

Right male inguinal region, anterior view. *Removed:* Cribriform fascia over the saphenous opening.

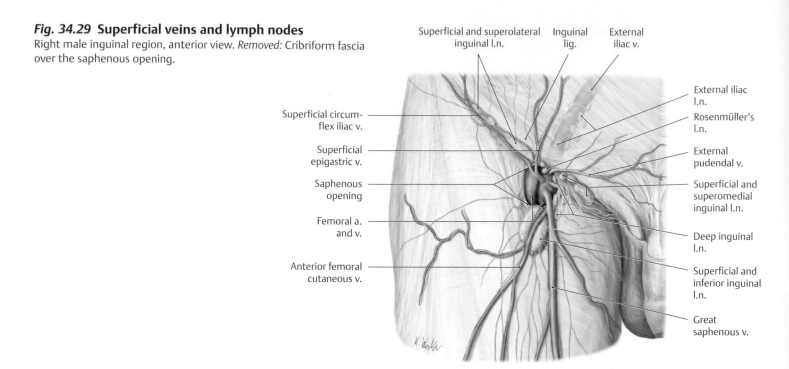

Superficial and superolateral inguinal l.n.

Inguinal lig.

External iliac v.

Superficial circumflex iliac v.

Superficial epigastric v.

Saphenous opening

Femoral a. and v.

Anterior femoral cutaneous v.

External iliac l.n.

Rosenmüller's l.n.

External pudendal v.

Superficial and superomedial inguinal l.n.

Deep inguinal l.n.

Superficial and inferior inguinal l.n.

Great saphenous v.

Fig. 34.30 Inguinal region

Right male inguinal region, anterior view.

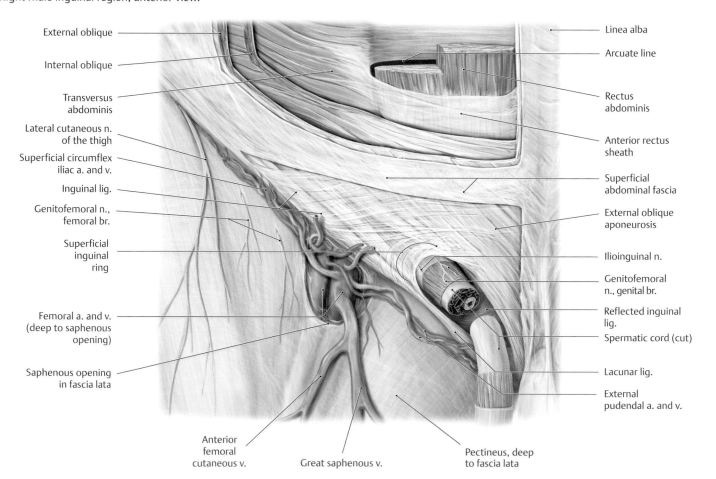

External oblique

Internal oblique

Transversus abdominis

Lateral cutaneous n. of the thigh

Superficial circumflex iliac a. and v.

Inguinal lig.

Genitofemoral n., femoral br.

Superficial inguinal ring

Femoral a. and v. (deep to saphenous opening)

Saphenous opening in fascia lata

Anterior femoral cutaneous v.

Great saphenous v.

Pectineus, deep to fascia lata

Linea alba

Arcuate line

Rectus abdominis

Anterior rectus sheath

Superficial abdominal fascia

External oblique aponeurosis

Ilioinguinal n.

Genitofemoral n., genital br.

Reflected inguinal lig.

Spermatic cord (cut)

Lacunar lig.

External pudendal a. and v.

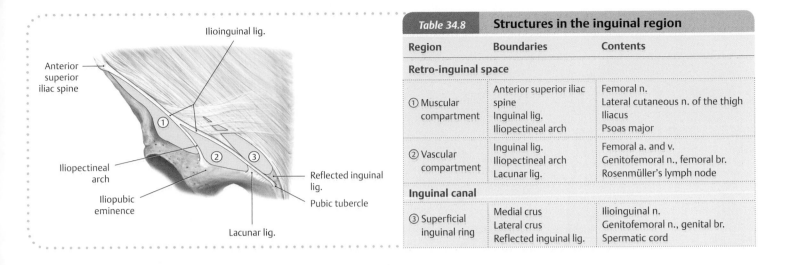

Table 34.8	Structures in the inguinal region	
Region	**Boundaries**	**Contents**
Retro-inguinal space		
① Muscular compartment	Anterior superior iliac spine Inguinal lig. Iliopectineal arch	Femoral n. Lateral cutaneous n. of the thigh Iliacus Psoas major
② Vascular compartment	Inguinal lig. Iliopectineal arch Lacunar lig.	Femoral a. and v. Genitofemoral n., femoral br. Rosenmüller's lymph node
Inguinal canal		
③ Superficial inguinal ring	Medial crus Lateral crus Reflected inguinal lig.	Ilioinguinal n. Genitofemoral n., genital br. Spermatic cord

**Fig. 34.31 Retro-inguinal space:
Muscular and vascular compartments**
Right inguinal region, anterior view.

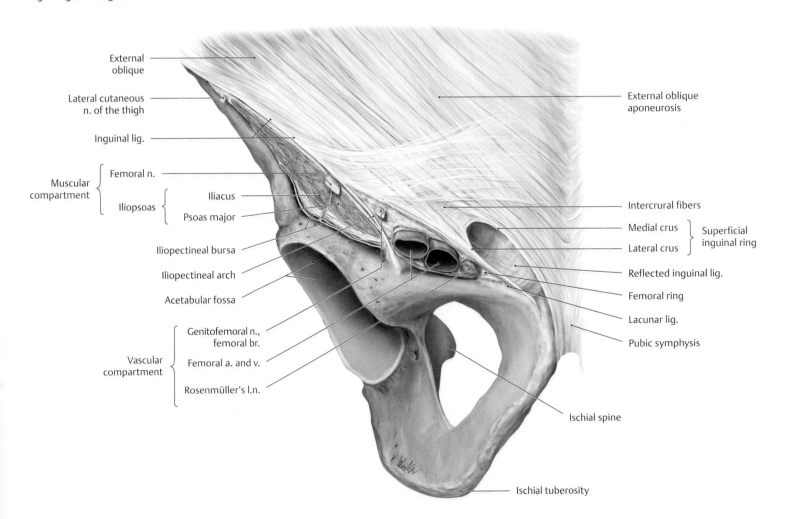

Topography of the Gluteal Region

***Fig. 34.32* Gluteal region**
Right gluteal region, posterior view.

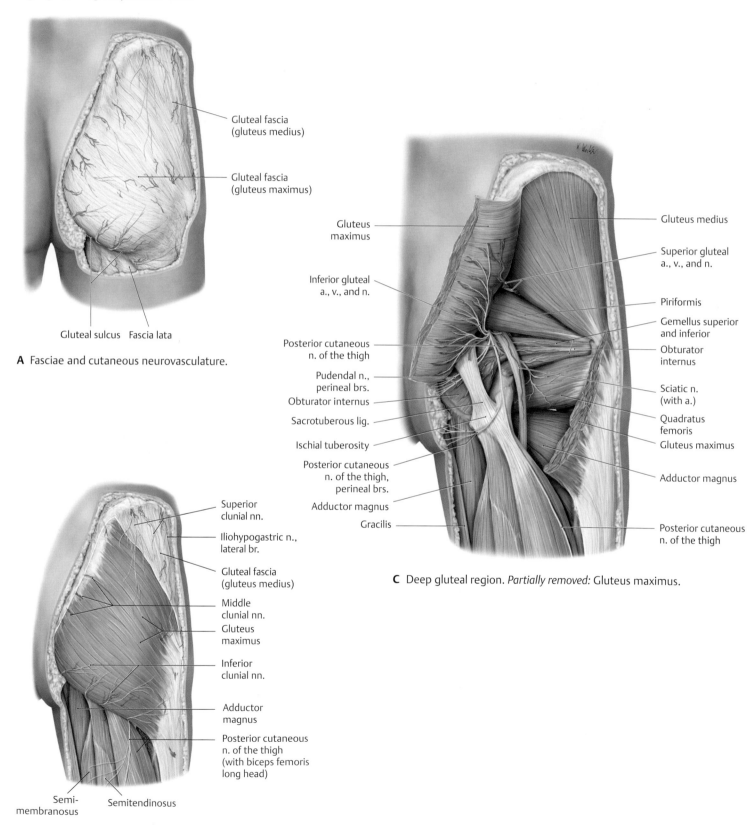

Gluteal fascia
(gluteus medius)

Gluteal fascia
(gluteus maximus)

Gluteal sulcus   Fascia lata

A Fasciae and cutaneous neurovasculature.

Gluteus
maximus

Gluteus medius

Superior gluteal
a., v., and n.

Inferior gluteal
a., v., and n.

Piriformis

Gemellus superior
and inferior

Posterior cutaneous
n. of the thigh

Obturator
internus

Pudendal n.,
perineal brs.

Obturator internus

Sacrotuberous lig.

Ischial tuberosity

Sciatic n.
(with a.)

Quadratus
femoris

Gluteus maximus

Posterior cutaneous
n. of the thigh,
perineal brs.

Adductor magnus

Adductor magnus

Gracilis

Posterior cutaneous
n. of the thigh

C Deep gluteal region. *Partially removed:* Gluteus maximus.

Superior
clunial nn.

Iliohypogastric n.,
lateral br.

Gluteal fascia
(gluteus medius)

Middle
clunial nn.

Gluteus
maximus

Inferior
clunial nn.

Adductor
magnus

Posterior cutaneous
n. of the thigh
(with biceps femoris
long head)

Semi-
membranosus   Semitendinosus

B Gluteal region. *Removed:* Fascia lata.

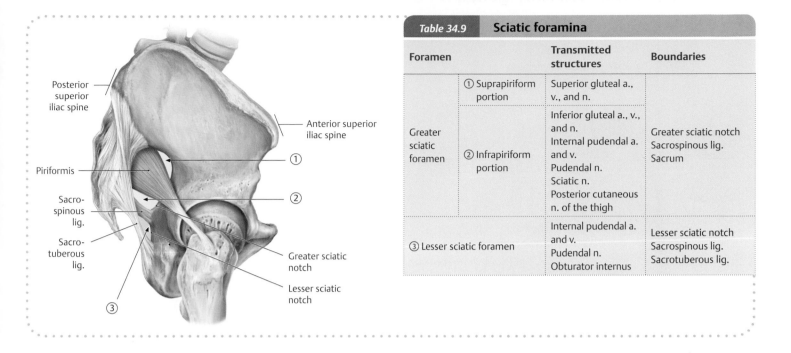

Table 34.9 Sciatic foramina

Foramen		Transmitted structures	Boundaries
Greater sciatic foramen	① Suprapiriform portion	Superior gluteal a., v., and n.	Greater sciatic notch Sacrospinous lig. Sacrum
	② Infrapiriform portion	Inferior gluteal a., v., and n. Internal pudendal a. and v. Pudendal n. Sciatic n. Posterior cutaneous n. of the thigh	
③ Lesser sciatic foramen		Internal pudendal a. and v. Pudendal n. Obturator internus	Lesser sciatic notch Sacrospinous lig. Sacrotuberous lig.

Fig. 34.33 **Gluteal region and ischioanal fossa**

Right gluteal region, posterior view.
Removed: Gluteus maximus and medius.

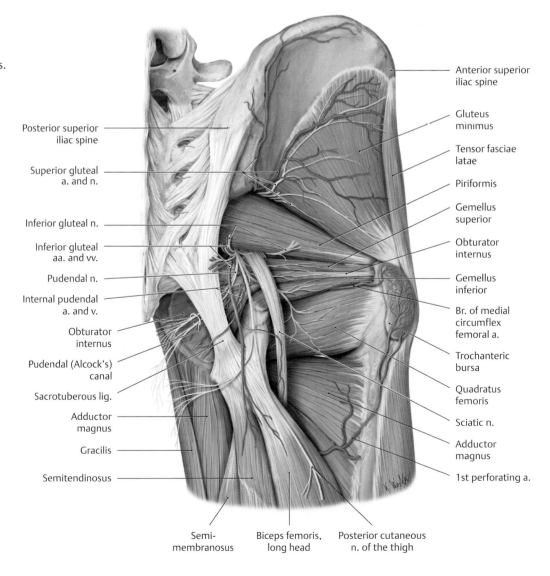

Topography of the Anterior, Medial & Posterior Thigh

Fig. 34.34 **Anterior and medial thigh**
Right thigh, anterior view.

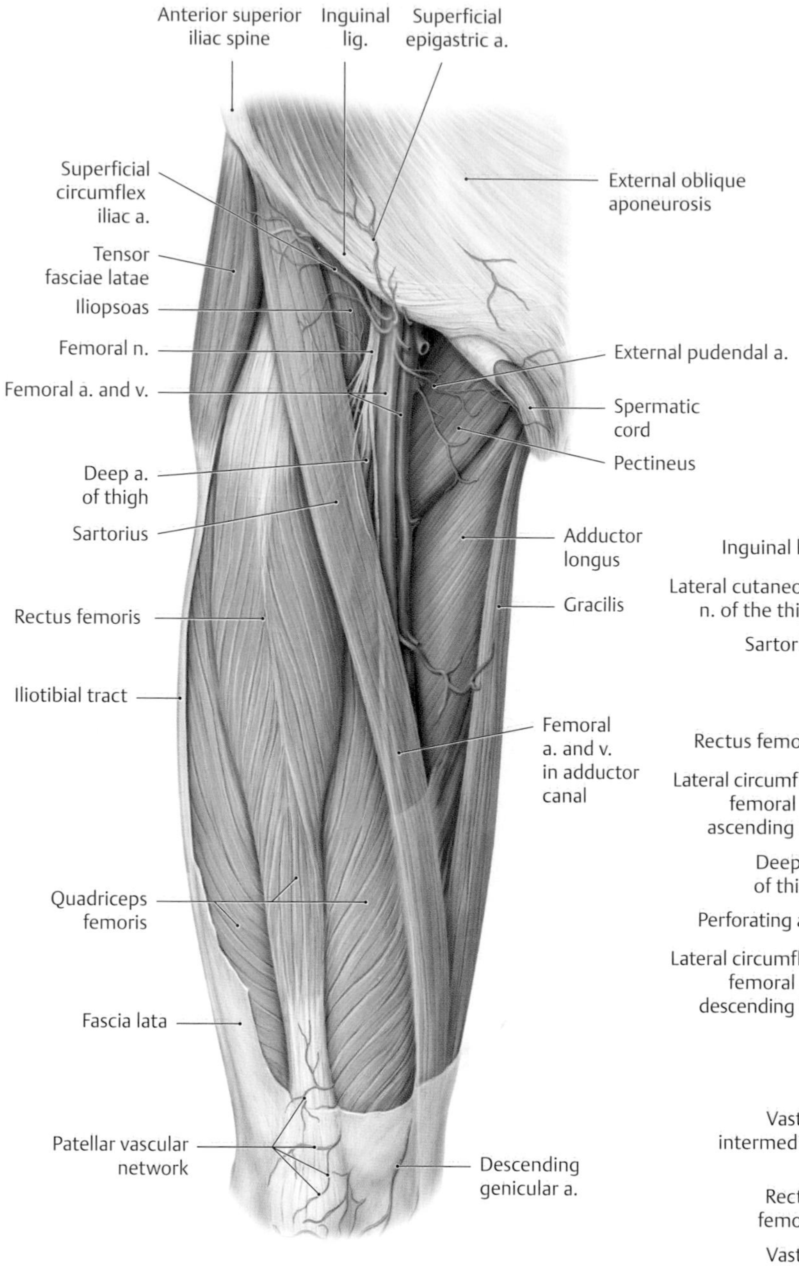

Anterior superior iliac spine
Inguinal lig.
Superficial epigastric a.
Superficial circumflex iliac a.
Tensor fasciae latae
Iliopsoas
Femoral n.
Femoral a. and v.
Deep a. of thigh
Sartorius
Rectus femoris
Iliotibial tract
Quadriceps femoris
Fascia lata
Patellar vascular network

External oblique aponeurosis
External pudendal a.
Spermatic cord
Pectineus
Adductor longus
Gracilis
Femoral a. and v. in adductor canal
Descending genicular a.

A Femoral triangle. *Removed:* Skin, subcutaneous tissue, and fascia lata. *Partially transparent:* Sartorius.

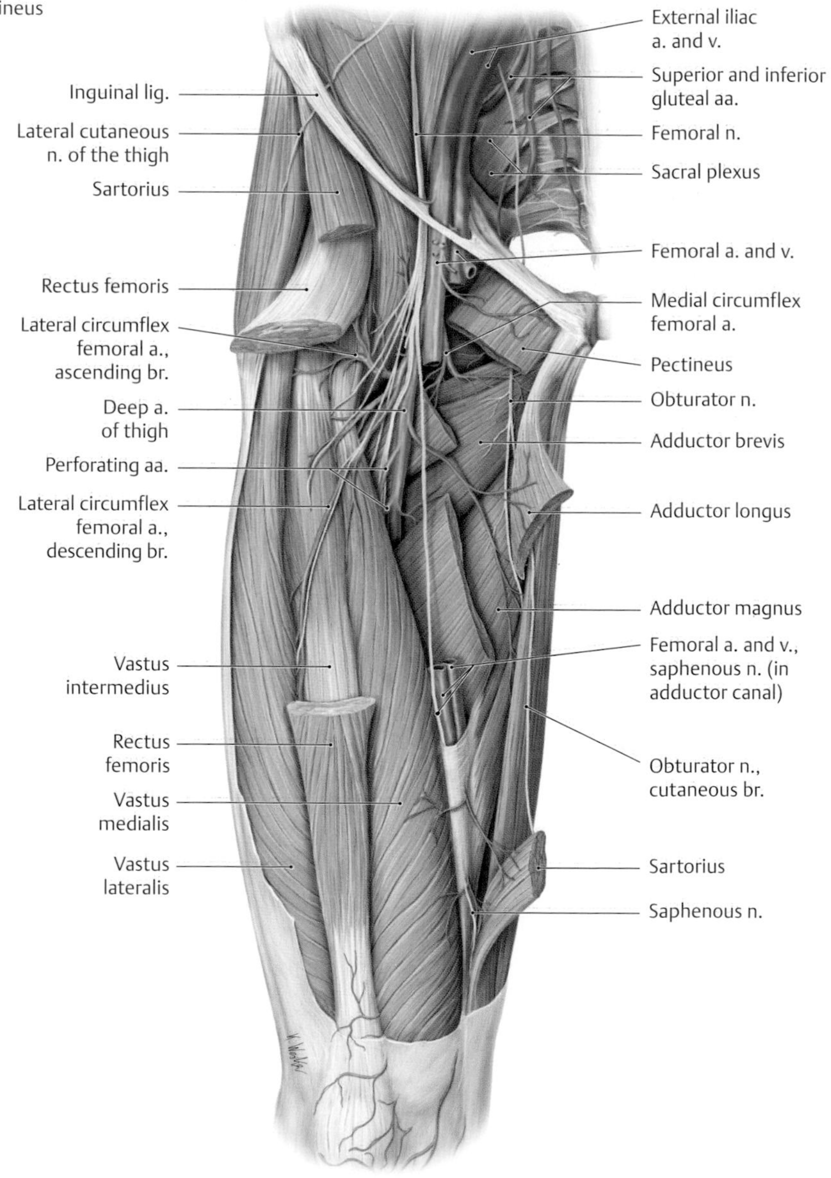

Inguinal lig.
Lateral cutaneous n. of the thigh
Sartorius
Rectus femoris
Lateral circumflex femoral a., ascending br.
Deep a. of thigh
Perforating aa.
Lateral circumflex femoral a., descending br.
Vastus intermedius
Rectus femoris
Vastus medialis
Vastus lateralis

External iliac a. and v.
Superior and inferior gluteal aa.
Femoral n.
Sacral plexus
Femoral a. and v.
Medial circumflex femoral a.
Pectineus
Obturator n.
Adductor brevis
Adductor longus
Adductor magnus
Femoral a. and v., saphenous n. (in adductor canal)
Obturator n., cutaneous br.
Sartorius
Saphenous n.

B Neurovasculature of the anterior thigh. *Removed:* Anterior abdominal wall. *Partially removed:* Sartorius, rectus femoris, adductor longus, and pectineus.

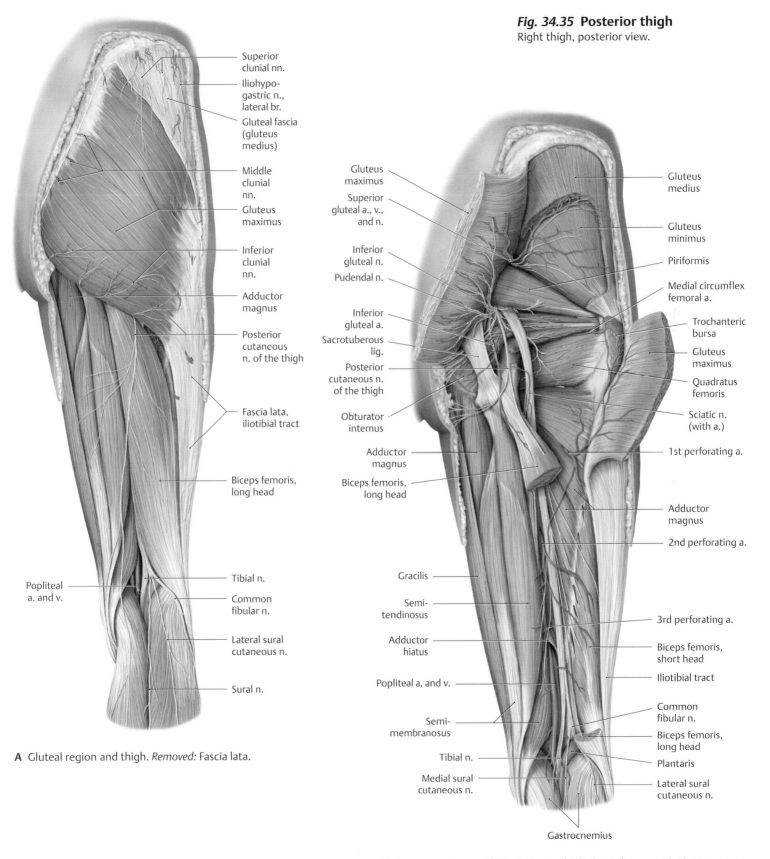

Fig. 34.35 Posterior thigh
Right thigh, posterior view.

Superior
clunial nn.

Iliohypo-
gastric n.,
lateral br.

Gluteal fascia
(gluteus
medius)

Middle
clunial
nn.

Gluteus
maximus

Inferior
clunial
nn.

Adductor
magnus

Posterior
cutaneous
n. of the thigh

Fascia lata,
iliotibial tract

Biceps femoris,
long head

Popliteal
a. and v.

Tibial n.

Common
fibular n.

Lateral sural
cutaneous n.

Sural n.

A Gluteal region and thigh. *Removed:* Fascia lata.

Gluteus
maximus

Superior
gluteal a., v.,
and n.

Inferior
gluteal n.

Pudendal n.

Inferior
gluteal a.

Sacrotuberous
lig.

Posterior
cutaneous n.
of the thigh

Obturator
internus

Adductor
magnus

Biceps femoris,
long head

Gracilis

Semi-
tendinosus

Adductor
hiatus

Popliteal a. and v.

Semi-
membranosus

Tibial n.

Medial sural
cutaneous n.

Gastrocnemius

Gluteus
medius

Gluteus
minimus

Piriformis

Medial circumflex
femoral a.

Trochanteric
bursa

Gluteus
maximus

Quadratus
femoris

Sciatic n.
(with a.)

1st perforating a.

Adductor
magnus

2nd perforating a.

3rd perforating a.

Biceps femoris,
short head

Iliotibial tract

Common
fibular n.

Biceps femoris,
long head

Plantaris

Lateral sural
cutaneous n.

B Neurovasculature of the posterior thigh. *Partially removed:* Gluteus maximus, gluteus medius, and biceps femoris. *Retracted:* Semimembranosus.

493

Topography of the Posterior Compartment of the Leg & Foot

Fig. 34.36 **Posterior compartment of leg**
Right leg, posterior view.

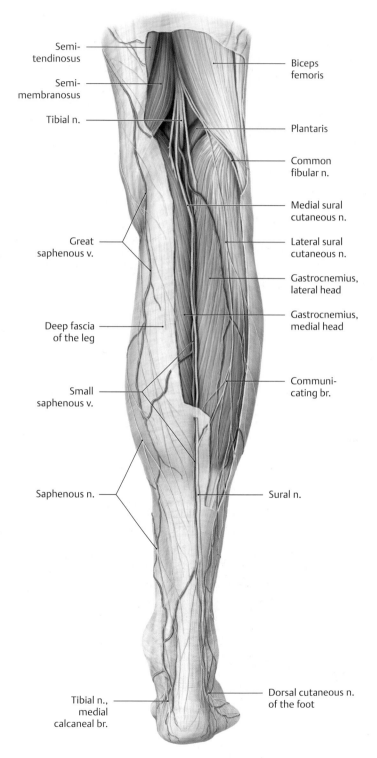

Semi-
tendinosus

Semi-
membranosus

Tibial n.

Biceps
femoris

Plantaris

Common
fibular n.

Medial sural
cutaneous n.

Great
saphenous v.

Lateral sural
cutaneous n.

Gastrocnemius,
lateral head

Gastrocnemius,
medial head

Deep fascia
of the leg

Small
saphenous v.

Communi-
cating br.

Saphenous n.

Sural n.

Tibial n.,
medial
calcaneal br.

Dorsal cutaneous n.
of the foot

A Superficial neurovascular structures.

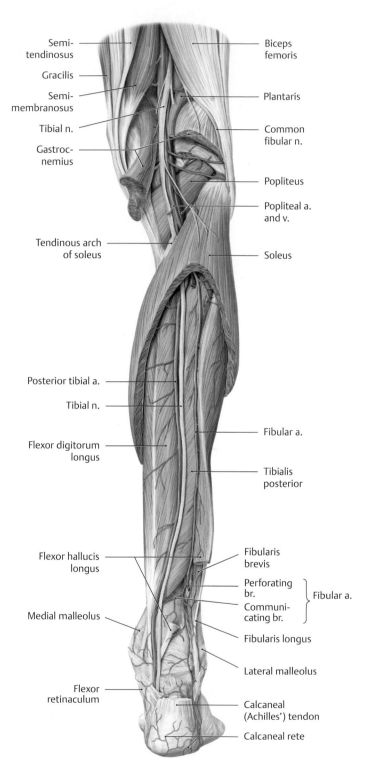

Semi-
tendinosus

Gracilis

Semi-
membranosus

Tibial n.

Gastroc-
nemius

Biceps
femoris

Plantaris

Common
fibular n.

Popliteus

Popliteal a.
and v.

Tendinous arch
of soleus

Soleus

Posterior tibial a.

Tibial n.

Flexor digitorum
longus

Fibular a.

Tibialis
posterior

Flexor hallucis
longus

Fibularis
brevis

Perforating
br.

Fibular a.

Communi-
cating br.

Medial malleolus

Fibularis longus

Lateral malleolus

Flexor
retinaculum

Calcaneal
(Achilles') tendon

Calcaneal rete

B Deep neurovascular structures. *Removed:*
Gastrocnemius. *Windowed:* Soleus.

Fig. 34.37 Popliteal region
Right leg, posterior view.

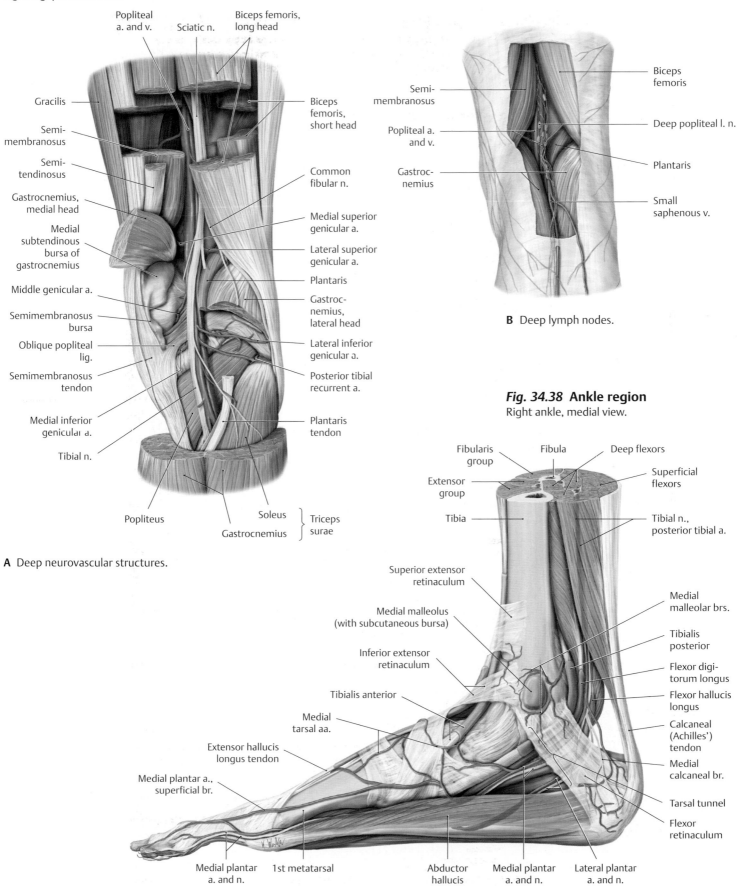

Popliteal a. and v.
Sciatic n.
Biceps femoris, long head
Gracilis
Semi-membranosus
Semi-tendinosus
Gastrocnemius, medial head
Medial subtendinous bursa of gastrocnemius
Middle genicular a.
Semimembranosus bursa
Oblique popliteal lig.
Semimembranosus tendon
Medial inferior genicular a.
Tibial n.
Biceps femoris, short head
Common fibular n.
Medial superior genicular a.
Lateral superior genicular a.
Plantaris
Gastroc-nemius, lateral head
Lateral inferior genicular a.
Posterior tibial recurrent a.
Plantaris tendon
Popliteus
Soleus
Gastrocnemius
Triceps surae

A Deep neurovascular structures.

Semi-membranosus
Popliteal a. and v.
Gastroc-nemius
Biceps femoris
Deep popliteal l. n.
Plantaris
Small saphenous v.

B Deep lymph nodes.

Fig. 34.38 Ankle region
Right ankle, medial view.

Fibularis group
Fibula
Deep flexors
Extensor group
Superficial flexors
Tibia
Tibial n., posterior tibial a.
Superior extensor retinaculum
Medial malleolus (with subcutaneous bursa)
Inferior extensor retinaculum
Tibialis anterior
Medial tarsal aa.
Extensor hallucis longus tendon
Medial plantar a., superficial br.
Medial plantar a. and n.
1st metatarsal
Abductor hallucis
Medial plantar a. and n.
Lateral plantar a. and n.
Medial malleolar brs.
Tibialis posterior
Flexor digi-torum longus
Flexor hallucis longus
Calcaneal (Achilles') tendon
Medial calcaneal br.
Tarsal tunnel
Flexor retinaculum

Topography of the Lateral & Anterior Compartments of the Leg & Dorsum of the Foot

Fig. 34.39 **Neurovasculature of the lateral compartment of the leg**

Right limb. *Removed:* Origins of the fibularis longus and extensor digitorum longus.

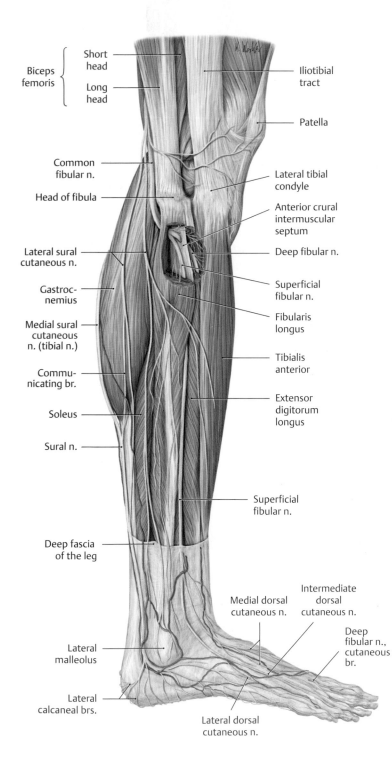

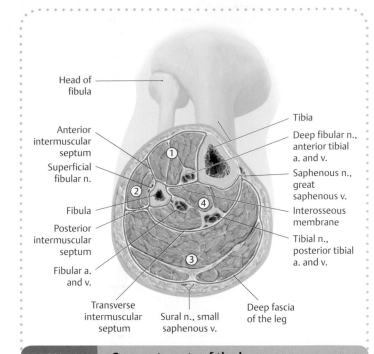

Table 34.10 | Compartments of the leg

Compartment		Muscular contents	Neurovascular contents
① Anterior compartment		Tibialis anterior	Deep fibular n. Anterior tibial a. and v.
		Extensor digitorum longus	
		Extensor hallucis longus	
		Fibularis tertius	
② Lateral compartment		Fibularis longus	Superficial fibular n.
		Fibularis brevis	
Posterior compartment	③ Superficial part	Triceps surae (gastrocnemius and soleus)	—
		Plantaris	
	④ Deep part	Tibialis posterior	Tibial n. Posterior tibial a. and v. Fibular a. and v.
		Flexor digitorum longus	
		Flexor hallucis longus	

Clinical box 34.5

Compartment syndrome
Muscle edema or hematoma can lead to a rise in tissue fluid pressure in the compartments of the leg. Subsequent compression of neurovascular structures due to this increased pressure may cause ischemia and irreversible muscle and nerve damage. Patients with *anterior* compartment syndrome, the most common form, suffer excruciating pain and cannot dorsiflex the toes. Emergency incision of the fascia of the leg may be performed to relieve compression.

Fig. 34.40 Neurovasculature of the anterior compartment of the leg and foot
Right limb with foot in plantar flexion.

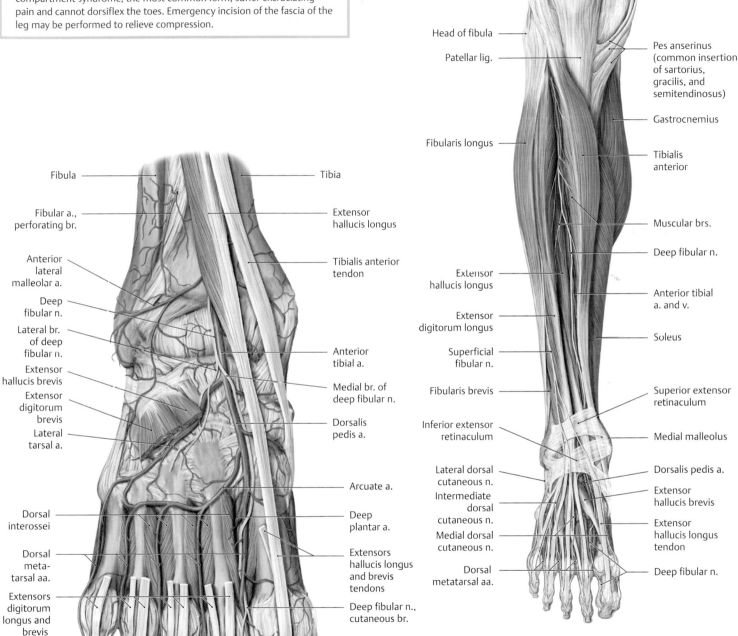

A Neurovasculature of the dorsum of the foot.

B Neurovasculature of the leg. *Removed:* Skin, subcutaneous tissue, and fasciae. *Retracted:* Tibialis anterior and extensor hallucis longus.

35 Sectional & Radiographic Anatomy
Sectional Anatomy of the Lower Limb

Fig. 35.1 **Windowed dissection of the thigh and leg**
Right limb, posterior view.

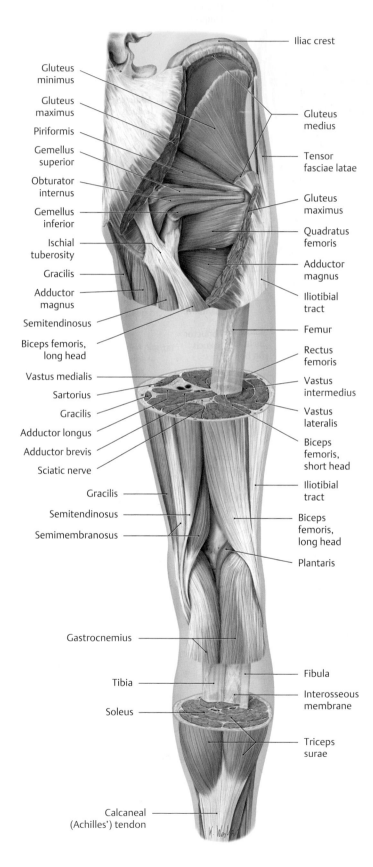

Fig. 35.2 **Cross-section through the thigh and leg**
Right limb, proximal view.

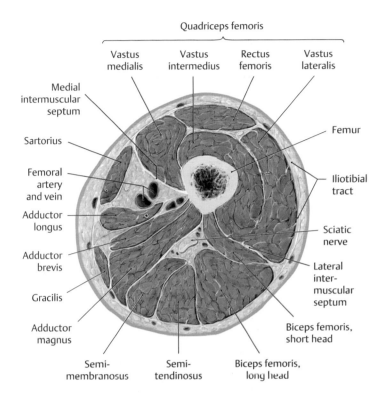

Quadriceps femoris

Vastus medialis
Vastus intermedius
Rectus femoris
Vastus lateralis

Medial intermuscular septum

Sartorius

Femoral artery and vein

Adductor longus

Adductor brevis

Gracilis

Adductor magnus

Femur

Iliotibial tract

Sciatic nerve

Lateral inter-muscular septum

Biceps femoris, short head

Semi-membranosus
Semi-tendinosus
Biceps femoris, long head

A Thigh (plane of upper section in **Fig. 35.1A**)

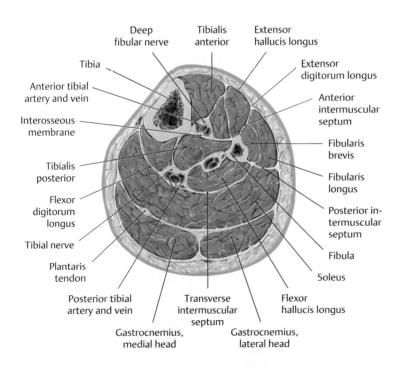

Deep fibular nerve
Tibialis anterior
Extensor hallucis longus

Tibia

Anterior tibial artery and vein

Interosseous membrane

Tibialis posterior

Flexor digitorum longus

Tibial nerve

Plantaris tendon

Extensor digitorum longus

Anterior intermuscular septum

Fibularis brevis

Fibularis longus

Posterior in-termuscular septum

Fibula

Soleus

Posterior tibial artery and vein
Transverse intermuscular septum
Flexor hallucis longus

Gastrocnemius, medial head
Gastrocnemius, lateral head

B Leg (plane of lower section in **Fig. 35.1B**)

Radiographic Anatomy of the Lower Limb (IV)

Fig. 35.14 Radiograph of the ankle

(Reproduced from Moeller TB, Reif E. Taschenatlas der Roentgenanatomie, 2nd ed. Stuttgart: Thieme; 1998.)

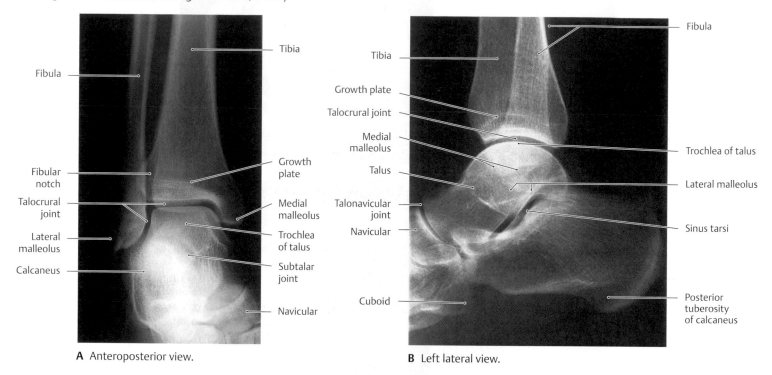

A Anteroposterior view.

B Left lateral view.

Fig. 35.15 Anterior-posterior view of the forefoot

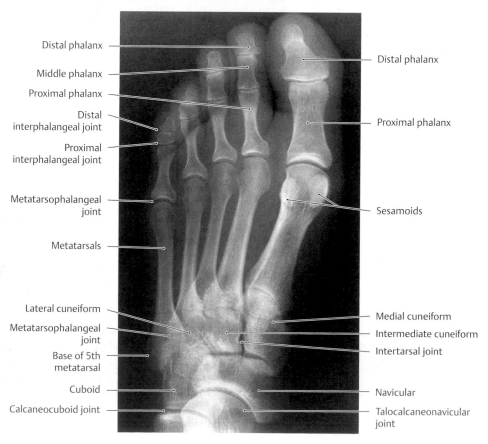

Fig. 35.16 MRI of the right ankle

Coronal section, anterior view. (Reproduced from Moeller TB, Reif E. Atlas of Sectional Anatomy: The Musculoskeletal System. New York, NY: Thieme; 2009.)

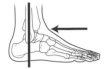

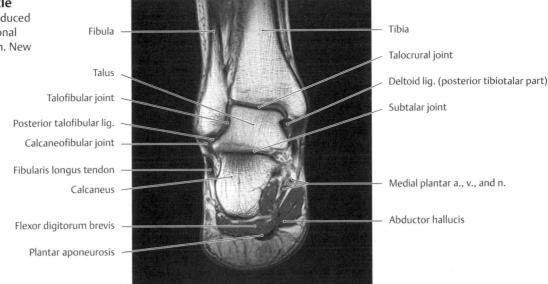

Fibula

Talus

Talofibular joint

Posterior talofibular lig.

Calcaneofibular joint

Fibularis longus tendon

Calcaneus

Flexor digitorum brevis

Plantar aponeurosis

Tibia

Talocrural joint

Deltoid lig. (posterior tibiotalar part)

Subtalar joint

Medial plantar a., v., and n.

Abductor hallucis

Fig. 35.17 MRI of the right foot

Coronal section, anterior (distal) view. (Reproduced from Moeller TB, Reif E. Atlas of Sectional Anatomy: The Musculoskeletal System. New York, NY: Thieme; 2009.)

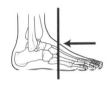

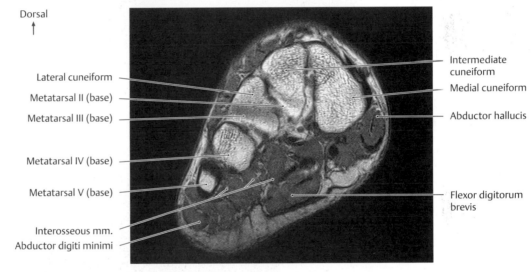

Dorsal

Lateral cuneiform

Metatarsal II (base)

Metatarsal III (base)

Metatarsal IV (base)

Metatarsal V (base)

Interosseous mm.

Abductor digiti minimi

Intermediate cuneiform

Medial cuneiform

Abductor hallucis

Flexor digitorum brevis

Fig. 35.18 MRI of the right foot and ankle

Sagittal section. (Reproduced from Moeller TB, Reif E. Atlas of Sectional Anatomy: The Musculoskeletal System. New York, NY: Thieme; 2009.)

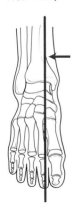

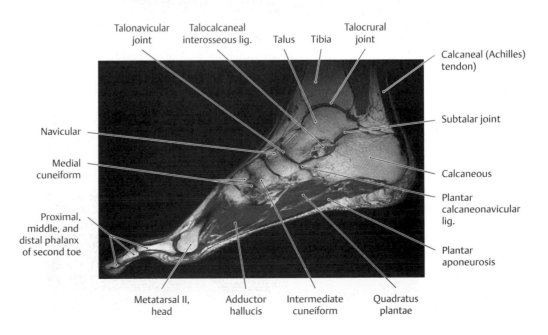

Talonavicular joint

Talocalcaneal interosseous lig.

Talus   Tibia

Talocrural joint

Calcaneal (Achilles) tendon)

Navicular

Medial cuneiform

Proximal, middle, and distal phalanx of second toe

Subtalar joint

Calcaneous

Plantar calcaneonavicular lig.

Plantar aponeurosis

Metatarsal II, head

Adductor hallucis

Intermediate cuneiform

Quadratus plantae

36 Surface Anatomy

Surface Anatomy

Fig. 36.1 **Regions of the head and neck**

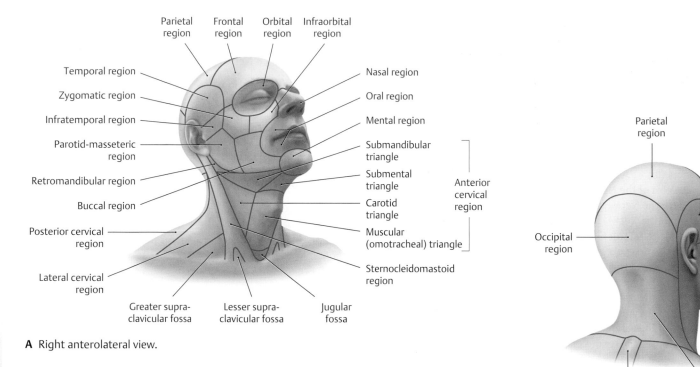

Parietal region

Frontal region

Orbital region

Infraorbital region

Temporal region

Zygomatic region

Infratemporal region

Parotid-masseteric region

Retromandibular region

Buccal region

Posterior cervical region

Lateral cervical region

Greater supra-clavicular fossa

Lesser supra-clavicular fossa

Jugular fossa

Nasal region

Oral region

Mental region

Submandibular triangle

Submental triangle

Carotid triangle

Muscular (omotracheal) triangle

Anterior cervical region

Sternocleidomastoid region

A Right anterolateral view.

Parietal region

Temporal region

Occipital region

Vertebra prominens

Posterior cervical region

B Right posterolateral view.

Fig. 36.2 **Surface anatomy of the head and neck**

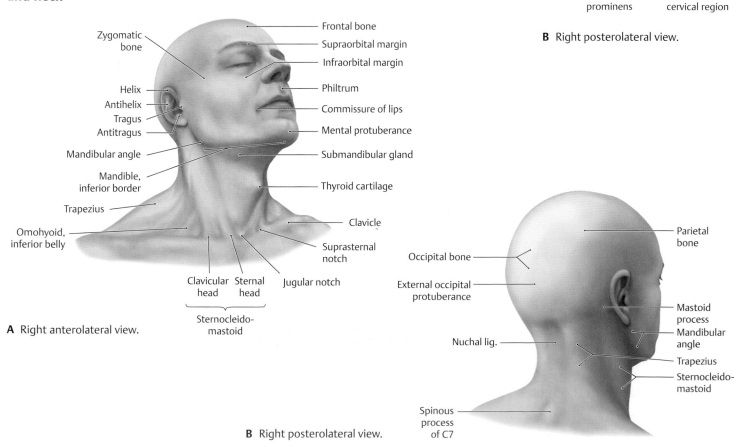

Zygomatic bone

Helix

Antihelix

Tragus

Antitragus

Mandibular angle

Mandible, inferior border

Trapezius

Omohyoid, inferior belly

Clavicular head

Sternal head

Sternocleido-mastoid

Frontal bone

Supraorbital margin

Infraorbital margin

Philtrum

Commissure of lips

Mental protuberance

Submandibular gland

Thyroid cartilage

Clavicle

Suprasternal notch

Jugular notch

A Right anterolateral view.

Occipital bone

External occipital protuberance

Nuchal lig.

Spinous process of C7

Parietal bone

Mastoid process

Mandibular angle

Trapezius

Sternocleido-mastoid

B Right posterolateral view.

Fig. 36.3 **Palpable bony prominences of the head and neck**

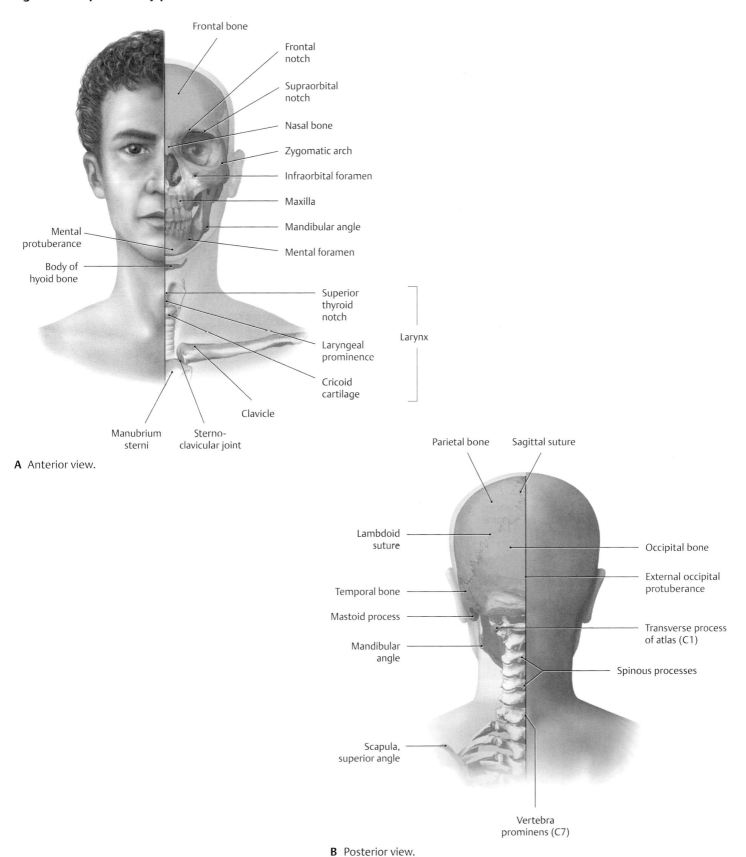

Frontal bone

Frontal notch

Supraorbital notch

Nasal bone

Zygomatic arch

Infraorbital foramen

Maxilla

Mandibular angle

Mental foramen

Mental protuberance

Body of hyoid bone

Superior thyroid notch

Laryngeal prominence

Cricoid cartilage

Larynx

Clavicle

Manubrium sterni

Sterno-clavicular joint

A Anterior view.

Parietal bone

Sagittal suture

Lambdoid suture

Occipital bone

External occipital protuberance

Temporal bone

Mastoid process

Transverse process of atlas (C1)

Mandibular angle

Spinous processes

Scapula, superior angle

Vertebra prominens (C7)

B Posterior view.

Table 37.8	Branches of the spinal nerves in the neck		
Posterior (dorsal) ramus			
	Nerve	Sensory function	Motor function
C1	Suboccipital n.	No C1 dermatome	Innervate intrinsic nuchal muscles
C2	Greater occipital n.	Innervate C2 dermatome	
C3	3rd occipital n.	Innervate C3 dermatome	
Anterior (ventral) ramus			
	Sensory branches	Sensory function	Motor branches	Motor function
C1	—	—		
C2	Lesser occipital n.			
C2–C3	Great auricular n.	Form sensory part of cervical plexus, innervate anterior and lateral neck	Form ansa cervicalis (motor part of cervical plexus)	Innervate infrahyoid muscles (except thyrohyoid)
	Transverse cervical n.			
C3–C4	Supraclavicular nn.		Contribute to phrenic n.*	Innervate diaphragm and pericardium*

*The anterior roots of C3–C5 combine to form the phrenic nerve (see **p. 66**).

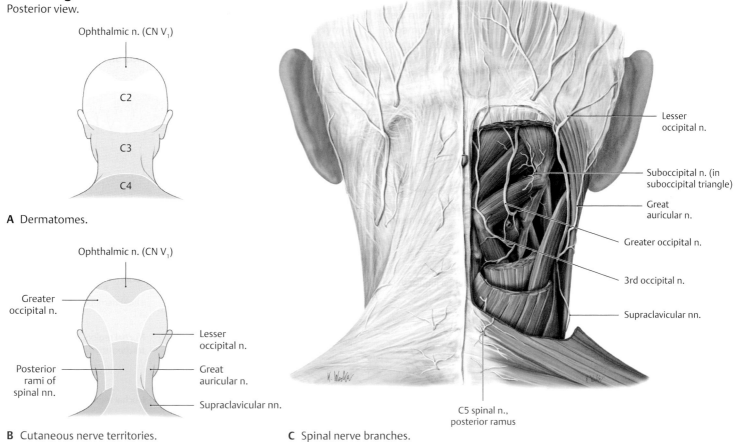

Branching of the cervical plexus.

Fig. 37.14 Sensory innervation of the nuchal region
Posterior view.

A Dermatomes.

B Cutaneous nerve territories.

C Spinal nerve branches.

Fig. 37.15 Sensory innervation of the anterolateral neck
Left lateral view.

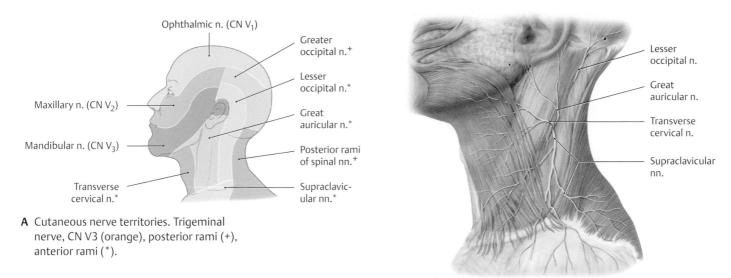

A Cutaneous nerve territories. Trigeminal nerve, CN V3 (orange), posterior rami (+), anterior rami (*).

B Sensory branches of the cervical plexus.

Fig. 37.16 Motor innervation of the anterolateral neck
Left lateral view.

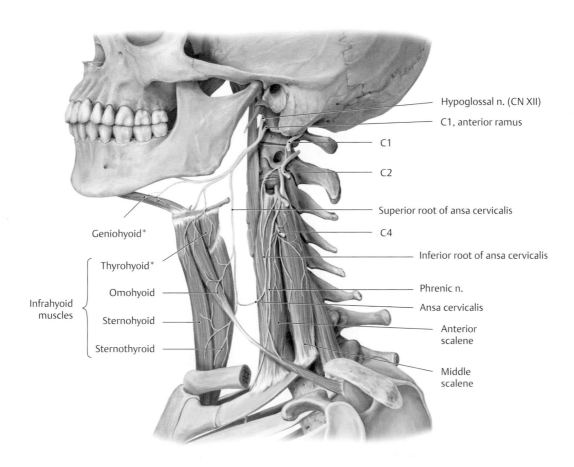

* Innervated by the anterior ramus of C1 (distributed by the hypoglossal n.).

Larynx: Cartilage & Structure

Fig. 37.17 Laryngeal cartilages

Left lateral view. The larynx consists of five laryngeal cartilages: epiglottic, thyroid, cricoid, and the paired arytenoid and corniculate cartilages. They are connected to each other, the trachea, and the hyoid bone by elastic ligaments.

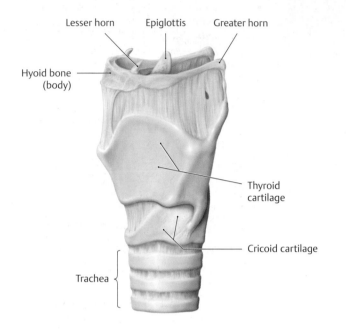

Lesser horn — Epiglottis — Greater horn

Hyoid bone (body)

Thyroid cartilage

Cricoid cartilage

Trachea

Fig. 37.18 Epiglottic cartilage

The elastic epiglottic cartilage comprises the internal skeleton of the epiglottis, providing resilience to return it to its initial position after swallowing.

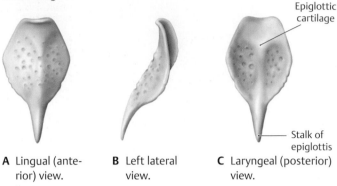

Epiglottic cartilage

Stalk of epiglottis

A Lingual (anterior) view.   **B** Left lateral view.   **C** Laryngeal (posterior) view.

Fig. 37.19 Thyroid cartilage

Left oblique view.

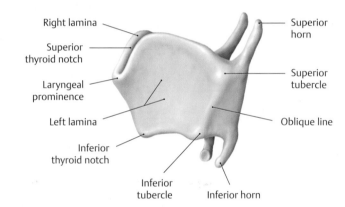

Right lamina — Superior horn
Superior thyroid notch — Superior tubercle
Laryngeal prominence — Oblique line
Left lamina
Inferior thyroid notch — Inferior horn
Inferior tubercle

Fig. 37.20 Cricoid cartilage

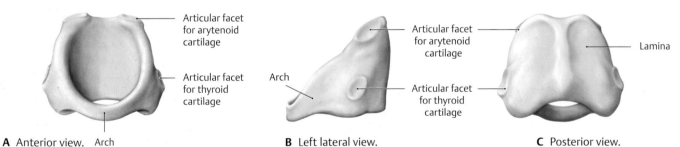

Articular facet for arytenoid cartilage
Articular facet for thyroid cartilage
Arch

A Anterior view.   Arch

Articular facet for arytenoid cartilage
Arch
Articular facet for thyroid cartilage

B Left lateral view.

Lamina

C Posterior view.

Fig. 37.21 Arytenoid and corniculate cartilages

Right cartilages.

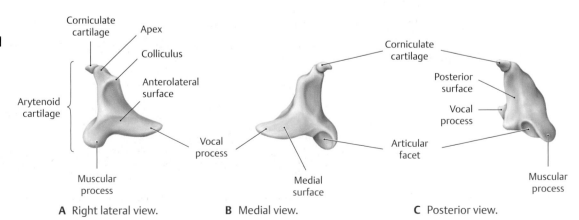

Corniculate cartilage — Apex
Colliculus
Anterolateral surface
Arytenoid cartilage
Vocal process
Muscular process

A Right lateral view.

Medial surface

B Medial view.

Corniculate cartilage
Posterior surface
Vocal process
Articular facet
Muscular process

C Posterior view.

Fig. 37.22 **Structure of the larynx**

The larynx is suspended from the hyoid bone, primarily by the thyro-hyoid membrane. The hyoid bone provides the sites for attachment of the suprahyoid and infrahyoid muscles.

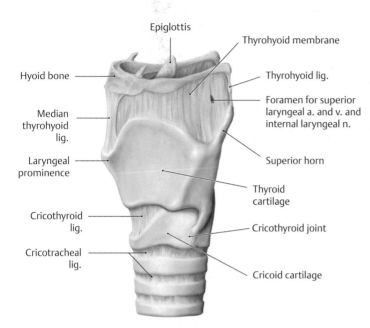

A Left anterior oblique view.

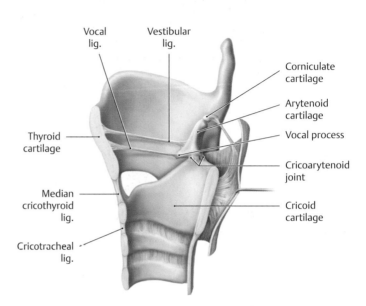

B Sagittal section, viewed from the left medial aspect. The arytenoid cartilage alters the position of the vocal folds during phonation.

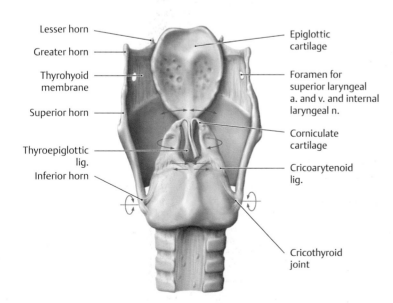

C Posterior view. Arrows indicate the directions of movement in the various joints.

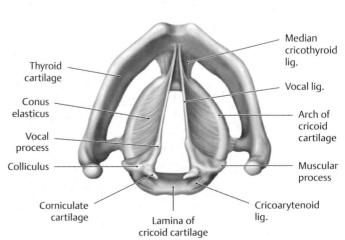

D Superior view.

Larynx: Muscles & Levels

Fig. 37.23 Laryngeal muscles

The laryngeal muscles move the laryngeal cartilages relative to one another, affecting the tension and/or position of the vocal folds. Muscles that move the larynx as a whole (infra- and suprahyoid muscles) are described on **p. 516**.

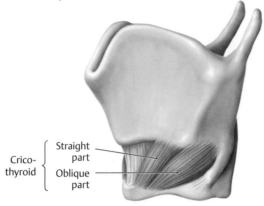

A Intrinsic laryngeal muscles, left lateral oblique view.

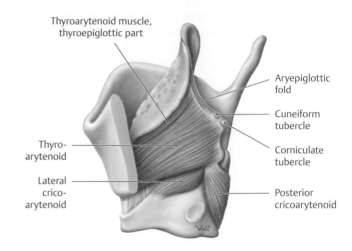

B Intrinsic laryngeal muscles, left lateral view. *Removed:* Thyroid cartilage (left half). *Revealed:* Epiglottis and thyroarytenoid muscle.

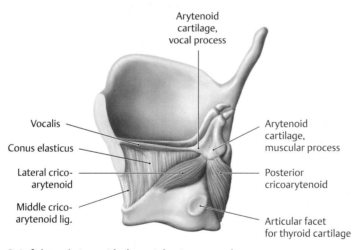

C Left lateral view with the epiglottis removed.

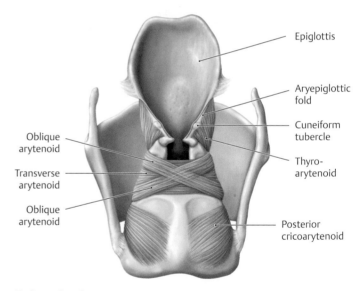

D Posterior view.

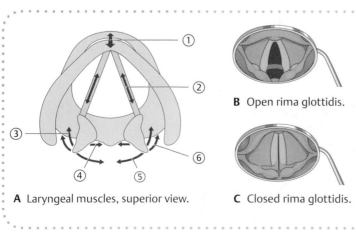

A Laryngeal muscles, superior view.

B Open rima glottidis.

C Closed rima glottidis.

Table 37.9	Actions of the laryngeal muscles	
Muscle	Action	Effect on rima glottidis
① Cricothyroid m.*	Tightens the vocal folds	None
② Vocalis m.		
③ Thyroarytenoid m.	Adducts the vocal folds	Closes
④ Transverse arytenoid m.		
⑤ Posterior cricoarytenoid m.	Abducts the vocal folds	Opens
⑥ Lateral cricoarytenoid m.	Adducts the vocal folds	Closes

* The cricothyroid is innervated by the external laryngeal n. All other intrinsic laryngeal mm. are innervated by the recurrent laryngeal n.

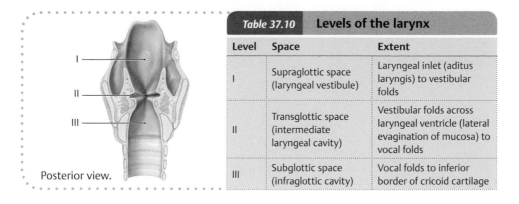

Table 37.10		Levels of the larynx
Level	Space	Extent
I	Supraglottic space (laryngeal vestibule)	Laryngeal inlet (aditus laryngis) to vestibular folds
II	Transglottic space (intermediate laryngeal cavity)	Vestibular folds across laryngeal ventricle (lateral evagination of mucosa) to vocal folds
III	Subglottic space (infraglottic cavity)	Vocal folds to inferior border of cricoid cartilage

Posterior view.

Fig. 37.24 **Cavity of the larynx**

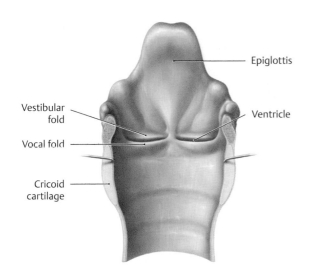

A Posterior view with the larynx splayed open.

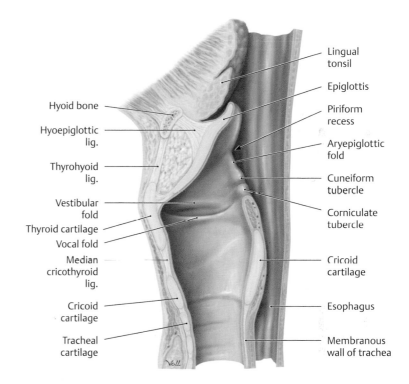

B Midsagittal section viewed from the left side.

Fig. 37.25 **Vestibular and vocal folds**
Coronal section, superior view.

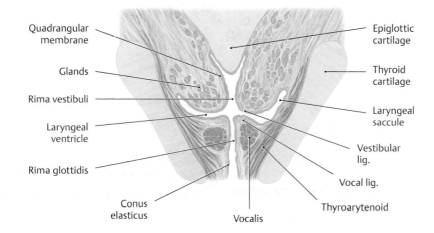

Neurovasculature of the Larynx, Thyroid & Parathyroids

Fig. 37.26 **Thyroid and parathyroid glands**

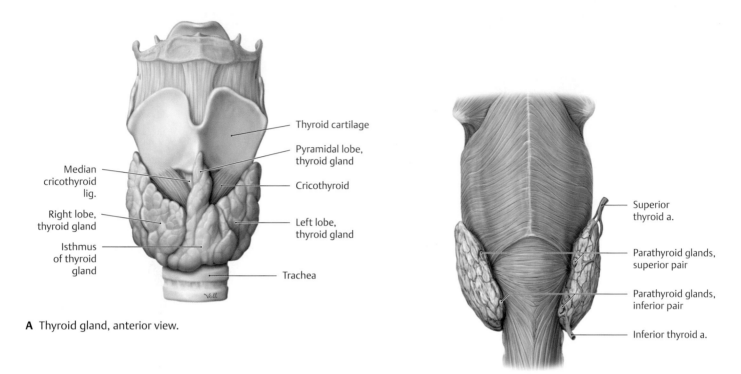

A Thyroid gland, anterior view.

Thyroid cartilage

Pyramidal lobe, thyroid gland

Median cricothyroid lig.

Cricothyroid

Right lobe, thyroid gland

Left lobe, thyroid gland

Isthmus of thyroid gland

Trachea

Superior thyroid a.

Parathyroid glands, superior pair

Parathyroid glands, inferior pair

Inferior thyroid a.

B Thyroid and parathyroid glands, posterior view.

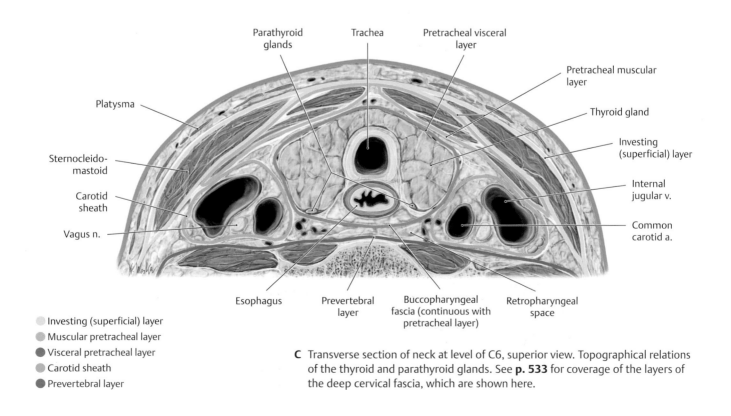

Parathyroid glands

Trachea

Pretracheal visceral layer

Pretracheal muscular layer

Thyroid gland

Investing (superficial) layer

Internal jugular v.

Common carotid a.

Platysma

Sternocleido-mastoid

Carotid sheath

Vagus n.

Esophagus

Prevertebral layer

Buccopharyngeal fascia (continuous with pretracheal layer)

Retropharyngeal space

- Investing (superficial) layer
- Muscular pretracheal layer
- Visceral pretracheal layer
- Carotid sheath
- Prevertebral layer

C Transverse section of neck at level of C6, superior view. Topographical relations of the thyroid and parathyroid glands. See **p. 533** for coverage of the layers of the deep cervical fascia, which are shown here.

Fig. 37.27 Arteries and nerves of the larynx

Anterior view. *Removed:* Thyroid gland (right half).

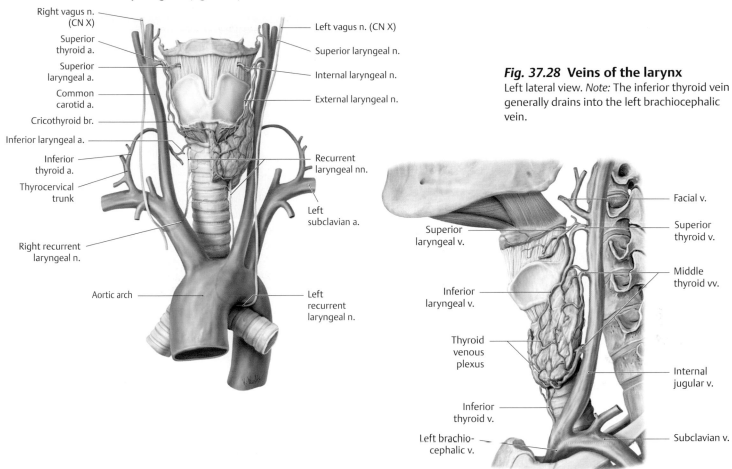

Right vagus n. (CN X)
Superior thyroid a.
Superior laryngeal a.
Common carotid a.
Cricothyroid br.
Inferior laryngeal a.
Inferior thyroid a.
Thyrocervical trunk
Right recurrent laryngeal n.
Aortic arch

Left vagus n. (CN X)
Superior laryngeal n.
Internal laryngeal n.
External laryngeal n.
Recurrent laryngeal nn.
Left subclavian a.
Left recurrent laryngeal n.

Fig. 37.28 Veins of the larynx

Left lateral view. *Note:* The inferior thyroid vein generally drains into the left brachiocephalic vein.

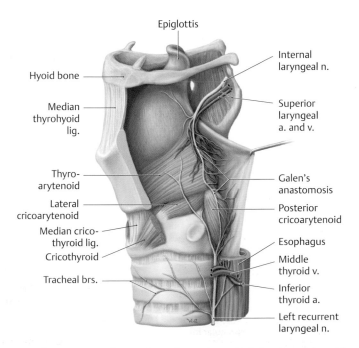

Superior laryngeal v.
Inferior laryngeal v.
Thyroid venous plexus
Inferior thyroid v.
Left brachio-cephalic v.

Facial v.
Superior thyroid v.
Middle thyroid vv.
Internal jugular v.
Subclavian v.

Fig. 37.29 Neurovasculature of the larynx

Left lateral view.

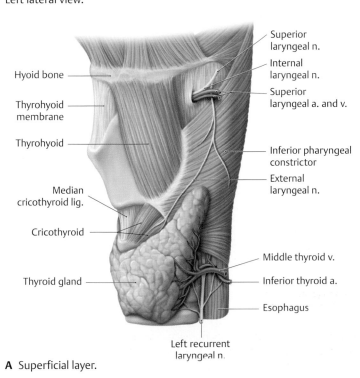

Hyoid bone
Thyrohyoid membrane
Thyrohyoid
Median cricothyroid lig.
Cricothyroid
Thyroid gland

Superior laryngeal n.
Internal laryngeal n.
Superior laryngeal a. and v.
Inferior pharyngeal constrictor
External laryngeal n.
Middle thyroid v.
Inferior thyroid a.
Esophagus
Left recurrent laryngeal n.

A Superficial layer.

Epiglottis
Hyoid bone
Median thyrohyoid lig.
Thyro-arytenoid
Lateral cricoarytenoid
Median crico-thyroid lig.
Cricothyroid
Tracheal brs.

Internal laryngeal n.
Superior laryngeal a. and v.
Galen's anastomosis
Posterior cricoarytenoid
Esophagus
Middle thyroid v.
Inferior thyroid a.
Left recurrent laryngeal n.

B Deep layer. *Removed:* Cricothyroid muscle and left lamina of thyroid cartilage. *Retracted:* Pharyngeal mucosa.

Topography of the Neck: Regions & Fascia

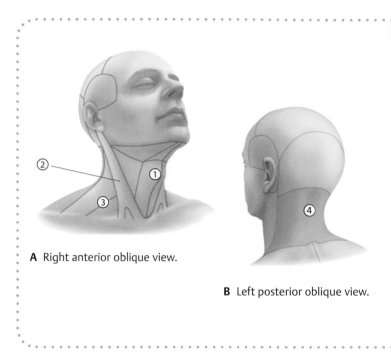

A Right anterior oblique view.

B Left posterior oblique view.

Table 37.11	Regions of the neck	
Region	**Divisions**	**Contents**
① Anterior cervical region (triangle)	Submandibular (digastric) triangle	Submandibular gland and l.n., hypoglossal n. (CN XII), facial a. and v.
	Submental triangle	Submental l.n.
	Muscular triangle	Sternothyroid and sternohyoid mm., thyroid and parathyroid glands
	Carotid triangle	Carotid bifurcation, carotid body, hypoglossal (CN XII) and vagus (CN X) nn.
② Sternocleidomastoid region*		Sternocleidomastoid, common carotid a., internal jugular v., vagus n. (CN X), jugular l.n.
③ Lateral cervical region (posterior triangle)	Omoclavicular (subclavian) triangle	Subclavian a., subscapular a., supraclavicular l.n.
	Occipital triangle	Accessory n. (CN XI), trunks of brachial plexus, transverse cervical a., cervical plexus (posterior branches)
④ Posterior cervical region		Nuchal mm., vertebral a., cervical plexus

* The sternocleidomastoid region also contains the lesser supraclavicular fossa.

Fig. 37.30 **Cervical regions**

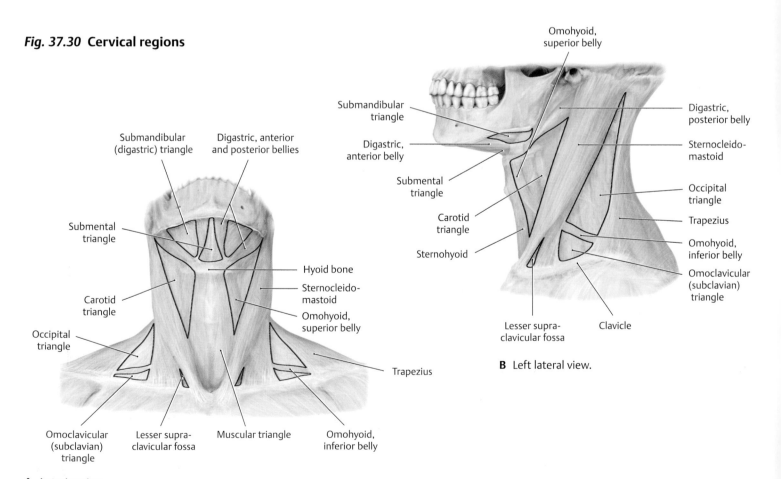

A Anterior view.

B Left lateral view.

Table 37.12	Deep cervical fascia		

The deep cervical fascia is divided into four layers that enclose the structures of the neck.

Layer		Type of fascia	Description
● ① Investing (superficial) layer		Muscular	Envelopes entire neck; splits to enclose sternocleidomastoid and trapezius muscles
Pretracheal layer	● ② Muscular		Encloses infrahyoid muscles
	● ③ Visceral		Surrounds thyroid gland, larynx, trachea, pharynx, and esophagus
● ④ Prevertebral layer		Muscular	Surrounds cervical vertebral column and associated muscles
● ⑤ Carotid sheath		Neurovascular	Encloses common carotid artery, internal jugular vein, and vagus nerve

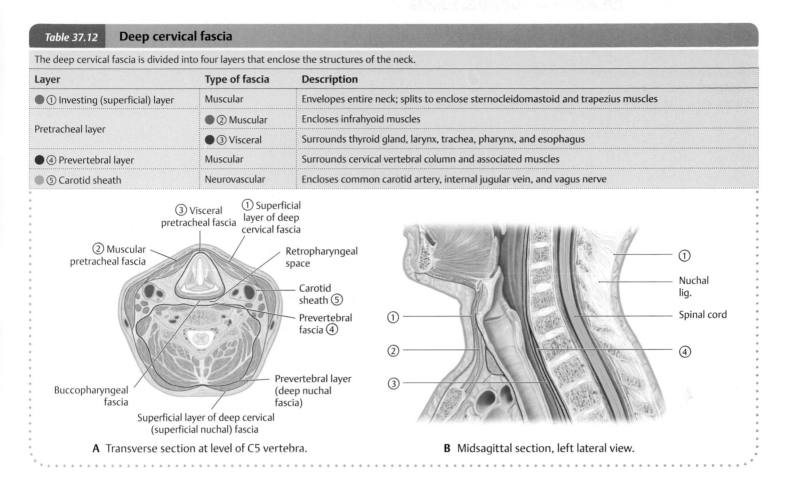

A Transverse section at level of C5 vertebra.

B Midsagittal section, left lateral view.

Fig. 37.31 **Deep cervical fascial layers**
Anterior view.

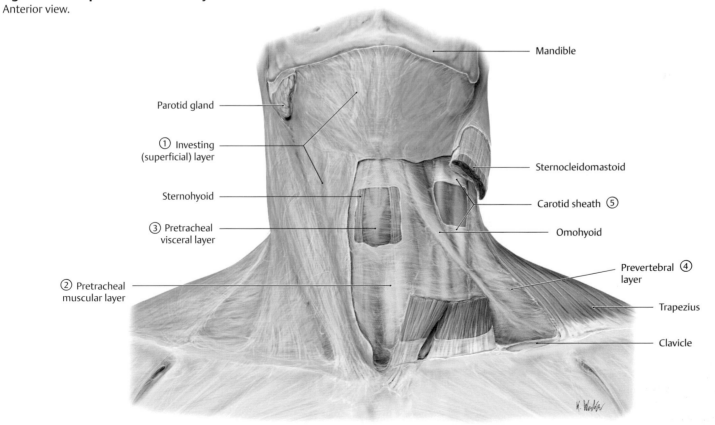

Topography of the Anterior Cervical Region

***Fig. 37.32* Anterior cervical triangle**
Anterior view.

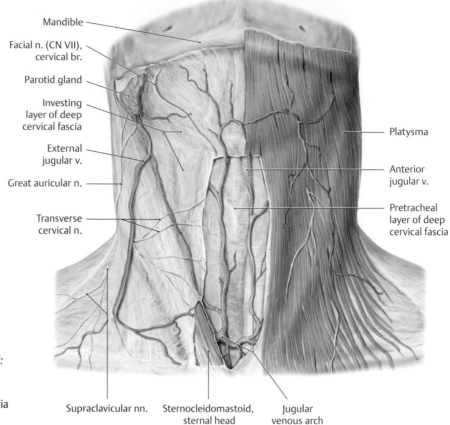

Mandible

Facial n. (CN VII), cervical br.

Parotid gland

Investing layer of deep cervical fascia

External jugular v.

Great auricular n.

Transverse cervical n.

Platysma

Anterior jugular v.

Pretracheal layer of deep cervical fascia

Supraclavicular nn.

Sternocleidomastoid, sternal head

Jugular venous arch

A Superficial layer. *Removed:* Subcutaneous platysma (right side) and investing layer of deep cervical fascia (center).

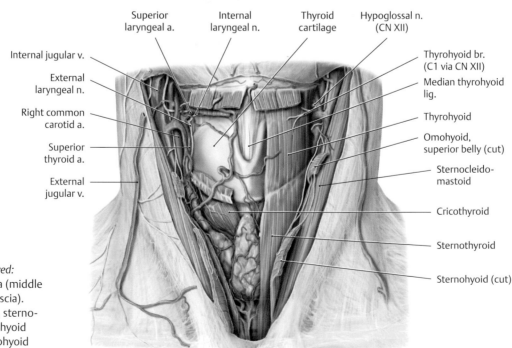

Superior laryngeal a.

Internal laryngeal n.

Thyroid cartilage

Hypoglossal n. (CN XII)

Internal jugular v.

External laryngeal n.

Right common carotid a.

Superior thyroid a.

External jugular v.

Thyrohyoid br. (C1 via CN XII)

Median thyrohyoid lig.

Thyrohyoid

Omohyoid, superior belly (cut)

Sternocleido-mastoid

Cricothyroid

Sternothyroid

Sternohyoid (cut)

B Deep layer. *Removed:* Pretracheal lamina (middle layer of cervical fascia). *Cuts:* Sternohyoid, sternothyroid, and thyrohyoid (right side); sternohyoid (left side).

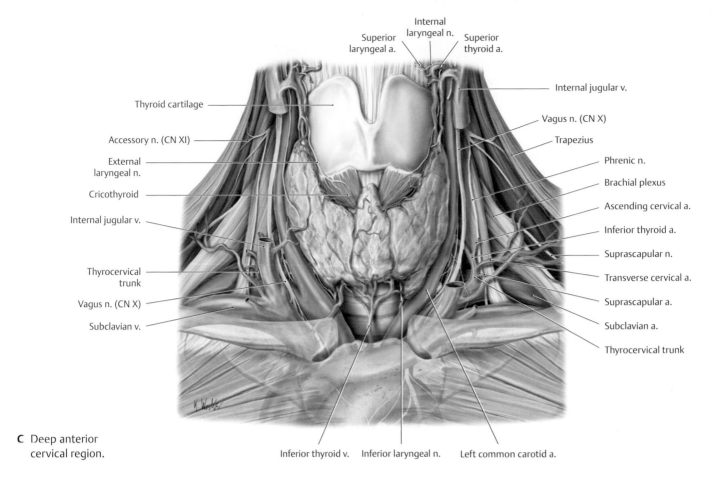

Internal
laryngeal n.

Superior
laryngeal a.

Superior
thyroid a.

Thyroid cartilage

Internal jugular v.

Accessory n. (CN XI)

Vagus n. (CN X)

External
laryngeal n.

Trapezius

Cricothyroid

Phrenic n.

Internal jugular v.

Brachial plexus

Ascending cervical a.

Inferior thyroid a.

Suprascapular n.

Thyrocervical
trunk

Transverse cervical a.

Vagus n. (CN X)

Suprascapular a.

Subclavian v.

Subclavian a.

Thyrocervical trunk

C Deep anterior
cervical region.

Inferior thyroid v.   Inferior laryngeal n.   Left common carotid a.

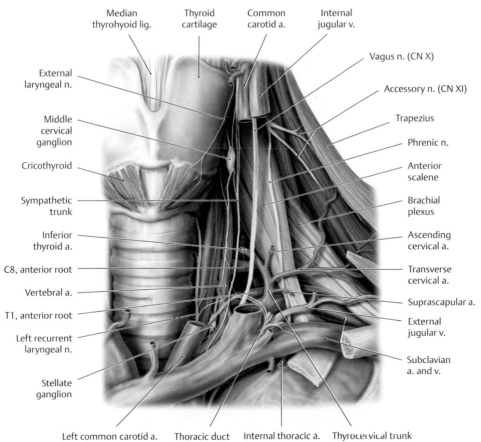

Median
thyrohyoid lig.

Thyroid
cartilage

Common
carotid a.

Internal
jugular v.

External
laryngeal n.

Vagus n. (CN X)

Accessory n. (CN XI)

Middle
cervical
ganglion

Trapezius

Cricothyroid

Phrenic n.

Sympathetic
trunk

Anterior
scalene

Inferior
thyroid a.

Brachial
plexus

C8, anterior root

Ascending
cervical a.

Vertebral a.

Transverse
cervical a.

T1, anterior root

Suprascapular a.

Left recurrent
laryngeal n.

External
jugular v.

Stellate
ganglion

Subclavian
a. and v.

D Root of the neck.

Left common carotid a.   Thoracic duct   Internal thoracic a.   Thyrocervical trunk

Topography of the Anterior & Lateral Cervical Regions

Fig. 37.33 Deep anterior cervical region

The deep midline viscera of the anterior cervical region are the larynx and thyroid gland. The two lateral neurovascular pathways primarily supply these organs.

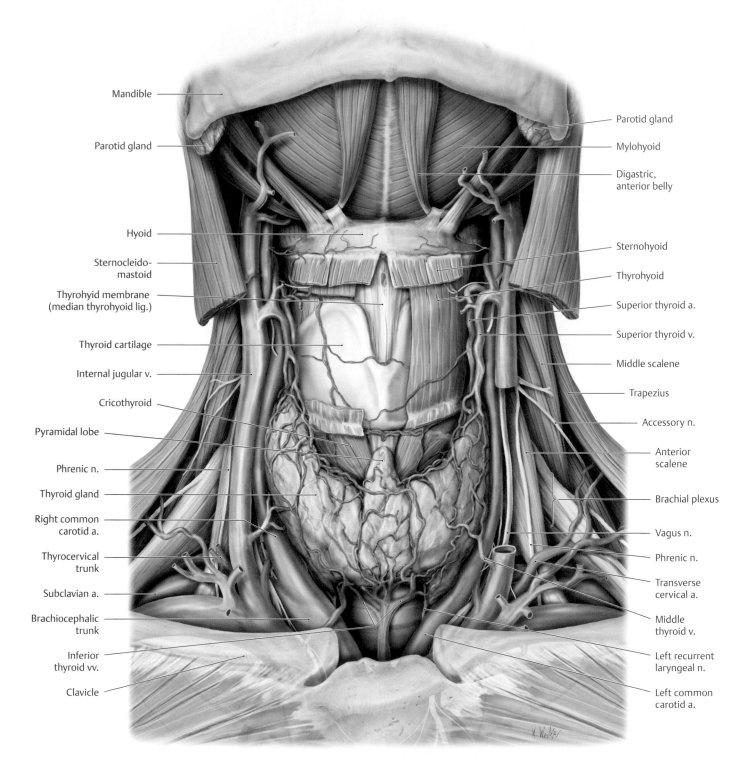

Mandible

Parotid gland

Hyoid

Sternocleido-mastoid

Thyrohyid membrane (median thyrohyoid lig.)

Thyroid cartilage

Internal jugular v.

Cricothyroid

Pyramidal lobe

Phrenic n.

Thyroid gland

Right common carotid a.

Thyrocervical trunk

Subclavian a.

Brachiocephalic trunk

Inferior thyroid vv.

Clavicle

Parotid gland

Mylohyoid

Digastric, anterior belly

Sternohyoid

Thyrohyoid

Superior thyroid a.

Superior thyroid v.

Middle scalene

Trapezius

Accessory n.

Anterior scalene

Brachial plexus

Vagus n.

Phrenic n.

Transverse cervical a.

Middle thyroid v.

Left recurrent laryngeal n.

Left common carotid a.

Fig. 37.34 Carotid triangle

Right lateral view. Internal jugular and facial veins removed.

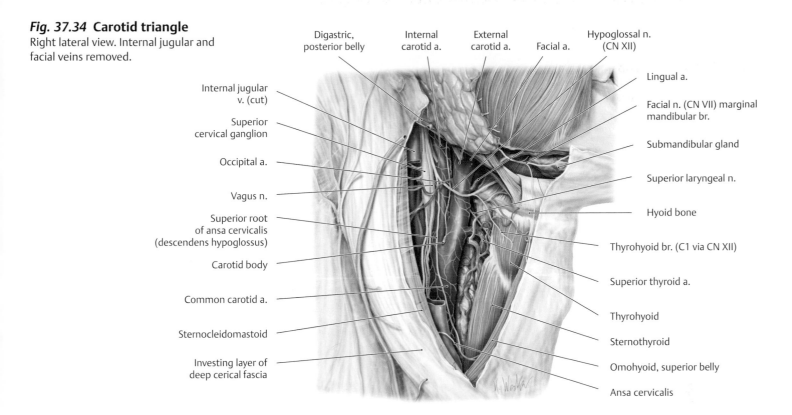

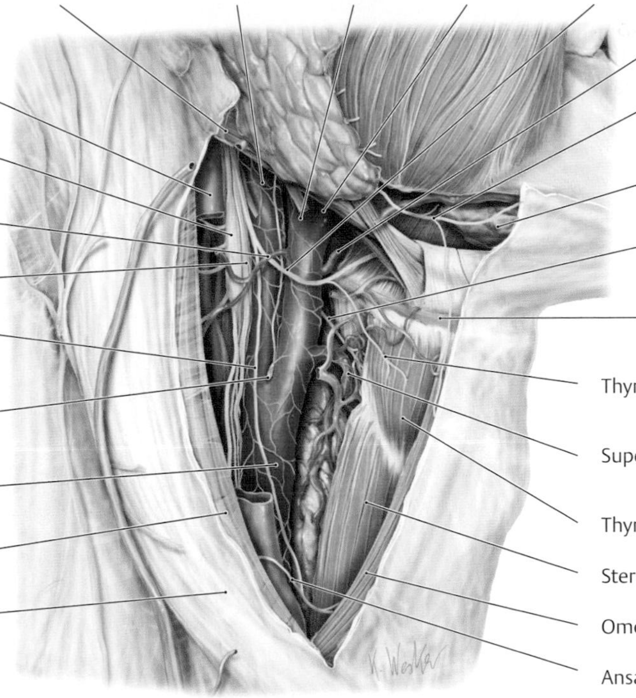
Digastric, posterior belly
Internal carotid a.
External carotid a.
Facial a.
Hypoglossal n. (CN XII)
Lingual a.
Facial n. (CN VII) marginal mandibular br.
Submandibular gland
Superior laryngeal n.
Hyoid bone
Thyrohyoid br. (C1 via CN XII)
Superior thyroid a.
Thyrohyoid
Sternothyroid
Omohyoid, superior belly
Ansa cervicalis
Internal jugular v. (cut)
Superior cervical ganglion
Occipital a.
Vagus n.
Superior root of ansa cervicalis (descendens hypoglossus)
Carotid body
Common carotid a.
Sternocleidomastoid
Investing layer of deep cerical fascia

Fig. 37.35 Deep lateral cervical region

Right lateral view with sternocleidomastoid windowed.

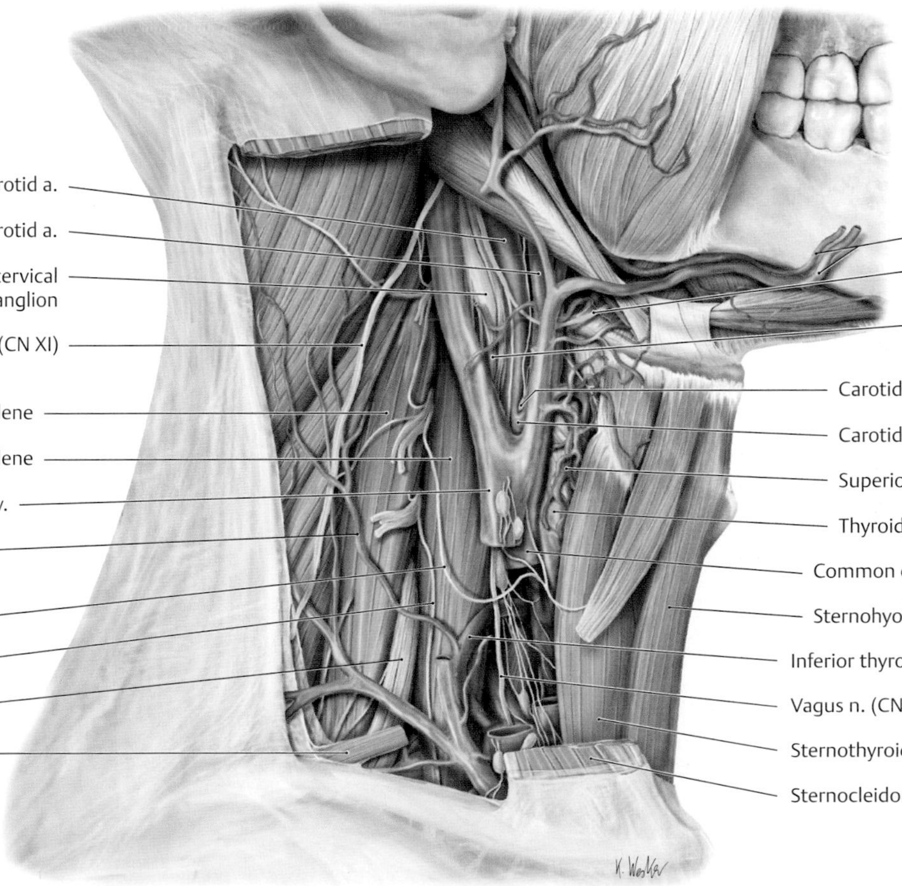
Internal carotid a.
External carotid a.
Superior cervical ganglion
Accessory n. (CN XI)
Middle scalene
Anterior scalene
Internal jugular v.
Superficial cervical a.
Ansa cervicalis
Phrenic n.
Brachial plexus
Omohyoid, inferior belly
Facial a. and v.
Hypoglossal n. (CN XII)
Sympathetic trunk
Carotid body
Carotid bifurcation
Superior thyroid a.
Thyroid gland
Common carotid a.
Sternohyoid
Inferior thyroid a.
Vagus n. (CN X)
Sternothyroid
Sternocleidomastoid

Topography of the Lateral Cervical Region

***Fig. 37.36* Lateral cervical region**
Right lateral view. The contents of the deep lateral cervical region are found in **Fig. 37.34.**

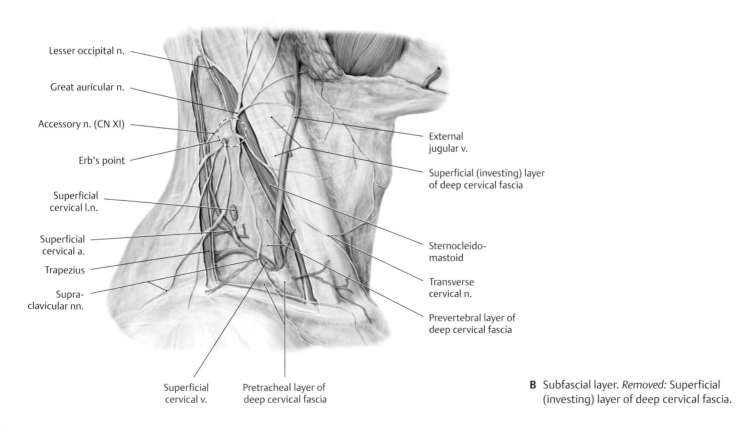

Parotid gland — Facial n. (CN VII), cervical br. — Masseter

Lesser occipital n.

Great auricular n.

Erb's point

Lateral supra-clavicular nn.

Trapezius, anterior border

External jugular v.

Sternocleido-mastoid, posterior border

Transverse cervical and CN VII anastomosis

Superficial (investing) layer of deep cervical fascia

Transverse cervical n.

Clavicle

A Subcutaneous layer.

Intermediate supra-clavicular nn.

Medial supra-clavicular nn.

Lesser occipital n.

Great auricular n.

Accessory n. (CN XI)

Erb's point

Superficial cervical l.n.

Superficial cervical a.

Trapezius

Supra-clavicular nn.

External jugular v.

Superficial (investing) layer of deep cervical fascia

Sternocleido-mastoid

Transverse cervical n.

Prevertebral layer of deep cervical fascia

Superficial cervical v.

Pretracheal layer of deep cervical fascia

B Subfascial layer. *Removed:* Superficial (investing) layer of deep cervical fascia.

538

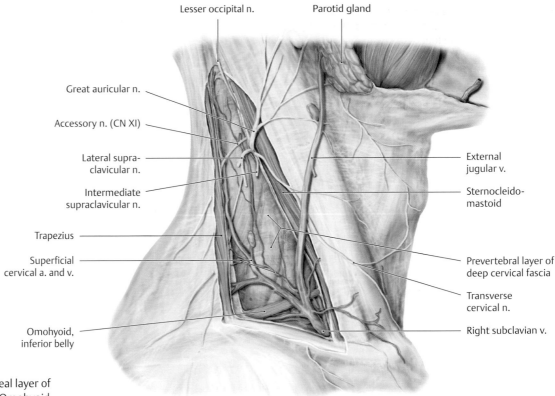

Lesser occipital n.

Parotid gland

Great auricular n.

Accessory n. (CN XI)

Lateral supra-
clavicular n.

Intermediate
supraclavicular n.

Trapezius

Superficial
cervical a. and v.

Omohyoid,
inferior belly

External
jugular v.

Sternocleido-
mastoid

Prevertebral layer of
deep cervical fascia

Transverse
cervical n.

Right subclavian v.

C Deep layer. *Removed:* Pretracheal layer of
deep cervical fascia. *Revealed:* Omohyoid,
omoclavicular (subclavian) triangle.

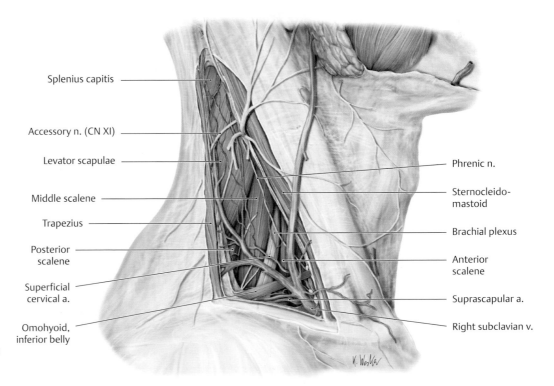

Splenius capitis

Accessory n. (CN XI)

Levator scapulae

Middle scalene

Trapezius

Posterior
scalene

Superficial
cervical a.

Omohyoid,
inferior belly

Phrenic n.

Sternocleido-
mastoid

Brachial plexus

Anterior
scalene

Suprascapular a.

Right subclavian v.

D Deepest layer. *Removed:* Prevertebral
layer of deep cervical fascia. *Revealed:*
Muscular floor of posterior triangle,
brachial plexus, and phrenic nerve.

Topography of the Posterior Cervical Region

Fig. 37.37 Occipital and posterior cervical regions
Posterior view. Subcutaneous layer (left), subfascial layer (right). The occiput is technically a region of the head, but it is included here due to the continuity of the vessels and nerves from the neck. *Removed on right side:* Investing layer of deep cervical fascia.

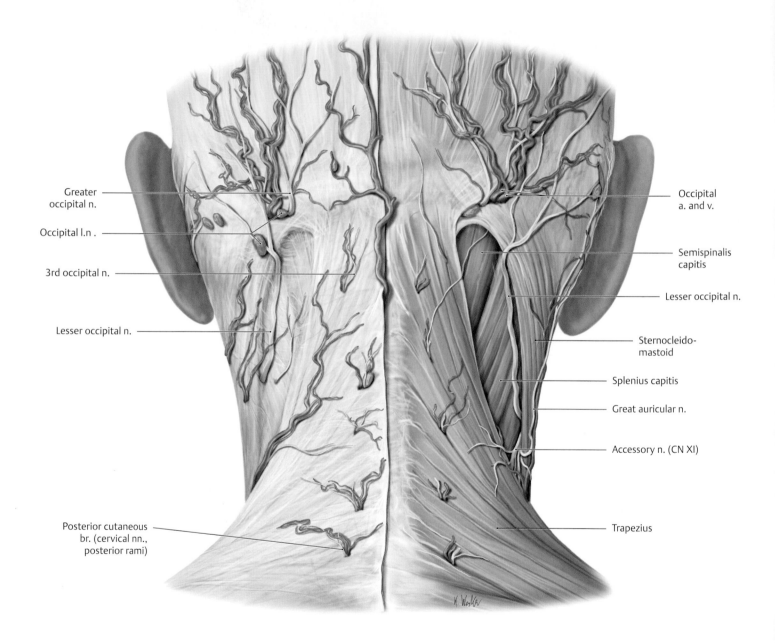

Greater occipital n.

Occipital l.n .

3rd occipital n.

Lesser occipital n.

Posterior cutaneous br. (cervical nn., posterior rami)

Occipital a. and v.

Semispinalis capitis

Lesser occipital n.

Sternocleido-mastoid

Splenius capitis

Great auricular n.

Accessory n. (CN XI)

Trapezius

Fig. 37.38 **Suboccipital triangle**

Right side, posterior view, windowed. The suboccipital triangle is bounded by the suboccipital muscles (rectus capitis posterior major and obliquus capitis superior and inferior) and contains the vertebral artery. The left and right vertebral arteries pass through the atlanto-occipital membrane and combine to form the basilar artery.

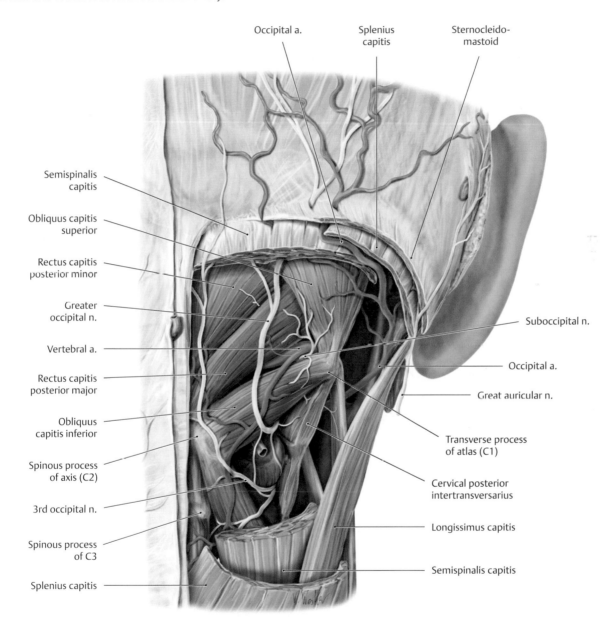

Occipital a.

Splenius capitis

Sternocleido-mastoid

Semispinalis capitis

Obliquus capitis superior

Rectus capitis posterior minor

Greater occipital n.

Vertebral a.

Rectus capitis posterior major

Obliquus capitis inferior

Spinous process of axis (C2)

3rd occipital n.

Spinous process of C3

Splenius capitis

Suboccipital n.

Occipital a.

Great auricular n.

Transverse process of atlas (C1)

Cervical posterior intertransversarius

Longissimus capitis

Semispinalis capitis

38 Bones of the Head
Anterior & Lateral Skull

Fig. 38.1 Lateral skull
Left lateral view.

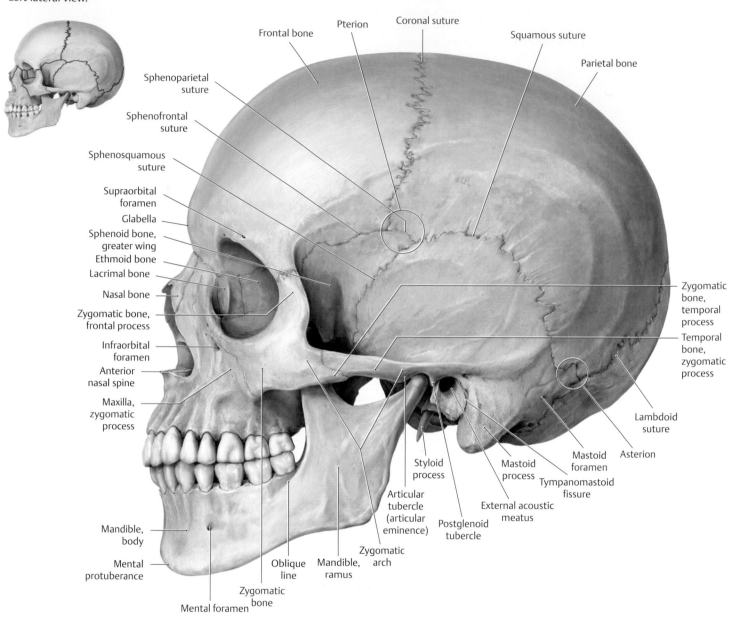

Labels (clockwise from top):
- Frontal bone
- Pterion
- Coronal suture
- Squamous suture
- Parietal bone
- Sphenoparietal suture
- Sphenofrontal suture
- Sphenosquamous suture
- Supraorbital foramen
- Glabella
- Sphenoid bone, greater wing
- Ethmoid bone
- Lacrimal bone
- Nasal bone
- Zygomatic bone, frontal process
- Infraorbital foramen
- Anterior nasal spine
- Maxilla, zygomatic process
- Mandible, body
- Mental protuberance
- Mental foramen
- Zygomatic bone
- Oblique line
- Mandible, ramus
- Zygomatic arch
- Articular tubercle (articular eminence)
- Styloid process
- Postglenoid tubercle
- External acoustic meatus
- Mastoid process
- Tympanomastoid fissure
- Mastoid foramen
- Asterion
- Lambdoid suture
- Temporal bone, zygomatic process
- Zygomatic bone, temporal process

Table 38.1   Bones of the skull

The skull is subdivided into the neurocranium (gray) and viscerocranium (orange). The neurocranium protects the brain, while the viscerocranium houses and protects the facial regions.

Neurocranium	Viscerocranium	
• Ethmoid bone (cribriform plate)*	• Ethmoid bone	• Mandible
• Frontal bone	• Hyoid bone	• Maxilla
• Occipital bone	• Inferior nasal concha	• Nasal bone
• Parietal bone	• Lacrimal bone	• Palatine bone
• Sphenoid bone	• Sphenoid bone (pterygoid process)	
• Temporal bone (petrous and squamous parts)	• Temporal bone	
	• Vomer	

*Most of the ethmoid bone is in the viscerocranium; most of the sphenoid bone is in the neurocranium. The temporal bone is divided between the two.

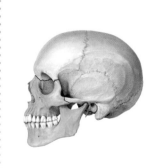

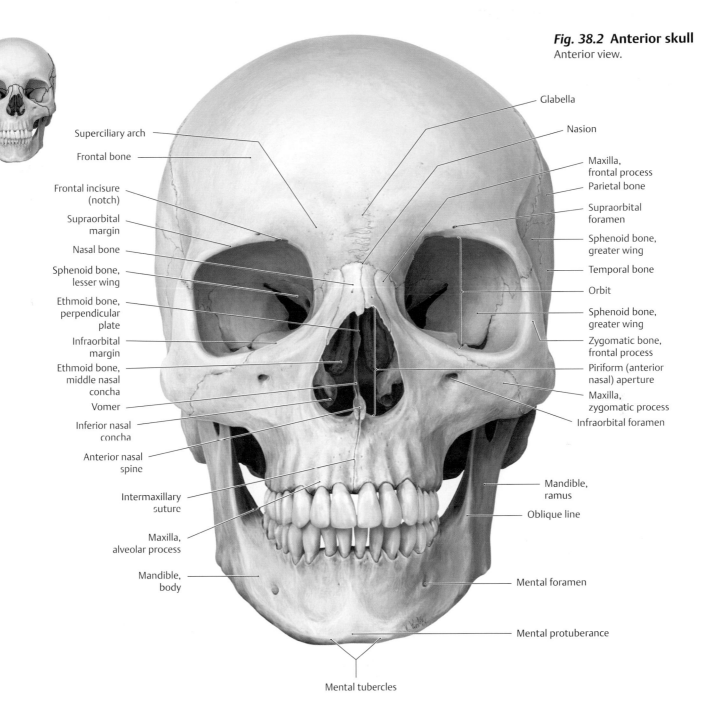

Fig. 38.2 Anterior skull
Anterior view.

Superciliary arch

Frontal bone

Frontal incisure (notch)

Supraorbital margin

Nasal bone

Sphenoid bone, lesser wing

Ethmoid bone, perpendicular plate

Infraorbital margin

Ethmoid bone, middle nasal concha

Vomer

Inferior nasal concha

Anterior nasal spine

Intermaxillary suture

Maxilla, alveolar process

Mandible, body

Glabella

Nasion

Maxilla, frontal process

Parietal bone

Supraorbital foramen

Sphenoid bone, greater wing

Temporal bone

Orbit

Sphenoid bone, greater wing

Zygomatic bone, frontal process

Piriform (anterior nasal) aperture

Maxilla, zygomatic process

Infraorbital foramen

Mandible, ramus

Oblique line

Mental foramen

Mental protuberance

Mental tubercles

Clinical box 38.1

Fractures of the face
The framelike construction of the facial skeleton leads to characteristic patterns for fracture lines (classified as Le Fort I, II, and III fractures).

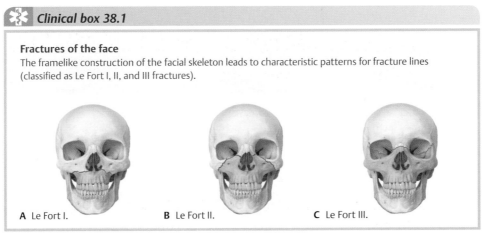

A Le Fort I.

B Le Fort II.

C Le Fort III.

Posterior Skull & Calvaria

Fig. 38.3 Posterior skull
Posterior view.

Parietal foramina

Lambda

Sagittal suture

Parietal bone

Parietal eminence

Lambdoid suture

Occipital bone

Temporal bone, squamous part

Supreme nuchal line

Temporal bone, petrous part

Asterion

External occipital protuberance (inion)

Superior nuchal line

Mastoid foramina

Median nuchal line (external occipital crest)

Mastoid notch

Inferior nuchal line

Temporal bone, mastoid process

Vomer

Temporal bone, styloid process

Occipital condyle

Sphenoid bone, pterygoid process

Palatine bone

Mandibular foramen

Mandible, ramus

Mylohyoid groove

Maxilla, palatine process

Incisive foramen

Mandible, body

Submandibular fossa

Mylohyoid line

Digastric fossa

Genial (mental) spines

✳ *Clinical box 38.2*

Cranial Fontanelles

In the neonate, there are areas between still-growing cranial bones not occupied by bone: the fontanelles. While these regions close at different times, they have clinical implications. The *posterior fontanelle* provides a reference point for describing the position of the fetal head during childbirth, and the *anterior fontanelle* provides a potential access site for drawing cerebrospinal fluid in infants (e.g., in suspected meningitis).

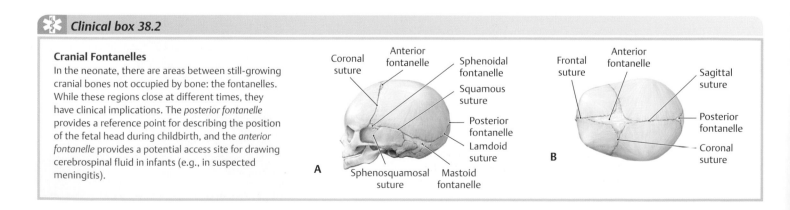

Coronal suture
Anterior fontanelle
Sphenoidal fontanelle
Squamous suture
Posterior fontanelle
Lamdoid suture
Mastoid fontanelle
Sphenosquamosal suture

A

Frontal suture
Anterior fontanelle
Sagittal suture
Posterior fontanelle
Coronal suture

B

Fig. 38.4 Calvaria

Fig. 38.5 Structure of the calvaria
Cross section.

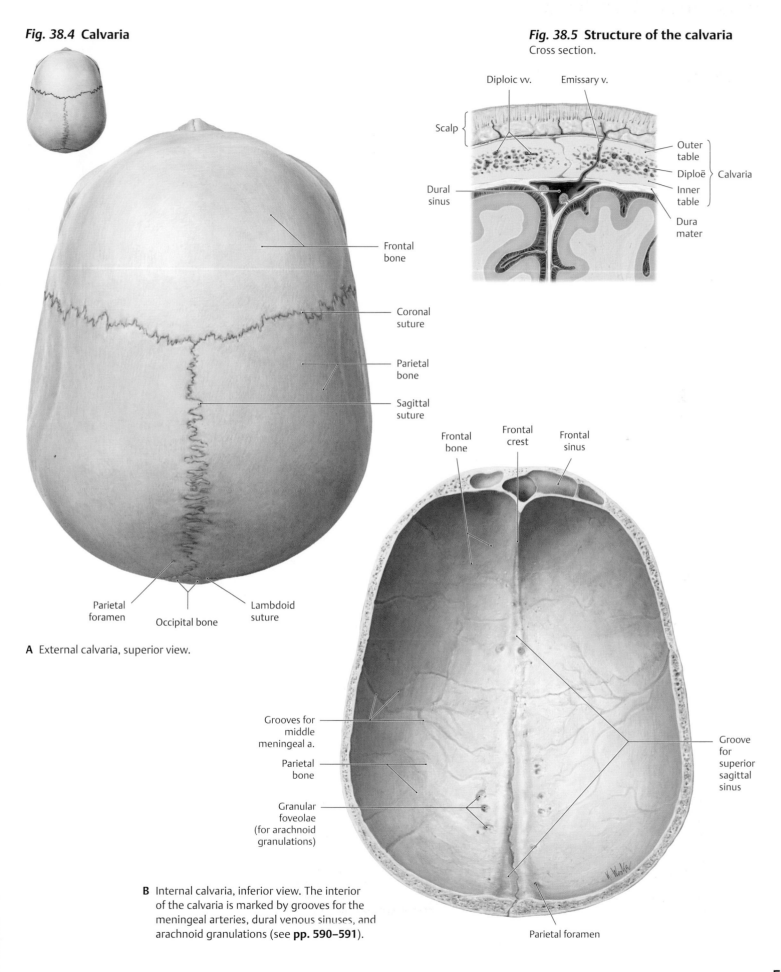

A External calvaria, superior view.

B Internal calvaria, inferior view. The interior of the calvaria is marked by grooves for the meningeal arteries, dural venous sinuses, and arachnoid granulations (see **pp. 590–591**).

Fig. 38.6 **Base of the skull: Exterior**
Inferior view. *Revealed:* Foramina and canals for blood vessels (see **p. 582**) and cranial nerves. *Note:* This view allows visual access into the posterior region of the nasal cavity.

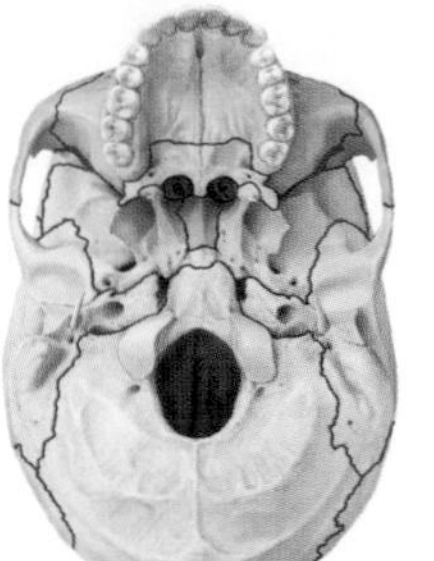

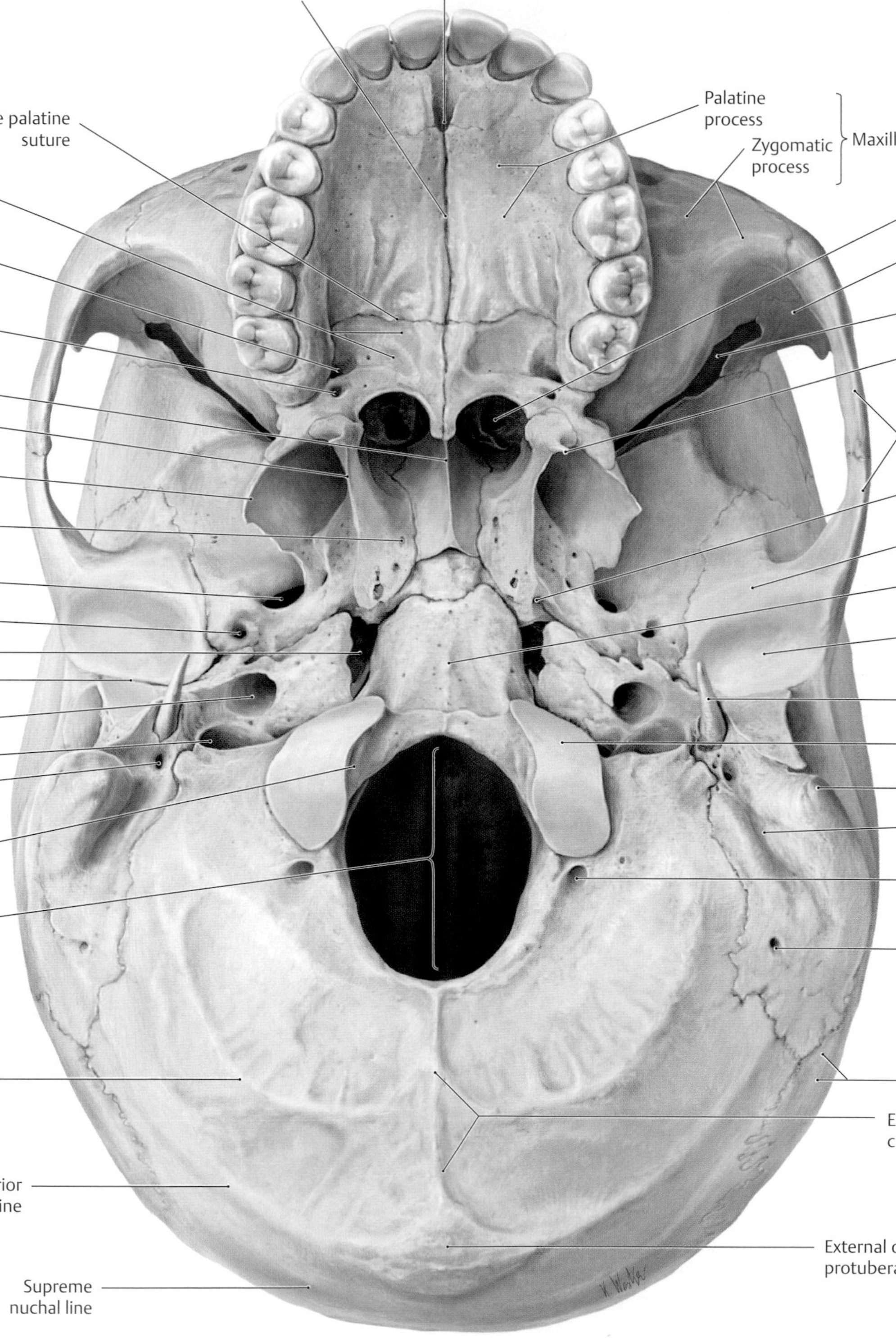

Median palatine suture

Incisive foramen

Transverse palatine suture

Palatine bone

Greater palatine foramen

Lesser palatine foramen

Vomer

Pterygoid process — Medial plate / Lateral plate

Palatovaginal (pharyngeal) canal

Foramen ovale

Foramen spinosum

Foramen lacerum

Petrotympanic fissure

Carotid canal

Jugular foramen

Stylomastoid foramen

Hypoglossal canal

Foramen magnum

Inferior nuchal line

Superior nuchal line

Supreme nuchal line

Palatine process

Zygomatic process — Maxilla

Choana

Zygomatic bone, temporal surface

Inferior orbital fissure

Hamulus (of medial pterygoid plate)

Zygomatic arch

Fossa of pterygoid canal

Articular tubercle

Pharyngeal tubercle

Mandibular fossa

Styloid process

Occipital condyle

Mastoid process

Mastoid notch (for digastric belly)

Condylar canal

Mastoid foramen

Parietal bone

External occipital crest

External occipital protuberance (inion)

Fig. 38.7 **Cranial fossae**

The interior of the skull base consists of three successive fossae that become progressively deeper in the frontal-to-occipital direction.

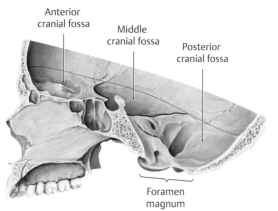

A Midsagittal section, left lateral view.

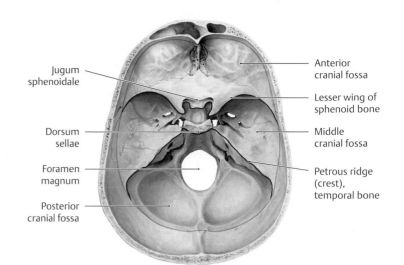

B Superior view of opened skull.

Fig. 38.8 **Base of the skull: Interior**

Superior view.

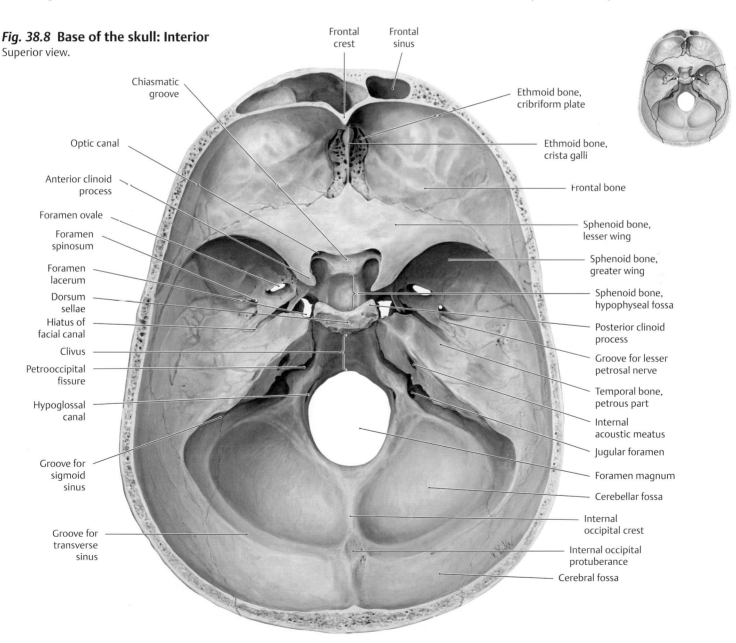

Neurovascular Pathways Exiting or Entering the Cranial Cavity

Fig. 38.9 Summary of the neurovascular structures exiting or entering the cranial cavity

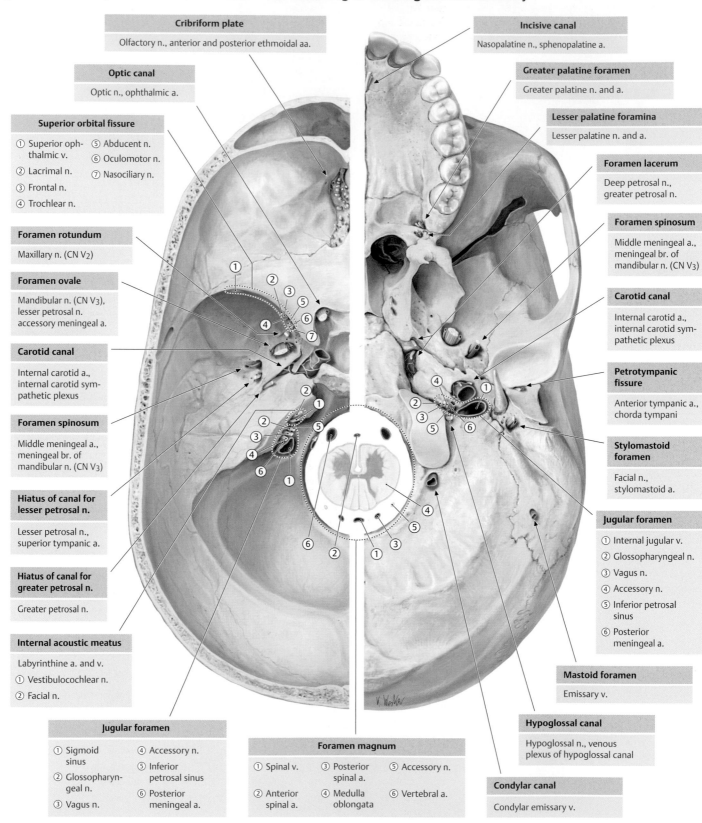

Cribriform plate

Olfactory n., anterior and posterior ethmoidal aa.

Incisive canal

Nasopalatine n., sphenopalatine a.

Optic canal

Optic n., ophthalmic a.

Greater palatine foramen

Greater palatine n. and a.

Superior orbital fissure

① Superior oph-   ⑤ Abducent n.
   thalmic v.   ⑥ Oculomotor n.
② Lacrimal n.   ⑦ Nasociliary n.
③ Frontal n.
④ Trochlear n.

Lesser palatine foramina

Lesser palatine n. and a.

Foramen lacerum

Deep petrosal n., greater petrosal n.

Foramen rotundum

Maxillary n. (CN V₂)

Foramen spinosum

Middle meningeal a., meningeal br. of mandibular n. (CN V₃)

Foramen ovale

Mandibular n. (CN V₃), lesser petrosal n. accessory meningeal a.

Carotid canal

Internal carotid a., internal carotid sympathetic plexus

Carotid canal

Internal carotid a., internal carotid sympathetic plexus

Petrotympanic fissure

Anterior tympanic a., chorda tympani

Foramen spinosum

Middle meningeal a., meningeal br. of mandibular n. (CN V₃)

Stylomastoid foramen

Facial n., stylomastoid a.

Hiatus of canal for lesser petrosal n.

Lesser petrosal n., superior tympanic a.

Jugular foramen

① Internal jugular v.
② Glossopharyngeal n.
③ Vagus n.
④ Accessory n.
⑤ Inferior petrosal sinus
⑥ Posterior meningeal a.

Hiatus of canal for greater petrosal n.

Greater petrosal n.

Internal acoustic meatus

Labyrinthine a. and v.
① Vestibulocochlear n.
② Facial n.

Mastoid foramen

Emissary v.

Hypoglossal canal

Hypoglossal n., venous plexus of hypoglossal canal

Condylar canal

Condylar emissary v.

Jugular foramen

① Sigmoid sinus   ④ Accessory n.
② Glossopharyn-   ⑤ Inferior petrosal sinus
   geal n.   ⑥ Posterior meningeal a.
③ Vagus n.

Foramen magnum

① Spinal v.   ③ Posterior spinal a.   ⑤ Accessory n.
② Anterior spinal a.   ④ Medulla oblongata   ⑥ Vertebral a.

A Cranial cavity (interior of skull base), left side, superior view.

B Exterior of skull base, left side, inferior view

Fig. 38.10 **Cranial nerves exiting the cranial cavity**

Cranial cavity (interior of skull base), right side, superior view. *Removed:* Brain and tentorium cerebelli. The ends of the cranial nerves have been cut to reveal the fissures, fossae, or dural cave where they pass through the cranial fossa.

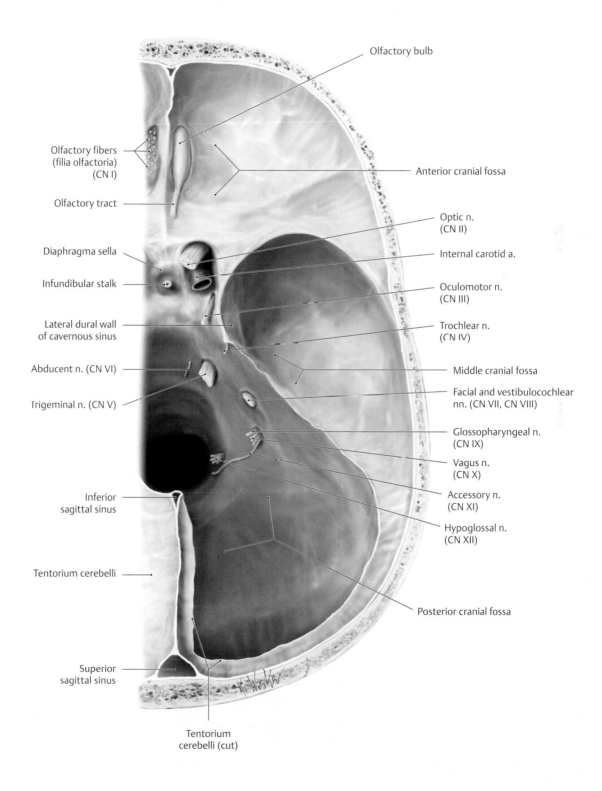

Olfactory bulb

Olfactory fibers (filia olfactoria) (CN I)

Anterior cranial fossa

Olfactory tract

Optic n. (CN II)

Diaphragma sella

Internal carotid a.

Infundibular stalk

Oculomotor n. (CN III)

Lateral dural wall of cavernous sinus

Trochlear n. (CN IV)

Abducent n. (CN VI)

Middle cranial fossa

Trigeminal n. (CN V)

Facial and vestibulocochlear nn. (CN VII, CN VIII)

Glossopharyngeal n. (CN IX)

Vagus n. (CN X)

Accessory n. (CN XI)

Inferior sagittal sinus

Hypoglossal n. (CN XII)

Tentorium cerebelli

Posterior cranial fossa

Superior sagittal sinus

Tentorium cerebelli (cut)

Ethmoid & Sphenoid Bones

The structurally complex ethmoid and sphenoid bones are shown here in isolation. The other bones of the skull are shown in their respective regions: orbit (see **pp. 602–603**), nasal cavity (see **pp. 616–617**), oral cavity (see **pp. 636–637**), and ear (see **pp. 624–625**).

Fig. 38.11 Ethmoid bone

The ethmoid bone is the central bone of the nose and paranasal air sinuses (see **pp. 616–619**).

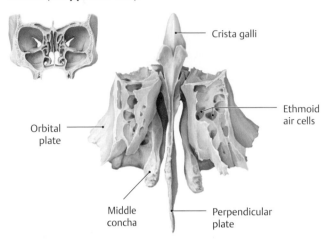

Crista galli

Ethmoid air cells

Orbital plate

Middle concha

Perpendicular plate

A Anterior view.

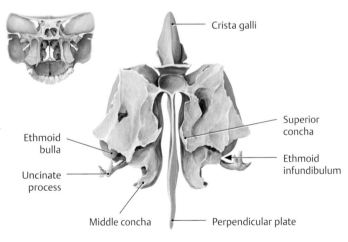

Crista galli

Ethmoid bulla

Uncinate process

Middle concha

Superior concha

Ethmoid infundibulum

Perpendicular plate

C Posterior view.

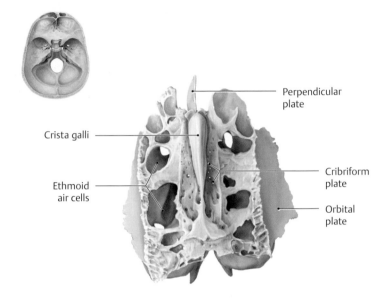

Perpendicular plate

Crista galli

Ethmoid air cells

Cribriform plate

Orbital plate

B Superior view.

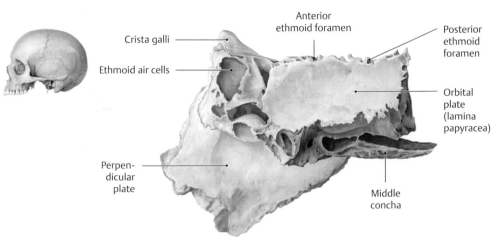

Crista galli

Ethmoid air cells

Anterior ethmoid foramen

Posterior ethmoid foramen

Orbital plate (lamina papyracea)

Perpendicular plate

Middle concha

D Left lateral view.

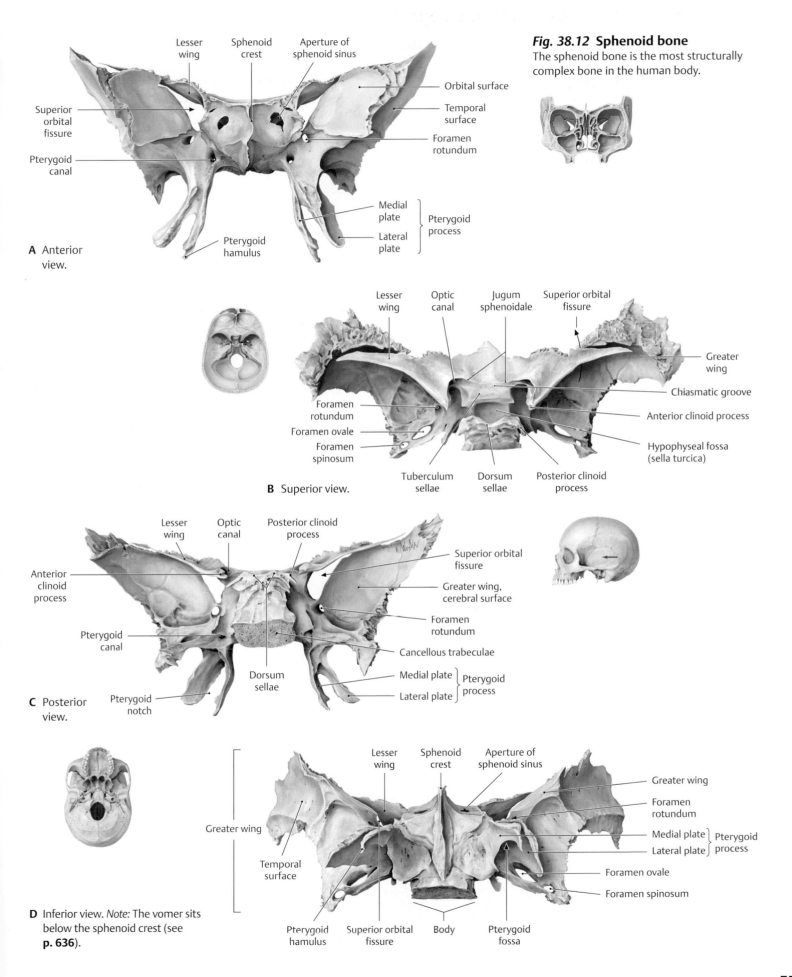

A Anterior view.

Lesser wing
Sphenoid crest
Aperture of sphenoid sinus
Superior orbital fissure
Pterygoid canal
Pterygoid hamulus
Orbital surface
Temporal surface
Foramen rotundum
Medial plate
Lateral plate
Pterygoid process

Fig. 38.12 **Sphenoid bone**
The sphenoid bone is the most structurally complex bone in the human body.

B Superior view.

Lesser wing
Optic canal
Jugum sphenoidale
Superior orbital fissure
Foramen rotundum
Foramen ovale
Foramen spinosum
Tuberculum sellae
Dorsum sellae
Posterior clinoid process
Greater wing
Chiasmatic groove
Anterior clinoid process
Hypophyseal fossa (sella turcica)

C Posterior view.

Lesser wing
Optic canal
Posterior clinoid process
Anterior clinoid process
Pterygoid canal
Dorsum sellae
Pterygoid notch
Superior orbital fissure
Greater wing, cerebral surface
Foramen rotundum
Cancellous trabeculae
Medial plate
Lateral plate
Pterygoid process

D Inferior view. *Note:* The vomer sits below the sphenoid crest (see **p. 636**).

Lesser wing
Sphenoid crest
Aperture of sphenoid sinus
Greater wing
Temporal surface
Greater wing
Foramen rotundum
Medial plate
Lateral plate
Pterygoid process
Foramen ovale
Foramen spinosum
Pterygoid hamulus
Superior orbital fissure
Body
Pterygoid fossa

39 Muscles of the Skull & Face

Muscles of Facial Expression & of Mastication

The muscles of the skull and face are divided into two groups. The muscles of facial expression make up the superficial muscle layer in the face. The muscles of mastication are responsible for the movement of the mandible during mastication (chewing).

Fig. 39.1 **Muscles of facial expression**

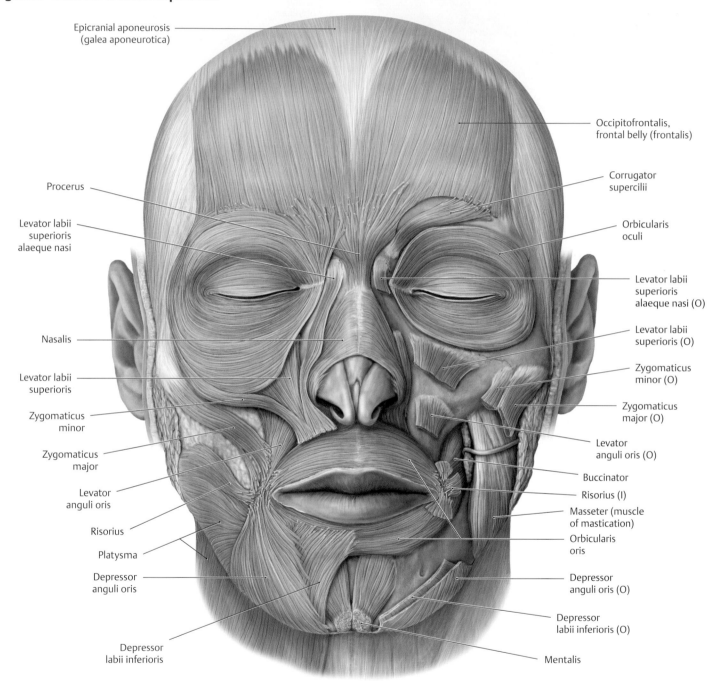

Epicranial aponeurosis (galea aponeurotica)

Occipitofrontalis, frontal belly (frontalis)

Procerus

Corrugator supercilii

Levator labii superioris alaeque nasi

Orbicularis oculi

Levator labii superioris alaeque nasi (O)

Nasalis

Levator labii superioris (O)

Levator labii superioris

Zygomaticus minor (O)

Zygomaticus minor

Zygomaticus major (O)

Zygomaticus major

Levator anguli oris (O)

Levator anguli oris

Buccinator

Risorius

Risorius (I)

Platysma

Masseter (muscle of mastication)

Depressor anguli oris

Orbicularis oris

Depressor labii inferioris

Depressor anguli oris (O)

Depressor labii inferioris (O)

Mentalis

A Anterior view. Muscle origins (O) and insertions (I) indicated on left side of face.

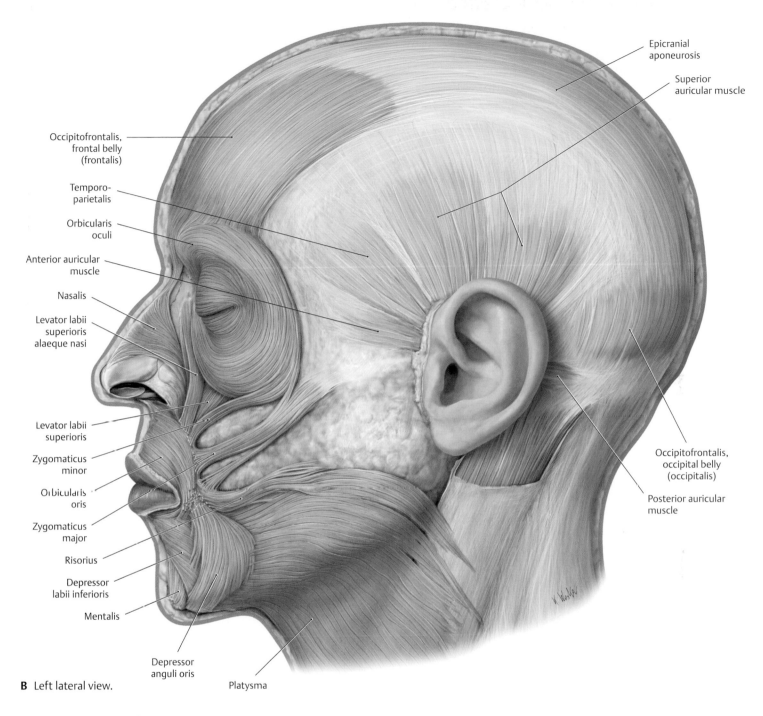

Epicranial aponeurosis

Superior auricular muscle

Occipitofrontalis, frontal belly (frontalis)

Temporo-parietalis

Orbicularis oculi

Anterior auricular muscle

Nasalis

Levator labii superioris alaeque nasi

Levator labii superioris

Zygomaticus minor

Orbicularis oris

Zygomaticus major

Risorius

Depressor labii inferioris

Mentalis

Occipitofrontalis, occipital belly (occipitalis)

Posterior auricular muscle

Depressor anguli oris

Platysma

B Left lateral view.

Fig. 39.2 **Muscles of mastication**
Left lateral view.

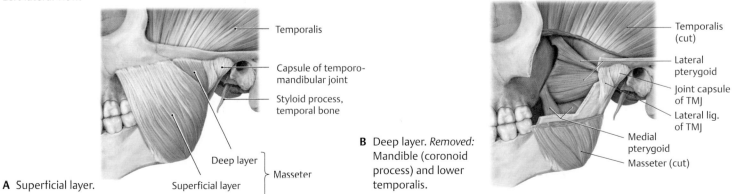

Temporalis

Capsule of temporo-mandibular joint

Styloid process, temporal bone

Deep layer

Superficial layer

Masseter

A Superficial layer.

B Deep layer. *Removed:* Mandible (coronoid process) and lower temporalis.

Temporalis (cut)

Lateral pterygoid

Joint capsule of TMJ

Lateral lig. of TMJ

Medial pterygoid

Masseter (cut)

Muscle Origins & Insertions on the Skull

Fig. 39.3 Lateral skull: Origins and insertions

Left lateral view. Muscle origins are shown in red, insertions in blue. *Note*: There are generally no bony insertions for the muscles of facial expression. These muscles insert into skin and other muscles of facial expression.

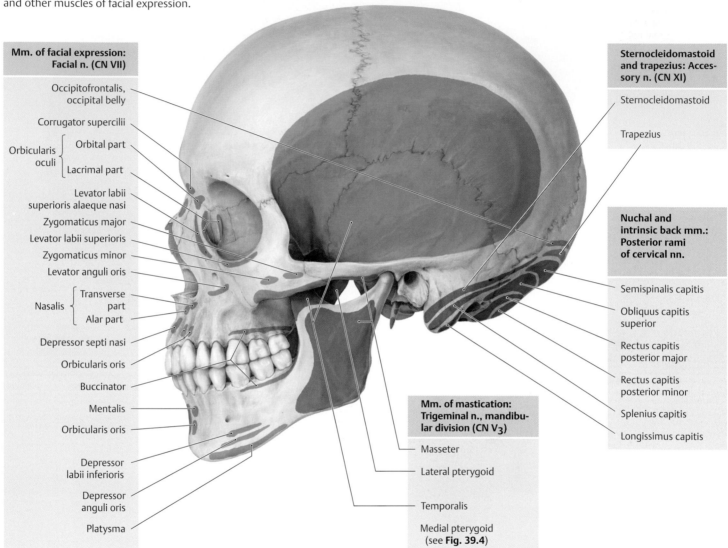

Mm. of facial expression: Facial n. (CN VII)

- Occipitofrontalis, occipital belly
- Corrugator supercilii
- Orbicularis oculi
  - Orbital part
  - Lacrimal part
- Levator labii superioris alaeque nasi
- Zygomaticus major
- Levator labii superioris
- Zygomaticus minor
- Levator anguli oris
- Nasalis
  - Transverse part
  - Alar part
- Depressor septi nasi
- Orbicularis oris
- Buccinator
- Mentalis
- Orbicularis oris
- Depressor labii inferioris
- Depressor anguli oris
- Platysma

Sternocleidomastoid and trapezius: Accessory n. (CN XI)

- Sternocleidomastoid
- Trapezius

Nuchal and intrinsic back mm.: Posterior rami of cervical nn.

- Semispinalis capitis
- Obliquus capitis superior
- Rectus capitis posterior major
- Rectus capitis posterior minor
- Splenius capitis
- Longissimus capitis

Mm. of mastication: Trigeminal n., mandibular division (CN V₃)

- Masseter
- Lateral pterygoid
- Temporalis
- Medial pterygoid (see **Fig. 39.4**)

Fig. 39.4 Mandible: Origins and insertions

Medial view of right hemimandible (inner surface). Muscle origins are shown in red, insertions in blue.

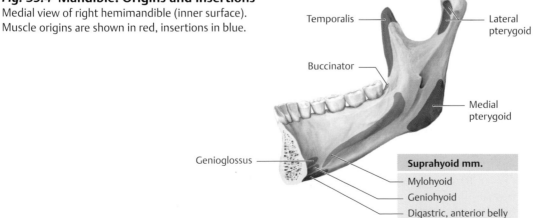

- Temporalis
- Lateral pterygoid
- Buccinator
- Medial pterygoid
- Genioglossus

Suprahyoid mm.

- Mylohyoid
- Geniohyoid
- Digastric, anterior belly

Fig. 39.5 Skull base: Origins and insertions

Inferior view of external skull.
Muscle origins are shown in red, insertions in blue.

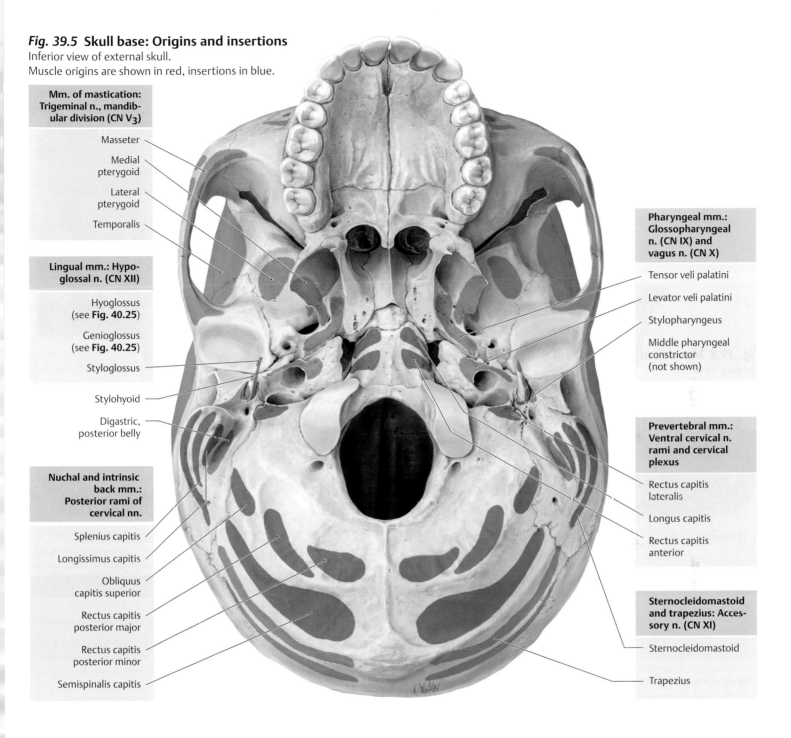

Mm. of mastication: Trigeminal n., mandibular division (CN V₃)

Masseter

Medial pterygoid

Lateral pterygoid

Temporalis

Lingual mm.: Hypoglossal n. (CN XII)

Hyoglossus (see **Fig. 40.25**)

Genioglossus (see **Fig. 40.25**)

Styloglossus

Stylohyoid

Digastric, posterior belly

Nuchal and intrinsic back mm.: Posterior rami of cervical nn.

Splenius capitis

Longissimus capitis

Obliquus capitis superior

Rectus capitis posterior major

Rectus capitis posterior minor

Semispinalis capitis

Pharyngeal mm.: Glossopharyngeal n. (CN IX) and vagus n. (CN X)

Tensor veli palatini

Levator veli palatini

Stylopharyngeus

Middle pharyngeal constrictor (not shown)

Prevertebral mm.: Ventral cervical n. rami and cervical plexus

Rectus capitis lateralis

Longus capitis

Rectus capitis anterior

Sternocleidomastoid and trapezius: Accessory n. (CN XI)

Sternocleidomastoid

Trapezius

Fig. 39.6 Hyoid bone: Origins and insertions

The larynx is suspended from the hyoid bone, primarily by the thyrohyoid membrane. The hyoid bone is the site for attachment for the suprahyoid and infrahyoid muscles. Muscle insertions are shown in blue.

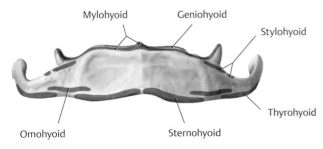

Mylohyoid

Geniohyoid

Stylohyoid

Thyrohyoid

Omohyoid

Sternohyoid

A Anterior view.

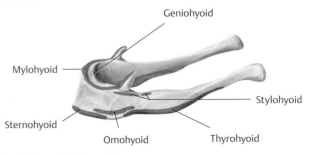

Geniohyoid

Mylohyoid

Stylohyoid

Sternohyoid

Omohyoid

Thyrohyoid

B Oblique left lateral view.

Muscle Facts (II)

The muscles of mastication are located at various depths in the parotid and infratemporal regions of the face. They attach to the mandible and receive their motor innervation from the mandibular division of the trigeminal nerve (CN V₃). The muscles of the oral floor that aid in opening the mouth are found on in **Table 37.3** on **p. 516**.

Table 39.3	Muscles of mastication: Masseter and temporalis			
Muscle	**Origin**	**Insertion**	**Innervation**	**Action**
① Masseter	Superficial layer: zygomatic arch (anterior two thirds)	Mandibular angle (masseteric tuberosity)	Mandibular n. (CN V₃) via masseteric n.	Elevates (entire muscle) and protrudes (superficial fibers) the mandible
	Deep layer: zygomatic arch (posterior one third)			
② Temporalis	Temporal fossa (inferior temporal line)	Coronoid process of mandible (apex and medial surface)	Mandibular n. (CN V₃) via deep temporal nn.	*Vertical fibers:* Elevate mandible *Horizontal fibers:* Retract (retrude) mandible *Unilateral:* Lateral movement of mandible (chewing)

Fig. 39.11 Masseter muscle
Left lateral view.

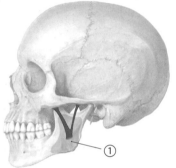

A Schematic.

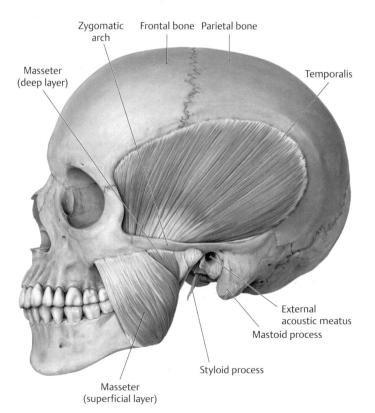

B Masseter with temporalis muscle.

Labels: Zygomatic arch — Frontal bone — Parietal bone — Temporalis — Masseter (deep layer) — External acoustic meatus — Mastoid process — Styloid process — Masseter (superficial layer)

Fig. 39.12 Temporalis muscle
Left lateral view.

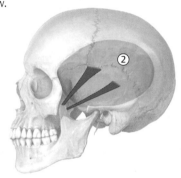

A Schematic.

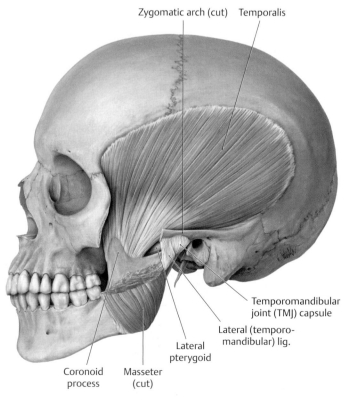

B Temporalis muscle. *Removed:* Masseter and zygomatic arch.

Labels: Zygomatic arch (cut) — Temporalis — Temporomandibular joint (TMJ) capsule — Lateral (temporomandibular) lig. — Lateral pterygoid — Masseter (cut) — Coronoid process

Table 39.4	Muscles of mastication: Pterygoid muscles				
Muscle		Origin	Insertion	Innervation	Action
Lateral pterygoid	③ Superior head	Greater wing of sphenoid bone (infratemporal crest)	Temporomandibular joint (articular disk)	Mandibular n. (CN V₃) via lateral pterygoid n.	*Bilateral:* Protrudes mandible (pulls articular disk forward) *Unilateral:* Lateral movements of mandible (chewing)
	④ Inferior head	Lateral pterygoid plate (lateral surface)	Mandible (condylar process)		
Medial pterygoid	⑤ Superficial head	Maxilla (tuberosity)	Pterygoid tuberosity on medial surface of the mandibular angle	Mandibular n. (CN V₃) via medial pterygoid n.	*Bilateral:* Elevates mandible with masseter; contributes to protrusion. *Unilateral:* small grinding movements.
	⑥ Deep head	Medial surface of lateral pterygoid plate and pterygoid fossa			

Fig. 39.13 Lateral pterygoid muscle
Left lateral view.

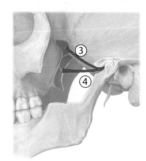

A Schematic.

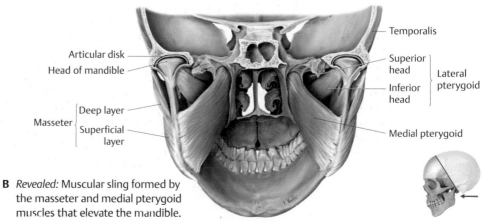

B Left lateral pterygoid muscle. *Removed:* Coronoid process and part of ramus of mandible.

Fig. 39.14 Medial pterygoid muscle
Left lateral view.

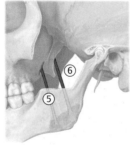

A Schematic.

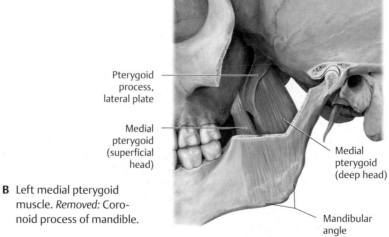

B Left medial pterygoid muscle. *Removed:* Coronoid process of mandible.

Fig. 39.15 Masticatory muscle sling
Oblique posterior view.

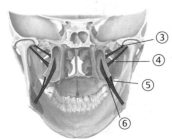

A Schematic.

B *Revealed:* Muscular sling formed by the masseter and medial pterygoid muscles that elevate the mandible.

40 Cranial Nerves

Cranial Nerves: Overview

Fig. 40.1 Cranial nerves

Inferior (basal) view. The 12 pairs of cranial nerves (CN) are numbered according to the order of their emergence from the brainstem. *Note:* The sensory and motor fibers of the cranial nerves enter and exit the brainstem at the same sites (in contrast to spinal nerves, whose sensory and motor fibers enter and leave through posterior and anterior roots, respectively). For fiber color code, see **Table 40.1.**

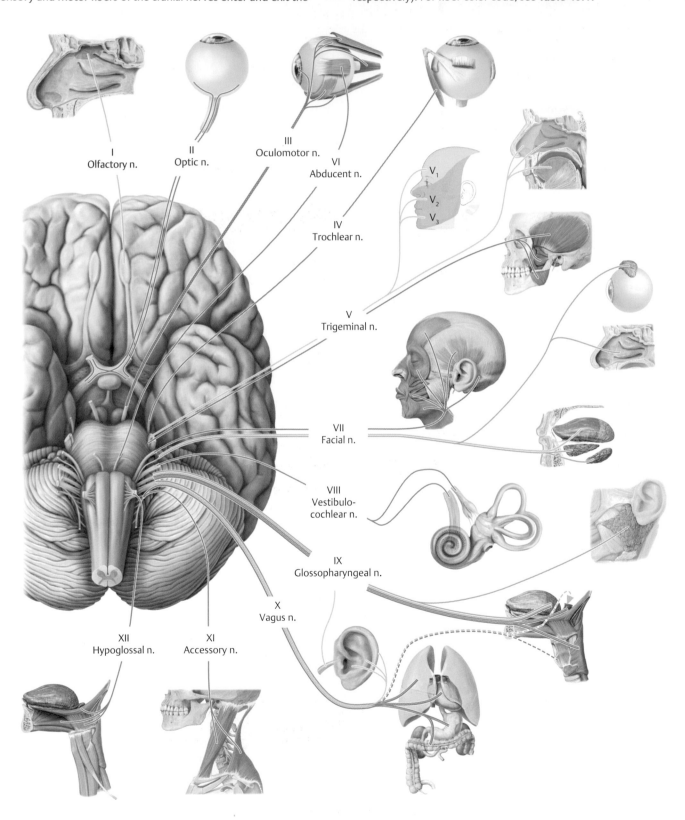

I Olfactory n.

II Optic n.

III Oculomotor n.

VI Abducent n.

IV Trochlear n.

V Trigeminal n.

VII Facial n.

VIII Vestibulo-cochlear n.

IX Glossopharyngeal n.

X Vagus n.

XI Accessory n.

XII Hypoglossal n.

Head & Neck

V_1 V_2 V_3

The cranial nerves contain both afferent (sensory) and efferent (motor) axons that belong to either the somatic or the autonomic (visceral) nervous system (see **pp. 694–695**). The somatic fibers allow interaction with the environment, whereas the visceral fibers regulate the autonomic activity of internal organs. In addition to the general fiber types, the cranial nerves may contain special fiber types associated with particular structures (e.g., auditory apparatus and taste buds). The cranial nerve fibers originate or terminate at specific nuclei, which are similarly classified as either general or special, somatic or visceral, and afferent or efferent.

Table 40.1	Classification of cranial nerve fibers and nuclei		
This color coding is used in subsequent chapters to indicate fiber and nuclei classifications.			
Fiber type	**Example**	**Fiber type**	**Example**
General somatic efferent (somatomotor function)	Innervate skeletal muscles	General somatic afferent (somatic sensation)	Conduct impulses from skin, skeletal muscle spindles
General visceral efferent (visceromotor function)	Innervate smooth muscle of the viscera, intraocular muscles, heart, salivary glands, etc.	Special somatic afferent	Conduct impulses from retina, auditory and vestibular apparatuses
Special visceral efferent	Innervate skeletal muscles derived from branchial arches	General visceral afferent (visceral sensation)	Conduct impulses from viscera, blood vessels
		Special visceral afferent	Conduct impulses from taste buds, olfactory mucosa

Fig. 40.2 Cranial nerve nuclei

The sensory and motor fibers of cranial nerves III to XII originate and terminate in the brainstem at specific nuclei.

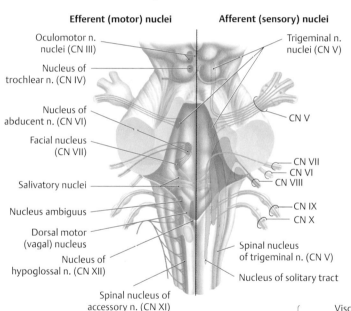

Efferent (motor) nuclei

Oculomotor n. nuclei (CN III)
Nucleus of trochlear n. (CN IV)
Nucleus of abducent n. (CN VI)
Facial nucleus (CN VII)
Salivatory nuclei
Nucleus ambiguus
Dorsal motor (vagal) nucleus
Nucleus of hypoglossal n. (CN XII)
Spinal nucleus of accessory n. (CN XI)

Afferent (sensory) nuclei

Trigeminal n. nuclei (CN V)
CN V
CN VII
CN VI
CN VIII
CN IX
CN X
Spinal nucleus of trigeminal n. (CN V)
Nucleus of solitary tract

A Posterior view with the cerebellum removed.

Table 40.2	Cranial nerves	
Cranial nerve	**Origin**	**Functional fiber types**
CN I: Olfactory n.	Telencephalon*	●
CN II: Optic n.	Diencephalon*	●
CN III: Oculomotor n.	Mesencephalon	● ●
CN IV: Trochlear n.		●
CN V: Trigeminal n.	Pons	● ●
CN VI: Abducent n.		●
CN VII: Facial n.		● ● ● ●
CN VIII: Vestibulocochlear n.		●
CN IX: Glossopharyngeal n.	Medulla oblongata	● ● ● ● ●
CN X: Vagus n.		● ● ● ● ●
CN XI: Accessory n.		●
CN XII: Hypoglossal n.		●

* The olfactory and optic nerves are extensions of the brain rather than true nerves; they are therefore not associated with nuclei in the brainstem.

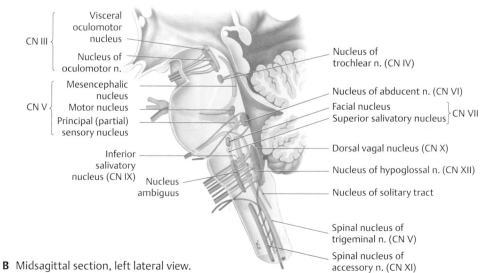

CN III
— Visceral oculomotor nucleus
— Nucleus of oculomotor n.

CN V
— Mesencephalic nucleus
— Motor nucleus
— Principal (partial) sensory nucleus

Inferior salivatory nucleus (CN IX)
Nucleus ambiguus

Nucleus of trochlear n. (CN IV)
Nucleus of abducent n. (CN VI)
Facial nucleus — CN VII
Superior salivatory nucleus — CN VII
Dorsal vagal nucleus (CN X)
Nucleus of hypoglossal n. (CN XII)
Nucleus of solitary tract
Spinal nucleus of trigeminal n. (CN V)
Spinal nucleus of accessory n. (CN XI)

B Midsagittal section, left lateral view.

CN III, IV & VI: Oculomotor, Trochlear & Abducent Nerves

Cranial nerves III, IV, and VI innervate the extraocular muscles (see **p. 605**). Of the three, only the oculomotor nerve (CN III) contains both somatic and visceral efferent fibers; it is also the only cranial nerve of the extraocular muscles to innervate multiple extra- and intraocular muscles.

Fig. 40.5 Nuclei of the oculomotor, trochlear, and abducent nerves

The trochlear nerve (CN IV) is the only cranial nerve in which all the fibers cross to the opposite side. It is also the only cranial nerve to emerge from the dorsal side of the brainstem and, consequently, has the longest intradural (intracranial) course of any cranial nerve.

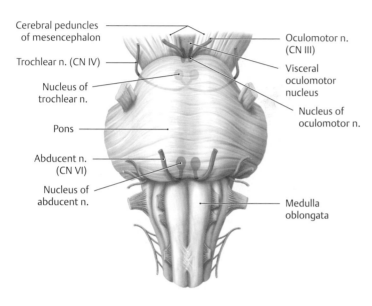

A Emergence of the cranial nerves of the extraocular muscles. Anterior view of the brainstem.

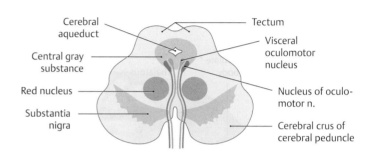

B Oculomotor nerve nuclei. Transverse section, superior view.

Table 40.3	Cranial nerves of the extraocular muscles			
Course*	**Fibers**	**Nuclei**	**Function**	**Effects of nerve injury**
Oculomotor nerve (CN III)				
Runs anteriorly from mesencephalon	Somatic efferent	Oculomotor nucleus	Innervates: • Levator palpebrae superioris • Superior, medial, and inferior rectus • Inferior oblique	Complete oculomotor palsy (paralysis of extra- and intraocular muscles): • Ptosis (drooping of eyelid) • Downward and lateral gaze deviation • Diplopia (double vision) • Mydriasis (pupil dilation) • Accommodation difficulties (ciliary paralysis)
	Visceral efferent	Visceral oculomotor (Edinger-Westphal) nucleus	Synapse with neurons in ciliary ganglia. Innervates: • Pupillary sphincter • Ciliary muscle	
Trochlear nerve (CN IV)				
Emerges from posterior surface of brainstem near midline, courses anteriorly around the cerebral peduncle	Somatic efferent	Nucleus of the trochlear n.	Innervates: • Superior oblique	• Diplopia • Affected eye is higher and deviated medially (dominance of inferior oblique)
Abducent nerve (CN VI)				
Follows a long extradural path**	Somatic efferent	Nucleus of the abducent n.	Innervates: • Lateral rectus	• Diplopia • Medial strabismus (sp.) (due to unopposed action of medial rectus)

* All three nerves enter the orbit through the superior orbital fissure; CN III and CN VI pass through the common tendinous ring of the extraocular muscles.
** The abducent nerve follows an extradural course; abducent nerve palsy may atherefore develop in association with meningitis and subarachnoid hemorrhage.

Note: The oculomotor nerve supplies parasympathetic innervation to the intraocular muscles and somatic motor innervation to most of the extraocular muscles (also the levator palpebrae superioris). Its parasympathetic fibers synapse in the ciliary ganglion. Oculomotor nerve palsy may affect exclusively the parasympathetic or somatic fibers, or both concurrently.

Fig. 40.6 Course of the nerves innervating the extraocular muscles

Right orbit.

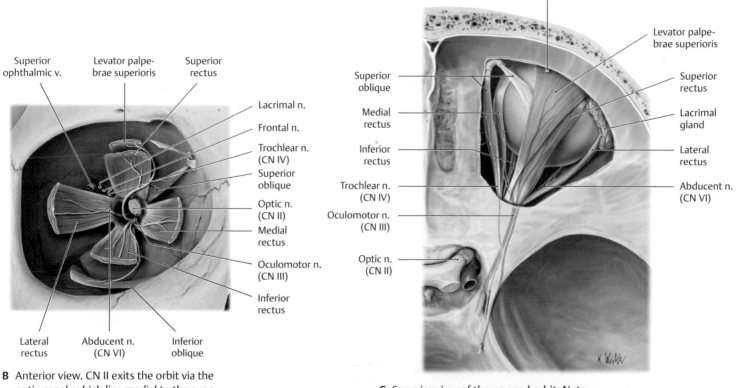

A Lateral view.

B Anterior view. CN II exits the orbit via the optic canal, which lies medial to the superior orbital fissure (site of emergence of CN III, IV, and VI).

C Superior view of the opened orbit. Note the relationship between the optic canal and the superior orbital fissure.

CN V: Trigeminal Nerve

The trigeminal nerve, the sensory nerve of the head, has three somatic afferent nuclei: the mesencephalic nucleus, which receives proprioceptive fibers from the muscles of mastication; the principal (pontine) sensory nucleus, which chiefly mediates touch; and the spinal nucleus, which mediates pain and temperature sensation. The motor nucleus supplies motor innervation to the muscles of mastication.

Fig. 40.7 Trigeminal nerve nuclei

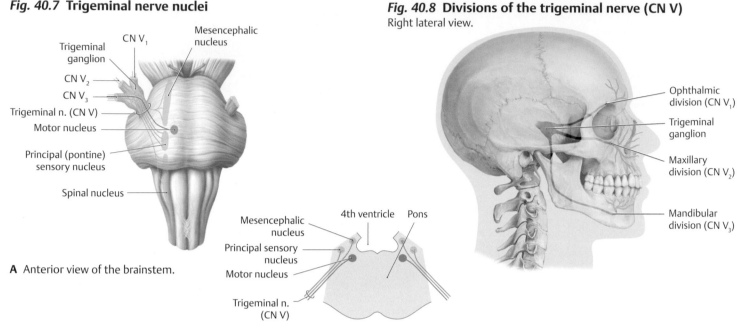

A Anterior view of the brainstem.

B Cross section through the pons, superior view.

Fig. 40.8 Divisions of the trigeminal nerve (CN V)
Right lateral view.

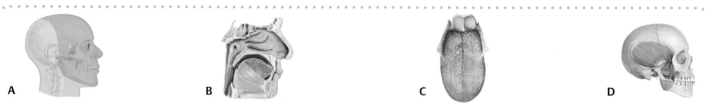

	Table 40.4	Trigeminal nerve (CN V)

Course	Fibers	Nuclei	Function	Effects of nerve injury
Exits from the middle cranial fossa. **Ophthalmic division (CN V₁):** Enters orbit through superior orbital fissure **Maxillary division (CN V₂):** Enters pterygopalatine fossa through foramen rotundum **Mandibular division (CN V₃):** Passes through foramen ovale into infratemporal fossa	Somatic afferent	• Principal (pontine) sensory nucleus of the trigeminal n. • Mesencephalic nucleus of the trigeminal n. • Spinal nucleus of the trigeminal n.	Innervates: • Facial skin (**A**) • Nasopharyngeal mucosa (**B**) • Tongue (anterior two thirds) (**C**) Involved in the corneal reflex (reflex closure of eyelid)	• Sensory loss (traumatic nerve lesions) • Herpes zoster ophthalmicus (varicella-zoster virus); herpes zoster of the face
	Special visceral efferent	Motor nucleus of the trigeminal n.	Innervates (via CN V₃): • Muscles of mastication (temporalis, masseter, medial and lateral pterygoids (**D**)) • Oral floor muscles (mylohyoid, anterior digastric) • Tensor tympani • Tensor veli palatini	
	Visceral efferent pathway*	• Lacrimal n. (CN V₁) conveys parasympathetic fibers from CN VII along the zygomatic n. (CN V₂) to the lacrimal gland • Lingual n. (CN V₃) conveys parasympathetic fibers from CN VII (via the chorda tympani) to the submandibular and sublingual glands • Auriculotemporal n. (CN V₃) conveys parasympathetic fibers from CN IX to the parotid gland		
	Visceral afferent pathway*	Gustatory (taste) fibers from CN VII (via chorda tympani) travel with the lingual n. (CN V₃) to the anterior two thirds of the tongue		

* Fibers of certain cranial nerves adhere to divisions or branches of the trigeminal nerve, by which they travel to their destination.
** All three divisions contribute to dural innervation in the anterior and middle cranial fossae.

Fig. 40.9 **Course of the trigeminal nerve divisions**
Right lateral view.

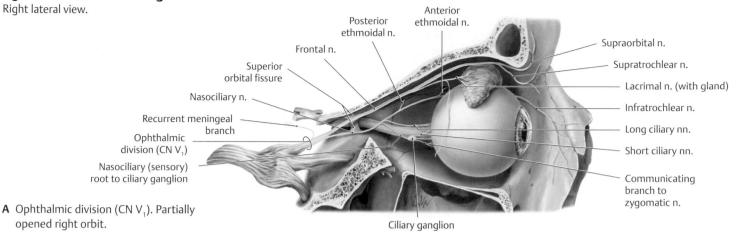

Posterior ethmoidal n.
Anterior ethmoidal n.
Frontal n.
Supraorbital n.
Supratrochlear n.
Superior orbital fissure
Lacrimal n. (with gland)
Nasociliary n.
Infratrochlear n.
Recurrent meningeal branch
Long ciliary nn.
Ophthalmic division (CN V₁)
Short ciliary nn.
Nasociliary (sensory) root to ciliary ganglion
Communicating branch to zygomatic n.
Ciliary ganglion

A Ophthalmic division (CN V₁). Partially opened right orbit.

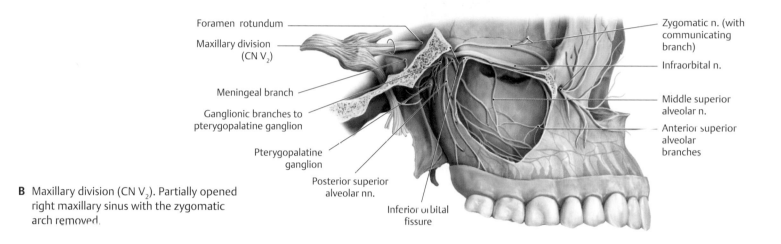

Foramen rotundum
Zygomatic n. (with communicating branch)
Maxillary division (CN V₂)
Infraorbital n.
Meningeal branch
Middle superior alveolar n.
Ganglionic branches to pterygopalatine ganglion
Anterior superior alveolar branches
Pterygopalatine ganglion
Posterior superior alveolar nn.
Inferior orbital fissure

B Maxillary division (CN V₂). Partially opened right maxillary sinus with the zygomatic arch removed.

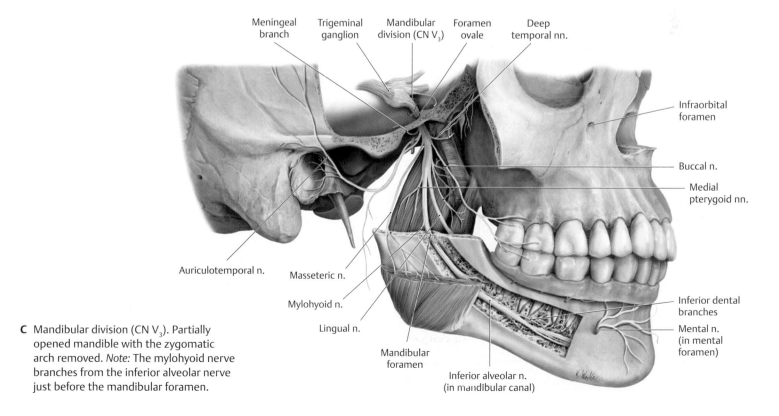

Meningeal branch
Trigeminal ganglion
Mandibular division (CN V₃)
Foramen ovale
Deep temporal nn.
Infraorbital foramen
Buccal n.
Medial pterygoid nn.
Auriculotemporal n.
Masseteric n.
Mylohyoid n.
Lingual n.
Inferior dental branches
Mental n. (in mental foramen)
Mandibular foramen
Inferior alveolar n. (in mandibular canal)

C Mandibular division (CN V₃). Partially opened mandible with the zygomatic arch removed. *Note:* The mylohyoid nerve branches from the inferior alveolar nerve just before the mandibular foramen.

CN VII: Facial Nerve

The facial nerve mainly conveys special visceral efferent (branchiogenic) fibers from the facial nerve nucleus to the muscles of facial expression. The other visceral efferent (parasympathetic) fibers from the superior salivatory nucleus are grouped with the visceral afferent (gustatory) fibers to form the nervus intermedius.

Fig. 40.10 Facial nerve nuclei

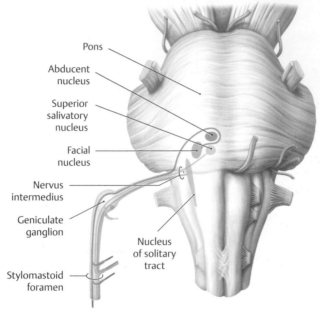

A Anterior view of the brainstem.

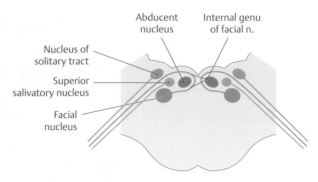

B Cross section through the pons, superior view.

Fig. 40.11 Branches of the facial nerve
Right lateral view.

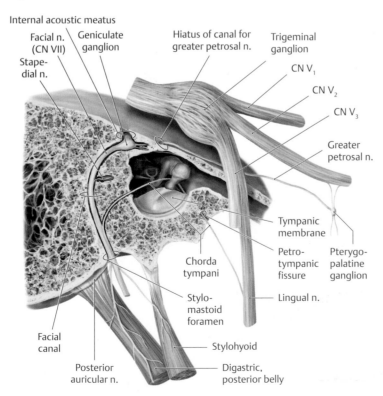

A Facial nerve in the temporal bone.

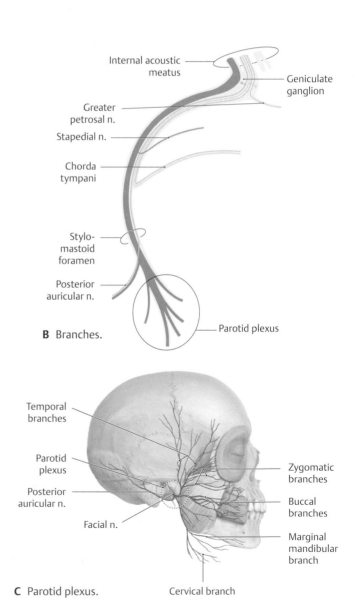

B Branches.

C Parotid plexus.

Table 40.5	Facial nerve (CN VII)				
Course	Fibers	Nuclei	Function		Effects of nerve injury
Emerges in the cerebellopontine angle between the pons and olive; passes through the internal acoustic meatus into the temporal bone (petrous part), where it divides into: • Greater petrosal n. • Stapedial n. • Chorda tympani Certain special visceral efferent fibers pass through the stylomastoid foramen to the skull base, forming the intraparotid plexus	Special visceral efferent	Facial nucleus	Innervate: • Muscles of facial expression • Stylohyoid • Digastric (posterior belly) • Stapedius		Peripheral facial nerve injury: paralysis of muscles of facial expression on affected side Associated disturbances of taste, lacrimation, salivation, hyperacusis, etc.
	Visceral efferent (para-sympathetic)*	Superior salivatory nucleus	Synapse with neurons in the pterygopalatine or submandibular ganglion. Innervate: • Lacrimal gland • Small glands of nasal mucosa, hard and soft palate • Submandibular gland • Sublingual gland • Small salivary glands of tongue (dorsum)		
	Special visceral afferent*	Nucleus of the solitary tract	Peripheral processes of fibers from geniculate ganglion form the chorda tympani (gustatory fibers from tongue)		
	Somatic afferent		Sensory fibers from the auricle, skin of the auditory canal, and outer surface of the tympanic membrane travel via CN VII to the principal sensory nucleus of the trigeminal n.		

* Grouped to form nervus intermedius, which aggregates with the visceral efferent fibers from the facial n. nucleus.

Fig. 40.12 Course of the facial nerve

Right lateral view. This figure shows the distribution of all the fiber types in **Table 40.5**. Visceral efferent (parasympathetic) and special visceral afferent (taste) fibers shown in blue and green respectively. Postganglionic sympathetic fibers are shown in black.

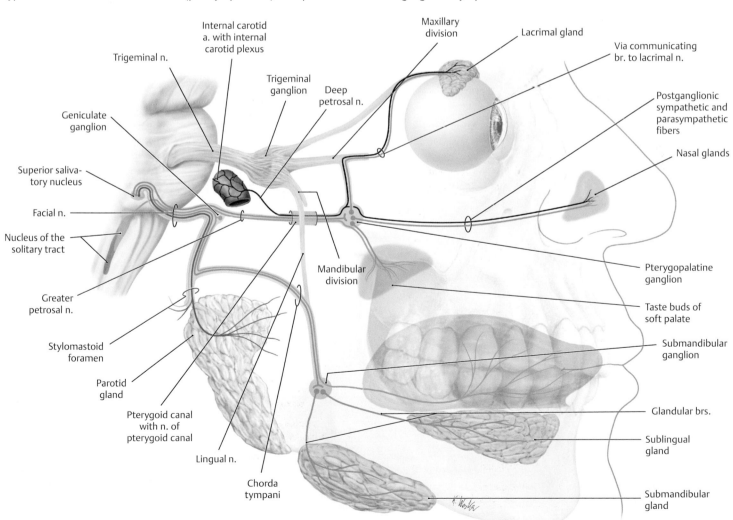

CN VIII: Vestibulocochlear Nerve

The vestibulochochlear nerve is a special somatic afferent nerve that consists of two roots. The vestibular root transmits impulses from the vestibular apparatus; the cochlear root transmits impulses from the auditory apparatus.

Fig. 40.13 **Vestibulocochlear nerve: Vestibular part**

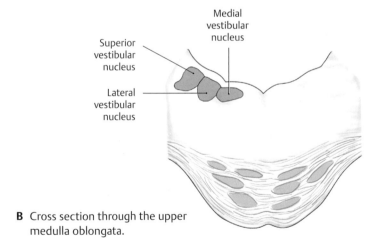

A Anterior view of the medulla oblongata and pons with cerebellum.

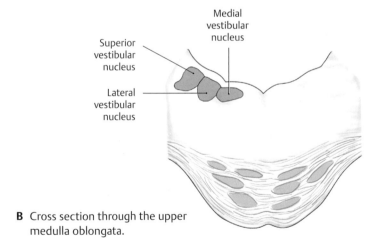

B Cross section through the upper medulla oblongata.

Fig. 40.14 **Vestibulocochlear nerve: Cochlear part**

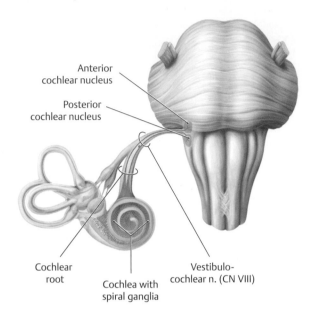

A Anterior view of the medulla oblongata and pons.

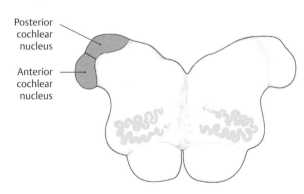

B Cross section through the upper medulla oblongata.

Table 40.6	Vestibulocochlear nerve (CN VIII)				
Part	**Course**	**Fibers**	**Nuclei**	**Function**	**Effects of nerve injury**
Vestibular part	Pass from the inner ear through the internal acoustic meatus to the cerebellopontine angle, where they enter the brain	Special somatic afferent	Superior, lateral, medial, and inferior vestibular nuclei	Peripheral processes from the semicircular canals, saccule, and utricle pass to the vestibular ganglion and then to the four vestibular nuclei	Dizziness
Cochlear part			Anterior and posterior cochlear nuclei	Peripheral processes beginning at the hair cells of the organ of Corti pass to the spiral ganglion and then to the two cochlear nuclei	Hearing loss

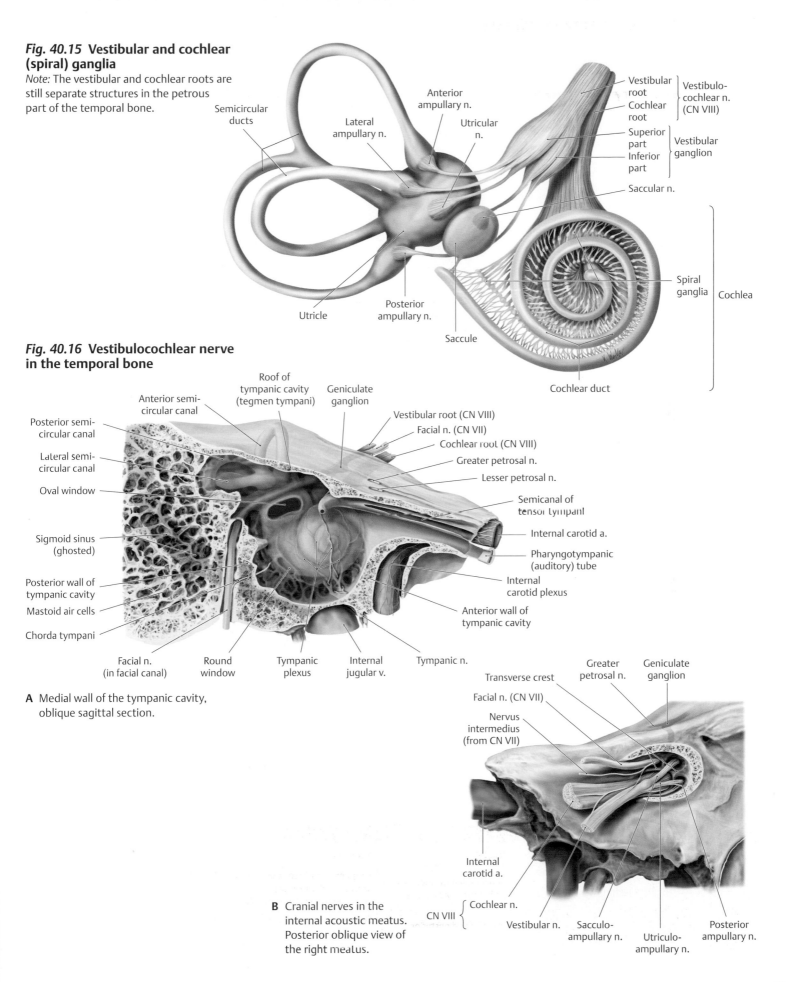

Fig. 40.15 Vestibular and cochlear (spiral) ganglia

Note: The vestibular and cochlear roots are still separate structures in the petrous part of the temporal bone.

Semicircular ducts

Anterior ampullary n.

Lateral ampullary n.

Utricular n.

Vestibular root

Cochlear root

Vestibulo-cochlear n. (CN VIII)

Superior part

Inferior part

Vestibular ganglion

Saccular n.

Spiral ganglia

Cochlea

Utricle

Posterior ampullary n.

Saccule

Cochlear duct

Fig. 40.16 Vestibulocochlear nerve in the temporal bone

Posterior semi-circular canal

Lateral semi-circular canal

Oval window

Sigmoid sinus (ghosted)

Posterior wall of tympanic cavity

Mastoid air cells

Chorda tympani

Anterior semi-circular canal

Roof of tympanic cavity (tegmen tympani)

Geniculate ganglion

Vestibular root (CN VIII)

Facial n. (CN VII)

Cochlear root (CN VIII)

Greater petrosal n.

Lesser petrosal n.

Semicanal of tensor tympani

Internal carotid a.

Pharyngotympanic (auditory) tube

Internal carotid plexus

Anterior wall of tympanic cavity

Facial n. (in facial canal)

Round window

Tympanic plexus

Internal jugular v.

Tympanic n.

A Medial wall of the tympanic cavity, oblique sagittal section.

Greater petrosal n.

Geniculate ganglion

Transverse crest

Facial n. (CN VII)

Nervus intermedius (from CN VII)

Internal carotid a.

B Cranial nerves in the internal acoustic meatus. Posterior oblique view of the right meatus.

CN VIII { Cochlear n. Vestibular n.

Sacculo-ampullary n.

Utriculo-ampullary n.

Posterior ampullary n.

CN IX: Glossopharyngeal Nerve

Fig. 40.17 Glossopharyngeal nerve nuclei

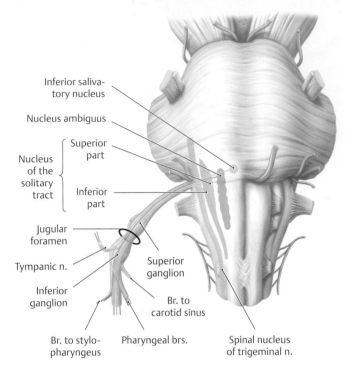

A Anterior view of the medulla oblongata.

B Cross section through the medulla oblongata, superior view. *Not shown:* Nuclei of the trigeminal nerve.

Fig. 40.18 Course of the glossopharyngeal nerve

Left lateral view. *Note:* Fibers from the vagus nerve (CN X) combine with fibers from the glossopharyngeal nerve (CN IX) to form the pharyngeal plexus and supply the carotid sinus.

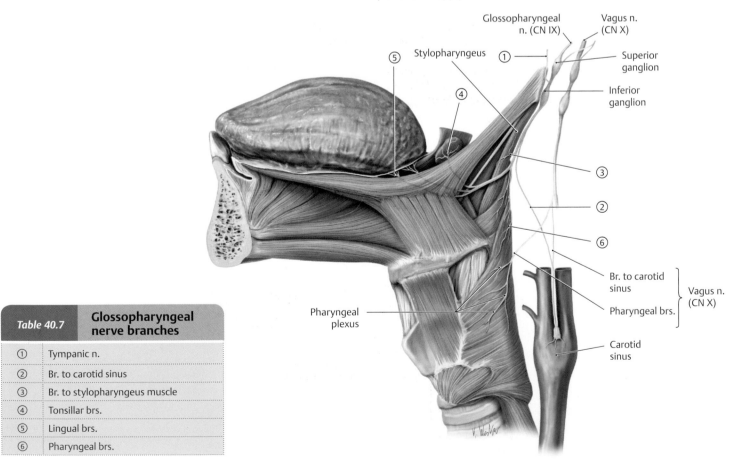

Table 40.7	Glossopharyngeal nerve branches
①	Tympanic n.
②	Br. to carotid sinus
③	Br. to stylopharyngeus muscle
④	Tonsillar brs.
⑤	Lingual brs.
⑥	Pharyngeal brs.

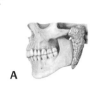   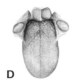 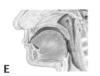 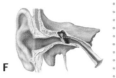

A B C D E F

Table 40.8	Glossopharyngeal nerve (CN IX)

Course	Fibers	Nuclei	Function	Effects of nerve injury
Emerges from the medulla oblongata; leaves cranial cavity through the jugular foramen	Visceral efferent (parasympathetic)	Inferior salivatory nucleus	Parasympathetic presynaptic fibers are sent to the otic ganglion; postsynaptic fibers are distributed to • Parotid gland (**A**) • Buccal gland • Labial gland	Isolated lesions of CN IX are rare. Lesions are generally accompanied by lesions of CN X and CN XI (cranial part), as all three emerge jointly from the jugular foramen and are susceptible to injury in basal skull fractures.
	Special visceral efferent (branchiogenic)	Nucleus ambiguus	Innervate: • Constrictor muscles of the pharynx (pharyngeal branches join with the vagus nerve to form the pharyngeal plexus) • Stylopharyngeus	
	Visceral afferent	Nucleus of the solitary tract (inferior part)	Receive sensory information from • Chemoreceptors in the carotid body (**B**) • Pressure receptors in the carotid sinus	
	Special visceral afferent	Nucleus of the solitary tract (superior part)	Receives sensory information from the posterior third of the tongue (via the inferior ganglion) (**C**)	
	Somatic afferent	Spinal nucleus of trigeminal nerve	Peripheral processes of the intracranial superior ganglion or the extracranial inferior ganglion arise from • Tongue, soft palate, pharyngeal mucosa, and tonsils (**D, E**) • Mucosa of the tympanic cavity, internal surface of the tympanic membrane, pharyngotympanic tube (tympanic plexus) (**F**) • Skin of the external ear and auditory canal (blends with the vagus n.)	

Fig. 40.19 Glossopharyngeal nerve in the tympanic cavity

Left anterolateral view. The tympanic nerve contains visceral efferent (presynaptic parasympathetic) fibers for the otic ganglion, as well as somatic afferent fibers for the tympanic cavity and pharyngotympanic tube. It joins with sympathetic fibers from the internal carotid plexus (via the caroticotympanic nerve) to form the tympanic plexus.

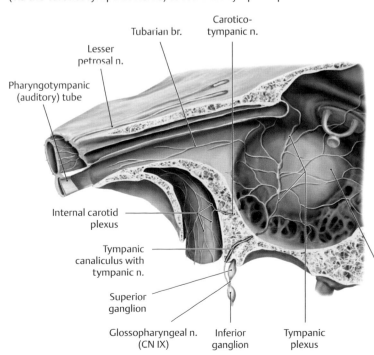

Fig. 40.20 Visceral efferent (parasympathetic) fibers of CN IX

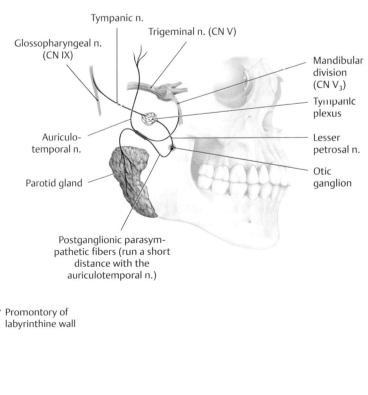

CN XI & XII: Accessory & Hypoglossal Nerves

The traditional "cranial root" of the accessory nerve (CN XI), with its cell bodies found in the nucleus ambiguus, is now considered a part of the vagus nerve (CN X) that travels with the spinal root of CN XI for a short distance before splitting off. The cranial fibers are therefore part of CN X distributed via the vagus nerve after traveling briefly with the spinal root of CN XI. The spinal root fibers, arising from the spinal nucleus of the accessory nerve are now considered to be the accessory nerve, continue on as the accessory nerve (CN XI).

Fig. 40.23 Accessory nerve
Posterior view of the brainstem with the cerebellum removed. *Note:* For didactic reasons, the muscles are displayed from the right side.

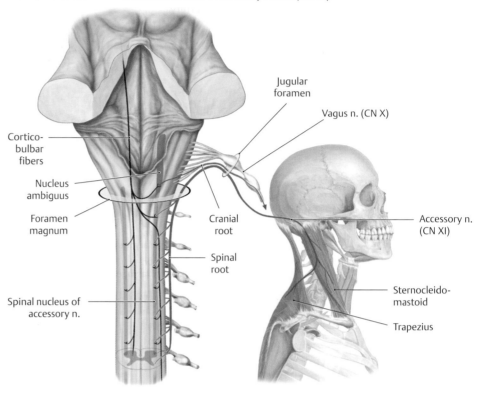

Fig. 40.24 Accessory nerve lesions
Lesion of the right accessory nerve.

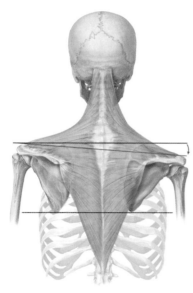

A Trapezius paralysis, posterior view. See **Table 40.11** (below) for clinical correlation explanation.

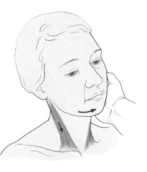

B Sternocleidomastoid paralysis, right anterolateral view. See **Table 40.11** (below) for clinical correlation explanation.

Table 40.11	Accessory nerve (CN XI)*				
Course	**Fibers**	**Nuclei**	**Function**	**Effects of nerve injury**	
The spinal root emerges from the spinal cord (at the level of C1–C5/6), passes superiorly, and enters the skull through the foramen magnum, where it joins with the cranial root arising from the medulla oblongata. Both roots leave the skull through the jugular foramen. Within the jugular foramen, fibers from the cranial root pass to the vagus n. (internal branch). The spinal portion descends to the nuchal region as the external branch.	Special visceral efferent	Nucleus ambiguus (caudal part)	Join CN X and are distributed with the recurrent laryngeal n. Innervate: • All laryngeal muscles (except cricothyroid)	*Trapezius paralysis:* drooping of shoulder on affected side and difficulty raising arm above horizontal plane. This paralysis is a concern during neck operations (e.g., lymph node biopsies). An injury of the accessory n. will not result in complete trapezius paralysis (the muscle is also innervated by segments C3 and C4). *Sternocleidomastoid paralysis:* torticollis (wry neck, i.e., difficulty turning head). Unilateral lesions cause flaccid paralysis (the muscle is supplied exclusively by the accessory n.). Bilateral lesions make it difficult to hold the head upright.	
	Somatic efferent	Spinal nucleus of accessory n.	Form the external branch of the accessory n. Innervate: • Trapezius • Sternocleidomastoid		

*See text at top of page, and **Table 40.2**, regarding new data on cranial fibers of CN XI.

Fig. 40.25 Hypoglossal nerve

Posterior view of the brainstem with the cerebellum removed.
Note: C1, which innervates the thyrohyoid and geniohyoid, runs briefly with the hypoglossal nerve.

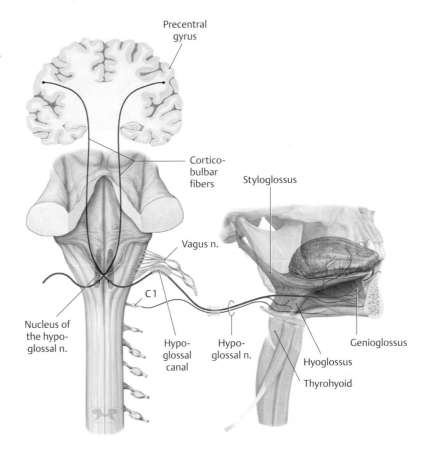

Precentral gyrus

Cortico-bulbar fibers

Styloglossus

Vagus n.

C1

Nucleus of the hypo-glossal n.

Hypo-glossal canal

Hypo-glossal n.

Genioglossus

Hyoglossus

Thyrohyoid

Fig. 40.26 Hypoglossal nerve nuclei

Note: The nucleus of the hypoglossal nerve is innervated by cortical neurons from the contralateral side.

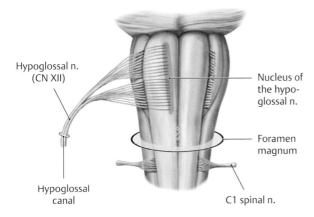

Hypoglossal n. (CN XII)

Nucleus of the hypo-glossal n.

Foramen magnum

Hypoglossal canal

C1 spinal n.

A Anterior view.

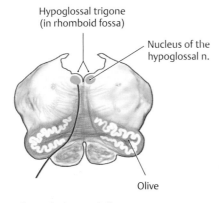

Hypoglossal trigone (in rhomboid fossa)

Nucleus of the hypoglossal n.

Olive

B Cross section through the medulla oblongata.

Fig. 40.27 Hypoglossal nerve lesions

Superior view. See **Table 40.12** below for clinical correlation explanation.

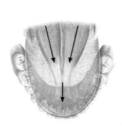

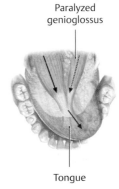

Paralyzed genioglossus

A Normal genioglossus muscles.

Tongue

B Unilateral nuclear or peripheral lesion.

Table 40.12	Hypoglossal nerve (CN XII)			
Course	**Fibers**	**Nuclei**	**Function**	**Effects of nerve injury**
Emerges from the medulla oblongata, leaves the cranial cavity through the hypoglossal canal, and descends laterally to the vagus nerve. CN XII enters the root of the tongue above the hyoid bone.	Somatic efferent	Nucleus of the hypo-glossal n.	Innervates: • Intrinsic and extrinsic muscles of the tongue (except the palatoglossus, supplied by CN X)	Central hypoglossal paralysis (supranuclear): tongue deviates *away* from the side of the lesion. Nuclear or peripheral paralysis: tongue deviates *toward* the affected side (due to preponderance of muscle on healthy side) Flaccid paralysis: both nuclei injured; tongue cannot be protruded.

Autonomic Innervation

Fig. 40.28 Parasympathetic nervous system (cranial part): Overview

There are four parasympathetic nuclei in the brainstem. The visceral efferent fibers of these nuclei travel along particular cranial nn., listed below.

- Visceral oculomotor (Edinger–Westphal) nucleus: oculomotor n. (CN III)
- Superior salivatory nucleus: facial n. (CN VII)
- Inferior salivatory nucleus: glossopharyngeal n. (CN IX)
- Dorsal vagal nucleus: vagus n. (CN X)

The preganglionic parasympathetic fibers often travel with multiple cranial nn. to reach their target organs. The vagus n. supplies all of the thoracic and abdominal organs as far as a point near the left colic flexure.

Note: The sympathetic fibers to the head travel along the arteries to their target organs.

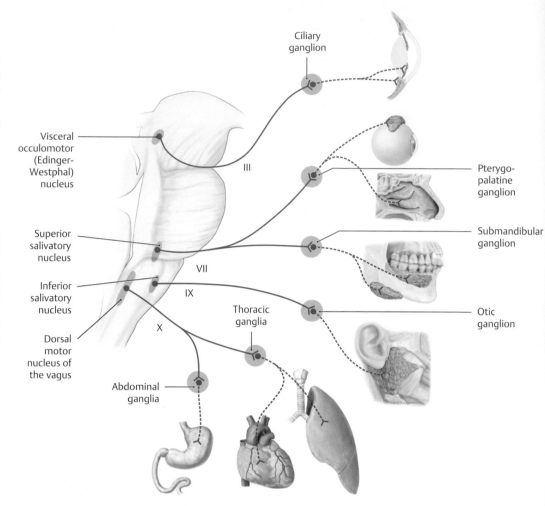

—— Parasympathetic preganglionic fibers
---- Parasympathetic postganglionic fibers

Table 40.13	Parasympathetic ganglia in the head			
Nucleus	**Path of presynaptic fibers**	**Ganglion**	**Postsynaptic fibers**	**Target organs**
Edinger-Westphal nucleus	Oculomotor n. (CN III)	Ciliary ganglion	Short ciliary nn. (CN V$_1$)	Ciliary muscle (accommodation) Pupillary sphincter (miosis)
Superior salivatory nucleus	Nervus intermedius (CN VII root) → greater petrosal n. → n. of pterygoid canal	Pterygopalatine ganglion	• Maxillary n. (CN V$_2$) → zygomatic n. → anastomosis → lacrimal n. (CN V$_1$) • Orbital branches • Posterior superior nasal brs. • Nasopalatine nn. • Greater and lesser palatine nn.	• Lacrimal gland • Glands of nasal cavity and paranasal sinuses • Glands of gingiva • Glands of hard and soft palate • Glands of pharynx
	Nervus intermedius (CN VII root) → chorda tympani → lingual n. (CN V$_3$)	Submandibular ganglion	Glandular branches	Submandibular gland Sublingual gland
Inferior salivatory nucleus	Glossopharyngeal n. (CN IX) → tympanic n. → lesser petrosal n.	Otic ganglion	Auriculotemporal n. (CN V$_3$)	Parotid gland
Dorsal motor (vagal) nucleus	Vagus n. (X)	Ganglia near organs	Fine fibers in organs, not individually named	Thoracic and abdominal viscera
→ = is continuous with				

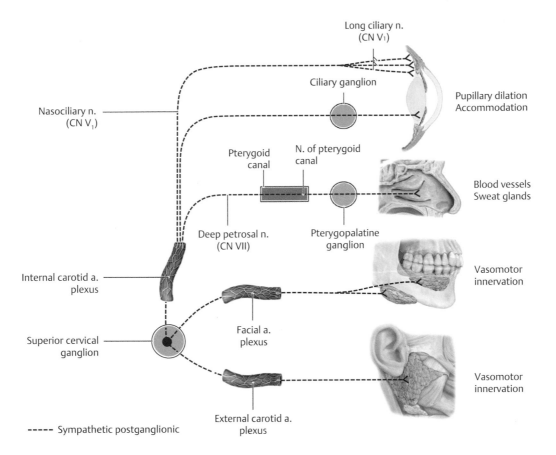

Fig. 40.29 Sympathetic innervation of the head

Sympathetic preganglionic neurons of the head originate in the lateral horn of the spinal cord (TI–T3). They exit into the sympathetic trunk and ascend to synapse in the superior cervical ganglion. Postganglionic neurons then travel with arterial plexuses. Postganglionic fibers that travel with the carotid plexus (on the internal carotid artery) join with the nasociliary nerves (of CN V₁) and then the long ciliary nerves to reach the dilator pupillae muscle (pupillary dilation); other postganglionic fibers travel through the ciliary ganglion (without synapsing) to reach the ciliary muscle to participate in accomodation. Still other postganglionic fibers from the carotid plexus leave with the deep petrosal nerve, which joins with the greater petrosal nerve (CN VII), to form the nerve of the pterygoid canal (vidian nerve). This nerve travels to the pterygopalatine ganglion where it distributes fibers via branches of the maxillary nerve to the glands of the nasal cavity, maxillary sinus, hard and soft palate, gingiva, and pharynx, and to sweat glands and blood vessels in the head. Postganglionic fibers from the superior cervical ganglion that travel with the facial artery plexus pass through the submandibular ganglion (without synapsing) to the submandibular and sublingual glands. Other postganglionic fibers travel with the middle meningeal plexus, through the otic ganglion (without synapsing), to the parotid gland.

Table 40.14	Sympathetic fibers in the head			
Nucleus	**Path of presynaptic fibers**	**Ganglion**	**Postsynaptic fibers**	**Target organs**
Lateral horn of spinal cord (TI–L2)	Enter sympathetic trunk and ascend to superior cervical ganglion	Superior cervical ganglion	ICA plexus → nasociliary n. (CN V₁) → long ciliary nn. (CN V₁)	Dilator pupillae muscle (mydriasis)
			Postganglionic fibers → ciliary ganglion* → short ciliary nn. (limited number of fibers)	Ciliary muscle (sparse sympathetic fibers contributing to accommodation)
			ICA plexus → deep petrosal n. → n. of pterygoid canal → pterygopalatine ganglion* → branches of maxillary n. (CN V₂)	Glands of nasal cavity Sweat glands Blood vessels
			Facial a. plexus → submandibular ganglion*	Submandibular gland Sublingual gland
			External carotid a. plexus	Parotid gland

*passes through without synpasing; → = is continuous with
ICA, internal carotid a.

41 Neurovasculature of the Skull & Face

Innervation of the Face

Fig. 41.1 Motor innervation of the face

Left lateral view. Five branches of the facial nerve (CN VII) provide motor innervation to the muscles of facial expression. The mandibular division of the trigeminal nerve (CN V₃) supplies motor innervation to the muscles of mastication.

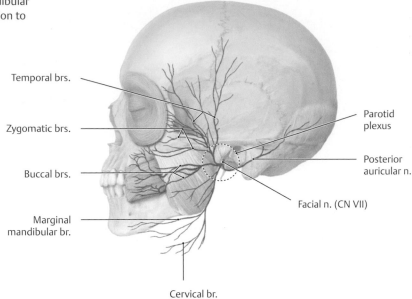

Temporal brs.
Zygomatic brs.
Buccal brs.
Marginal mandibular br.
Parotid plexus
Posterior auricular n.
Facial n. (CN VII)
Cervical br.

A Motor innervation of the muscles of facial expression.

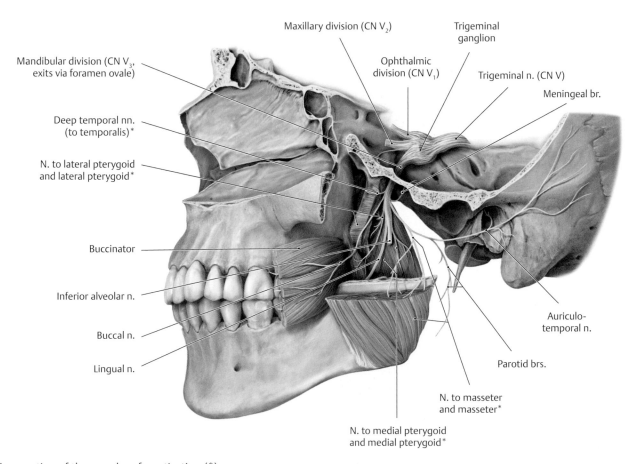

Maxillary division (CN V₂)
Trigeminal ganglion
Mandibular division (CN V₃, exits via foramen ovale)
Ophthalmic division (CN V₁)
Trigeminal n. (CN V)
Meningeal br.
Deep temporal nn. (to temporalis)*
N. to lateral pterygoid and lateral pterygoid*
Buccinator
Inferior alveolar n.
Buccal n.
Lingual n.
Auriculo-temporal n.
Parotid brs.
N. to masseter and masseter*
N. to medial pterygoid and medial pterygoid*

B Motor innervation of the muscles of mastication (*).

Fig. 41.2 Sensory innervation of the face

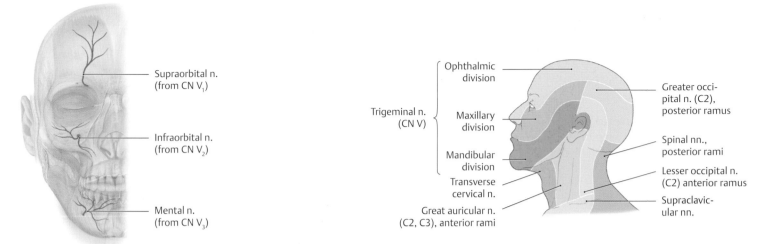

A Sensory branches of the trigeminal nerve, anterior view. The sensory branches of the three divisions emerge from the supraorbital, infraorbital, and mental foramina, respectively.

B Cutaneous innervation of the head and neck, left lateral view. The occiput and nuchal regions are supplied by the posterior rami (blue) of the spinal nerves (the greater occipital nerve is the posterior ramus of C2).

Supraorbital n. (from CN V₁)

Infraorbital n. (from CN V₂)

Mental n. (from CN V₃)

Ophthalmic division

Maxillary division

Mandibular division

Trigeminal n. (CN V)

Transverse cervical n.

Great auricular n. (C2, C3), anterior rami

Greater occipital n. (C2), posterior ramus

Spinal nn., posterior rami

Lesser occipital n. (C2) anterior ramus

Supraclavicular nn.

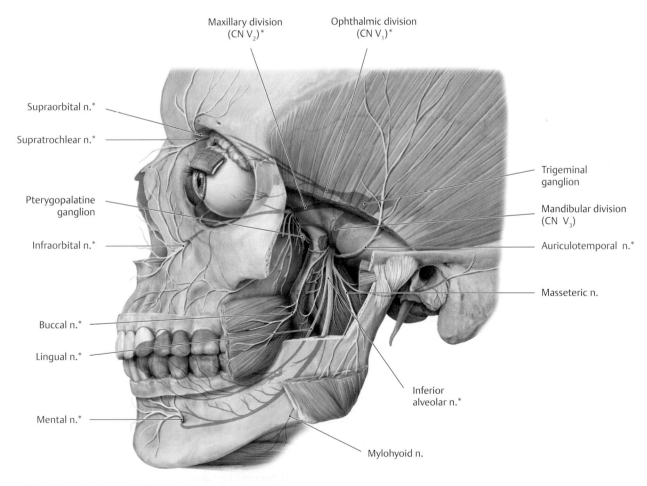

Maxillary division (CN V₂)*

Ophthalmic division (CN V₁)*

Supraorbital n.*

Supratrochlear n.*

Pterygopalatine ganglion

Infraorbital n.*

Buccal n.*

Lingual n.*

Mental n.*

Inferior alveolar n.*

Mylohyoid n.

Trigeminal ganglion

Mandibular division (CN V₃)

Auriculotemporal n.*

Masseteric n.

C Divisions of the trigeminal nerve, left lateral view.

*Indicates sensory nn.

Arteries of the Head & Neck

The head and neck are supplied by branches of the common carotid artery. The common carotid splits at the carotid bifurcation into two branches: the internal and external carotid arteries. The internal carotid chiefly supplies the brain (**p. 688**), although its branches anastomose with the external carotid in the orbit and nasal septum. The external carotid is the major supplier of structures of the head and neck.

Fig. 41.3 Internal carotid artery

Left lateral view. The most important extra-cerebral branch of the internal carotid artery is the ophthalmic artery, which supplies the upper nasal septum (**p. 620**) and the orbit (**p. 608**). See **pp. 688–689** for the arteries of the brain.

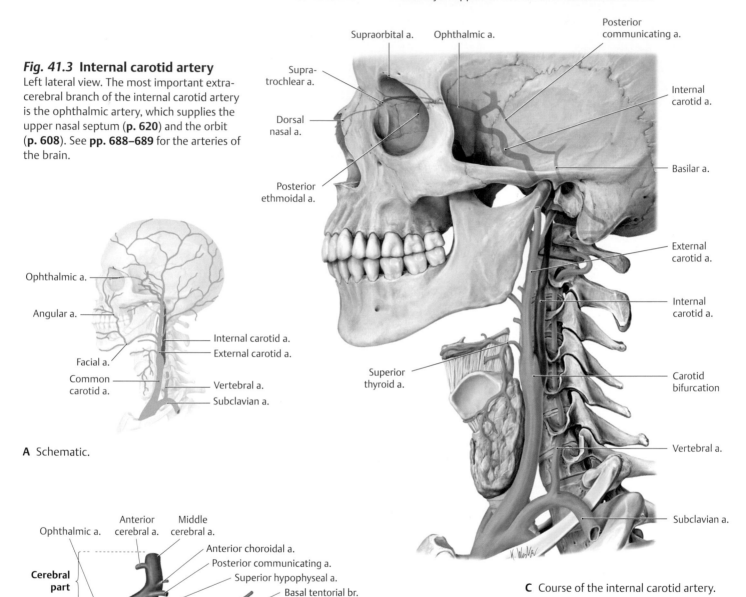

A Schematic.

C Course of the internal carotid artery.

B Parts and branches of the internal carotid artery.

Carotid artery atherosclerosis

The carotid artery is often affected by atherosclerosis, a hardening of arterial walls due to plaque formation. The examiner can determine the status of the arteries using ultrasound. *Note:* The absence of atherosclerosis in the carotid artery does not preclude coronary heart disease or atherosclerotic changes in other locations.

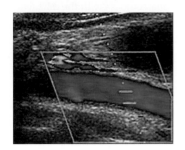

A Common carotid artery with "normal" flow.

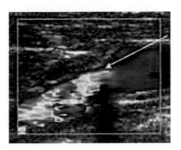

B Calcified plaque in the carotid bulb.

Fig. 41.4 **External carotid artery: Overview**

Left lateral view.

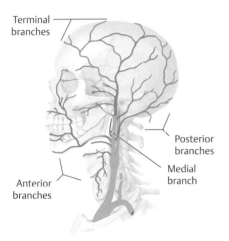

Terminal branches

Posterior branches

Medial branch

Anterior branches

A Schematic of the external carotid artery.

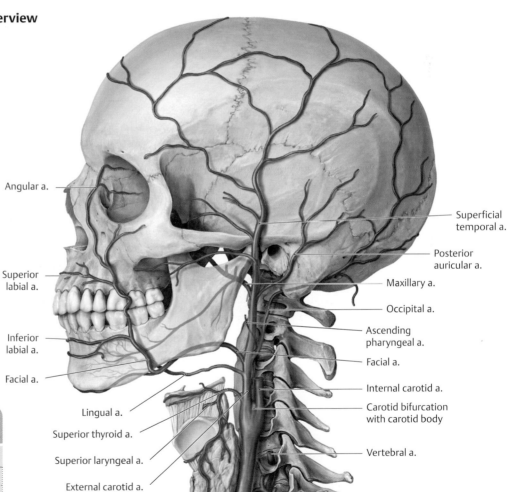

Angular a.

Superior labial a.

Inferior labial a.

Facial a.

Lingual a.

Superior thyroid a.

Superior laryngeal a.

External carotid a.

Left common carotid a.

Superficial temporal a.

Posterior auricular a.

Maxillary a.

Occipital a.

Ascending pharyngeal a.

Facial a.

Internal carotid a.

Carotid bifurcation with carotid body

Vertebral a.

Thyrocervical a.

Left subclavian a.

B Course of the external carotid artery.

Table 41.1	Branches of the external carotid artery
Group	**Artery**
Anterior (**p. 584**)	Superior thyroid a.
	Lingual a.
	Facial a.
Medial (**p. 584**)	Ascending pharyngeal a.
Posterior (**p. 585**)	Occipital a.
	Posterior auricular a.
Terminal (**p. 585**)	Maxillary a.
	Superficial temporal a.

External Carotid Artery: Anterior, Medial & Posterior Branches

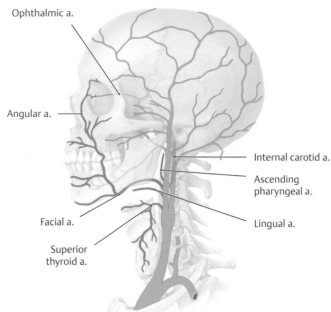

- Ophthalmic a.
- Angular a.
- Facial a.
- Superior thyroid a.
- Internal carotid a.
- Ascending pharyngeal a.
- Lingual a.

Fig. 41.5 Anterior and medial branches

Left lateral view. The arteries of the anterior aspect supply the anterior structures of the head and neck, including the orbit (**p. 606**), ear (**p. 632**), larynx (**p. 530**), pharynx (**p. 654**), and oral cavity. *Note:* The angular artery anastomoses with the dorsal nasal artery of the internal carotid (via the ophthalmic artery).

A Arteries of the anterior and medial branches. The copious blood supply to the face makes facial injuries bleed profusely but heal quickly. There are extensive anastomoses between branches of the external carotid artery and between the external carotid artery and branches of the ophthalmic artery.

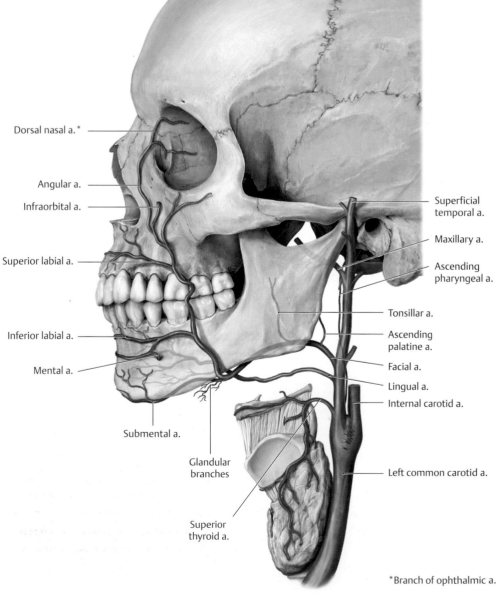

- Dorsal nasal a.*
- Angular a.
- Infraorbital a.
- Superior labial a.
- Inferior labial a.
- Mental a.
- Submental a.
- Glandular branches
- Superior thyroid a.
- Superficial temporal a.
- Maxillary a.
- Ascending pharyngeal a.
- Tonsillar a.
- Ascending palatine a.
- Facial a.
- Lingual a.
- Internal carotid a.
- Left common carotid a.

B Course of the anterior and medial branches.

*Branch of ophthalmic a.

Fig. 41.6 Posterior branches

Left lateral view. The posterior branches of the external carotid artery supply the ear (**p. 632**), posterior skull (**p. 594**), and posterior neck muscles (**p. 541**).

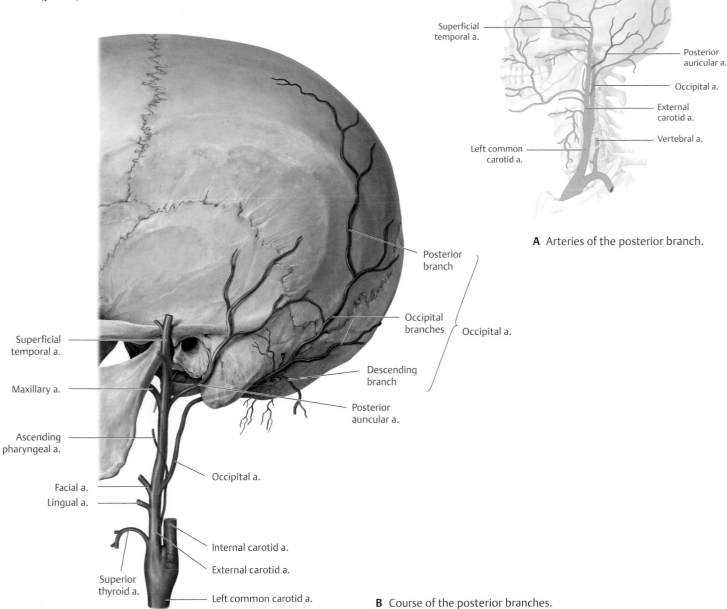

A Arteries of the posterior branch.

B Course of the posterior branches.

Table 41.2	Anterior, medial, and posterior branches of the external carotid artery	
Branch	**Artery**	**Divisions and distribution**
Anterior brs.	Superior thyroid a.	Glandular br. (to thyroid gland); superior laryngeal a.; sternocleidomastoid br.
	Lingual a.	Dorsal lingual brs. (to base of tongue, palatoglossal arch, tonsil, soft palate and epiglottis); sublingual a. (to sublingual gland, tongue, oral floor, oral cavity); sublingual br. to the sublingual gland; deep lingual a.
	Facial a.	Ascending palatine a. (to pharyngeal wall, soft palate, pharyngotympanic tube); tonsillar branch (to palatine tonsils); submental a. (to oral floor, submandibular gland); labial aa.; angular a. (to nasal root)
Medial br.	Ascending pharyngeal a.	Pharyngeal brs.; inferior tympanic a. (to mucosa of inner ear); posterior meningeal a.
Posterior brs.	Occipital a.	Occipital brs.; descending br. (to posterior neck muscles)
	Posterior auricular a.	Stylomastoid a. (to facial n. in facial canal); posterior tympanic a.; auricular br.; occipital br.; parotid br.
For terminal brs., see **Table 41.3 (p. 586)**.		

External Carotid Artery: Terminal Branches

The terminal branches of the external carotid artery consist of two major arteries: superficial temporal and maxillary. The superficial temporal artery supplies the lateral skull. The maxillary artery is a major artery for internal structures of the face.

Fig. 41.7 Superficial temporal artery

Left lateral view. Inflammation of the superficial temporal artery due to temporal arteritis can cause severe headaches. The course of the frontal branch of the artery can often be seen superficially under the skin of elderly patients.

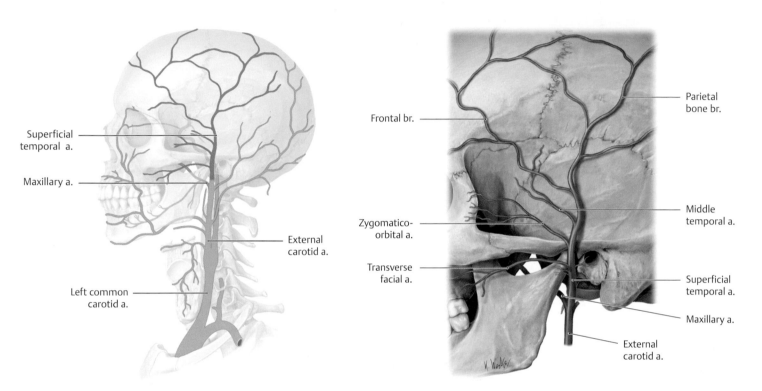

A Arteries of the terminal branch.

B Course of the superficial temporal artery.

Table 41.3	Terminal branches of the external carotid artery		
Branch	**Artery**	**Divisions and distribution**	
External carotid a.	Superficial temporal a.	Transverse facial a. (to soft tissues below the zygomatic arch); frontal brs.; parietal brs.; zygomatico-orbital a. (to lateral orbital wall)	
	Maxillary a.	Mandibular part	Inferior alveolar a. (to mandible, teeth, gingiva); middle meningeal a.; deep auricular a. (to temporomandibular joint, external auditory canal); anterior tympanic a.
		Pterygoid part	Masseteric a.; deep temporal brs.; pterygoid brs.; buccal a.
		Pterygopalatine part	Posterosuperior alveolar a. (to maxillary molars, maxillary sinus, gingiva); infraorbital a. (to maxillary alveoli)
			Descending palatine a. — Greater palatine a. (to hard palate)
			Descending palatine a. — Lesser palatine a. (to soft palate, palatine tonsil, pharyngeal wall)
			Sphenopalatine a. — Lateral posterior nasal aa. (to lateral wall of nasal cavity, conchae)
			Sphenopalatine a. — Posterior septal brs. (to nasal septum)

* Parts not shown here. See **Fig 41.27 (p. 599)** and **Table 41.8 (p. 601)**.

Fig. 41.8 **Maxillary artery**

Left lateral view. The maxillary artery consists of three parts: mandibular (blue), pterygoid (green), and pterygopalatine (yellow).

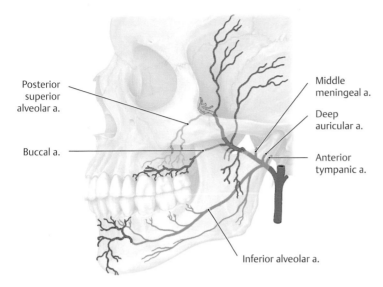

A Divisions of the maxillary artery.

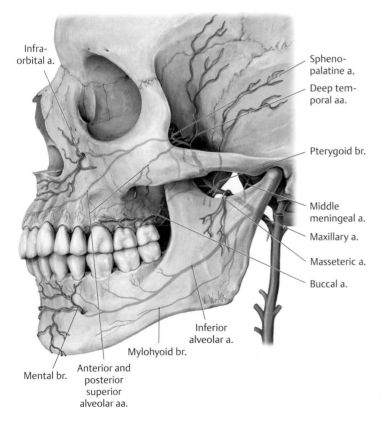

B Course of the maxillary artery.

 Clinical box 41.2

Middle meningeal artery

The middle meningeal artery supplies the meninges and overlying calvaria. Rupture of the artery (generally due to head trauma) results in an epidural hematoma.

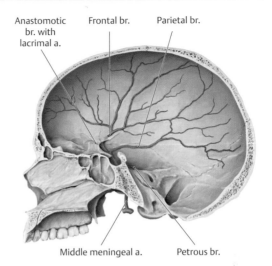

A Right middle meningeal artery, medial view of opened skull.

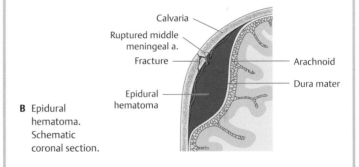

B Epidural hematoma. Schematic coronal section.

Sphenopalatine artery

The sphenopalatine artery supplies the wall of the nasal cavity. Excessive nasopharyngeal bleeding from the branches of the sphenopalatine artery may necessitate ligation of the maxillary artery in the pterygopalatine fossa.

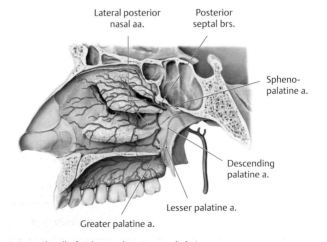

C Lateral wall of right nasal cavity, medial view.

Veins of the Head & Neck

Fig. 41.9 **Veins of the head and neck**

Left lateral view. The veins of the head and neck drain into the brachiocephalic vein. *Note:* The left and right brachiocephalic veins are not symmetrical.

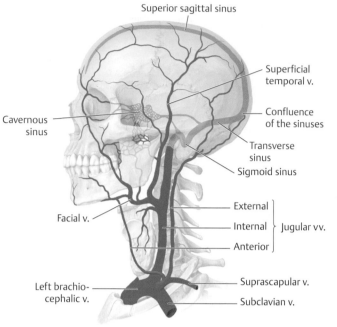

A Principal veins of the head and neck.

Table 41.4	Principal superficial veins	
Vein	**Region drained**	**Location**
Internal jugular v.	Interior of skull (including brain)	Within carotid sheath
External jugular v.	Superficial head	Within superficial cervical fascia
Anterior jugular v.	Neck, portions of head	

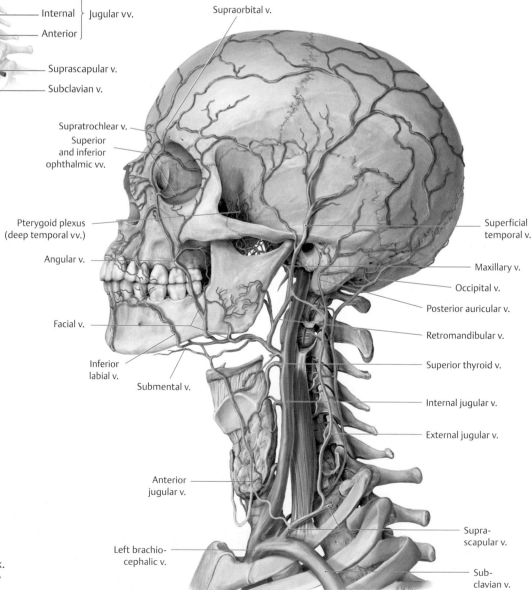

B Superficial veins of the head and neck. *Note*: The course of the veins is highly variable.

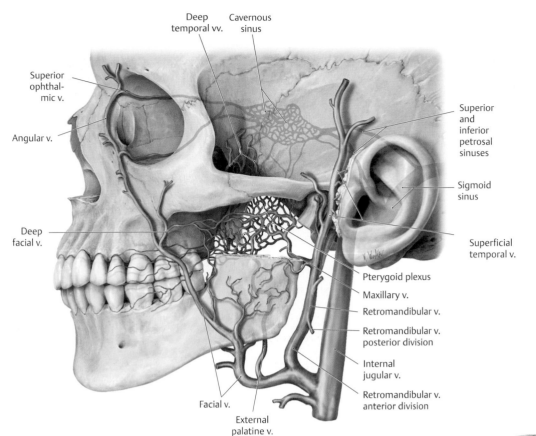

Fig. 41.10 Deep veins of the head

Left lateral view. *Removed:* Upper ramus, condylar and coronoid processes of mandible. The pterygoid plexus is a venous network situated between the mandibular ramus and the muscles of mastication. The cavernous sinus connects branches of the facial vein to the sigmoid sinuses.

Labels (Fig. 41.10): Deep temporal vv.; Cavernous sinus; Superior ophthalmic v.; Angular v.; Deep facial v.; Superior and inferior petrosal sinuses; Sigmoid sinus; Superficial temporal v.; Pterygoid plexus; Maxillary v.; Retromandibular v.; Retromandibular v. posterior division; Internal jugular v.; Retromandibular v. anterior division; Facial v.; External palatine v.

Fig. 41.11 Veins of the occiput

Posterior view. The superficial veins of the occiput communicate with the dural venous sinuses via emissary veins that drain to diploic veins (calvaria, **p. 545**). *Note:* The external vertebral venous plexus traverses the entire length of the spine (**p. 45**).

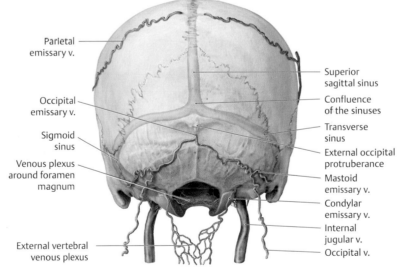

Labels (Fig. 41.11): Parietal emissary v.; Occipital emissary v.; Sigmoid sinus; Venous plexus around foramen magnum; External vertebral venous plexus; Superior sagittal sinus; Confluence of the sinuses; Transverse sinus; External occipital protruberance; Mastoid emissary v.; Condylar emissary v.; Internal jugular v.; Occipital v.

Table 41.5	Venous anastomoses	
The extensive venous anastomoses in this region provide routes for the spread of infections.		
Extracranial vein	**Connecting vein**	**Venous sinus**
Angular v.	Superior and inferior ophthalmic vv.	Cavernous sinus*
Vv. of palatine tonsil	Pterygoid plexus; inferior ophthalmic v.	
Superficial temporal v.	Parietal emissary vv.	Superior sagittal sinus
Occipital v.	Occipital emissary v.	Transverse sinus, confluence of the sinuses
Posterior auricular v.	Mastoid emissary v.	Sigmoid sinus
External vertebral venous plexus	Condylar emissary v.	
*Deep spread of bacterial infection from the facial region may result in cavernous sinus thrombosis.		

Meninges

The brain and spinal cord are covered by membranes called meninges. The meninges are composed of three layers: dura mater (dura), arachnoid mater (arachnoid membrane), and pia mater. The subarachnoid space, located between the arachnoid mater and pia mater, contains cerebrospinal fluid (CSF, see p. 684). See p. 40 for the coverings of the spinal cord.

Fig. 41.12 Layers of the meninges

See pp. 686–687 for the veins of the brain.

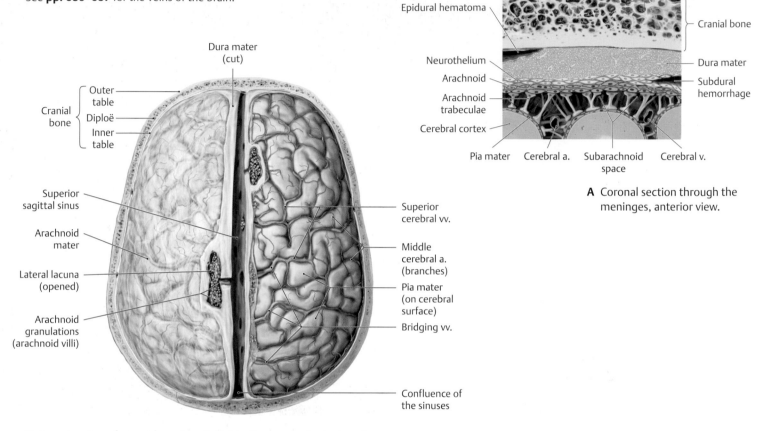

A Coronal section through the meninges, anterior view.

B Superior view of opened cranium. *Left side:* Dura mater (outer layer) cut to reveal arachnoid (middle layer). *Right side:* Dura mater and arachnoid removed to reveal pia mater (inner layer) lining the surface of the brain. *Note:* Arachnoid granulations, sites for reabsorption of cerebrospinal fluid into the venous blood, are protrusions of the arachnoid layer of the meninges into the venous sinus system.

Fig. 41.13 Dural folds (septa)

Left anterior oblique view. Two layers of meningeal dura come together, after separating from the periosteal dura during formation of a dural (venous) sinus, to form a dural fold or septum. These include the falx cerebri (separating right and left cerebral hemispheres); the tentorium cerebelli (supporting the cerebrum to keep it from crushing the underlying cerebellum); the falx cerebelli (not shown, separating right and left cerebellar lobes under the tentorium); and the diaphragma sellae (forming the roof over the hypophyseal fossa and invaginated by the hypophysis).

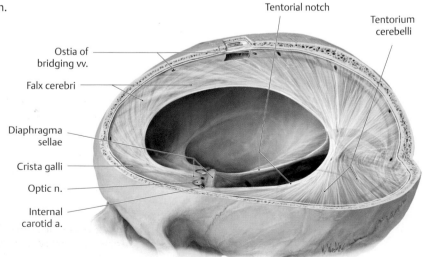

Clinical box 41.3

Extracerebral hemorrhages

Bleeding between the bony calvarium and the soft tissue of the brain (extracerebral hemorrhage) exerts pressure on the brain. A rise of intracranial pressure may damage brain tissue both at the bleeding site and in more remote brain areas. Three types of intracranial hemorrhage are distinguished based on the relationship to the dura mater. See **pp. 688–689** for the arteries and **pp. 686–687** for the veins of the brain.

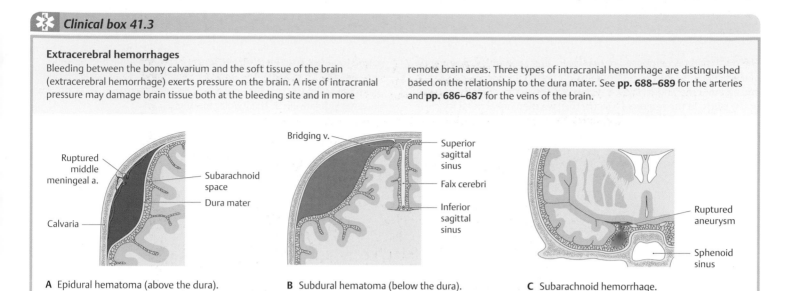

A Epidural hematoma (above the dura).

B Subdural hematoma (below the dura).

C Subarachnoid hemorrhage.

Fig. 41.14 Arteries of the dura mater

Midsagittal section, left lateral view. See **pp. 688–689** for the arteries of the brain.

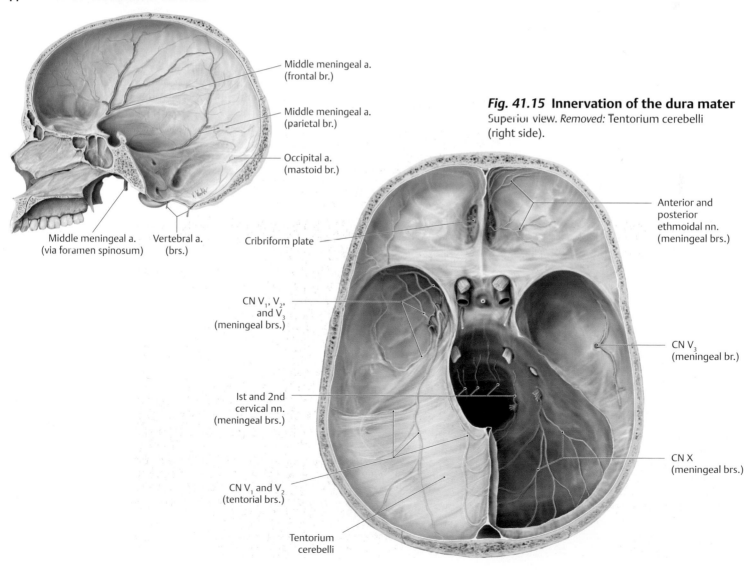

Fig. 41.15 Innervation of the dura mater

Superior view. *Removed:* Tentorium cerebelli (right side).

Dural Sinuses

The dura mater is composed of two layers that separate in the region of a venous sinus into an outer periosteal layer, which lines the calvaria and an inner meningeal layer, which forms the unattached boundaries of the sinus. In the region of a sinus, the two meningeal dural layers come together after forming the sinus to create a dural fold, or septa (see **Fig. 41.13, p. 590**). The network of venous sinuses collect blood from the scalp, the calvaria, and the brain and eventually drain into the internal jugular vein at the jugular foramen.

Fig. 41.16 Formation of a dural sinus

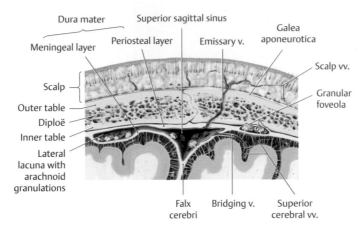

A Structure of a dural sinus. Superior sagittal sinus, coronal section, anterior view.

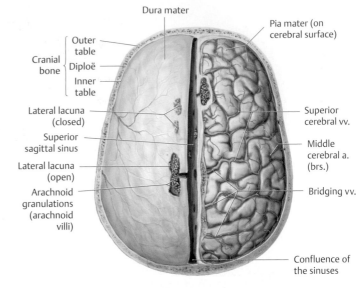

B Superior sagittal sinus in situ. Superior view of opened cranial cavity. The roof of the sinus (the periosteal layer of the dura attached to the calvaria) is removed. *Left side:* Areas of dura mater removed to show arachnoid granulations (protrusions of the arachnoid layer of the meninges) in the sinus. *Right side:* Dura mater and arachnoid layers removed to reveal pia mater adhering to the cerebral cortex.

Fig. 41.17 Dural sinuses in the cranial cavity

Superior view of opened cranial cavity. Dural sinus system ghosted in blue. *Removed:* Tentorium cerebelli (right side).

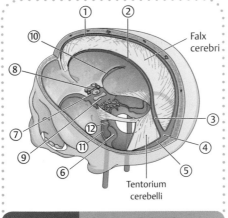

Table 41.6	Principal dural sinuses		
Upper group		**Lower group**	
①	Superior sagittal sinus	⑦	Cavernous sinus
②	Inferior sagittal sinus	⑧	Anterior inter-cavernous sinus
③	Straight sinus	⑨	Posterior inter-cavernous sinus
④	Confluence of the sinuses	⑩	Sphenoparietal sinus
⑤	Transverse sinus	⑪	Superior petrosal sinus
⑥	Sigmoid sinus	⑫	Inferior petrosal sinus

The occipital sinus is also included in the upper group (see **Fig. 49.1, p. 686**).

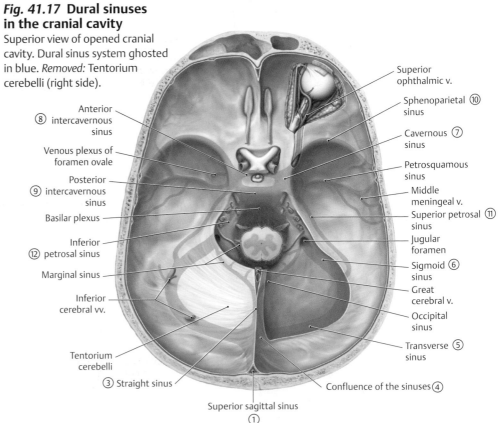

Fig. 41.18 Cavernous sinus and cranial nerves

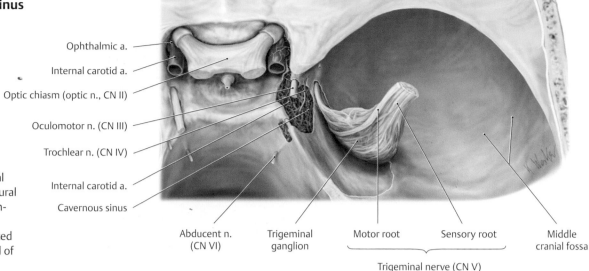

Ophthalmic a.

Internal carotid a.

Optic chiasm (optic n., CN II)

Oculomotor n. (CN III)

Trochlear n. (CN IV)

Internal carotid a.

Cavernous sinus

Abducent n. (CN VI)

Trigeminal ganglion

Motor root

Sensory root

Middle cranial fossa

Trigeminal nerve (CN V)

A Superior view of the right anterior and middle cranial fossae. *Removed:* Lateral dural wall and roof of the cavernous sinus. The trigeminal ganglion is cut and retracted laterally following removal of its dural covering

B Topography of the extradural course of the abducent nerve along the clivus and in the left cavernous sinus. Left lateral view. *Note* the long extradural path the abducent nerve follows along the clivus. It runs within the subarachnoid space, pierces the dura mater, passes under Gruber's ligament through Dorello's canal and enters the cavernous sinus at the tip of the petrous temporal bone (at the junction of the middle and posterior cranial fossae). It courses through the cavernous sinus lateral to the internal carotid artery to reach the orbit through the superior orbital fissure.

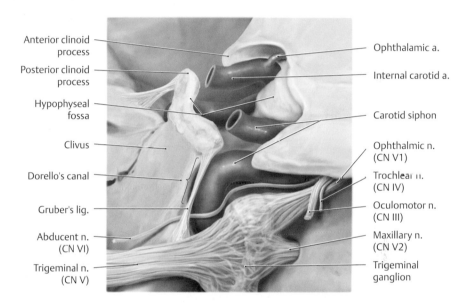

Anterior clinoid process

Posterior clinoid process

Hypophyseal fossa

Clivus

Dorello's canal

Gruber's lig.

Abducent n. (CN VI)

Trigeminal n. (CN V)

Ophthalamic a.

Internal carotid a.

Carotid siphon

Ophthalmic n. (CN V1)

Trochlear n. (CN IV)

Oculomotor n. (CN III)

Maxillary n. (CN V2)

Trigeminal ganglion

Fig. 41.19 Cavernous sinus, coronal section through middle cranial fossa

Anterior view. The right and left cavernous sinuses connect via the intercavernous sinuses that pass around the hypophysis, which sits in the hypophyseal fossa after invaginating the diaphragma sellae. On each side, this coronal section cuts through the internal carotid artery twice due to the presence of the carotid siphon, a 180 degree bend in the cavernous part of the artery. Of the five cranial nerves, or their divisions, associated with the sinus only the abducent nerve (CN VI) is not embedded in the lateral dural wall.

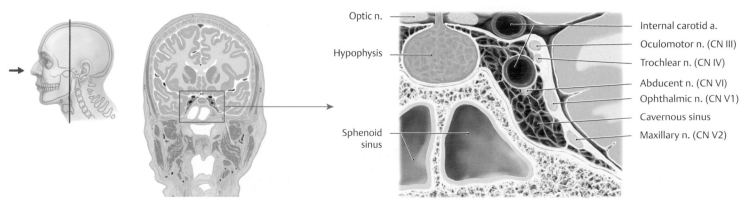

Optic n.

Hypophysis

Sphenoid sinus

Internal carotid a.

Oculomotor n. (CN III)

Trochlear n. (CN IV)

Abducent n. (CN VI)

Ophthalmic n. (CN V1)

Cavernous sinus

Maxillary n. (CN V2)

Topography of the Superficial Face

***Fig. 41.20* Superficial neurovasculature of the face**
Anterior view. *Removed:* Skin and fatty subcutaneous tissue; muscles of
facial expression (left side).

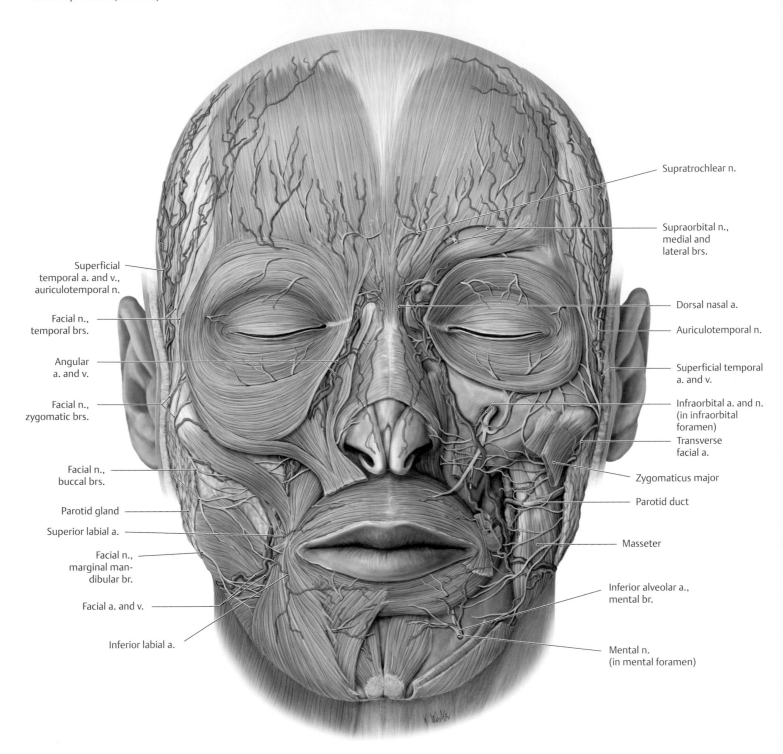

Supratrochlear n.

Supraorbital n.,
medial and
lateral brs.

Superficial
temporal a. and v.,
auriculotemporal n.

Facial n.,
temporal brs.

Angular
a. and v.

Facial n.,
zygomatic brs.

Facial n.,
buccal brs.

Parotid gland

Superior labial a.

Facial n.,
marginal man-
dibular br.

Facial a. and v.

Inferior labial a.

Dorsal nasal a.

Auriculotemporal n.

Superficial temporal
a. and v.

Infraorbital a. and n.
(in infraorbital
foramen)

Transverse
facial a.

Zygomaticus major

Parotid duct

Masseter

Inferior alveolar a.,
mental br.

Mental n.
(in mental foramen)

Fig. 41.21 Superficial neurovasculature of the head
Left lateral view.

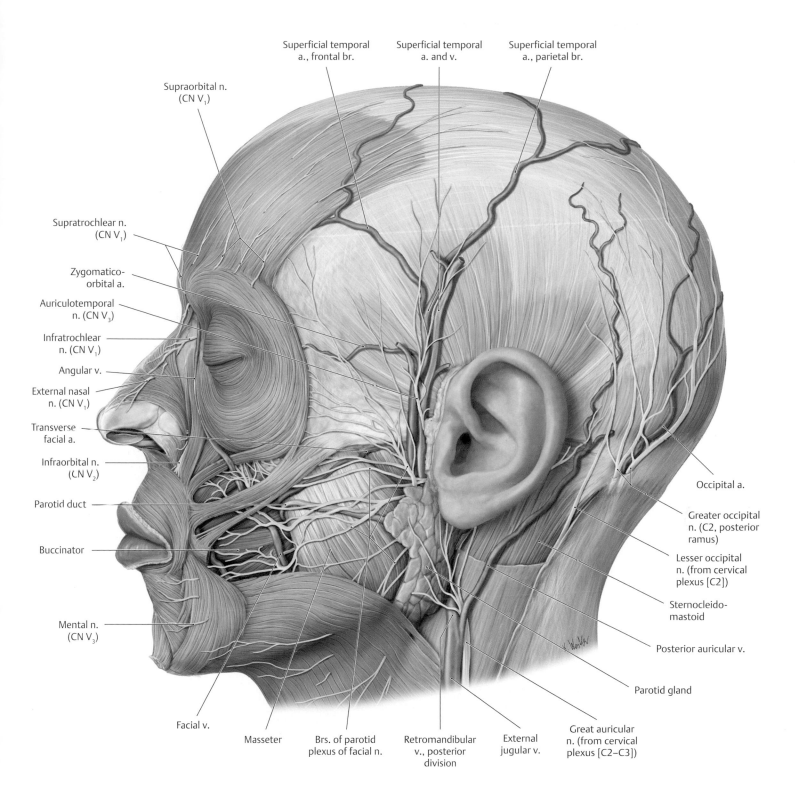

Supraorbital n. (CN V₁)

Supratrochlear n. (CN V₁)

Zygomatico-orbital a.

Auriculotemporal n. (CN V₃)

Infratrochlear n. (CN V₁)

Angular v.

External nasal n. (CN V₁)

Transverse facial a.

Infraorbital n. (CN V₂)

Parotid duct

Buccinator

Mental n. (CN V₃)

Superficial temporal a., frontal br.

Superficial temporal a. and v.

Superficial temporal a., parietal br.

Occipital a.

Greater occipital n. (C2, posterior ramus)

Lesser occipital n. (from cervical plexus [C2])

Sternocleido-mastoid

Posterior auricular v.

Parotid gland

Facial v.

Masseter

Brs. of parotid plexus of facial n.

Retromandibular v., posterior division

External jugular v.

Great auricular n. (from cervical plexus [C2–C3])

Topography of the Parotid Region & Temporal Fossa

Fig. 41.22 Parotid region
Left lateral view. *Removed:* Parotid gland,
sternocleidomastoid, and veins of the head.
Revealed: Parotid bed and carotid triangle.

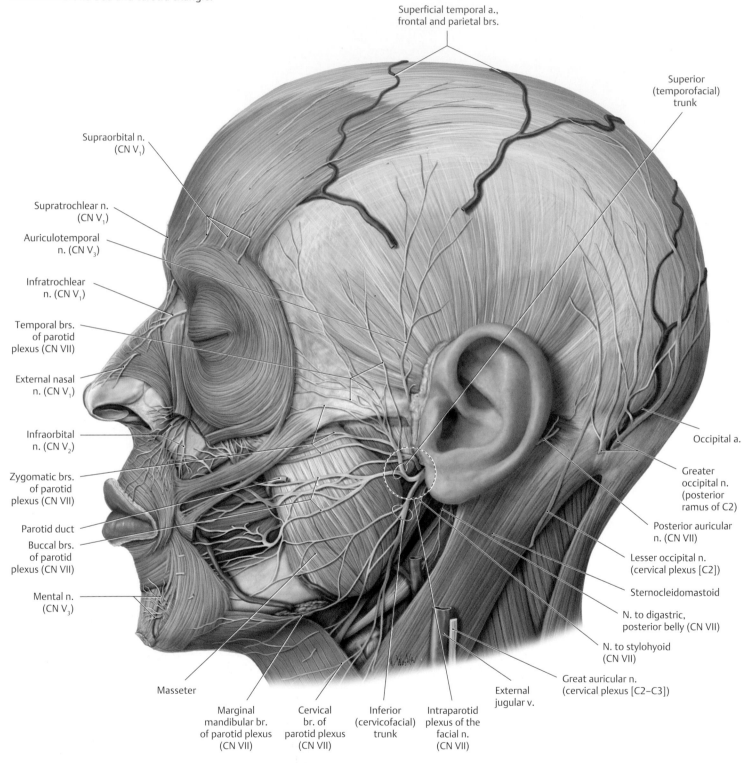

Superficial temporal a.,
frontal and parietal brs.

Superior
(temporofacial)
trunk

Supraorbital n.
(CN V₁)

Supratrochlear n.
(CN V₁)

Auriculotemporal
n. (CN V₃)

Infratrochlear
n. (CN V₁)

Temporal brs.
of parotid
plexus (CN VII)

External nasal
n. (CN V₁)

Infraorbital
n. (CN V₂)

Zygomatic brs.
of parotid
plexus (CN VII)

Parotid duct

Buccal brs.
of parotid
plexus (CN VII)

Mental n.
(CN V₃)

Occipital a.

Greater
occipital n.
(posterior
ramus of C2)

Posterior auricular
n. (CN VII)

Lesser occipital n.
(cervical plexus [C2])

Sternocleidomastoid

N. to digastric,
posterior belly (CN VII)

N. to stylohyoid
(CN VII)

Great auricular n.
(cervical plexus [C2–C3])

Masseter

Marginal
mandibular br.
of parotid plexus
(CN VII)

Cervical
br. of
parotid plexus
(CN VII)

Inferior
(cervicofacial)
trunk

Intraparotid
plexus of the
facial n.
(CN VII)

External
jugular v.

Fig. 41.23 Temporal fossa

Left lateral view. The temporal fossa is located on the lateral aspect of the skull. It communicates with the infratemporal fossa inferiorly (medial to the zygomatic arch). The main component of the fossa is the large temporalis muscle.

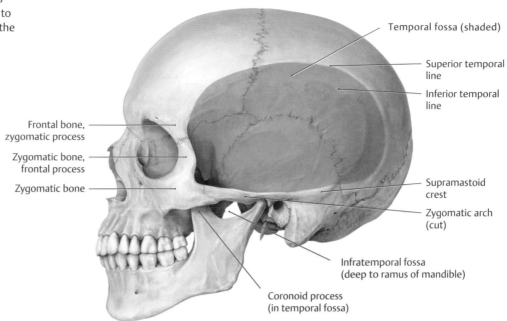

Temporal fossa (shaded)

Superior temporal line

Inferior temporal line

Frontal bone, zygomatic process

Zygomatic bone, frontal process

Zygomatic bone

Supramastoid crest

Zygomatic arch (cut)

Infratemporal fossa (deep to ramus of mandible)

Coronoid process (in temporal fossa)

Fig. 41.24 Temporal fossa

Left lateral view. *Removed:* Sternocleidomastoid and masseter. *Revealed:* Temporal fossa and temporomandibular joint (**p. 638**).

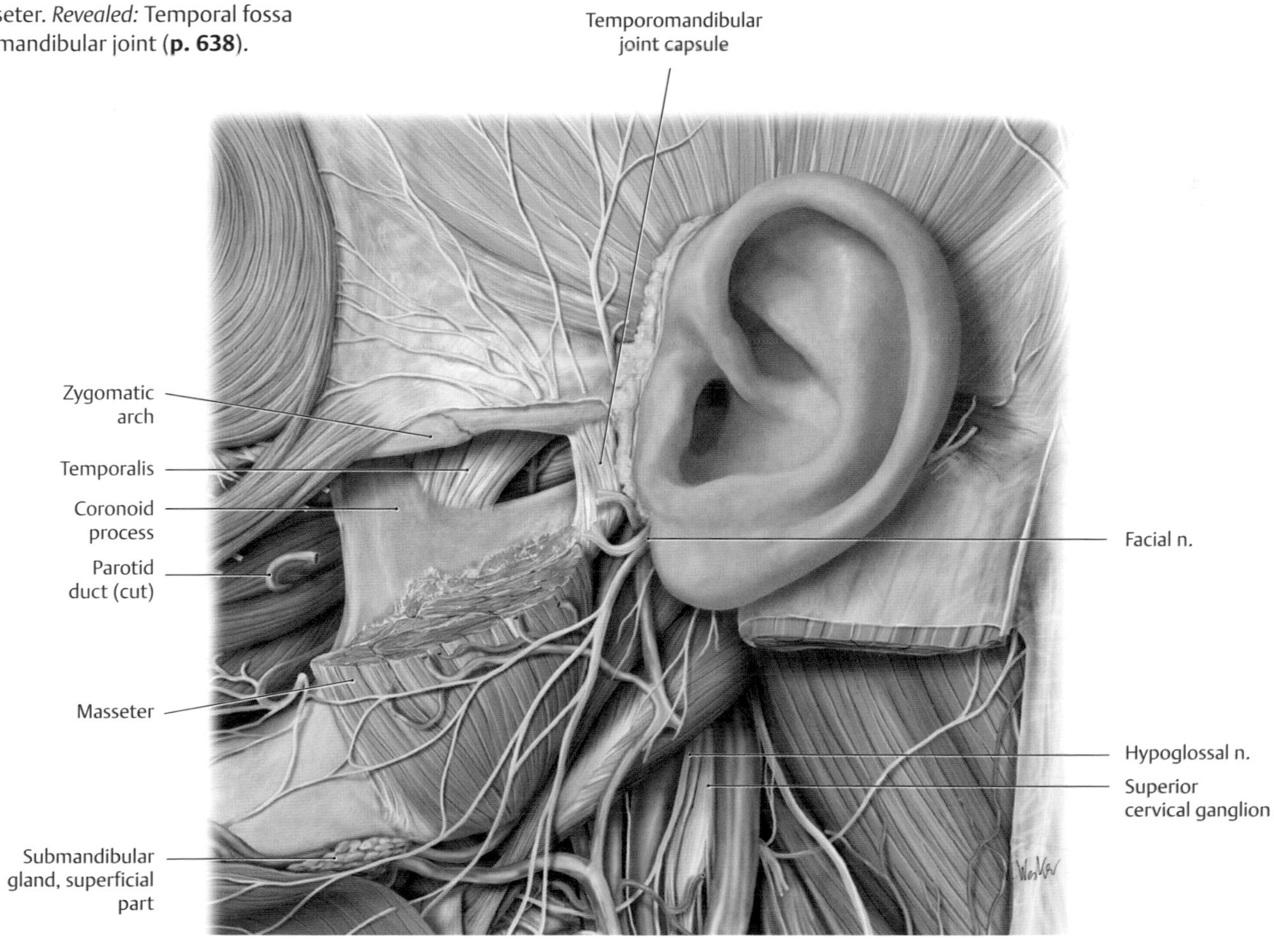

Temporomandibular joint capsule

Zygomatic arch

Temporalis

Coronoid process

Parotid duct (cut)

Masseter

Submandibular gland, superficial part

Facial n.

Hypoglossal n.

Superior cervical ganglion

Neurovasculature of the Infratemporal Fossa

***Fig. 41.28* Mandibular nerve (CN V$_3$) in the infratemporal fossa**

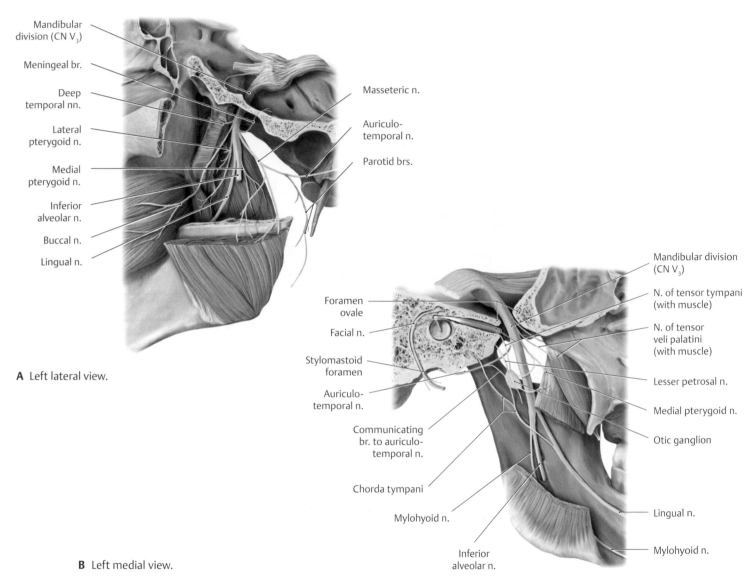

Mandibular division (CN V$_3$)

Meningeal br.

Deep temporal nn.

Lateral pterygoid n.

Medial pterygoid n.

Inferior alveolar n.

Buccal n.

Lingual n.

Masseteric n.

Auriculo-temporal n.

Parotid brs.

A Left lateral view.

Foramen ovale

Facial n.

Stylomastoid foramen

Auriculo-temporal n.

Communicating br. to auriculo-temporal n.

Chorda tympani

Mylohyoid n.

Inferior alveolar n.

Mandibular division (CN V$_3$)

N. of tensor tympani (with muscle)

N. of tensor veli palatini (with muscle)

Lesser petrosal n.

Medial pterygoid n.

Otic ganglion

Lingual n.

Mylohyoid n.

B Left medial view.

Table 41.7	Nerves of the infratemporal fossa	
Nerve	**Nerve Fibers**	**Distribution**
Muscular Branches (CN V$_3$)	Branchial motor	Muscles of mastication; mylohyoid; tensor tympani; tensor veli palatini, anterior belly of digastric
Auriculotemzporal (CN V$_3$)	General sensory	Auricle, temporal region, and temporomandibular joint
	Visceral motor from glossopharyngeal n. (CN IX)	Parotid gland
Inferior alveolar (CN V$_3$)	General sensory	Mandibular teeth; mental branch supplies skin of lower lip and chin
Lingual (CN V$_3$)	General sensory	Anterior two thirds of tongue, floor of mouth
Buccal (CN V$_3$)	General sensory	Skin and mucous membrane of cheek
Meningeal (CN V$_3$)	General sensory	Dura of middle cranial fossa
Chorda tympani (CN VII)	Special sensory taste	Anterior two thirds of tongue
	Visceral motor	Submandibular and sublingual glands via submandibular ganglion and lingual n (CN V$_3$)

Fig. 41.29 Arteries in the infratemporal fossa

Left lateral view into area. The maxillary artery passes either superficial or deep to the lateral pterygoid in the infratemporal fossa (see **Fig. 41.27, p. 599**) and passes medially into the pterygopalatine fossa through the pterygo-maxillary fissure.

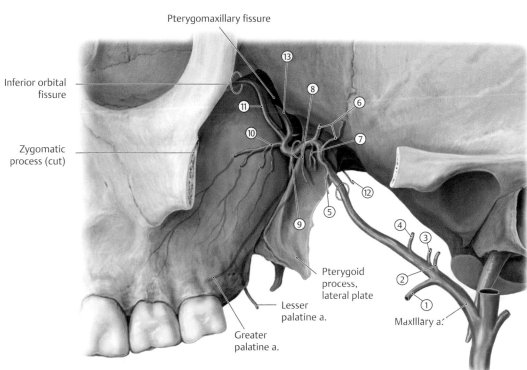

Pterygomaxillary fissure

Inferior orbital fissure

Zygomatic process (cut)

Pterygoid process, lateral plate

Lesser palatine a.

Greater palatine a.

Maxillary a.

Table 41.8	Branches of the maxillary artery		
Part	**Artery**		**Distribution**
Mandibular part (between the origin and the first circle around artery in **Fig. 41.29**)	① Inferior alveolar a.		Mandible, teeth, gingiva
	② Anterior tympanic a.		Tympanic cavity
	③ Deep auricular a.		Temporomandibular joint, external auditory canal
	④ Middle meningeal a.		Calvaria, dura, anterior and middle cranial fossae
Pterygoid part (between the first and second circles around the artery)	⑤ Masseteric a.		Masseter m.
	⑥ Deep temporal aa.		Temporalis m.
	⑦ Pterygoid brs.		Pterygoid mm.
	⑧ Buccal a.		Buccal mucosa
Pterygopalatine part (between the second and third circles around the artery)	⑨ Descending palatine a.	Greater palatine a.	Hard palate
		Lesser palatine a.	Soft palate, palatine tonsil, pharyngeal wall
	⑩ Posterior superior alveolar a.		Maxillary molars, maxillary sinus, gingiva
	⑪ Infraorbital a.		Maxillary alveoli
	⑫ A. of pterygoid canal		
	⑬ Sphenopalatine a.	Lateral posterior nasal aa.	Lateral wall of nasal cavity, choanae
		Posterior septal brs.	Nasal septum

Muscles of the Orbit

Fig. 42.2 Extraocular muscles

The eyeball is moved by six extrinsic muscles: four rectus (superior, inferior, medial, and lateral) and two oblique (superior and inferior).

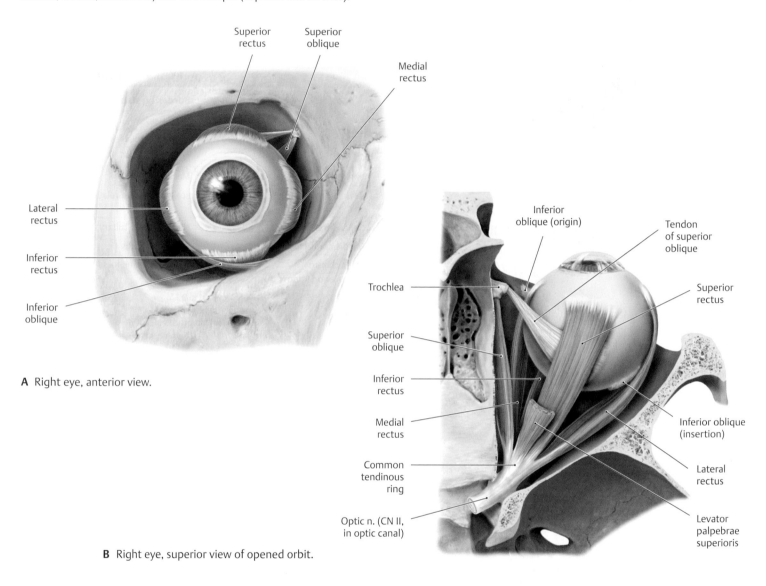

A Right eye, anterior view.

B Right eye, superior view of opened orbit.

Fig. 42.3 Testing the extraocular muscles

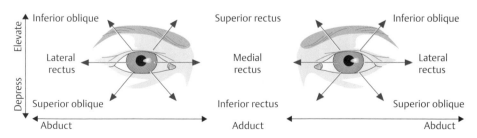

A Starting with the eyes directed anteriorly, movement to any of the cardinal directions of gaze (*arrows*) requires activation of two extraocular muscles, each of which is innervated by a different cranial nerve, thus testing the function of those pairs of muscles.

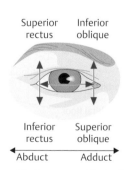

B Starting with the eyes adducted or abducted, elevating or lowering the eyes activates only the oblique or the rectus muscles, respectively, allowing for testing of the function of individual muscles.

Fig. 42.4 **Actions of the extraocular muscles**

Superior view of opened orbit. Vertical axis, red circle; horizontal axis, black; anteroposterior (visual/optical) axis, blue.

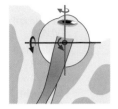 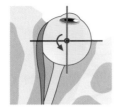 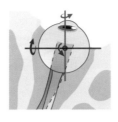 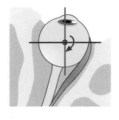 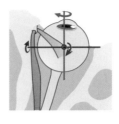 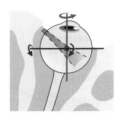

A Superior rectus. **B** Medial rectus. **C** Inferior rectus. **D** Lateral rectus. **E** Superior oblique. **F** Inferior oblique.

Table 42.3 **Extraocular muscles**

Muscle	Origin	Insertion	Action (see Fig. 42.4)* Vertical axis (red)	Horizontal axis (black)	Anteroposterior axis (blue)	Innervation
Superior rectus	Common tendinous ring (common annular tendon)	Sclera of the eye	Elevates	Adducts	Rotates medially	Oculomotor n. (CN III), superior branch
Medial rectus			—	Adducts	—	Oculomotor n. (CN III), inferior branch
Inferior rectus			Depresses	Adducts	Rotates laterally	
Lateral rectus			—	Abducts	—	Abducent n. (CN VI)
Superior oblique	Sphenoid bone⁺		Depresses	Abducts	Rotates medially	Trochlear n. (CN IV)
Inferior oblique	Medial orbital margin		Elevates	Abducts	Rotates laterally	Oculomotor n. (CN III), inferior branch

* Starting from gaze directed anteriorly
⁺ The tendon of the superior oblique passes through a tendinous loop (trochlea) attached to the superomedial orbital margin.

✳ *Clinical box 42.1*

Oculomotor palsies

Oculomotor palsies may result from a lesion involving an eye muscle or its associated cranial nerve (at the nucleus or along the course of the nerve). If one extraocular muscle is weak or paralyzed, deviation of the eye will be noted.

Impairment of the coordinated actions of the extraocular muscles may cause the visual axis of one eye to deviate from its normal position. The patient will therefore perceive a double image (diplopia).

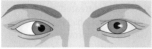

A Abducent nerve palsy. *Disabled:* Lateral rectus.

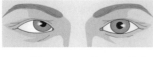

B Trochlear nerve palsy. *Disabled:* Superior oblique.

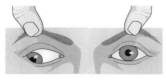

C Complete oculomotor palsy. *Disabled:* Superior, inferior, and medial recti and inferior oblique.

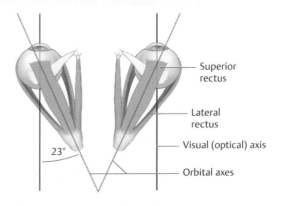

D Normal visual and orbital axes.

Superior rectus
Lateral rectus
Visual (optical) axis
Orbital axes
23°

Topography of the Orbit

Fig. 42.9 **Neurovascular structures of the orbit**

Anterior view. *Right side:* Orbicularis oculi removed. *Left side:* Orbital septum partially removed.

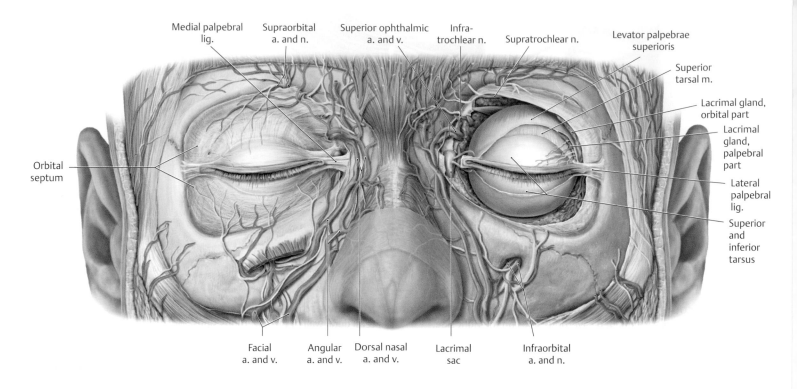

Medial palpebral lig. — Supraorbital a. and n. — Superior ophthalmic a. and v. — Infra-trochlear n. — Supratrochlear n. — Levator palpebrae superioris — Superior tarsal m. — Lacrimal gland, orbital part — Lacrimal gland, palpebral part — Lateral palpebral lig. — Superior and inferior tarsus — Orbital septum — Facial a. and v. — Angular a. and v. — Dorsal nasal a. and v. — Lacrimal sac — Infraorbital a. and n.

Fig. 42.10 **Passage of neurovascular structures through the orbit**

Anterior view. *Removed:* Orbital contents. *Note:* The optic nerve and ophthalmic artery travel in the optic canal. The remaining structures pass through the superior orbital fissure.

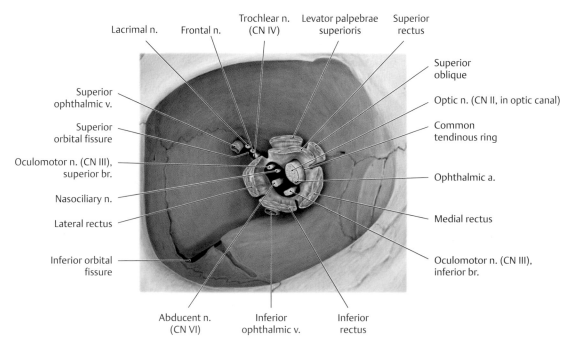

Lacrimal n. — Frontal n. — Trochlear n. (CN IV) — Levator palpebrae superioris — Superior rectus — Superior oblique — Optic n. (CN II, in optic canal) — Common tendinous ring — Ophthalmic a. — Medial rectus — Oculomotor n. (CN III), inferior br. — Superior ophthalmic v. — Superior orbital fissure — Oculomotor n. (CN III), superior br. — Nasociliary n. — Lateral rectus — Inferior orbital fissure — Abducent n. (CN VI) — Inferior ophthalmic v. — Inferior rectus

Fig. 42.11 Neurovascular contents of the orbit

Superior view. *Removed:* Bony roof of orbit, peritorbita, and retro-orbital fat.

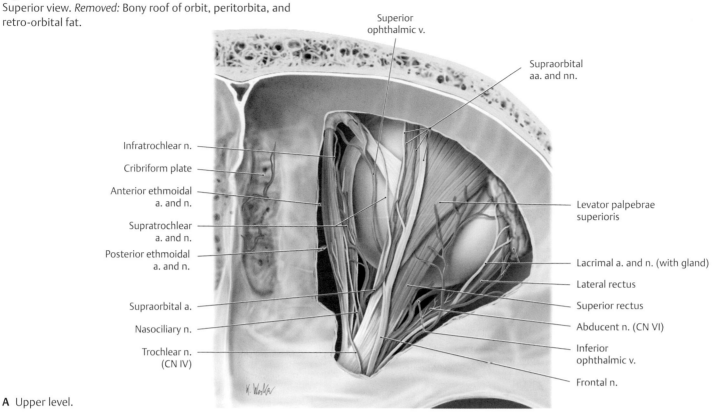

Infratrochlear n.
Cribriform plate
Anterior ethmoidal a. and n.
Supratrochlear a. and n.
Posterior ethmoidal a. and n.
Supraorbital a.
Nasociliary n.
Trochlear n. (CN IV)

Superior ophthalmic v.
Supraorbital aa. and nn.
Levator palpebrae superioris
Lacrimal a. and n. (with gland)
Lateral rectus
Superior rectus
Abducent n. (CN VI)
Inferior ophthalmic v.
Frontal n.

A Upper level.

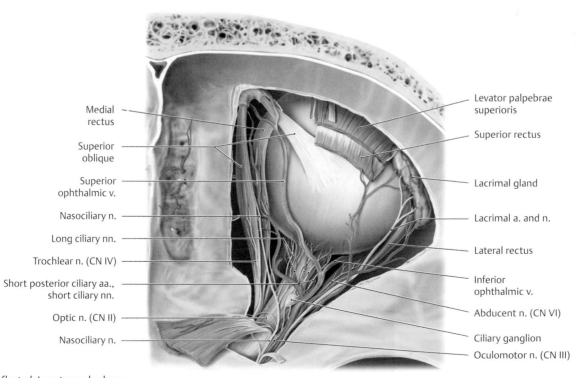

Medial rectus
Superior oblique
Superior ophthalmic v.
Nasociliary n.
Long ciliary nn.
Trochlear n. (CN IV)
Short posterior ciliary aa., short ciliary nn.
Optic n. (CN II)
Nasociliary n.

Levator palpebrae superioris
Superior rectus
Lacrimal gland
Lacrimal a. and n.
Lateral rectus
Inferior ophthalmic v.
Abducent n. (CN VI)
Ciliary ganglion
Oculomotor n. (CN III)

B Middle level. *Reflected:* Levator palpebrae superioris and superior rectus. *Revealed:* Optic nerve.

Eyeball

Fig. 42.15 **Structure of the eyeball**

Transverse section through right eyeball, superior view. *Note:* The orbital axis (running along the optic nerve through the optic disk) deviates from the optical axis (running through the center of the eye to the fovea centralis) by 23 degrees.

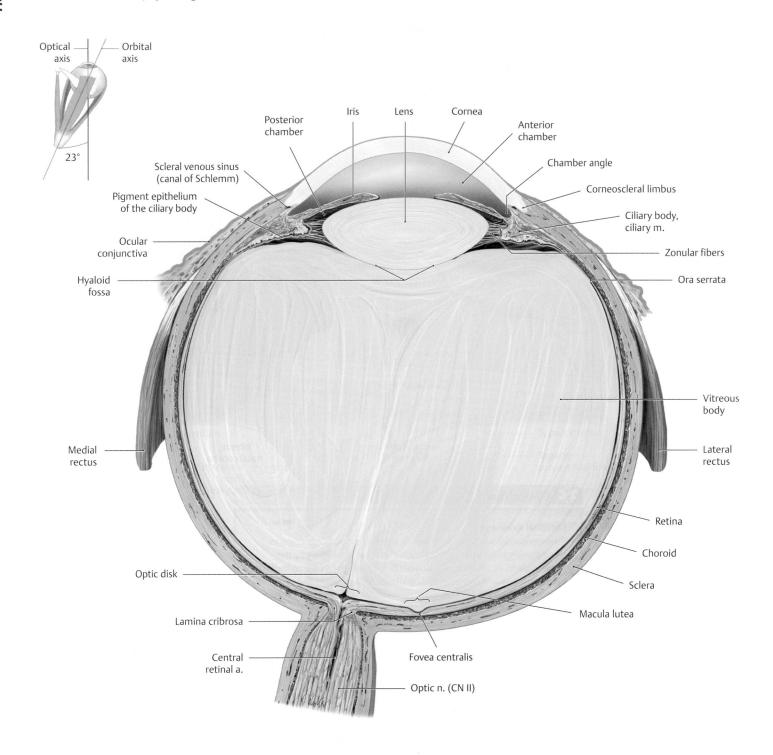

Fig. 42.16 Blood vessels of the eyeball

Transverse section through the right eyeball at the level of the optic nerve, superior view. The arteries of the eye arise from the ophthalmic artery, a terminal branch of the internal carotid artery. Blood is drained by four to eight vorticose veins that open into the superior and inferior ophthalmic veins.

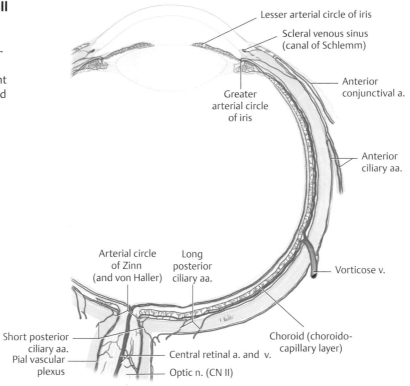

Lesser arterial circle of iris

Scleral venous sinus (canal of Schlemm)

Anterior conjunctival a.

Anterior ciliary aa.

Greater arterial circle of iris

Vorticose v.

Arterial circle of Zinn (and von Haller)

Long posterior ciliary aa.

Choroid (choroidocapillary layer)

Short posterior ciliary aa.

Pial vascular plexus

Central retinal a. and v.

Optic n. (CN II)

Clinical box 42.4

Optic fundus

The optic fundus is the only place in the body where capillaries can be examined directly. Examination of the optic fundus permits observation of vascular changes that may be caused by high blood pressure or diabetes. Examination of the optic disk is important in determining intracranial pressure and diagnosing multiple sclerosis.

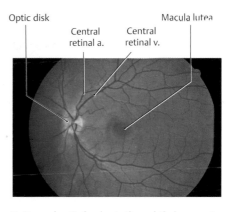

Optic disk

Macula lutea

Central retinal a.

Central retinal v.

B Normal optic fundus in the ophthalmoscopic examination.

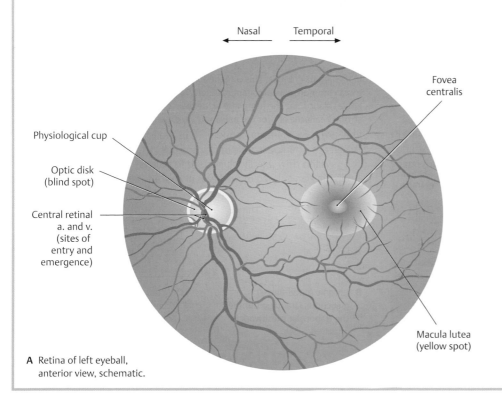

Nasal ← → Temporal

Physiological cup

Optic disk (blind spot)

Central retinal a. and v. (sites of entry and emergence)

Fovea centralis

Macula lutea (yellow spot)

A Retina of left eyeball, anterior view, schematic.

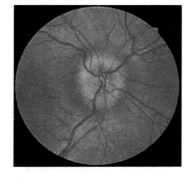

C High intracranial pressure; the edges of the optic disk appear less sharp.

43 Nasal Cavity & Nose
Bones of the Nasal Cavity

Fig. 43.1 Skeleton of the nose

The skeleton of the nose is composed of an upper bony portion and a lower cartilaginous portion. The proximal portions of the nostrils (alae) are composed of connective tissue with small embedded pieces of cartilage.

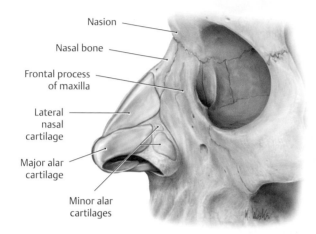

A Left lateral view.

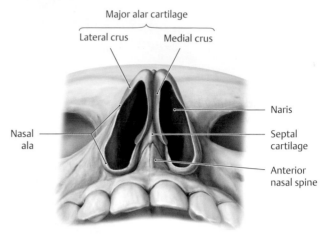

B Inferior view.

Fig. 43.2 Bones of the nasal cavity

The left and right nasal cavities are flanked by lateral walls and separated by the nasal septum. Air enters the nasal cavity through the anterior nasal aperture and travels through three passages: the superior, middle, and inferior meatuses (*arrows*). These passages are separated by the superior, middle, and inferior conchae. Air leaves the nose through the choanae, entering the nasopharynx.

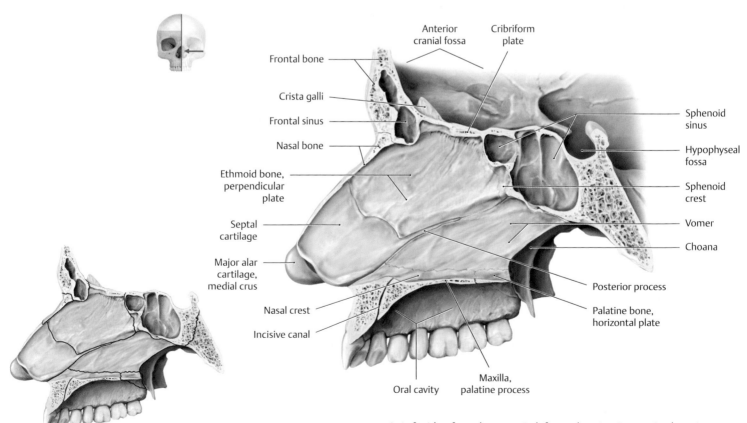

A Left side of nasal septum in left nasal cavity. Parasagittal section.

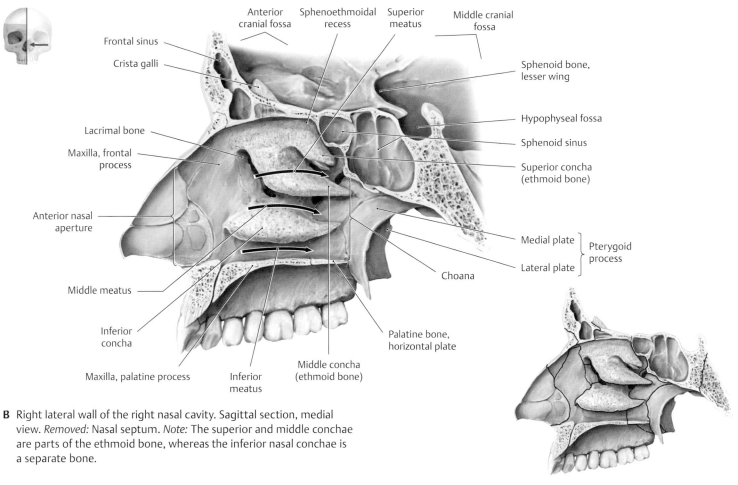

Frontal sinus

Crista galli

Anterior cranial fossa

Sphenoethmoidal recess

Superior meatus

Middle cranial fossa

Sphenoid bone, lesser wing

Hypophyseal fossa

Sphenoid sinus

Superior concha (ethmoid bone)

Lacrimal bone

Maxilla, frontal process

Anterior nasal aperture

Medial plate ⎱
Lateral plate ⎰ Pterygoid process

Choana

Middle meatus

Inferior concha

Maxilla, palatine process

Inferior meatus

Middle concha (ethmoid bone)

Palatine bone, horizontal plate

B Right lateral wall of the right nasal cavity. Sagittal section, medial view. *Removed:* Nasal septum. *Note:* The superior and middle conchae are parts of the ethmoid bone, whereas the inferior nasal conchae is a separate bone.

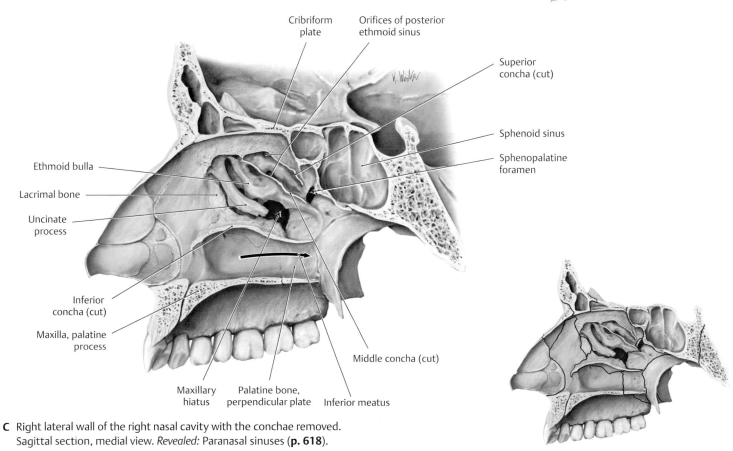

Cribriform plate

Orifices of posterior ethmoid sinus

Superior concha (cut)

Sphenoid sinus

Sphenopalatine foramen

Ethmoid bulla

Lacrimal bone

Uncinate process

Inferior concha (cut)

Maxilla, palatine process

Maxillary hiatus

Palatine bone, perpendicular plate

Inferior meatus

Middle concha (cut)

C Right lateral wall of the right nasal cavity with the conchae removed. Sagittal section, medial view. *Revealed:* Paranasal sinuses (**p. 618**).

Pterygopalatine Fossa

The pterygopalatine fossa is a small pyramidal space just inferior to the apex of the orbit. It is continuous with the infratemporal fossa laterally through the pterygomaxillary fissure. The pterygopalatine fossa is a crossroad for neurovascular structures traveling between the middle cranial fossa, orbit, nasal cavity, and oral cavity.

Fig. 43.10 Bony boundaries of pterygopalatine fossa

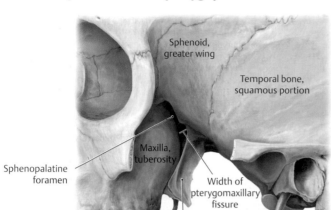

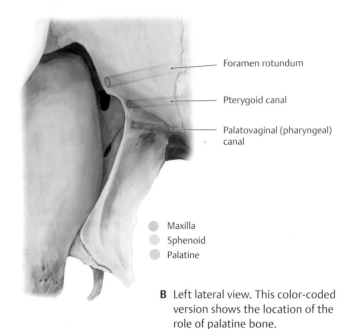

Foramen rotundum

Pterygoid canal

Palatovaginal (pharyngeal) canal

Sphenoid, greater wing

Temporal bone, squamous portion

Maxilla, tuberosity

Sphenopalatine foramen

Width of pterygomaxillary fissure

Lateral plate, pterygoid process

○ Maxilla
○ Sphenoid
○ Palatine

A Left lateral view. The lateral approach through the infratemporal fossa via the pterygomaxillary fissure.

B Left lateral view. This color-coded version shows the location of the role of palatine bone.

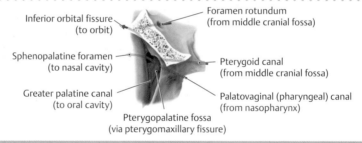

Inferior orbital fissure (to orbit)

Foramen rotundum (from middle cranial fossa)

Sphenopalatine foramen (to nasal cavity)

Pterygoid canal (from middle cranial fossa)

Greater palatine canal (to oral cavity)

Palatovaginal (pharyngeal) canal (from nasopharynx)

Pterygopalatine fossa (via pterygomaxillary fissure)

Table 43.2	**Communications of the Pterygopalatine Fossa**		
Communication	**Direction**	**Via**	**Transmitted structures**
Middle cranial fossa	Posterosuperiorly	Foramen rotundum	• Maxillary n. (CN V$_2$)
Middle cranial fossa	Posteriorly in anterior wall of foramen lacerum	Pterygoid (vidian) canal	• N. of pterygoid canal, formed from: ○ Greater petrosal n. (preganglionic parasympathetic fibers from CN VII) ○ Deep petrosal n. (postganglionic sympathetic fibers from internal carotid plexus) • A. of pterygoid canal • Vv. of pterygoid canal
Orbit	Anterosuperiorly	Inferior orbital fissure	• Branches of maxillary n. (CN V$_2$) ○ Infraorbital n. ○ Zygomatic n. • Infraorbital a. and vv. • Communicating vv. between inferior ophthalmic v. and pterygoid plexus of vv.
Nasal cavity	Medially	Sphenopalatine foramen	• Nasopalatine (sp) n. (CN V$_2$), lateral and medial superior posterior nasal branches • Sphenopalatine a. and vv.
Oral cavity	Inferiorly	Greater palatine canal (foramen)	• Greater (descending) palatine n. (CN V$_2$) and a. • Branches that emerge through lesser palatine canals: ○ Lesser palatine nn. (CN V$_2$) and aa.
Nasopharynx	Inferoposteriorly	Palatovaginal (pharyngeal) canal	• Pharyngeal branches of maxillary n. (CN V$_2$), and pharyngeal a.
Infratemporal fossa	Laterally	Pterygomaxillary fissure	• Maxillary a., pterygopalatine (third) part • Posterior superior alveolar n., a., and v.

The maxillary division of the trigeminal nerve (CN V$_2$, see **Fig. 40.9, p. 567**) passes from the middle cranial fossa through the foramen rotundum into the pterygopalatine fossa. The parasympathetic pterygopalatine ganglion receives postganglionic fibers from the greater petrosal nerve (the parasympathetic root of the nervus intermedius branch of the facial nerve). The preganglionic fibers of the pterygopalatine ganglion synapse with ganglion cells that innervate the lacrimal, small palatal, and small nasal glands. The sympathetic fibers of the deep petrosal nerve (sympathetic root) and sensory fibers of the maxillary nerve (sensory root) pass through the pterygopalatine ganglion without synapsing. The pterygopalatine structures can be seen from the medial view in **Fig. 43.8B, p. 621.**

Fig. 43.11 Nerves in the pterygopalatine fossa

Left lateral view. For simplicity in a small, structurally compressed area, numbers are used to identify the nerves. The key to these numbers is found in **Table 43.3** (below).

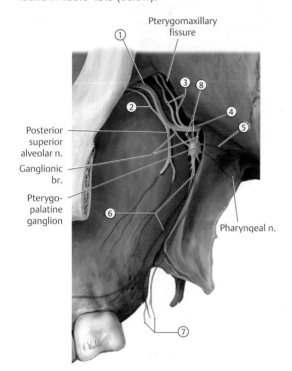

Pterygomaxillary fissure

Posterior superior alveolar n.

Ganglionic br.

Pterygopalatine ganglion

Pharyngeal n.

Fig. 43.12 Coronal view of the pterygopalatine fossa

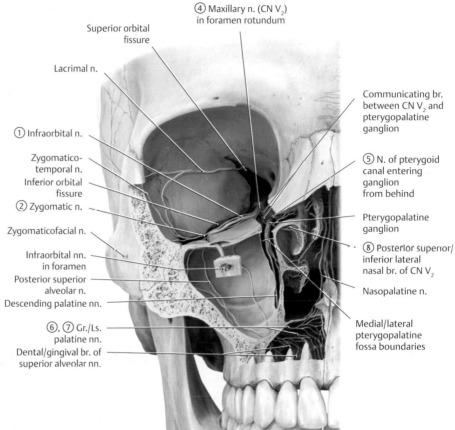

④ Maxillary n. (CN V$_2$) in foramen rotundum

Superior orbital fissure

Lacrimal n.

① Infraorbital n.

Zygomaticotemporal n.

Inferior orbital fissure

② Zygomatic n.

Zygomaticofacial n.

Infraorbital nn. in foramen

Posterior superior alveolar n.

Descending palatine nn.

⑥, ⑦ Gr./Ls. palatine nn.

Dental/gingival br. of superior alveolar nn.

Communicating br. between CN V$_2$ and pterygopalatine ganglion

⑤ N. of pterygoid canal entering ganglion from behind

Pterygopalatine ganglion

⑧ Posterior superior/ inferior lateral nasal br. of CN V$_2$

Nasopalatine n.

Medial/lateral pterygopalatine fossa boundaries

Table 43.3	Nerves of the pterygopalatine fossa	
Origin of structures	**Passageway**	**Transmitted nerves**
Orbit	Inferior orbital fissure	① Infraorbital n.
		② Zygomatic n.
		③ Orbital brs. (from CN V$_2$)
Middle cranial fossa	Foramen rotundum	④ Maxillary n. (CN V$_2$)
Base of skull	Pterygoid (Vidian) canal	⑤ N. of pterygoid canal
Palate	Greater palatine canal	⑥ Greater palatine n.
	Lesser palatine canals	⑦ Lesser palatine nn.
Nasal cavity	Sphenopalatine foramen	⑧ Medial and lateral posterior superior and posterior inferior nasal brs. (from nasopalatine n., CN V$_2$)

44 Temporal Bone & Ear
Temporal Bone

Fig. 44.1 **Temporal bone**
Left bone. The temporal bone consists of three major parts: squamous, petrous, and tympanic (see **Fig. 44.2**).

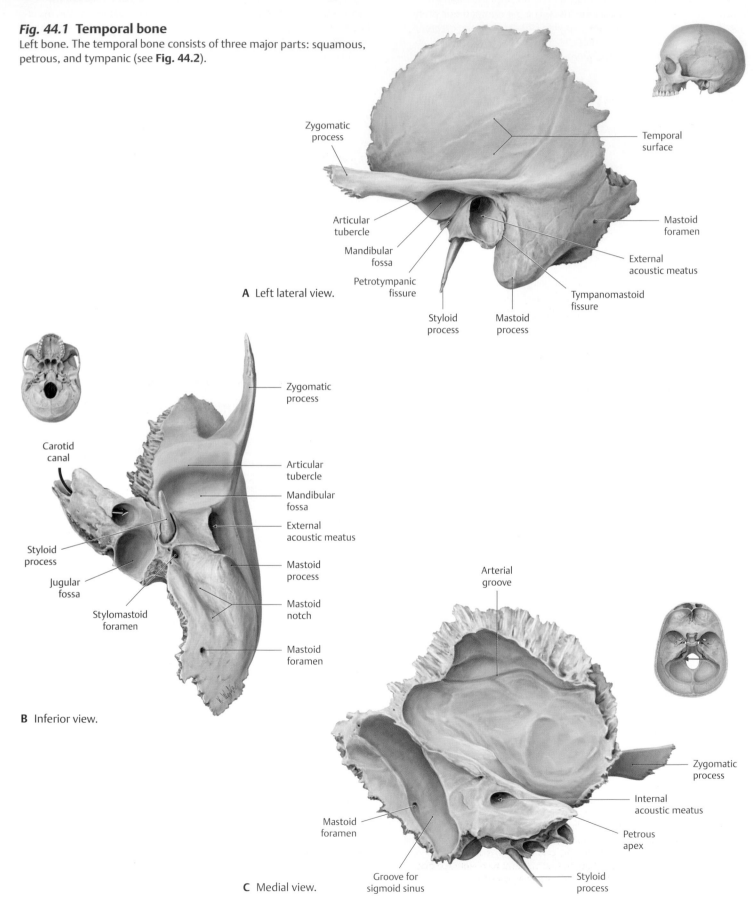

Zygomatic process

Temporal surface

Articular tubercle

Mandibular fossa

Petrotympanic fissure

Mastoid foramen

External acoustic meatus

Tympanomastoid fissure

Styloid process

Mastoid process

A Left lateral view.

Zygomatic process

Carotid canal

Articular tubercle

Mandibular fossa

External acoustic meatus

Styloid process

Mastoid process

Jugular fossa

Mastoid notch

Stylomastoid foramen

Mastoid foramen

B Inferior view.

Arterial groove

Zygomatic process

Internal acoustic meatus

Mastoid foramen

Petrous apex

Groove for sigmoid sinus

Styloid process

C Medial view.

Fig. 44.2 Parts of the temporal bone

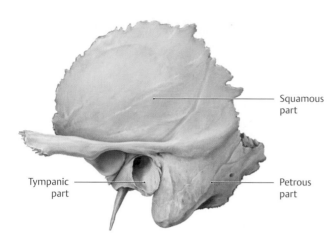

A Left lateral view.

Squamous part

Tympanic part

Petrous part

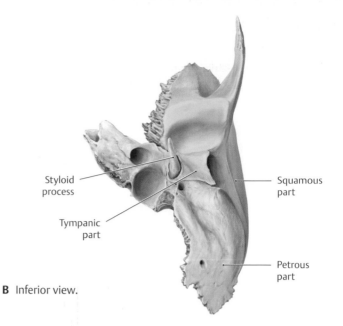

B Inferior view.

Styloid process

Squamous part

Tympanic part

Petrous part

Clinical box 44.1

Structures in the temporal bone

The mastoid process contains mastoid air cells that communicate with the middle ear; the middle ear in turn communicates with the nasopharynx via the pharyngotympanic (auditory) tube (**A**). Bacteria may use this pathway to move from the nasopharynx into the middle ear. In severe cases, bacteria may pass from the mastoid air cells into the cranial cavity, causing meningitis.

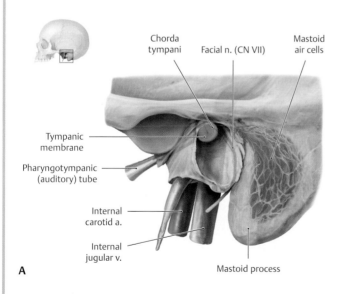

Chorda tympani

Facial n. (CN VII)

Mastoid air cells

Tympanic membrane

Pharyngotympanic (auditory) tube

Internal carotid a.

Internal jugular v.

Mastoid process

A

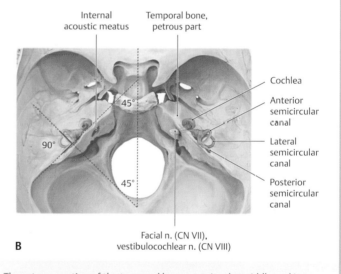

Internal acoustic meatus

Temporal bone, petrous part

Cochlea

Anterior semicircular canal

Lateral semicircular canal

Posterior semicircular canal

45°

90°

45°

Facial n. (CN VII), vestibulocochlear n. (CN VIII)

B

The petrous portion of the temporal bone contains the middle and inner ear as well as the tympanic membrane. The bony semicircular canals are oriented at an approximately 45-degree angle from the coronal, transverse, and sagittal planes (**B**).

Irrigation of the auditory canal with warm (44°C) or cool (30°C) water can induce a thermal current in the endolymph of the semicircular canal, causing the patient to manifest vestibular nystagmus (jerky eye movements, vestibulo-ocular reflex). This caloric testing is important in the diagnosis of unexplained vertigo. The patient must be oriented so that the semicircular canal of interest lies in the vertical plane (**C**).

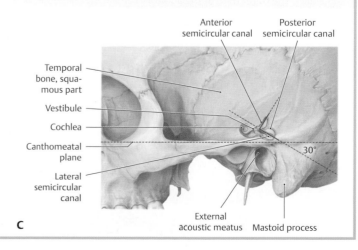

Anterior semicircular canal

Posterior semicircular canal

Temporal bone, squamous part

Vestibule

Cochlea

Canthomeatal plane

Lateral semicircular canal

External acoustic meatus

Mastoid process

30°

C

External Ear & Auditory Canal

The auditory apparatus is divided into three main parts: external, middle, and inner ear. The external and middle ear are part of the sound conduction apparatus, and the inner ear is the actual organ of hearing (see **p. 634**). The inner ear also contains the vestibular apparatus, the organ of balance (see **p. 634**).

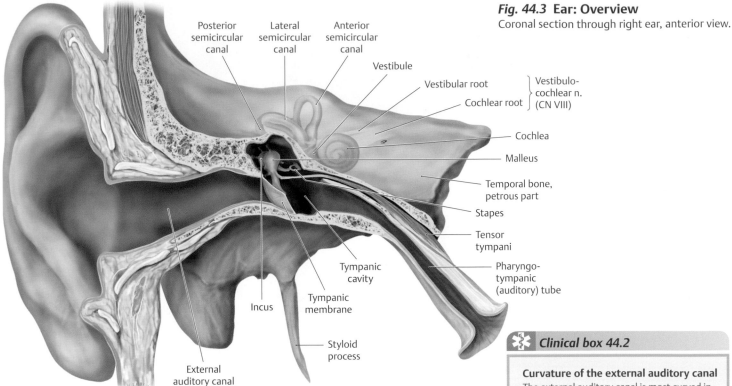

Fig. 44.3 **Ear: Overview**
Coronal section through right ear, anterior view.

Posterior semicircular canal
Lateral semicircular canal
Anterior semicircular canal
Vestibule
Vestibular root
Cochlear root
Vestibulo-cochlear n. (CN VIII)
Cochlea
Malleus
Temporal bone, petrous part
Stapes
Tensor tympani
Pharyngo-tympanic (auditory) tube
Tympanic cavity
Tympanic membrane
Incus
Styloid process
External auditory canal

Fig. 44.4 **External auditory canal**
Coronal section through right ear, anterior view. The tympanic membrane separates the external auditory canal from the tympanic cavity (middle ear). The outer third of the auditory canal is cartilaginous, and the inner two thirds are osseous (tympanic part of temporal bone).

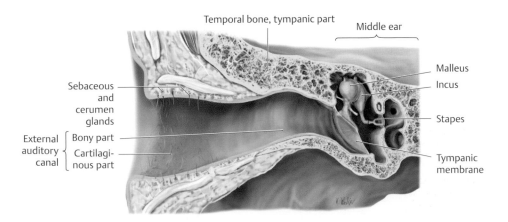

Temporal bone, tympanic part
Middle ear
Sebaceous and cerumen glands
Malleus
Incus
Stapes
External auditory canal { Bony part / Cartilaginous part }
Tympanic membrane

🩺 *Clinical box 44.2*

Curvature of the external auditory canal
The external auditory canal is most curved in its cartilaginous portion. When an otoscope is being inserted, the auricle should be pulled backward and upward so the speculum can be introduced into a straightened canal.

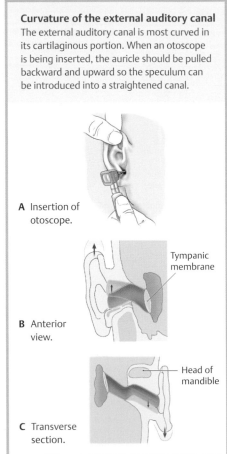

A Insertion of otoscope.

B Anterior view.

Tympanic membrane

C Transverse section.

Head of mandible

Fig. 44.5 Structure of the auricle

The auricle of the ear encloses a cartilaginous framework that forms a funnel-shaped receptor for acoustic vibrations. The muscles of the auricle are considered muscles of facial expression, although they are vestigial in humans.

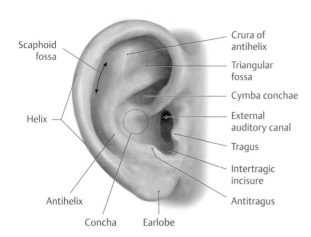

A Right auricle, right lateral view.

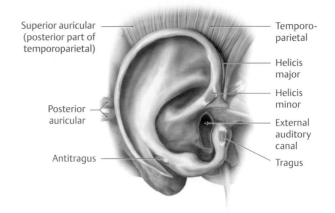

B Cartilage and muscles of the right auricle, right lateral view.

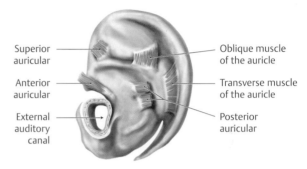

C Cartilage and muscles of the right auricle, medial view of posterior surface.

Fig. 44.6 Arteries of the auricle

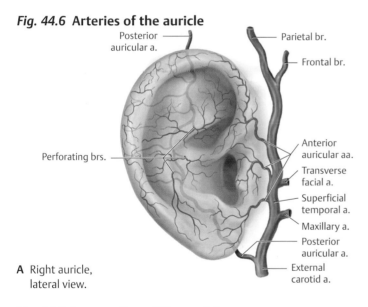

A Right auricle, lateral view.

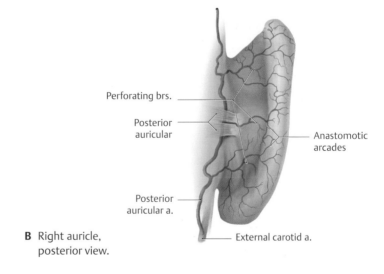

B Right auricle, posterior view.

Fig. 44.7 Innervation of the auricle

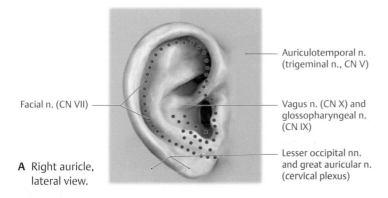

A Right auricle, lateral view.

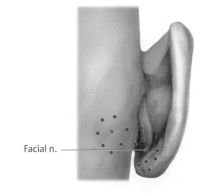

B Right auricle, posterior view.

Middle Ear: Tympanic Cavity

Fig. 44.8 Middle ear

Right petrous bone, superior view. The tympanic cavity of the middle ear communicates anteriorly with the pharynx via the pharyngotympanic (auditory) tube and posteriorly with the mastoid air cells.

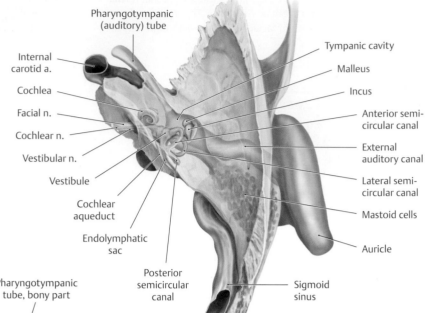

Fig. 44.9 Tympanic cavity and pharyngotympanic tube

Medial view of opened tympanic cavity.

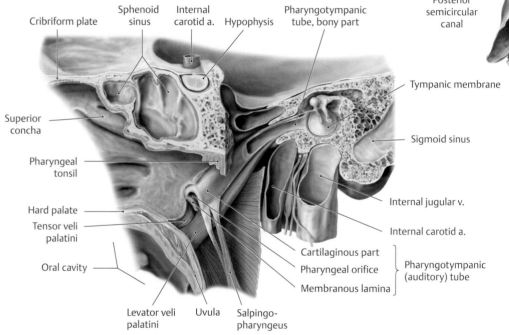

Table 44.1	Boundaries of the tympanic cavity			
During chronic suppurative otitis media (inflammation of the middle ear), pathogenic bacteria may spread to adjacent regions.				
Direction	**Wall**	**Anatomical boundary**	**Neighboring structures**	**Infection**
Anterior	Carotid	Opening to pharyngotympanic tube	Carotid canal	
Lateral	Membranous	Tympanic membrane	External ear	
Superior	Tegmental	Tegmen tympani	Middle cranial fossa	Meningitis, cerebral abscess (especially of temporal lobe)
Medial	Labyrinthine	Promontory overlying basal turn of cochlea	Inner ear	
			CSF space (via petrous apex)	Abducent paralysis, trigeminal nerve irritation, visual disturbances (Gradenigo's syndrome)
Inferior	Jugular	Temporal bone, tympanic part	Bulb of jugular v.	
			Sigmoid sinus	Sinus thrombosis
Posterior	Mastoid	Aditus to mastoid antrum	Air cells of mastoid process	Mastoiditis
			Facial n. canal	Facial paralysis
CSF, cerebrospinal fluid.				

Fig. 44.10 Tympanic cavity

A Levels of the tympanic cavity. Anterior view.
The tympanic cavity is divided into three
levels: epi-, meso-, and hypotympanum.

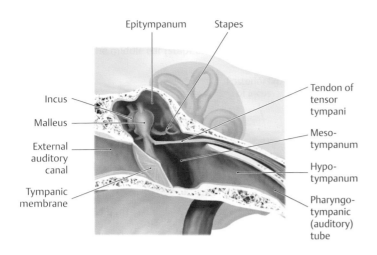

Epitympanum · Stapes
Incus
Malleus
External auditory canal
Tympanic membrane
Tendon of tensor tympani
Meso-tympanum
Hypo-tympanum
Pharyngo-tympanic (auditory) tube

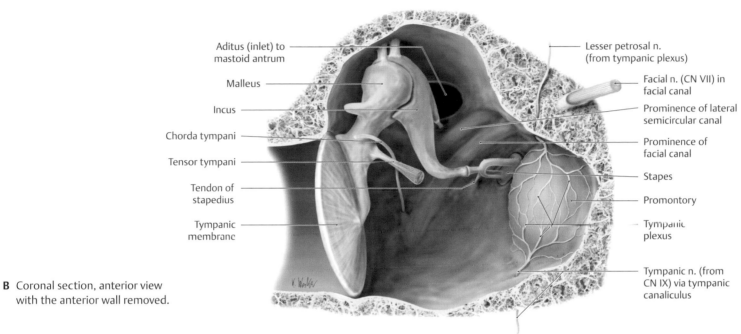

B Coronal section, anterior view
with the anterior wall removed.

Aditus (inlet) to mastoid antrum
Malleus
Incus
Chorda tympani
Tensor tympani
Tendon of stapedius
Tympanic membrane
Lesser petrosal n. (from tympanic plexus)
Facial n. (CN VII) in facial canal
Prominence of lateral semicircular canal
Prominence of facial canal
Stapes
Promontory
Tympanic plexus
Tympanic n. (from CN IX) via tympanic canaliculus

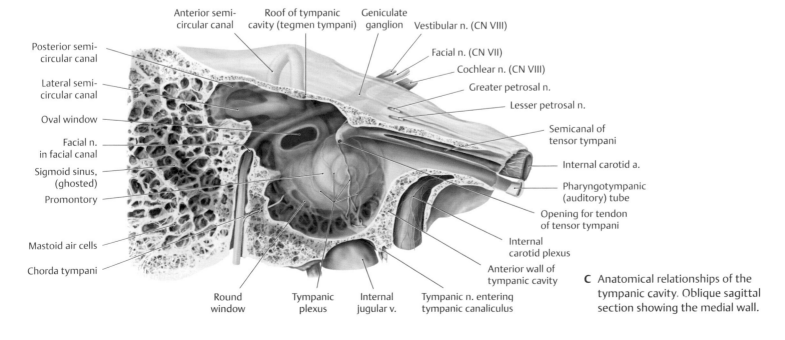

Anterior semi-circular canal
Roof of tympanic cavity (tegmen tympani)
Geniculate ganglion
Vestibular n. (CN VIII)
Posterior semi-circular canal
Lateral semi-circular canal
Oval window
Facial n. in facial canal
Sigmoid sinus, (ghosted)
Promontory
Mastoid air cells
Chorda tympani
Facial n. (CN VII)
Cochlear n. (CN VIII)
Greater petrosal n.
Lesser petrosal n.
Semicanal of tensor tympani
Internal carotid a.
Pharyngotympanic (auditory) tube
Opening for tendon of tensor tympani
Internal carotid plexus
Anterior wall of tympanic cavity
Tympanic n. entering tympanic canaliculus
Round window
Tympanic plexus
Internal jugular v.

C Anatomical relationships of the
tympanic cavity. Oblique sagittal
section showing the medial wall.

45 Oral Cavity & Pharynx
Bones of the Oral Cavity

The floor of the nasal cavity (the maxilla and palatine bone) forms the roof of the oral cavity, the hard palate. The two horizontal processes of the maxilla (the palatine processes) grow together during development, eventually fusing at the median palatine suture. Failure to fuse results in a cleft palate.

Fig. 45.1 Hard palate

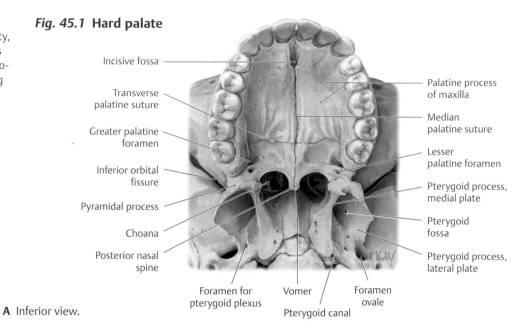

Incisive fossa
Transverse palatine suture
Greater palatine foramen
Inferior orbital fissure
Pyramidal process
Choana
Posterior nasal spine
Foramen for pterygoid plexus
Vomer
Pterygoid canal
Foramen ovale
Palatine process of maxilla
Median palatine suture
Lesser palatine foramen
Pterygoid process, medial plate
Pterygoid fossa
Pterygoid process, lateral plate

A Inferior view.

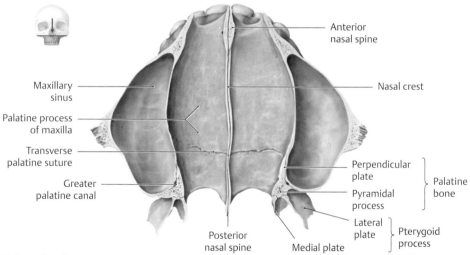

Maxillary sinus
Palatine process of maxilla
Transverse palatine suture
Greater palatine canal
Posterior nasal spine
Medial plate
Anterior nasal spine
Nasal crest
Perpendicular plate
Pyramidal process
Palatine bone
Lateral plate
Pterygoid process

B Superior view.
Removed: Maxilla (upper part).

Anterior clinoid process
Septum of sphenoid sinus
Optic canal
Sphenoid, lesser wing
Ostium of sphenoid sinus
Pterygoid fossa
Inferior orbital fissure
Choana
Vomer
Median palatine suture
Incisive foramen
Superior orbital fissure
Middle concha
Ethmoid bone, perpendicular plate
Inferior concha
Lateral plate
Medial plate
Pterygoid process
Palatine bone
Palatine process of maxilla

C Oblique posterior view.

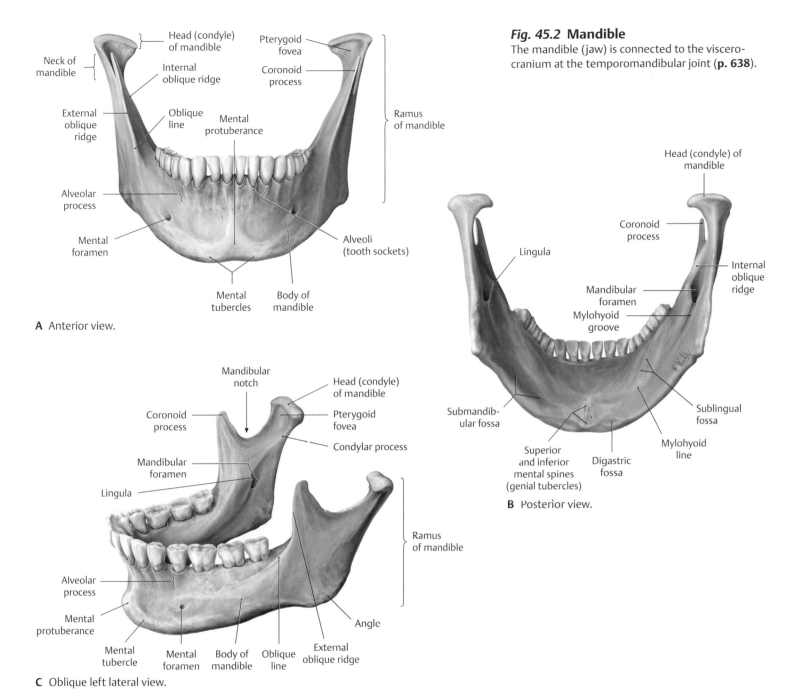

Fig. 45.2 Mandible

The mandible (jaw) is connected to the viscero-cranium at the temporomandibular joint (**p. 638**).

A Anterior view.

B Posterior view.

C Oblique left lateral view.

Fig. 45.3 Hyoid bone

The hyoid bone is suspended in the neck by muscles between the floor of the mouth and the larynx. Although not listed among the cranial bones, the hyoid bone gives attachment to the muscles of the oral floor. The greater horn and body of the hyoid are palpable in the neck.

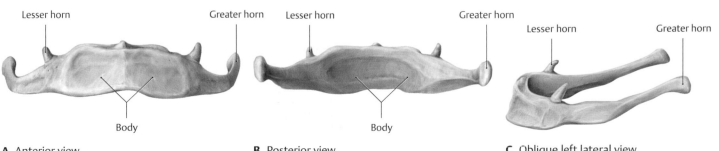

A Anterior view.

B Posterior view.

C Oblique left lateral view.

Teeth

Fig. 45.8 **Structure of a tooth**
Each tooth consists of hard tissue (enamel, dentin, cementum) and soft tissue (dental pulp) arranged into a crown, neck (cervix), and root.

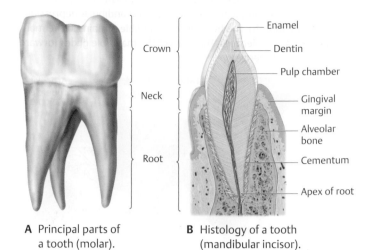

A Principal parts of a tooth (molar).

B Histology of a tooth (mandibular incisor).

Fig. 45.9 **Permanent teeth**
Each half of the maxilla and mandible contains a set of three anterior teeth (two incisors, one canine) and five posterior (postcanine) teeth (two premolars, three molars).

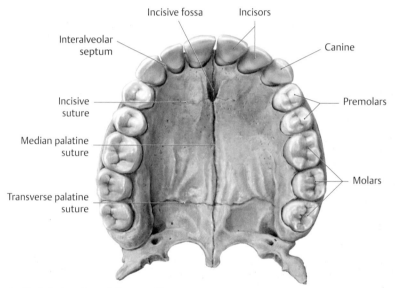

A Maxillary teeth. Inferior view of the maxilla.

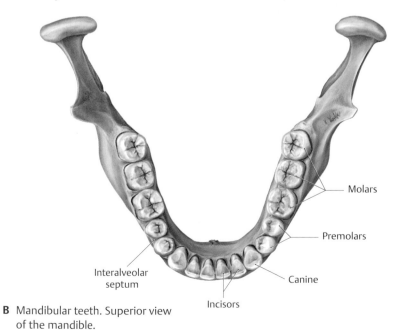

B Mandibular teeth. Superior view of the mandible.

Fig. 45.10 **Tooth surfaces**
The top of the tooth is known as the occlusal surface.

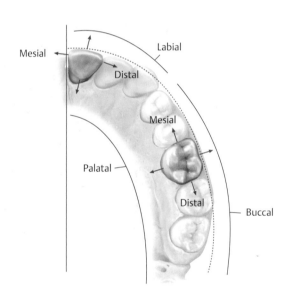

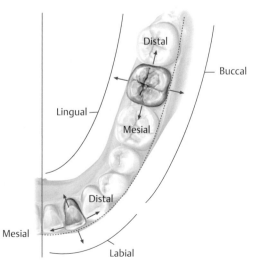

Fig. 45.11 Coding of the teeth

In the United States, the 32 permanent teeth are numbered sequentially (not assigned to quadrants). The 20 deciduous (baby) teeth are coded A to J (upper arch), and K to T (lower arch), in a similar clockwise fashion. The third upper right molar is 1; the second upper right premolar is A.

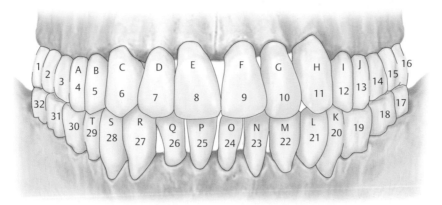

Fig. 45.12 Dental panoramic tomogram

The dental panoramic tomogram (DPT) is a survey radiograph that allows preliminary assessment of the temporomandibular joints, maxillary sinuses, maxillomandibular bone, and dental status (carious lesions, location of wisdom teeth, etc.). *DPT courtesy of Dr. U. J. Rother, Director of the Department of Diagnostic Radiology, Center for Dentistry and Oromaxillofacial Surgery, Eppendorf University Medical Center, Hamburg, Germany.*

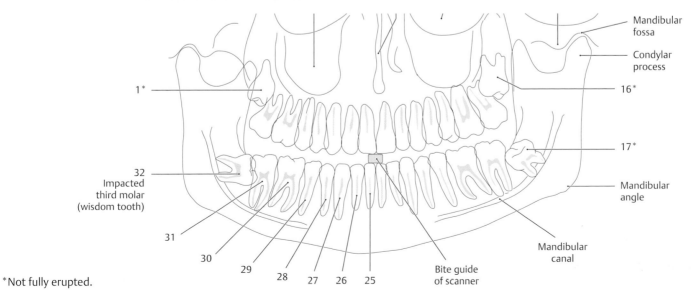

*Not fully erupted.

Oral Cavity Muscle Facts

Fig. 45.13 Muscles of the oral floor
See **pp. 516–517** for the infrahyoid muscles.

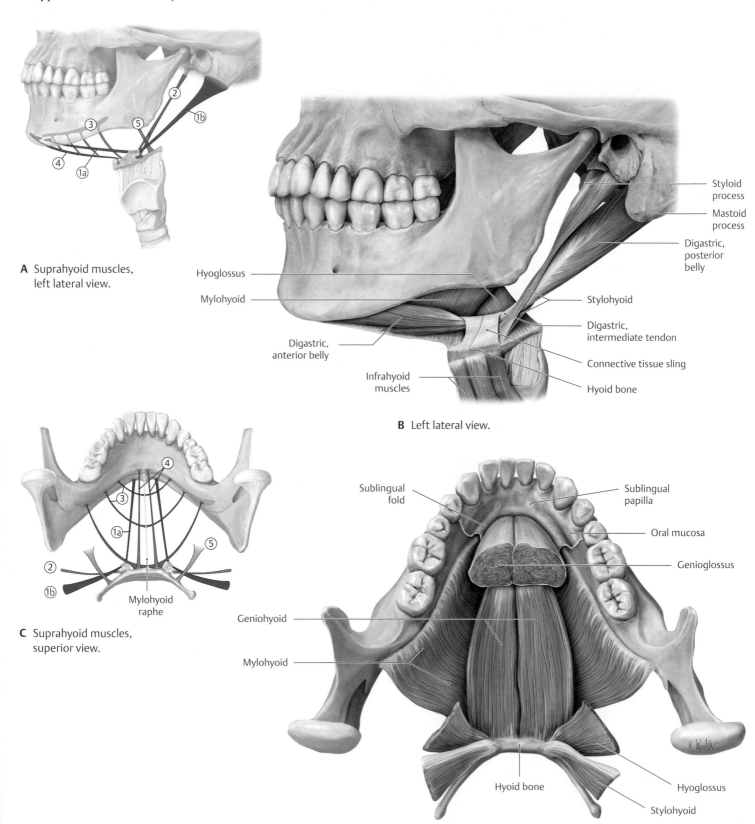

A Suprahyoid muscles, left lateral view.

B Left lateral view.

Styloid process

Mastoid process

Digastric, posterior belly

Hyoglossus

Mylohyoid

Stylohyoid

Digastric, intermediate tendon

Digastric, anterior belly

Connective tissue sling

Infrahyoid muscles

Hyoid bone

C Suprahyoid muscles, superior view.

Mylohyoid raphe

Sublingual fold

Sublingual papilla

Oral mucosa

Genioglossus

Geniohyoid

Mylohyoid

Hyoid bone

Hyoglossus

Stylohyoid

D Superior view of the mandible and hyoid bone.

Table 45.1 Suprahyoid muscles

Muscle		Origin	Insertion			Innervation	Action
① Digastric	①a Anterior belly	Mandible (digastric fossa)	Hyoid bone (body)	Via an intermediate tendon with a fibrous loop		Mylohyoid n. (from CN V₃)	Elevates hyoid bone (during swallowing), assists in opening mandible
	①b Posterior belly	Temporal bone (mastoid notch, medial to mastoid process)				Facial n. (CN VII)	
② Stylohyoid		Temporal bone (styloid process)		Via a split tendon			
③ Mylohyoid		Mandible (mylohyoid line)		Via median tendon of insertion (mylohyoid raphe)		Mylohyoid n. (from CN V₃)	Tightens and elevates oral floor, draws hyoid bone forward (during swallowing), assists in opening mandible and moving it side to side (mastication)
④ Geniohyoid		Mandible (inferior mental spine)	Body of hyoid bone			Anterior ramus of C1 via hypoglossal n. (CN XII)	Draws hyoid bone forward (during swallowing), assists in opening mandible
⑤ Hyoglossus		Hyoid bone (superior border of greater cornu)	Sides of tongue			Hypoglossal n. (CN XII)	Depresses and retracts the tongue

Fig. 45.14 Muscles of the soft palate

Inferior view. The soft palate forms the posterior boundary of the oral cavity, separating it from the oropharynx.

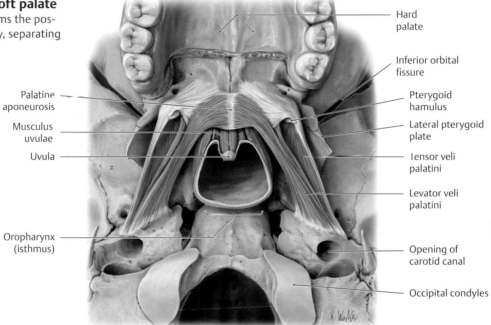

Labels: Hard palate; Inferior orbital fissure; Pterygoid hamulus; Lateral pterygoid plate; Tensor veli palatini; Levator veli palatini; Opening of carotid canal; Occipital condyles; Palatine aponeurosis; Musculus uvulae; Uvula; Oropharynx (isthmus)

Table 45.2 Muscles of the soft palate

Muscle	Origin	Insertion	Innervation	Action
Tensor veli palatini	Medial pterygoid plate (scaphoid fossa); sphenoid bone (spine); cartilage of pharyngotympanic tube	Palatine aponeurosis	Medial pterygoid n. (CN V₃)	Tightens soft palate; opens inlet to pharyngotympanic (auditory) tube (during swallowing, yawning)
Levator veli palatini	Cartilage of pharyngotympanic tube; temporal bone (petrous part)		Vagus n. via pharyngeal plexus	Raises soft palate to horizontal position
Musculus uvulae	Uvula (mucosa)	Palatine aponeurosis; posterior nasal spine		Shortens and raises uvula
Palatoglossus*	Tongue (side)	Palatine aponeurosis		Elevates tongue (posterior portion); pulls soft palate onto tongue
Palatopharyngeus*				Tightens soft palate; during swallowing pulls pharyngeal walls superiorly, anteriorly, and medially

*For the palatoglossus, see **Figs. 45.19, p. 646 and 45.24, p. 648**; and for the palatopharyngeus, see **Figs. 45.24, p. 648 and 45.29C, p. 653**.

Innervation of the Oral Cavity

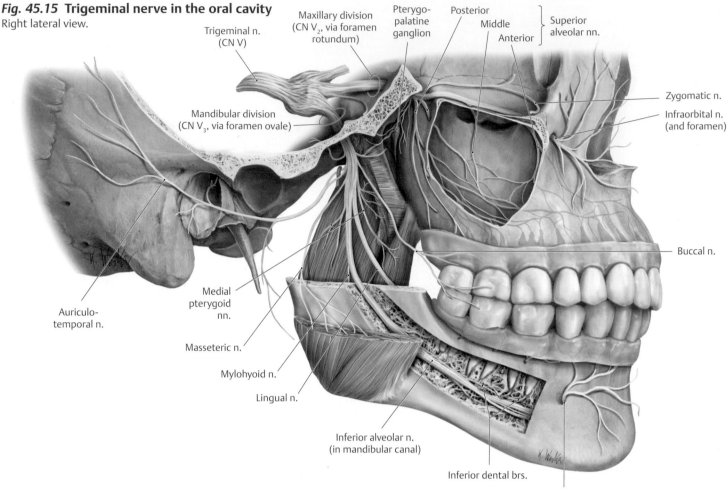

Fig. 45.15 Trigeminal nerve in the oral cavity
Right lateral view.

Fig. 45.16 Neurovasculature of the hard palate

Inferior view. The hard palate receives sensory innervation primarily from terminal branches of the maxillary division of the trigeminal nerve (CN V₂). The arteries of the hard palate arise from the maxillary artery.

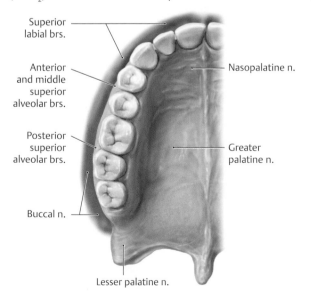

A Sensory innervation. *Note:* The buccal nerve is a branch of the mandibular division (CN V₃).

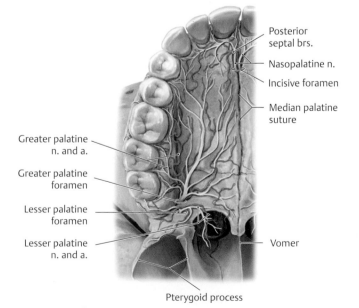

B Nerves and arteries.

The muscles of the oral floor have a complex nerve supply with contributions from the trigeminal nerve (CN V₃), facial nerve (CN VII), and C1 spinal nerve via the hypoglossal nerve (CN XII).

Fig. 45.17 **Innervation of the oral floor muscles**

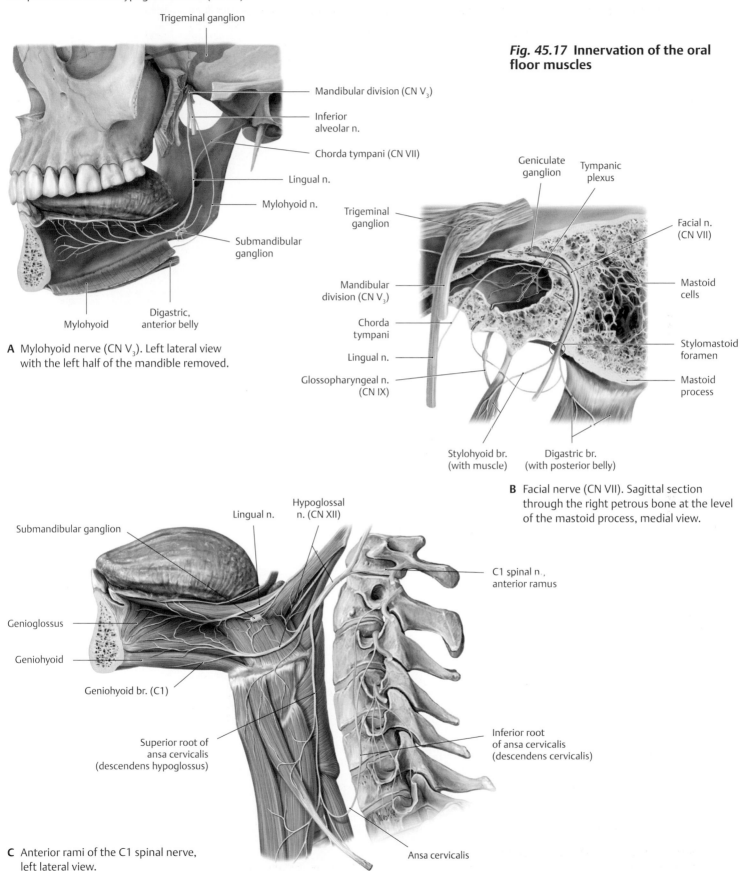

Trigeminal ganglion

Mandibular division (CN V₃)

Inferior alveolar n.

Chorda tympani (CN VII)

Lingual n.

Mylohyoid n.

Submandibular ganglion

Mylohyoid

Digastric, anterior belly

A Mylohyoid nerve (CN V₃). Left lateral view with the left half of the mandible removed.

Geniculate ganglion

Tympanic plexus

Trigeminal ganglion

Facial n. (CN VII)

Mandibular division (CN V₃)

Chorda tympani

Lingual n.

Glossopharyngeal n. (CN IX)

Mastoid cells

Stylomastoid foramen

Mastoid process

Stylohyoid br. (with muscle)

Digastric br. (with posterior belly)

B Facial nerve (CN VII). Sagittal section through the right petrous bone at the level of the mastoid process, medial view.

Submandibular ganglion

Lingual n.

Hypoglossal n. (CN XII)

C1 spinal n., anterior ramus

Genioglossus

Geniohyoid

Geniohyoid br. (C1)

Superior root of ansa cervicalis (descendens hypoglossus)

Inferior root of ansa cervicalis (descendens cervicalis)

Ansa cervicalis

C Anterior rami of the C1 spinal nerve, left lateral view.

Tongue

The dorsum of the tongue is covered by a highly specialized mucosa that supports its sensory functions (taste and fine tactile discrimination). The tongue is endowed with a very powerful muscular body to support its motor properties during mastication, swallowing, and speaking.

Fig. 45.18 Structure of the tongue

Superior view. The V-shaped sulcus terminalis divides the tongue into an anterior 2/3rds (oral, presulcal) and a posterior 1/3rd (pharyngeal, postsulcal).

Fig. 45.19 Muscles of the tongue

The extrinsic lingual muscles (genioglossus, hyoglossus, palatoglossus, and styloglossus) have bony attachments and move the tongue as a whole. The intrinsic lingual muscles (superior and inferior longitudinal muscles, transverse muscle, and vertical muscle) have no bony attachments and alter the shape of the tongue.

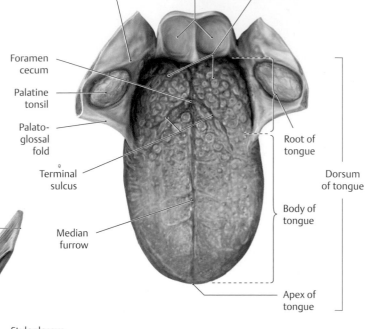

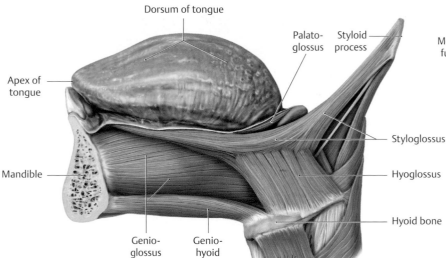

A Left lateral view.

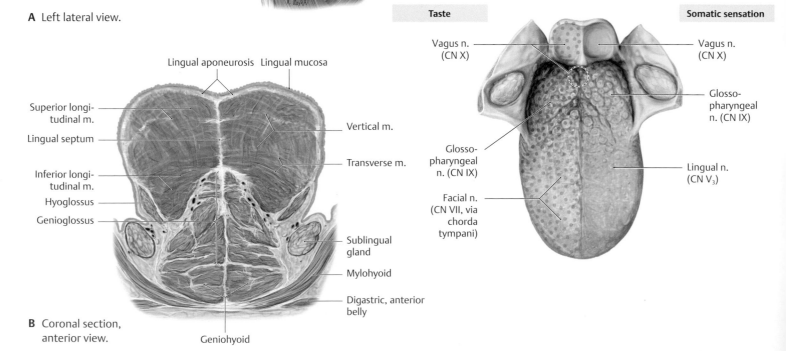

B Coronal section, anterior view.

Fig. 45.20 Somatosensory and taste innervation of the tongue

Superior view.

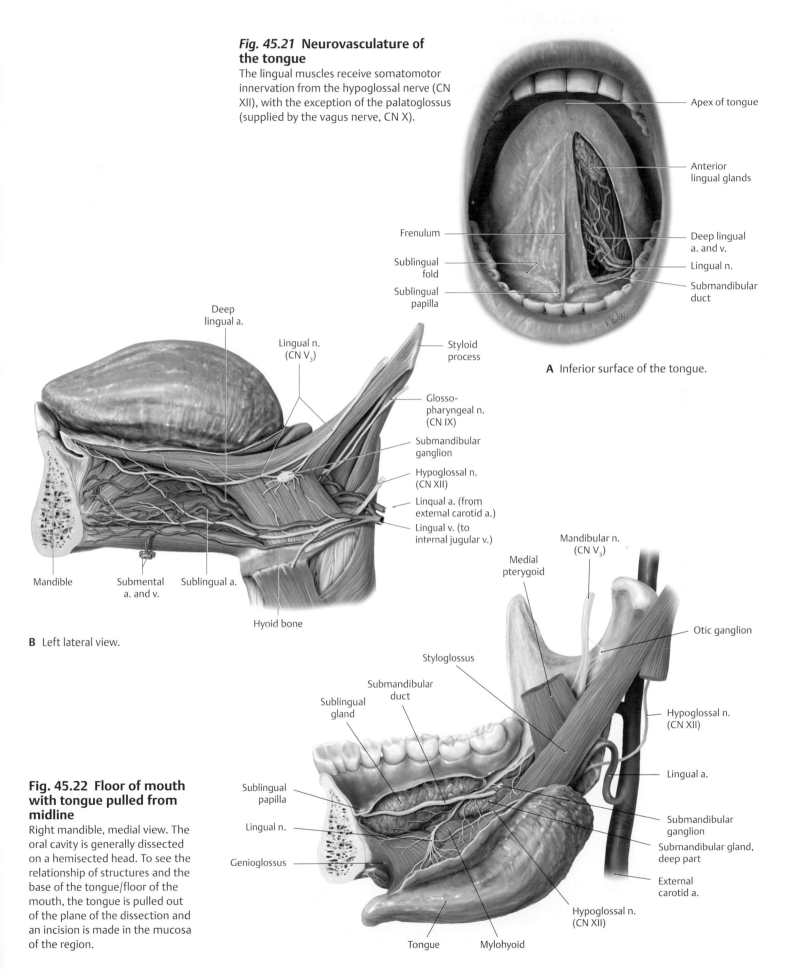

Fig. 45.21 Neurovasculature of the tongue

The lingual muscles receive somatomotor innervation from the hypoglossal nerve (CN XII), with the exception of the palatoglossus (supplied by the vagus nerve, CN X).

Apex of tongue

Anterior lingual glands

Frenulum

Deep lingual a. and v.

Sublingual fold

Lingual n.

Sublingual papilla

Submandibular duct

A Inferior surface of the tongue.

Deep lingual a.

Lingual n. (CN V₃)

Styloid process

Glosso-pharyngeal n. (CN IX)

Submandibular ganglion

Hypoglossal n. (CN XII)

Lingual a. (from external carotid a.)

Lingual v. (to internal jugular v.)

Mandible

Submental a. and v.

Sublingual a.

Hyoid bone

B Left lateral view.

Mandibular n. (CN V₃)

Medial pterygoid

Otic ganglion

Styloglossus

Submandibular duct

Sublingual gland

Hypoglossal n. (CN XII)

Fig. 45.22 Floor of mouth with tongue pulled from midline

Right mandible, medial view. The oral cavity is generally dissected on a hemisected head. To see the relationship of structures and the base of the tongue/floor of the mouth, the tongue is pulled out of the plane of the dissection and an incision is made in the mucosa of the region.

Sublingual papilla

Lingual n.

Genioglossus

Lingual a.

Submandibular ganglion

Submandibular gland, deep part

External carotid a.

Hypoglossal n. (CN XII)

Tongue

Mylohyoid

Topography of the Oral Cavity & Salivary Glands

The oral cavity is located below the nasal cavity and anterior to the pharynx. It is bounded by the hard and soft palates, the tongue and muscles of the oral floor, and the uvula.

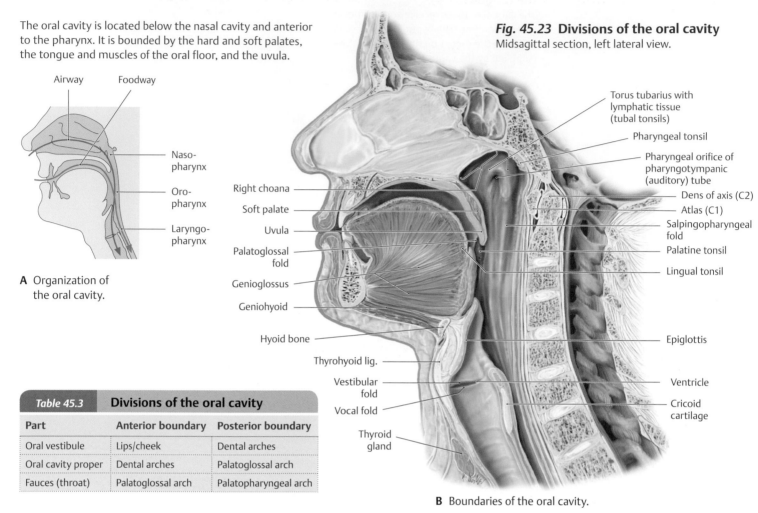

Fig. 45.23 **Divisions of the oral cavity**
Midsagittal section, left lateral view.

A Organization of the oral cavity.

Table 45.3	**Divisions of the oral cavity**	
Part	**Anterior boundary**	**Posterior boundary**
Oral vestibule	Lips/cheek	Dental arches
Oral cavity proper	Dental arches	Palatoglossal arch
Fauces (throat)	Palatoglossal arch	Palatopharyngeal arch

B Boundaries of the oral cavity.

Fig. 45.24 Oral cavity topography
Right side, anterior view.

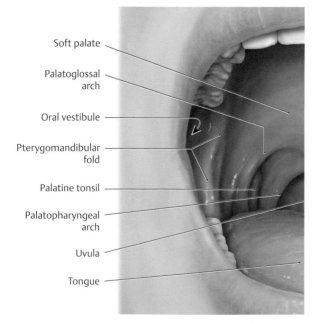

A Open oral cavity.

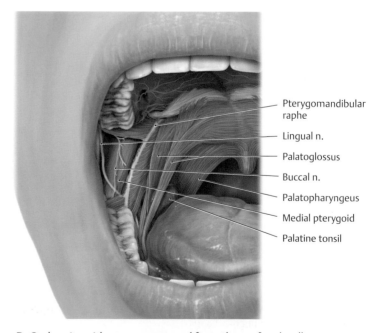

B Oral cavity with mucosa removed from the roof and walls.

The three large, paired salivary glands are the parotid, submandibular, and sublingual glands. The parotid gland is a purely serous (watery) salivary gland. The sublingual gland is predominantly mucous; the submandibular gland is a mixed seromucous gland.

Fig. 45.25 **Salivary glands**

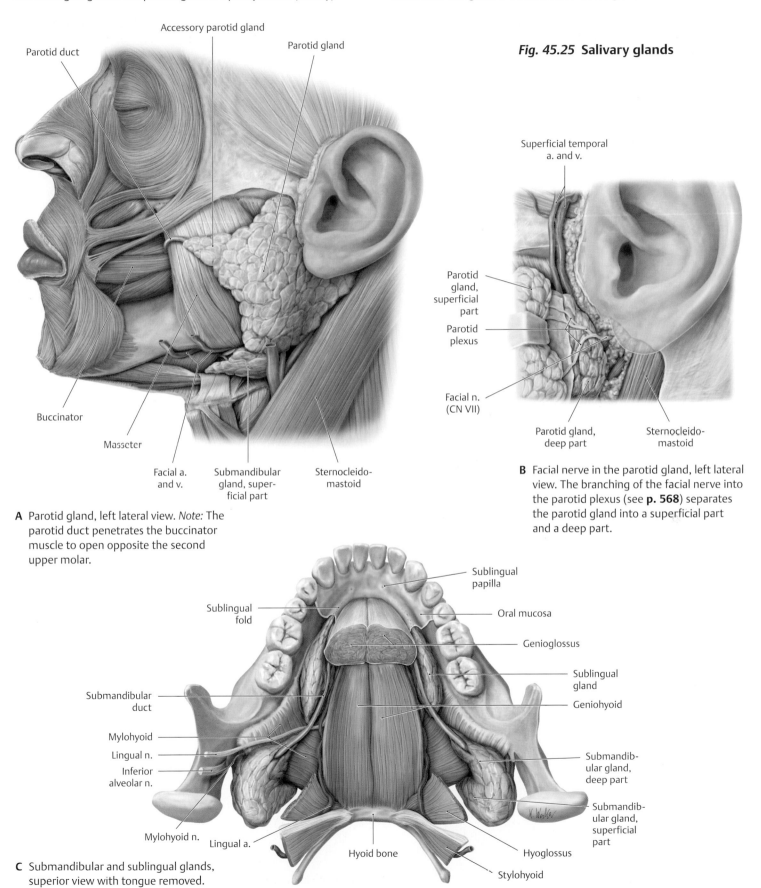

A Parotid gland, left lateral view. *Note:* The parotid duct penetrates the buccinator muscle to open opposite the second upper molar.

B Facial nerve in the parotid gland, left lateral view. The branching of the facial nerve into the parotid plexus (see **p. 568**) separates the parotid gland into a superficial part and a deep part.

C Submandibular and sublingual glands, superior view with tongue removed.

Tonsils & Pharynx

Fig. 45.26 Tonsils

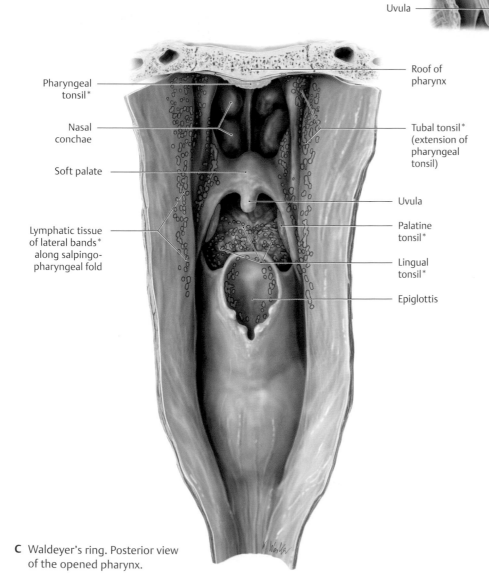

Soft palate

Palato-glossal arch

Palato-pharyngeal arch

Tonsillar fossa

Palatine tonsil

Uvula

A Palatine tonsils, anterior view.

Choana

Roof of pharynx

Nasal septum

Pharyngeal tonsil

Torus tubarius with lymphatic tissue (tubal tonsils)

Pharyngeal orifice of pharyngo-tympanic tube

Dens of axis (C2)

Soft palate

Salpingo-pharyngeal fold

Uvula

B Pharyngeal tonsils. Sagittal section through the roof of the pharynx.

Roof of pharynx

Pharyngeal tonsil*

Nasal conchae

Tubal tonsil* (extension of pharyngeal tonsil)

Soft palate

Uvula

Palatine tonsil*

Lymphatic tissue of lateral bands* along salpingo-pharyngeal fold

Lingual tonsil*

Epiglottis

C Waldeyer's ring. Posterior view of the opened pharynx.

Table 45.4	Structures in Waldeyer's ring
Tonsil*	**#**
Pharyngeal tonsil	1
Tubal tonsils	2
Palatine tonsils	2
Lingual tonsil	1
Lateral bands	2

Tonsil infections
Abnormal enlargement of the palatine tonsils due to severe viral or bacterial infection can result in obstruction of the oropharynx, causing difficulty swallowing.

Particularly well developed in young children, the pharyngeal tonsil begins to regress at 6 to 7 years of age. Abnormal enlargement is common, with the tonsil bulging into the nasopharynx and obstructing air passages, forcing the child to "mouth breathe."

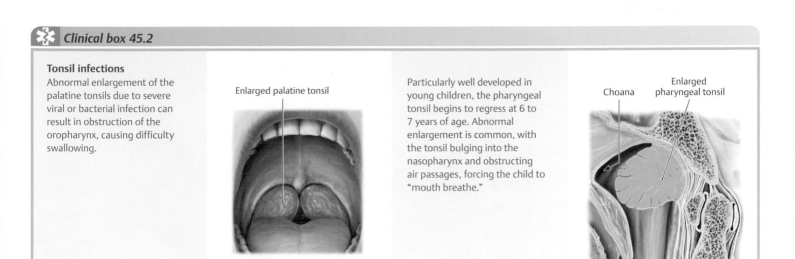

Enlarged palatine tonsil

Choana — Enlarged pharyngeal tonsil

Fig. 45.27 **Pharyngeal mucosa**

Posterior view of the opened pharynx. The anterior portion of the muscular tube contains three openings: choanae (to the nasal cavity), faucial isthmus (to the oral cavity), and aditus (to the laryngeal inlet).

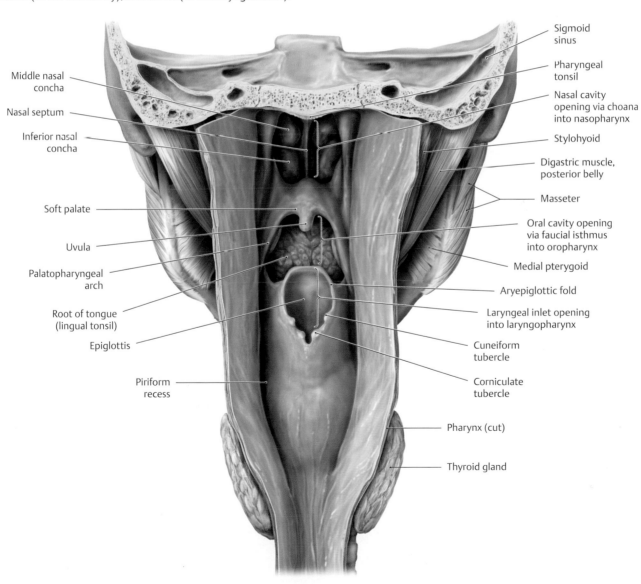

Middle nasal concha
Nasal septum
Inferior nasal concha
Soft palate
Uvula
Palatopharyngeal arch
Root of tongue (lingual tonsil)
Epiglottis
Piriform recess

Sigmoid sinus
Pharyngeal tonsil
Nasal cavity opening via choana into nasopharynx
Stylohyoid
Digastric muscle, posterior belly
Masseter
Oral cavity opening via faucial isthmus into oropharynx
Medial pterygoid
Aryepiglottic fold
Laryngeal inlet opening into laryngopharynx
Cuneiform tubercle
Corniculate tubercle
Pharynx (cut)
Thyroid gland

Pharyngeal Muscles

Fig. 45.28 **Pharyngeal muscles: Left lateral view**
The pharyngeal musculature consists of the pharyngeal constrictors and the relatively weak pharyngeal elevators.

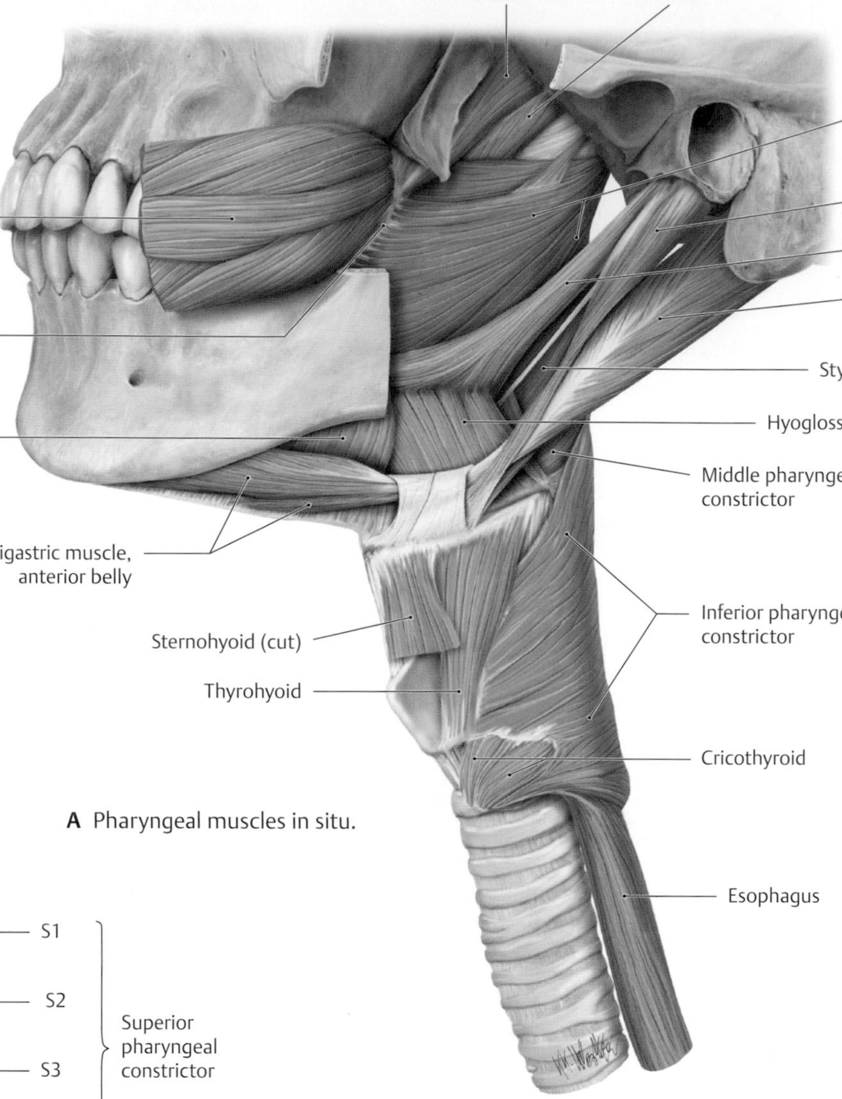

A Pharyngeal muscles in situ.

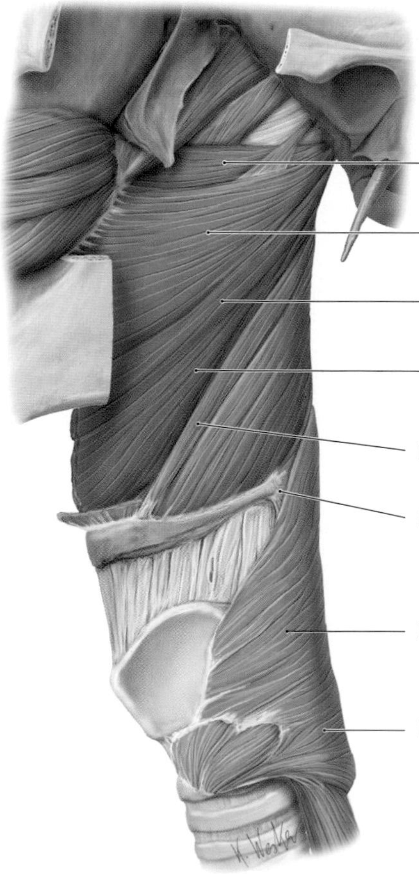

B Subdivisions of the pharyngeal constrictors.

Table 45.5	Pharyngeal constrictors
Superior pharyngeal constrictor	
S1	Pterygopharyngeal part
S2	Buccopharyngeal part
S3	Mylopharyngeal part
S4	Glossopharyngeal part
Middle pharyngeal constrictor	
M1	Chondropharyngeal part
M2	Ceratopharyngeal part
Inferior pharyngeal constrictor	
I1	Thyropharyngeal part
I2	Cricopharyngeal part

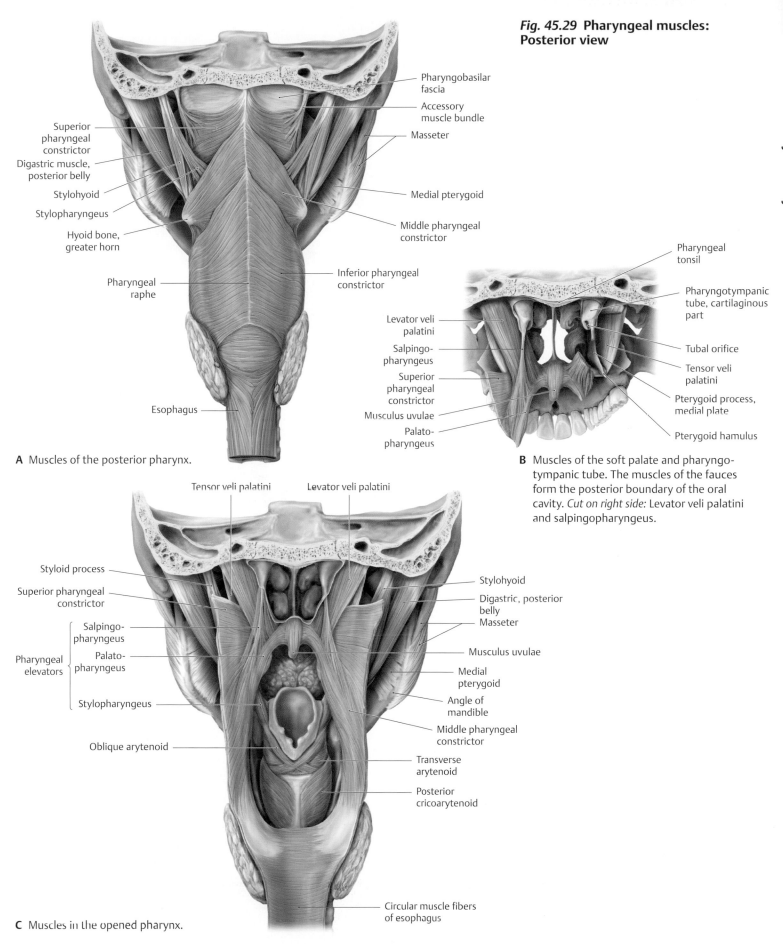

Fig. 45.29 Pharyngeal muscles: Posterior view

Pharyngobasilar fascia

Accessory muscle bundle

Masseter

Superior pharyngeal constrictor

Digastric muscle, posterior belly

Stylohyoid

Stylopharyngeus

Hyoid bone, greater horn

Medial pterygoid

Middle pharyngeal constrictor

Pharyngeal raphe

Inferior pharyngeal constrictor

Esophagus

A Muscles of the posterior pharynx.

Pharyngeal tonsil

Levator veli palatini

Pharyngotympanic tube, cartilaginous part

Salpingo-pharyngeus

Tubal orifice

Superior pharyngeal constrictor

Tensor veli palatini

Musculus uvulae

Pterygoid process, medial plate

Palato-pharyngeus

Pterygoid hamulus

B Muscles of the soft palate and pharyngo-tympanic tube. The muscles of the fauces form the posterior boundary of the oral cavity. *Cut on right side:* Levator veli palatini and salpingopharyngeus.

Tensor veli palatini

Levator veli palatini

Styloid process

Superior pharyngeal constrictor

Stylohyoid

Digastric, posterior belly

Masseter

Salpingo-pharyngeus

Pharyngeal elevators

Palato-pharyngeus

Musculus uvulae

Stylopharyngeus

Medial pterygoid

Angle of mandible

Oblique arytenoid

Middle pharyngeal constrictor

Transverse arytenoid

Posterior cricoarytenoid

Circular muscle fibers of esophagus

C Muscles in the opened pharynx.

Neurovasculature of the Pharynx

Fig. 45.30 Neurovasculature in the parapharyngeal space

Posterior view. *Removed:* Vertebral column and posterior structures.

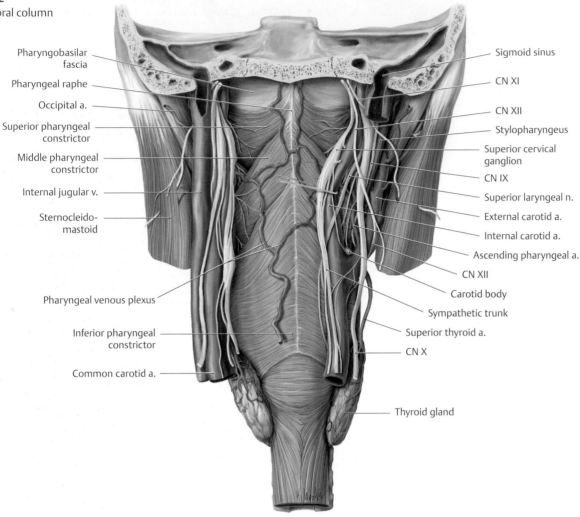

Pharyngobasilar fascia
Pharyngeal raphe
Occipital a.
Superior pharyngeal constrictor
Middle pharyngeal constrictor
Internal jugular v.
Sternocleido-mastoid
Pharyngeal venous plexus
Inferior pharyngeal constrictor
Common carotid a.

Sigmoid sinus
CN XI
CN XII
Stylopharyngeus
Superior cervical ganglion
CN IX
Superior laryngeal n.
External carotid a.
Internal carotid a.
Ascending pharyngeal a.
CN XII
Carotid body
Sympathetic trunk
Superior thyroid a.
CN X
Thyroid gland

Fig. 45.31 Fasciae and potential tissue spaces in the head

Transverse section at the level of the tonsillar fossa, superior view. Fascial boundaries are key to outlining pathways for the spread of infection. Potential spaces in the head, shown on this figure, become true spaces when they are infiltrated by products of infection. These spaces are defined by bones, muscles and fascia and initially confine an infection but eventually allow it to spread through communications between spaces.

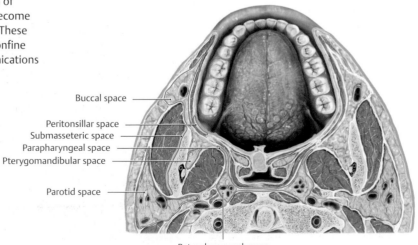

Buccal space
Peritonsillar space
Submasseteric space
Parapharyngeal space
Pterygomandibular space
Parotid space
Retropharyngeal space

Fig. 45.32 **Neurovasculature of the opened pharynx**
Posterior view.

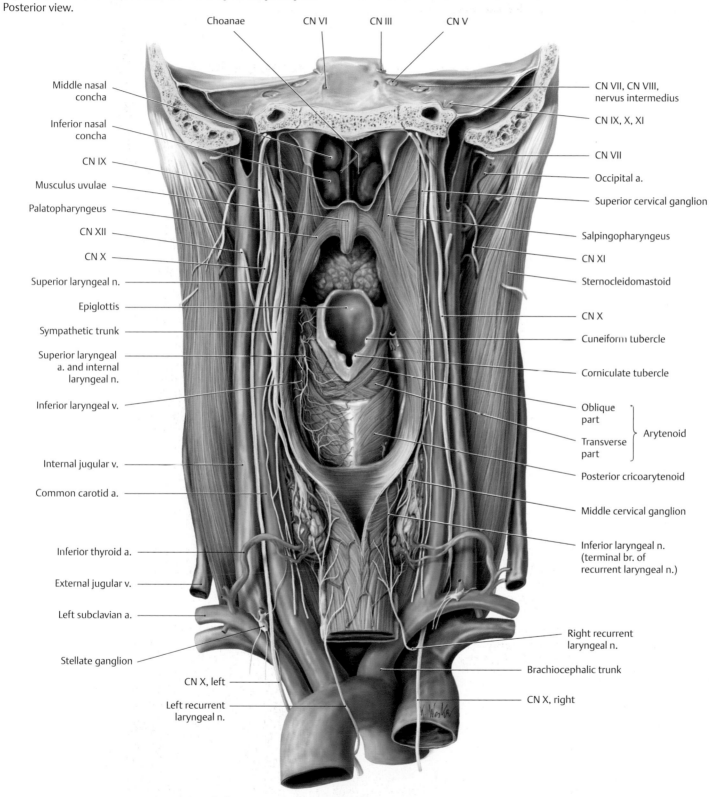

Choanae CN VI CN III CN V

Middle nasal concha

Inferior nasal concha

CN IX

Musculus uvulae

Palatopharyngeus

CN XII

CN X

Superior laryngeal n.

Epiglottis

Sympathetic trunk

Superior laryngeal a. and internal laryngeal n.

Inferior laryngeal v.

Internal jugular v.

Common carotid a.

Inferior thyroid a.

External jugular v.

Left subclavian a.

Stellate ganglion

CN X, left

Left recurrent laryngeal n.

CN VII, CN VIII, nervus intermedius

CN IX, X, XI

CN VII

Occipital a.

Superior cervical ganglion

Salpingopharyngeus

CN XI

Sternocleidomastoid

CN X

Cuneiform tubercle

Corniculate tubercle

Oblique part ⎫
                ⎬ Arytenoid
Transverse part ⎭

Posterior cricoarytenoid

Middle cervical ganglion

Inferior laryngeal n. (terminal br. of recurrent laryngeal n.)

Right recurrent laryngeal n.

Brachiocephalic trunk

CN X, right

CN III, oculomotor n.; CN V, trigeminal n.; CN VI, abducent n.;
CN VII, facial n.; CN VIII, vestibulocochlear n.; CN IX, glossopharyngeal n.;
CN X, vagus n.; CN XI, accessory n.; CN XII, hypoglossal n..
See Chapter 39 for the cranial nerves.

46 Sectional & Radiographic Anatomy

Sectional Anatomy of the Head & Neck (I)

Fig. 46.1 Coronal section through the anterior orbital margin

Anterior view. This section shows four regions of the head: the oral cavity, the nasal cavity and sinuses, the orbit, and the anterior cranial fossa. Muscles of the oral floor, the apex of the tongue, the hard palate, the neurovascular structures in the mandibular canal, and the first molar are all seen in the region of the oral cavity. This section reinforces the clinical implications of the relationship of the maxillary sinus with the maxillary teeth and the floor of the orbit and with the maxillary nerve in the infraorbital groove. The medial wall of the orbit shares a thin bony wall (orbital plate) with the ethmoid air cells (sinus). The section is enough anterior so that the lateral bony walls of the orbit are not included due to the lateral curvature of the skull.

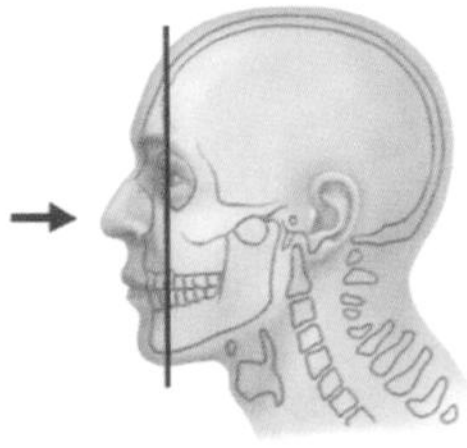

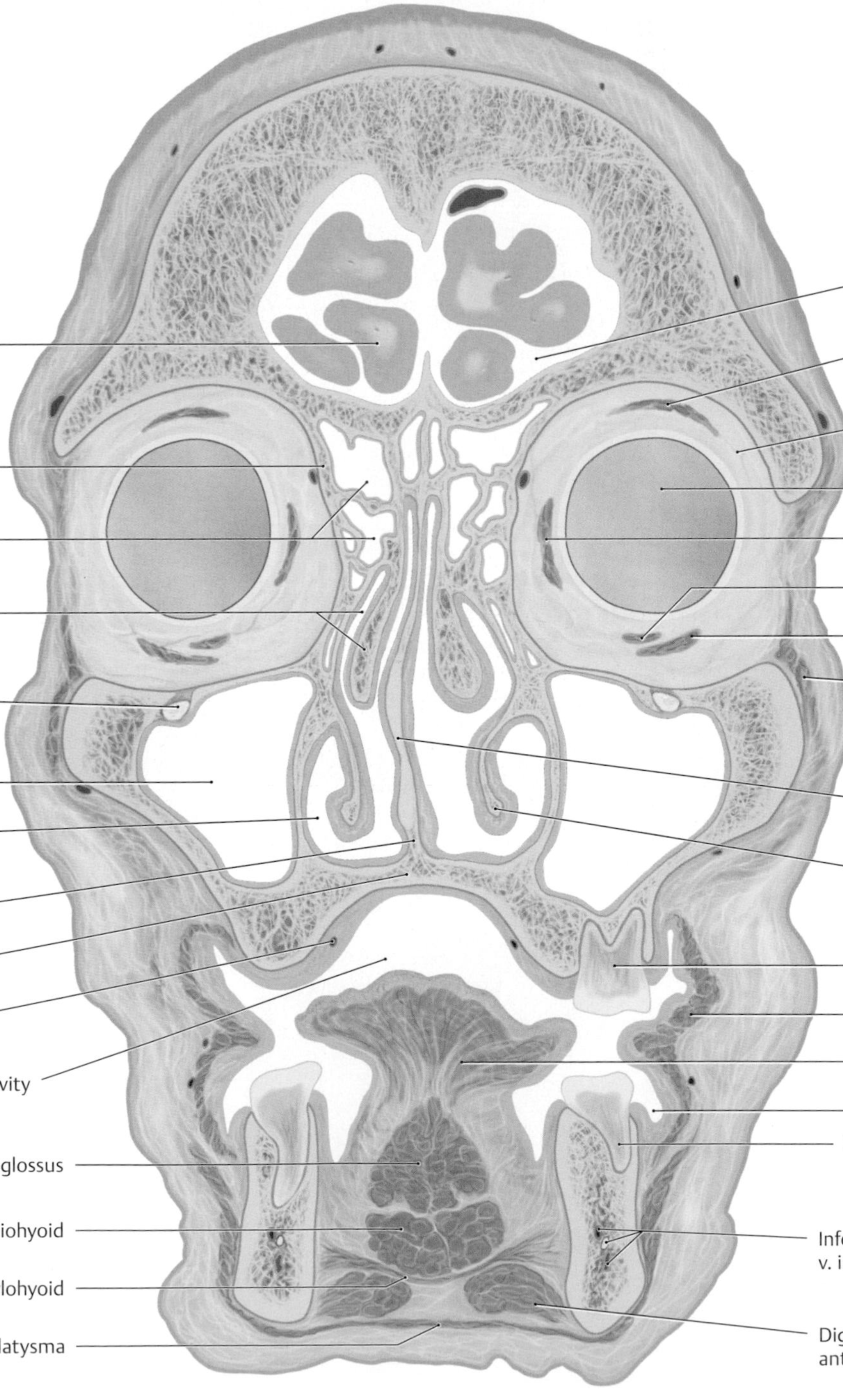

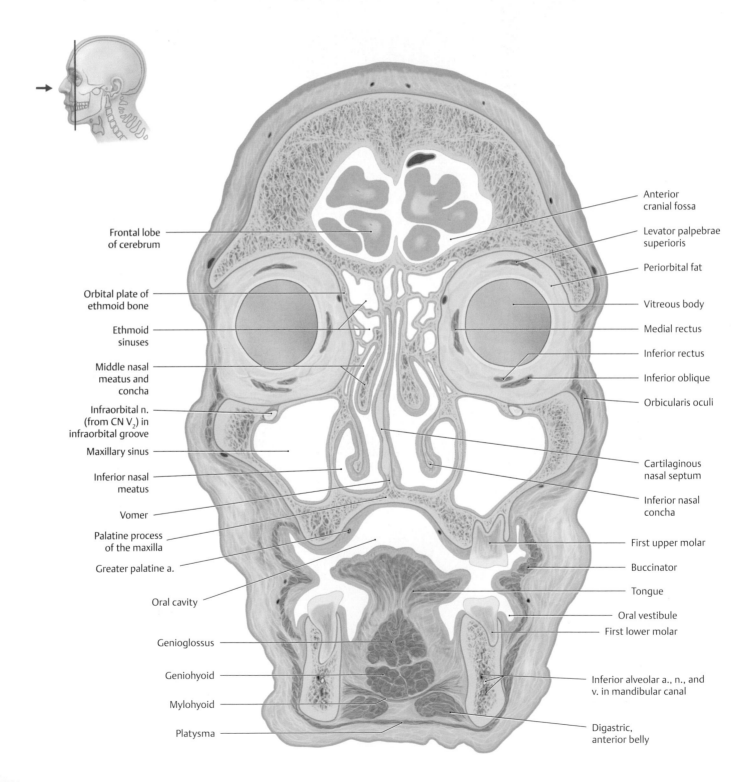

Frontal lobe of cerebrum
Orbital plate of ethmoid bone
Ethmoid sinuses
Middle nasal meatus and concha
Infraorbital n. (from CN V_2) in infraorbital groove
Maxillary sinus
Inferior nasal meatus
Vomer
Palatine process of the maxilla
Greater palatine a.
Oral cavity
Genioglossus
Geniohyoid
Mylohyoid
Platysma
Anterior cranial fossa
Levator palpebrae superioris
Periorbital fat
Vitreous body
Medial rectus
Inferior rectus
Inferior oblique
Orbicularis oculi
Cartilaginous nasal septum
Inferior nasal concha
First upper molar
Buccinator
Tongue
Oral vestibule
First lower molar
Inferior alveolar a., n., and v. in mandibular canal
Digastric, anterior belly

Fig. 46.2 Coronal section through the orbital apex

Anterior view. In this more posterior section than that of **Fig. 46.1**, the soft palate now separates the oral and nasal cavities. The buccal fat pad is also visible. The section is slightly angled, producing an apparent discontinuity in the mandibular ramus on the left side.

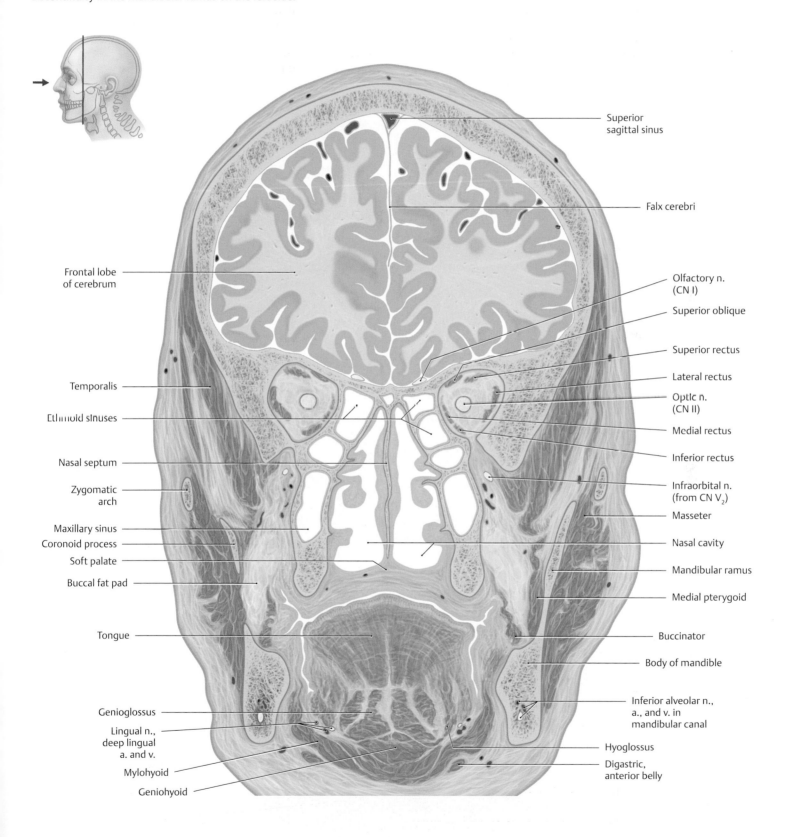

Superior sagittal sinus

Falx cerebri

Frontal lobe of cerebrum

Olfactory n. (CN I)

Superior oblique

Superior rectus

Temporalis

Lateral rectus

Ethmoid sinuses

Optic n. (CN II)

Medial rectus

Nasal septum

Inferior rectus

Zygomatic arch

Infraorbital n. (from CN V₂)

Masseter

Maxillary sinus

Coronoid process

Nasal cavity

Soft palate

Mandibular ramus

Buccal fat pad

Medial pterygoid

Tongue

Buccinator

Body of mandible

Genioglossus

Inferior alveolar n., a., and v. in mandibular canal

Lingual n., deep lingual a. and v.

Hyoglossus

Mylohyoid

Digastric, anterior belly

Geniohyoid

Sectional Anatomy of the Head & Neck (II)

Fig. 46.3 **Coronal section through the pituitary**
Anterior view.

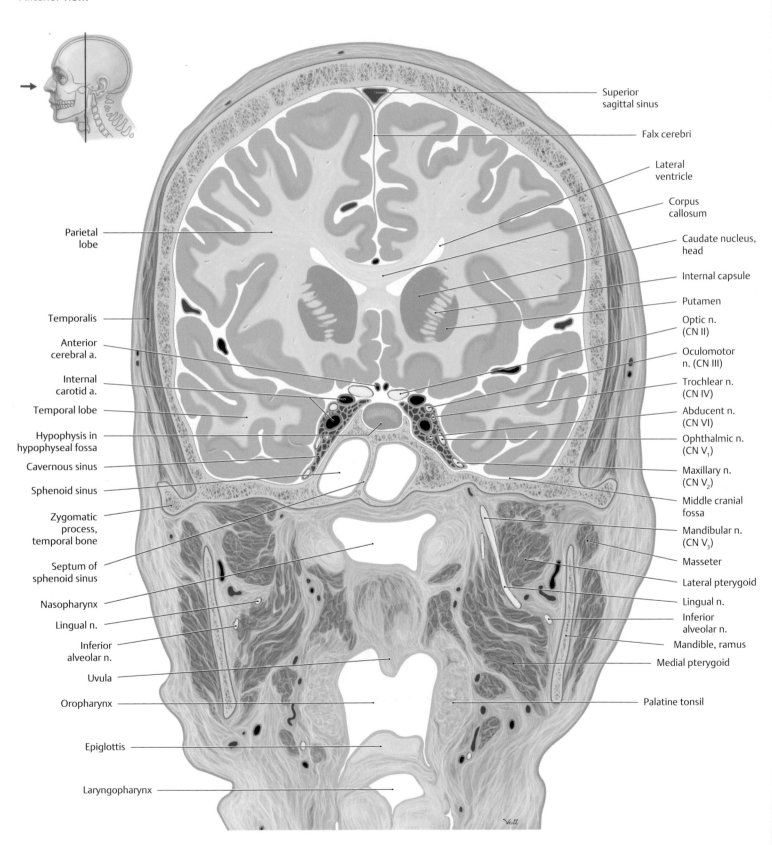

Superior sagittal sinus

Falx cerebri

Lateral ventricle

Corpus callosum

Caudate nucleus, head

Internal capsule

Putamen

Optic n. (CN II)

Oculomotor n. (CN III)

Trochlear n. (CN IV)

Abducent n. (CN VI)

Ophthalmic n. (CN V₁)

Maxillary n. (CN V₂)

Middle cranial fossa

Mandibular n. (CN V₃)

Masseter

Lateral pterygoid

Lingual n.

Inferior alveolar n.

Mandible, ramus

Medial pterygoid

Palatine tonsil

Parietal lobe

Temporalis

Anterior cerebral a.

Internal carotid a.

Temporal lobe

Hypophysis in hypophyseal fossa

Cavernous sinus

Sphenoid sinus

Zygomatic process, temporal bone

Septum of sphenoid sinus

Nasopharynx

Lingual n.

Inferior alveolar n.

Uvula

Oropharynx

Epiglottis

Laryngopharynx

Fig. 46.4 Midsagittal section through the nasal septum
Left lateral view.

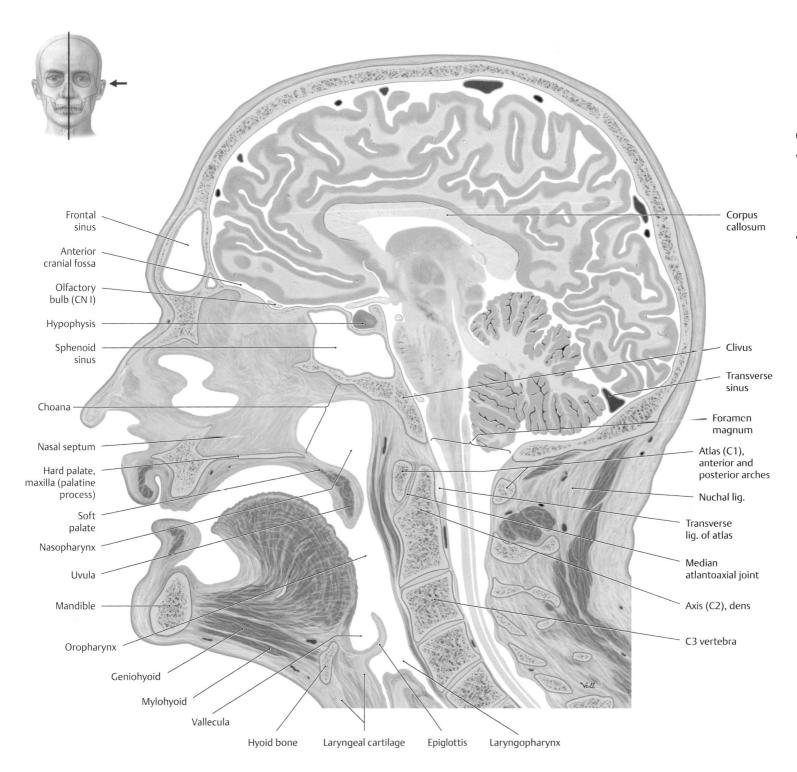

Frontal sinus

Anterior cranial fossa

Olfactory bulb (CN I)

Hypophysis

Sphenoid sinus

Choana

Nasal septum

Hard palate, maxilla (palatine process)

Soft palate

Nasopharynx

Uvula

Mandible

Oropharynx

Geniohyoid

Mylohyoid

Vallecula

Hyoid bone

Laryngeal cartilage

Epiglottis

Laryngopharynx

Corpus callosum

Clivus

Transverse sinus

Foramen magnum

Atlas (C1), anterior and posterior arches

Nuchal lig.

Transverse lig. of atlas

Median atlantoaxial joint

Axis (C2), dens

C3 vertebra

Sectional Anatomy of the Head & Neck (IV)

***Fig. 46.7* Transverse section through the optic nerve and pituitary**
Inferior view.

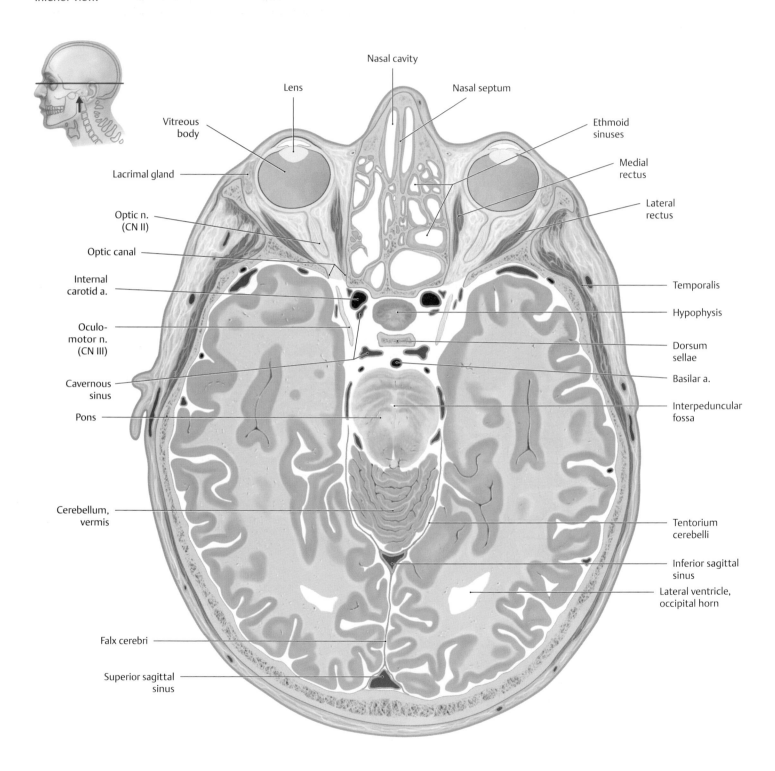

Nasal cavity

Lens

Nasal septum

Vitreous body

Ethmoid sinuses

Lacrimal gland

Medial rectus

Optic n. (CN II)

Lateral rectus

Optic canal

Temporalis

Internal carotid a.

Hypophysis

Oculo-motor n. (CN III)

Dorsum sellae

Cavernous sinus

Basilar a.

Pons

Interpeduncular fossa

Cerebellum, vermis

Tentorium cerebelli

Inferior sagittal sinus

Falx cerebri

Lateral ventricle, occipital horn

Superior sagittal sinus

Fig. 46.8 Transverse section of head through the median atlantoaxial joint

Superior view. This section passes through the soft palate and muco-periosteum of the hard palate. The articulation of the odontoid process (dens of C2) with the axis (C1) at the median atlantoaxial joint is shown, as well as the carotid sheath, containing the vertical neuro-vascular elements of the neck. The vertebral artery is sectioned as it prepares to enter the foramen magnum and fuse with its opposite to form the basilar artery.

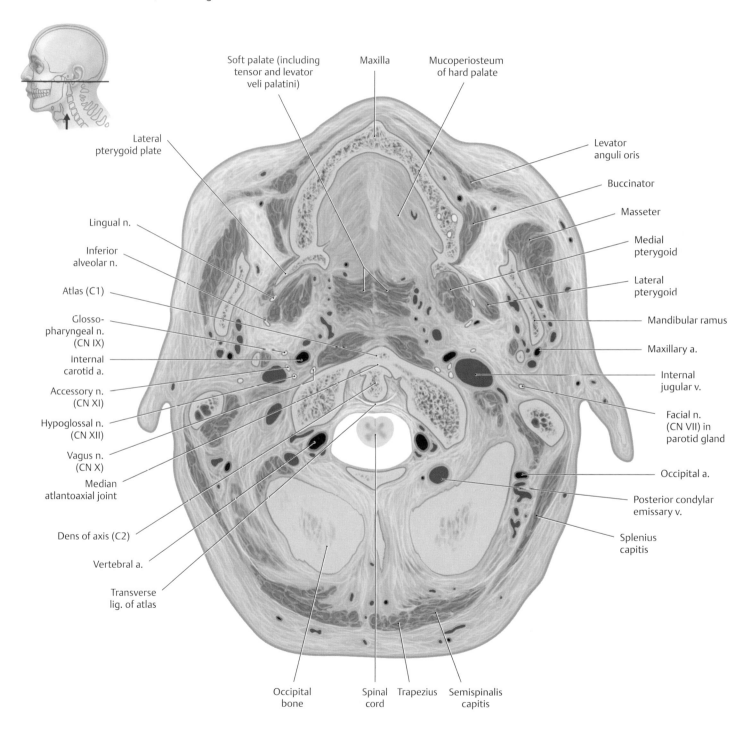

Soft palate (including tensor and levator veli palatini)

Maxilla

Mucoperiosteum of hard palate

Lateral pterygoid plate

Levator anguli oris

Buccinator

Masseter

Lingual n.

Medial pterygoid

Inferior alveolar n.

Lateral pterygoid

Atlas (C1)

Mandibular ramus

Glosso-pharyngeal n. (CN IX)

Maxillary a.

Internal carotid a.

Internal jugular v.

Accessory n. (CN XI)

Facial n. (CN VII) in parotid gland

Hypoglossal n. (CN XII)

Vagus n. (CN X)

Occipital a.

Median atlantoaxial joint

Posterior condylar emissary v.

Dens of axis (C2)

Splenius capitis

Vertebral a.

Transverse lig. of atlas

Occipital bone

Spinal cord

Trapezius

Semispinalis capitis

Radiographic Anatomy of the Head & Neck (I)

Fig. 46.12 Radiograph of the skull
Anteroposterior view. (Reproduced from Moeller TB, Reif E. Pocket Atlas of Radiographic Anatomy, 3rd ed. New York, NY: Thieme; 2010.)

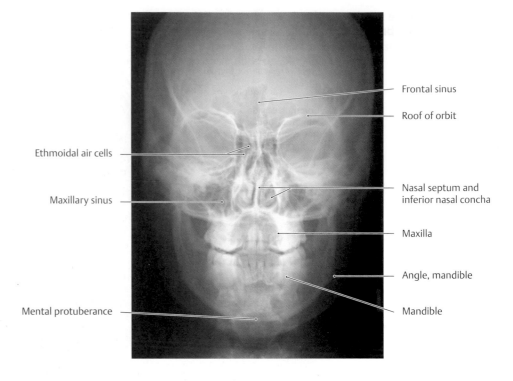

Frontal sinus

Roof of orbit

Ethmoidal air cells

Nasal septum and inferior nasal concha

Maxillary sinus

Maxilla

Angle, mandible

Mental protuberance

Mandible

Fig. 46.13 Coronal MRI through the eyeball
Anterior view.

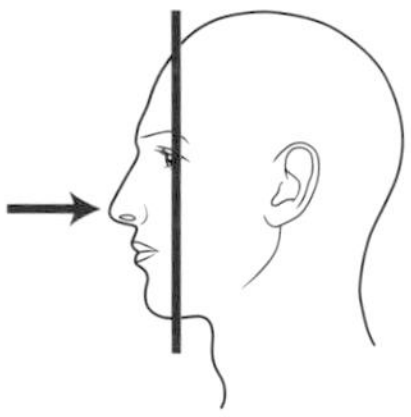

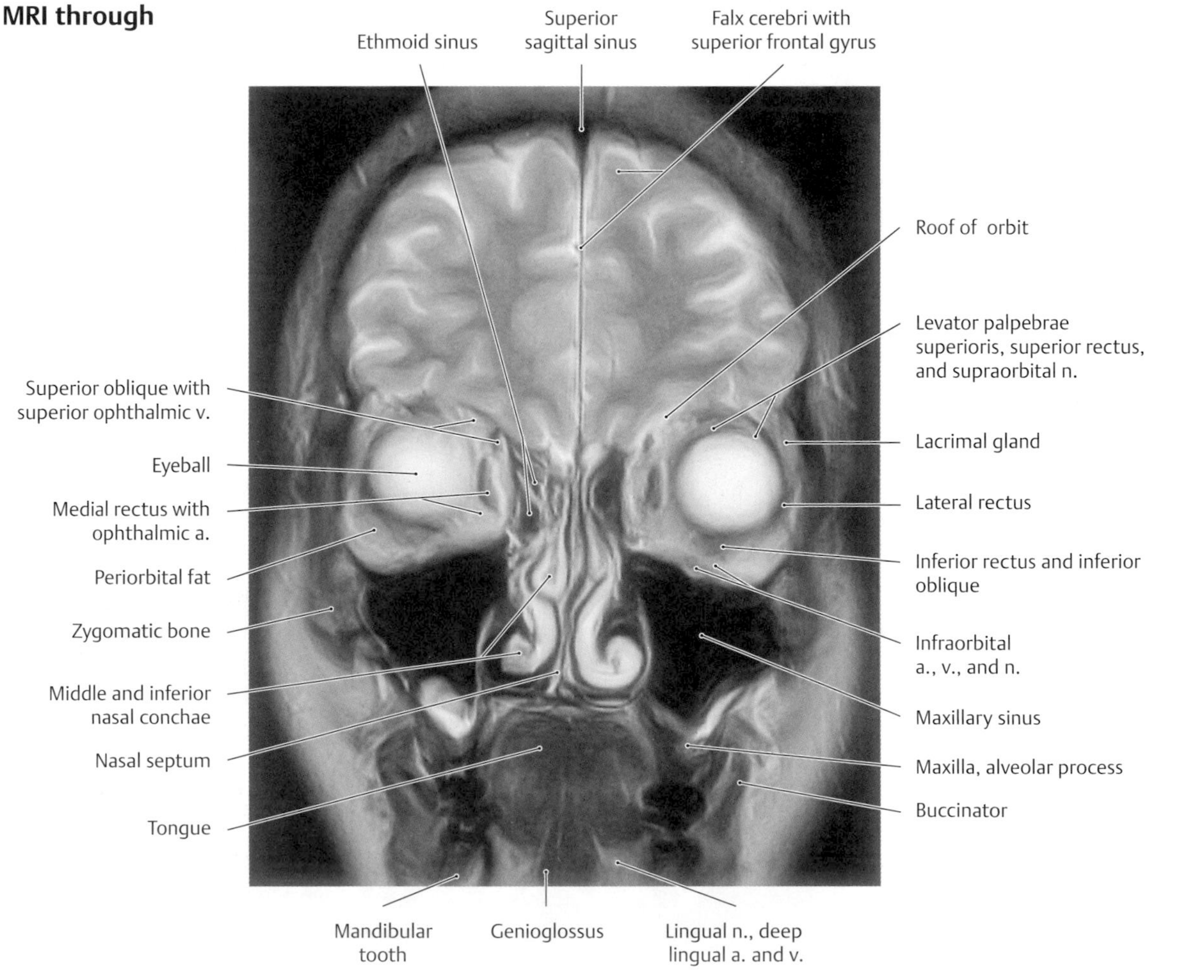

Ethmoid sinus

Superior sagittal sinus

Falx cerebri with superior frontal gyrus

Roof of orbit

Levator palpebrae superioris, superior rectus, and supraorbital n.

Superior oblique with superior ophthalmic v.

Lacrimal gland

Eyeball

Lateral rectus

Medial rectus with ophthalmic a.

Inferior rectus and inferior oblique

Periorbital fat

Zygomatic bone

Infraorbital a., v., and n.

Middle and inferior nasal conchae

Maxillary sinus

Nasal septum

Maxilla, alveolar process

Tongue

Buccinator

Mandibular tooth

Genioglossus

Lingual n., deep lingual a. and v.

Fig. 46.14 Radiograph of the skull

Left lateral view. (Reproduced from Moeller TB, Reif E. Pocket Atlas of Radiographic Anatomy, 3rd ed. New York, NY: Thieme; 2010.)

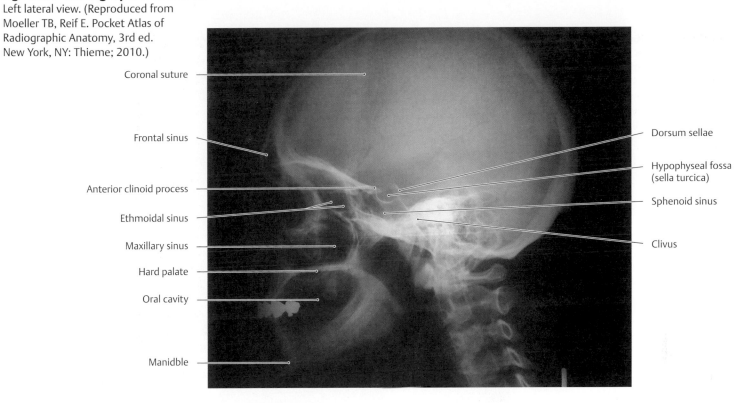

- Coronal suture
- Frontal sinus
- Anterior clinoid process
- Ethmoidal sinus
- Maxillary sinus
- Hard palate
- Oral cavity
- Manidble
- Dorsum sellae
- Hypophyseal fossa (sella turcica)
- Sphenoid sinus
- Clivus

Fig. 46.15 Midsagittal MRI through the nasal septum

Left lateral view. Boxed area represents the location of the ventricular system, thalamus, and pons. A more detail labeled version of this area can be seen in **Fig. 51.5, p. 700.** (Reproduced from Moeller TB, Reif E. Pocket Atlas of Sectional Anatomy, Vol 1, 4th ed. New York, NY: Thieme; 2014.)

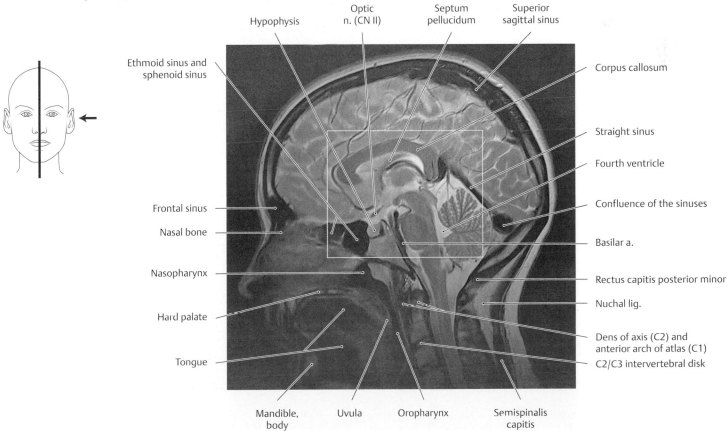

- Hypophysis
- Optic n. (CN II)
- Septum pellucidum
- Superior sagittal sinus
- Ethmoid sinus and sphenoid sinus
- Corpus callosum
- Straight sinus
- Fourth ventricle
- Confluence of the sinuses
- Frontal sinus
- Nasal bone
- Basilar a.
- Nasopharynx
- Rectus capitis posterior minor
- Nuchal lig.
- Hard palate
- Dens of axis (C2) and anterior arch of atlas (C1)
- Tongue
- C2/C3 intervertebral disk
- Mandible, body
- Uvula
- Oropharynx
- Semispinalis capitis

Radiographic Anatomy of the Head & Neck (II)

Fig. 46.16 Radiograph of the skull

Inferosuperior oblique view (Waters view). (Reproduced from Moeller TB, Reif E. Pocket Atlas of Radiographic Anatomy, 3rd ed. New York, NY: Thieme; 2010.)

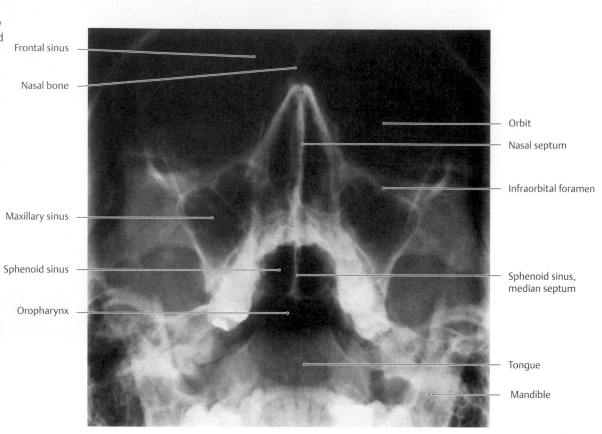

Frontal sinus

Nasal bone

Orbit

Nasal septum

Infraorbital foramen

Maxillary sinus

Sphenoid sinus

Sphenoid sinus, median septum

Oropharynx

Tongue

Mandible

Fig. 46.17 Radiograph of the mandible

Left lateral view. (Reproduced from Moeller TB, Reif E. Pocket Atlas of Radiographic Anatomy, 3rd ed. New York, NY: Thieme; 2010.)

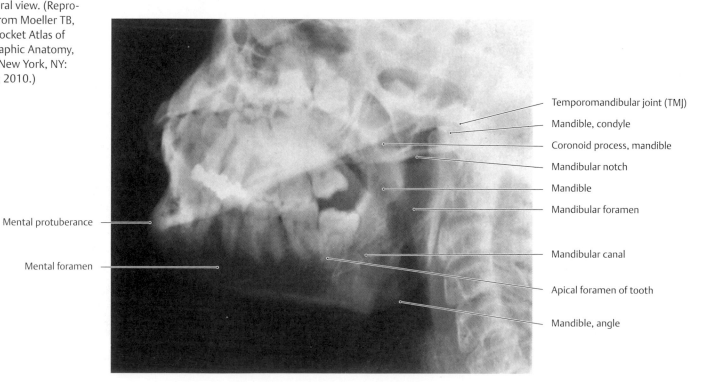

Temporomandibular joint (TMJ)

Mandible, condyle

Coronoid process, mandible

Mandibular notch

Mandible

Mandibular foramen

Mental protuberance

Mandibular canal

Mental foramen

Apical foramen of tooth

Mandible, angle

Fig. 46.18 Transverse MRI through the orbit and nasolacrimal duct

Inferior view. (Reproduced from Moeller TB, Reif E. Pocket Atlas of Sectional Anatomy, Vol 1, 4th ed. New York, NY: Thieme; 2014.)

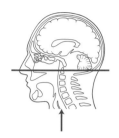

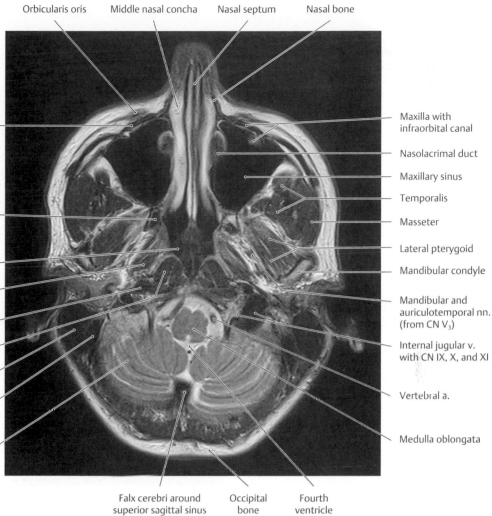

Orbicularis oris — Middle nasal concha — Nasal septum — Nasal bone

Levator labii superioris

Maxilla with infraorbital canal

Nasolacrimal duct

Maxillary sinus

Temporalis

Masseter

Medial pterygoid between medial and lateral pterygoid plates

Lateral pterygoid

Pharyngeal recess

Mandibular condyle

Levator and tensor veli palatini

Mandibular and auriculotemporal nn. (from CN V₃)

Internal carotid a.

Internal jugular v. with CN IX, X, and XI

Longus capitis

Mastoid air cells

Sigmoid sinus

Vertebral a.

Cerebellum, posterior lobe

Medulla oblongata

Falx cerebri around superior sagittal sinus — Occipital bone — Fourth ventricle

Fig. 46.19 Transverse MRI through the neck

Inferior view. (Reproduced from Moeller TB, Reif E. Pocket Atlas of Sectional Anatomy, Vol 1, 4th ed. New York, NY: Thieme; 2014.)

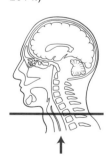

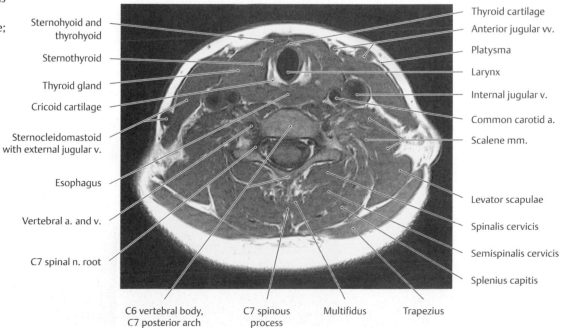

Sternohyoid and thyrohyoid

Thyroid cartilage

Anterior jugular vv.

Sternothyroid

Platysma

Thyroid gland

Larynx

Cricoid cartilage

Internal jugular v.

Sternocleidomastoid with external jugular v.

Common carotid a.

Scalene mm.

Esophagus

Vertebral a. and v.

Levator scapulae

Spinalis cervicis

C7 spinal n. root

Semispinalis cervicis

Splenius capitis

C6 vertebral body, C7 posterior arch — C7 spinous process — Multifidus — Trapezius

Radiographic Anatomy of the Head & Neck (III)

Fig. 46.20 CT scan of temporomandibular joint (TMJ)
Coronal section. (Reproduced from Moeller TB, Reif E. Atlas of Sectional Anatomy: The Musculoskeletal System. New York, NY: Thieme; 2009.)

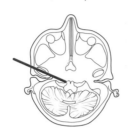

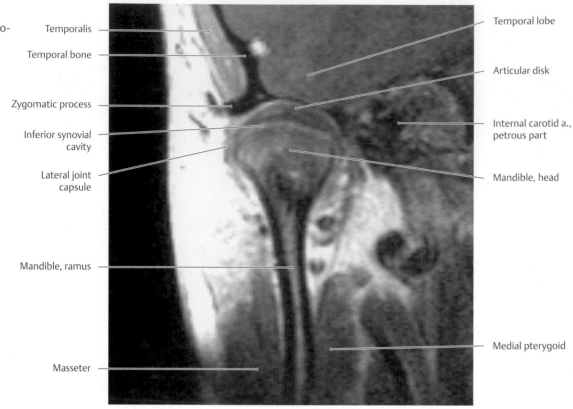

- Temporalis
- Temporal bone
- Zygomatic process
- Inferior synovial cavity
- Lateral joint capsule
- Mandible, ramus
- Masseter

- Temporal lobe
- Articular disk
- Internal carotid a., petrous part
- Mandible, head
- Medial pterygoid

Fig. 46.21 CT scan of temporomandibular joint (TMJ)
Sagittal section, mouth closed. (Reproduced from Moeller TB, Reif E. Atlas of Sectional Anatomy: The Musculoskeletal System. New York, NY: Thieme; 2009.)

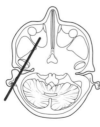

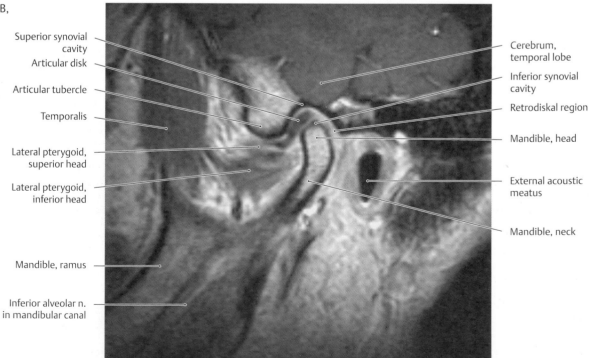

- Superior synovial cavity
- Articular disk
- Articular tubercle
- Temporalis
- Lateral pterygoid, superior head
- Lateral pterygoid, inferior head
- Mandible, ramus
- Inferior alveolar n. in mandibular canal

- Cerebrum, temporal lobe
- Inferior synovial cavity
- Retrodiskal region
- Mandible, head
- External acoustic meatus
- Mandible, neck

Fig. 46.22 Cranial MR angiography

Cranial view. In this angiogram note that the right posterior cerebral a. arises from the internal carotid artery instead of the basilar artery—a variant. The normal configuration is seen on the left side. (Reproduced from Moeller TB, Reif E. Pocket Atlas of Sectional Anatomy, Vol 1, 4th ed. New York, NY: Thieme; 2014.)

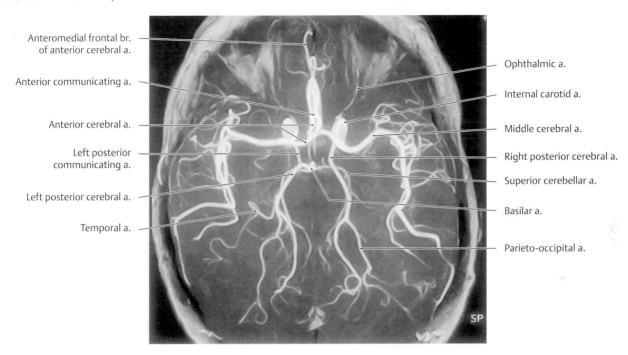

Anteromedial frontal br. of anterior cerebral a.

Anterior communicating a.

Anterior cerebral a.

Left posterior communicating a.

Left posterior cerebral a.

Temporal a.

Ophthalmic a.

Internal carotid a.

Middle cerebral a.

Right posterior cerebral a.

Superior cerebellar a.

Basilar a.

Parieto-occipital a.

Fig. 46.23 Dural venous sinus system of the head

Right lateral view. Lateral internal carotid arteriogram, venous phase.

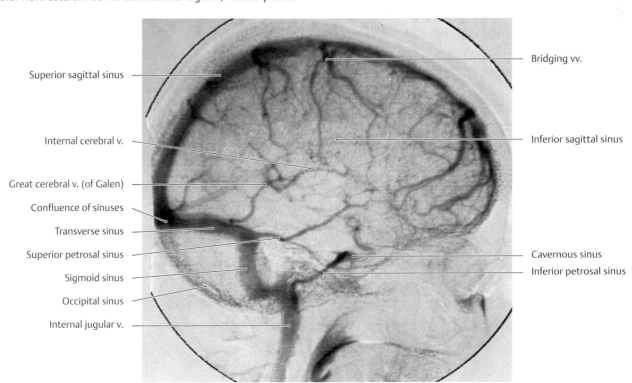

Superior sagittal sinus

Internal cerebral v.

Great cerebral v. (of Galen)

Confluence of sinuses

Transverse sinus

Superior petrosal sinus

Sigmoid sinus

Occipital sinus

Internal jugular v.

Bridging vv.

Inferior sagittal sinus

Cavernous sinus

Inferior petrosal sinus

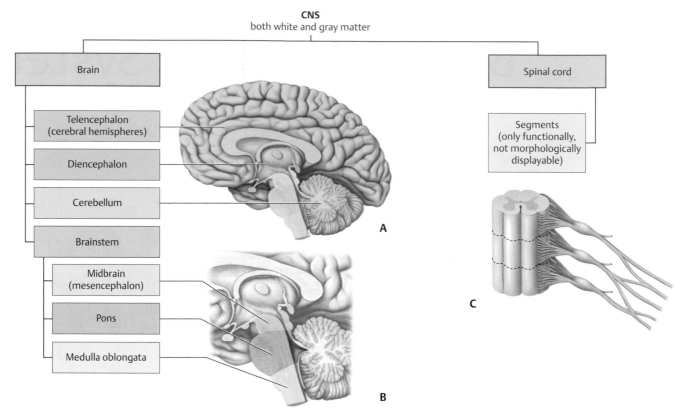

Fig. 47.1 Morphology of the Central Nervous System (CNS)

A and **B** Right side of the brain, medial view; **C** Section of the spinal cord, ventral view. A general morphological overview of the entire nervous system is necessary to help with understanding the material that follows. The CNS is divided into the brain and the spinal cord with the brain subdivided into the following regions:

- Cerebral hemispheres (telencephalon or endbrain)
- Interbrain (diencephalon)
- Cerebellum
- Brain stem composed of the midbrain (mesencephalon), pons (bridge) and medulla oblongata

In contrast, the other part of the CNS, the **spinal cord** appears morphologically rather as one homogenous structure. In terms of its functions, however, the spinal cord can also be divided into segments. The division of gray and white matter is clearly visible:

- Gray matter: centrally located, butterfly-shaped structure
- White matter: substance that surrounds the "butterfly"

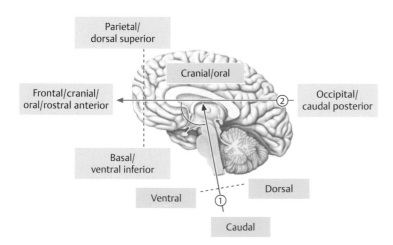

Fig. 47.2 Axes of the nervous system and directional terms

The same planes, axes and directional terms apply for both the entire body and the PNS. However, with the CNS, one differentiates between two axes:

- Axis No. 1: Meynert axis: It corresponds to the axes of the body and is used to designate locations in the spinal cord, brainstem (truncus encephali) and cerebellum.
- Axis No. 2: Forel axis. It turns horizontally through the diencephalon and telencephalon and forms an 80° angle to axis 1. As a result, the diencephalon and telencephalon lie "face down".

Note: In order to avoid topographical misunderstandings, the following directional terms for axis No. 2 (Forel axis) are used:

- basal instead of ventral
- parietal instead of dorsal
- frontal and oral/rostral respectively instead of cranial
- occipital instead of caudal

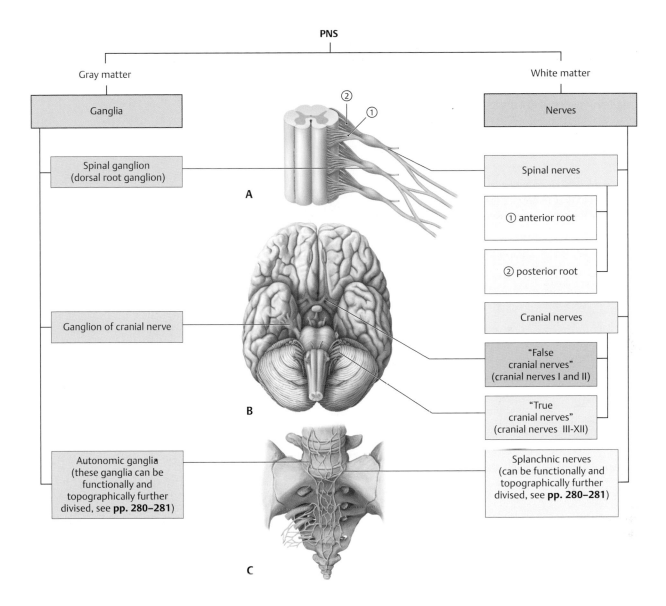

PNS

Gray matter | White matter

Ganglia | Nerves

Spinal ganglion (dorsal root ganglion)

A

Ganglion of cranial nerve

B

Autonomic ganglia (these ganglia can be functionally and topographically further divised, see **pp. 280–281**)

C

Spinal nerves

① anterior root

② posterior root

Cranial nerves

"False cranial nerves" (cranial nerves I and II)

"True cranial nerves" (cranial nerves III-XII)

Splanchnic nerves (can be functionally and topographically further divised, see **pp. 280–281**)

Fig. 47.3 Morphology of the peripheral nervous system

A Segment of the spinal cord, ventral view; **B** Base of the brain; **C** view of sympathetic ganglia and nerves located anterior to the sacrum.

The nerves and ganglia forming the peripheral nervous system are generally named for the part of the CNS with which they communicate:

- Spinal nerves (connect the periphery of the body with the spinal cord. Usually 31 or 32 pairs. Spinal nerves (except those related to vertebral levels T1 to T11 or T12) generally have their anterior rami form plexuses for reasons of functionality.
- Cranial nerves (connect the periphery of the body to the brain). 12 pairs.

Nerve cells found within ganglia (in the PNS) can be classified based on their affiliation with a particular functional division of the nervous system:

- Sensory neurons can be found within either division of the nervous system. In the PNS, sensory neurons are found within the sensory (dorsal root) ganglia on the posterior (dorsal) root of the spinal nerve.

In the CNS, sensory neurons are found within the sensory nuclei associated with the appropriate cranial nerves that contain sensory fibers.

- Ganglia of the autonomic nervous system contain postganglionic sympathetic and parasympathetic neurons that control the organs of the body. Autonomic ganglia are associated with splanchnic nerves that take vasomotor fibers to the viscera. The autonomic nervous system also demonstrates characteristic plexus formation.

Note: The distinction of sensory nerves in the CNS applies except for a few special cases. For instance, cranial nerves I (olfactory) and II (optic) are not true nerves but parts of the telencephalon or diencephalon, which clearly makes them part of the CNS. For historical reasons, they have been called "nerves", which is systematically false. These "bogus" cranial nerves (colored red on the brain in the figure above) are often contrasted with the 10 true cranial nerves (colored yellow on this figure), which are clearly part of the PNS. In the interest of clarity, further details are located within each region throughout the atlas.

Nervous System: Development

Fig. 47.4 **Central and peripheral nervous systems**

The CNS consists of the brain and spinal cord, which constitute a functional unit. The PNS consists of the nerves emerging from the brain and spinal cord (cranial and spinal nerves, respectively). Nerves emerging from the spinal canal after the end of the spinal cord, form the cauda equina (see **p. 41**)

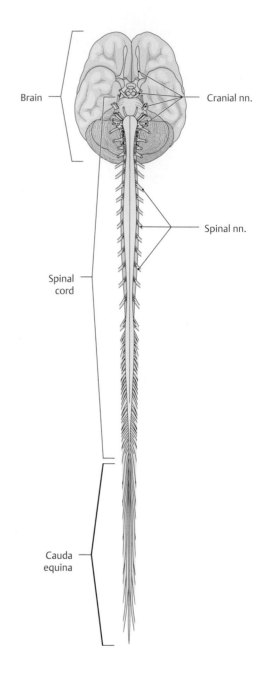

Fig. 47.5 **Gray and white matter in the CNS**

Nerve cell bodies appear gray in gross inspection, whereas nerve cell processes (axons) and their insulating myelin sheaths appear white.

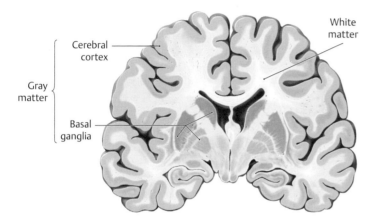

A Coronal section through the brain.

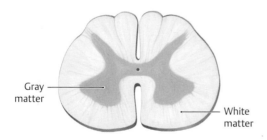

B Transverse section through the spinal cord.

Table 47.1	**Development of the brain**				
	Primary vesicle	**Region**			**Structure**
Neural tube	Prosencephalon (forebrain)	Telencephalon (cerebrum)			Cerebral cortex, white matter, and basal ganglia
		Diencephalon			Epithalamus (pineal), dorsal thalamus, subthalamus, and hypothalamus
	Mesencephalon (midbrain)*				Tectum, tegmentum, and cerebral peduncles
	Rhombencephalon (hindbrain)	Metencephalon	Cerebellum		Cerebellar cortex, nuclei, and peduncles
			Pons*		Nuclei and fiber tracts
		Myelencephalon	Medulla oblongata*		

* The mesencephalon, pons, and medulla oblongata are collectively known as the brainstem.

Fig. 47.6 Embryonic development of the brain
Left lateral view.

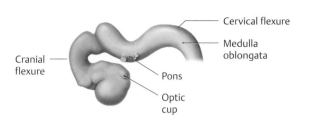

A Start of 2nd month.

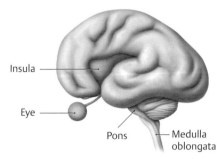

C 3rd month of development.

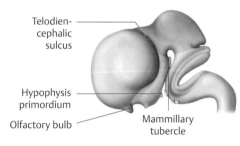

B End of 2nd month.

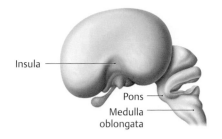

D 7th month.

Fig. 47.7 Adult brain
See **Fig. 47.10** for lobes of the cerebrum. CN, cranial nerve.

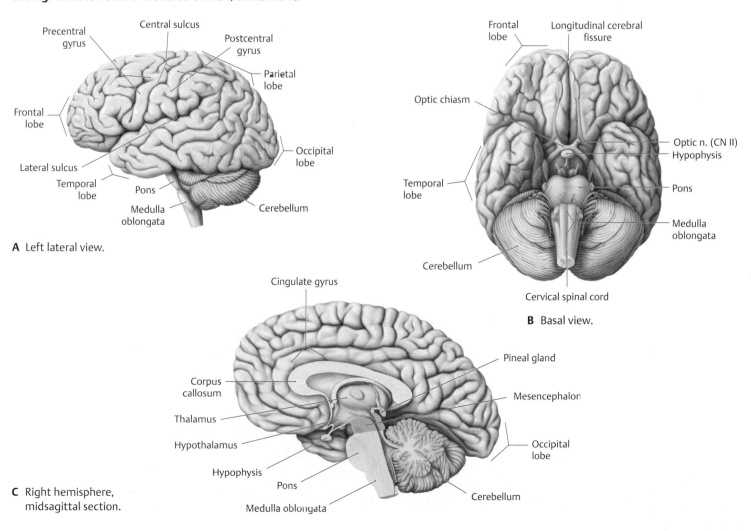

A Left lateral view.

B Basal view.

C Right hemisphere, midsagittal section.

Fig. 47.8 Cerebrum

Left lateral view. The cerebrum is part of the anterior subdivision of the embryonic forebrain (telencephalon)—the part of the adult forebrain that includes the cerebral hemispheres and associated structures. The surface anatomy of the cerebrum can be divided macroscopically into 4 lobes: frontal, parietal, temporal, and occipital. The surface contours of the cerebrum are defined by convolutions (gyri) and depressions (sulci).

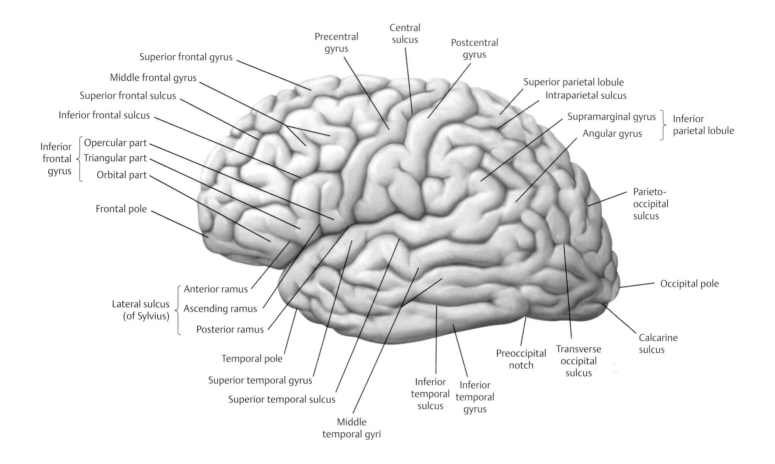

Fig. 47.9 Insular lobe

Lateral view of the retracted left cerebral hemisphere. Part of the cerebral cortex sinks below the surface during development forming the insula (or insular lobe). Those portions of the cerebral cortex that overlie this deeper cortical region are called opercula ("little lids").

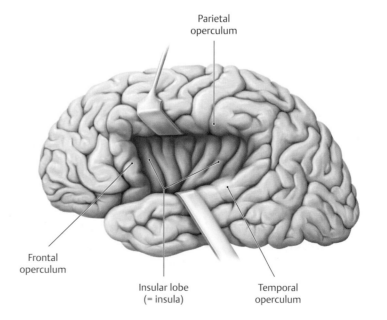

Fig. 47.10 Lobes in the cerebral hemispheres

The isocortex also may be functionally divided into association areas (lobes).

Frontal lobe
Parietal lobe
Temporal lobe
Occipital lobe
Insular lobe (insula)
Limbic lobe (limbus)

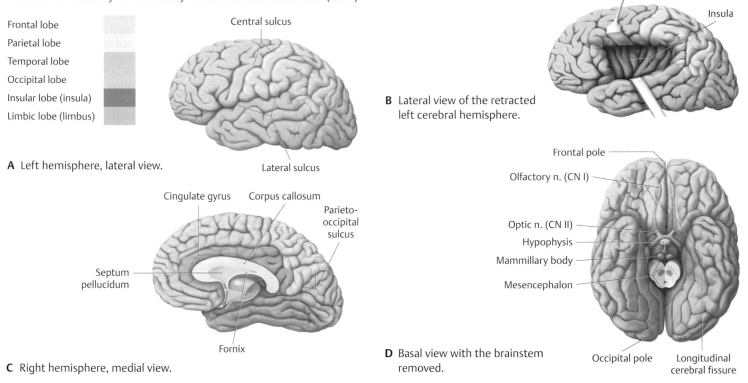

A Left hemisphere, lateral view.

Central sulcus

Lateral sulcus

B Lateral view of the retracted left cerebral hemisphere.

Insula

Cingulate gyrus   Corpus callosum

Parieto-occipital sulcus

Septum pellucidum

Fornix

C Right hemisphere, medial view.

Frontal pole

Olfactory n. (CN I)

Optic n. (CN II)

Hypophysis

Mammillary body

Mesencephalon

D Basal view with the brainstem removed.

Occipital pole   Longitudinal cerebral fissure

Fig. 47.11 Midsagittal section of the brain showing the medial surface of the right hemisphere

The brain has been split along the longitudinal cerebral fissure.

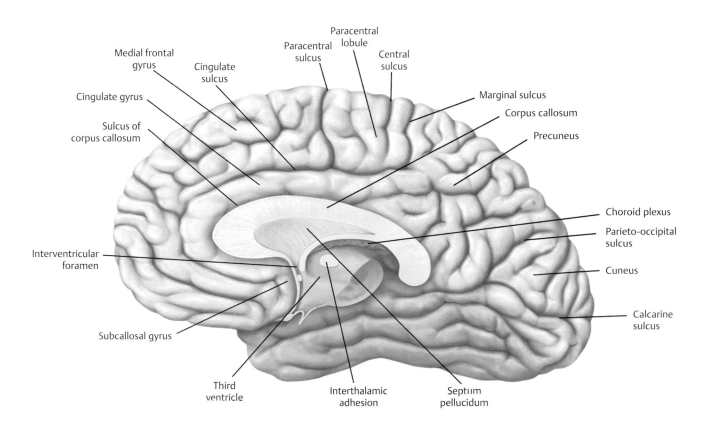

Medial frontal gyrus
Cingulate sulcus
Paracentral sulcus
Paracentral lobule
Central sulcus
Cingulate gyrus
Marginal sulcus
Sulcus of corpus callosum
Corpus callosum
Precuneus
Choroid plexus
Parieto-occipital sulcus
Interventricular foramen
Cuneus
Subcallosal gyrus
Calcarine sulcus
Third ventricle
Interthalamic adhesion
Septum pellucidum

Brainstem & Cerebellum

The stalk-like region of the brain connecting the cerebral hemispheres to the cerebellum and spinal cord consists of the diencephalon (thalamus and associated structures) and the brainstem—composed of the mesencephalon or midbrain, pons and medulla oblongata moving sequentially caudal. Fiber bundles pass through this region from the spinal cord on their way to and from the cerebrum; thick fiber bundles pass contralaterally from the cerebrum into the cerebellar hemispheres; and 10 of the 12 cranial nerves are associated with the brainstem.

Fig. 47.16 Diencephalon, brainstem, and cerebellum
Left lateral view.

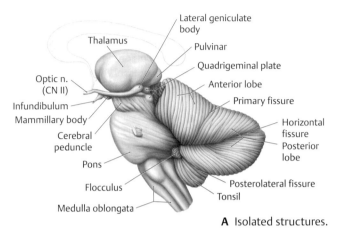

Lateral geniculate body
Thalamus
Pulvinar
Quadrigeminal plate
Optic n. (CN II)
Anterior lobe
Infundibulum
Primary fissure
Mammillary body
Cerebral peduncle
Horizontal fissure
Posterior lobe
Pons
Flocculus
Posterolateral fissure
Medulla oblongata
Tonsil

A Isolated structures.

Corpus callosum
Fornix
Choroid plexus
Pineal
Tectal
Anterior commissure
Hypothalamus
Optic chiasm
Infundibulum
Adenohypophysis
Neurohypophysis
Central lobule
Primary fissure
Lingula
Horizontal fissure
Superior medullary velum
Pyramid
4th ventricle
Choroid plexus
Nodule
Prebiventral fissure

B Midsagittal section.

Fig. 47.17 Cerebellum

Anterior lobe
Primary fissure
Culmen
Quadrangular lobule
Simple lobule
Superior semilunar lobule
Vermis
Posterior lobe
Folium of vermis
Horizontal fissure
Inferior semilunar lobule

Median part
Lateral parts

A Superior view.

Superior medullary velum
Central lobule
Lingula
Superior cerebellar peduncle
Middle cerebellar peduncle
4th ventricle
Inferior cerebellar peduncle
Horizontal fissure
Uvula vermis
Nodule — Flocculo-
Flocculus — nodular lobe
Pyramid of vermis
Vallecula
Tonsil
Peduncle of flocculus

Intermediate parts

B Anterior view.

Fig. 47.18 Cerebellar peduncles
Tracts of afferent (sensory) or efferent (motor) axons enter or leave the cerebellum through cerebellar peduncles. Afferent axons originate in the spinal cord, vestibular organs, inferior olive, and pons. Efferent axons originate in the cerebellar nuclei.

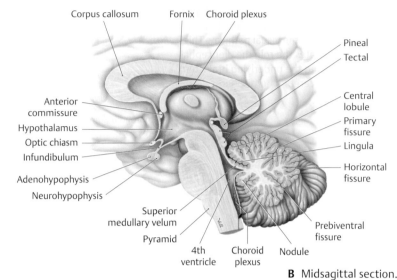

Superior cerebellar peduncle
Inferior cerebellar peduncle
Anterior spinocerebellar tract
Middle cerebellar peduncle
Trigeminal n. (CN V)
Vestibulocochlear n. (CN VIII)
Facial n. (CN VII)
Central tegmental tract
Olive

Fig. 47.19 Brainstem

The brainstem is the site of emergence and entry of the 10 pairs of true cranial nerves (CN III–XII). See **pp. 560–561** for an overview of the cranial nerves and their nuclei.

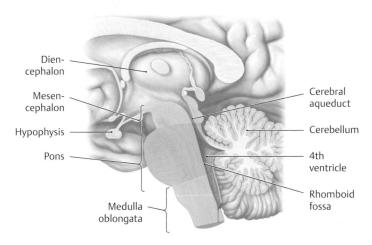

A Levels of the brainstem.

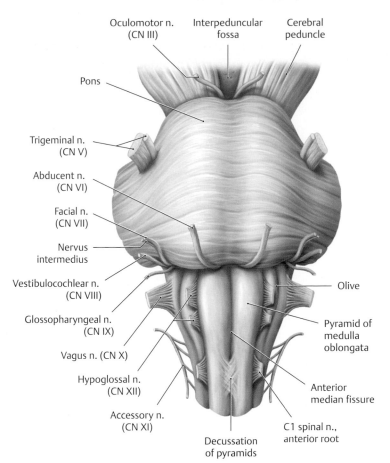

B Anterior view.

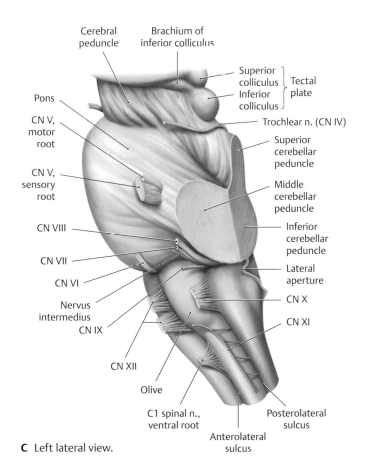

C Left lateral view.

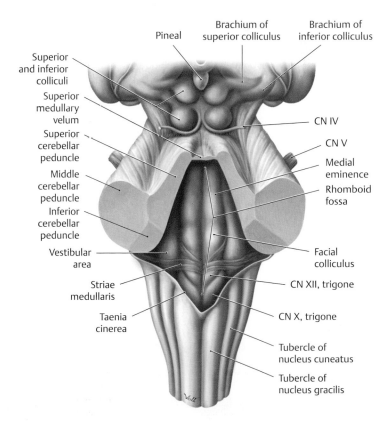

D Posterior view.

Ventricles & CSF Spaces

Fig. 47.20 **Circulation of cerebrospinal fluid (CSF)**

The brain and spinal cord are suspended in CSF. Produced continually in the choroid plexus, CSF occupies the subarachnoid space and ventricles of the brain and drains through arachnoid granulations into the dural venous sinus system (primarily the superior sagittal sinus) of the cranial cavity. Smaller amounts drain along proximal portions of the spinal nerves into venous plexuses or lymphatic pathways.

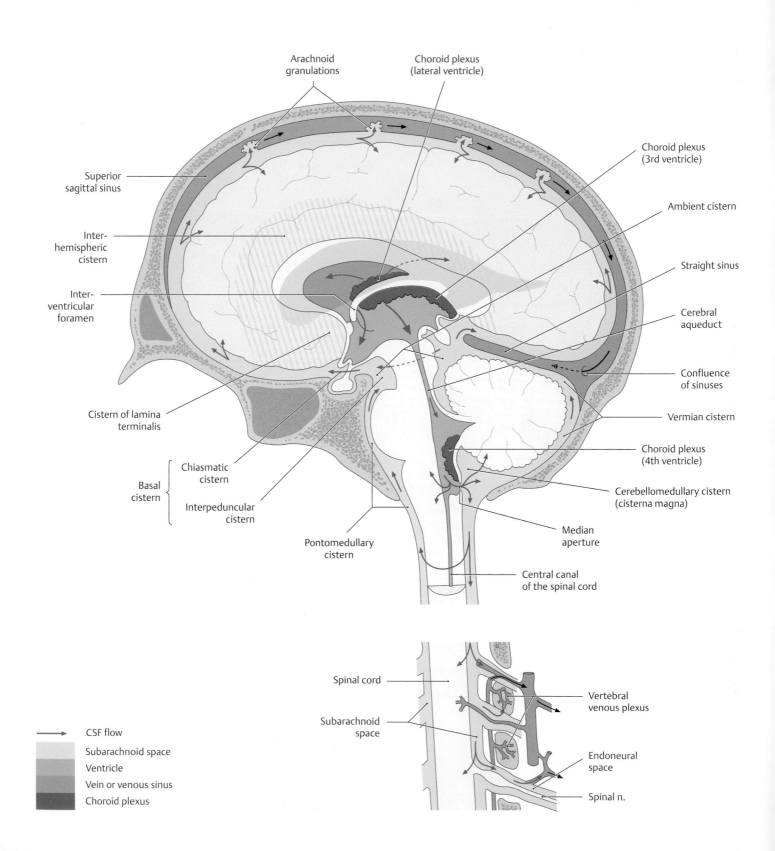

Fig. 47.21 **Ventricular system**

The ventricular system is a continuation of the central spinal canal into the brain. Cast specimens are used to demonstrate the connections between the four ventricular cavities.

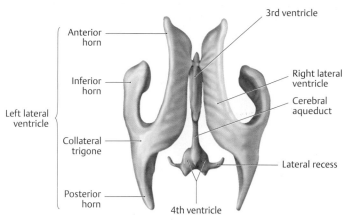

A Superior view.

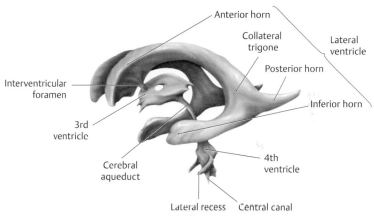

B Lateral ventricles in transverse section.

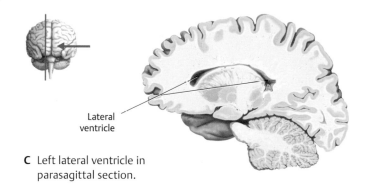

C Left lateral ventricle in parasagittal section.

D Left lateral view.

Fig. 47.22 **Ventricular system in situ**

Left lateral view.

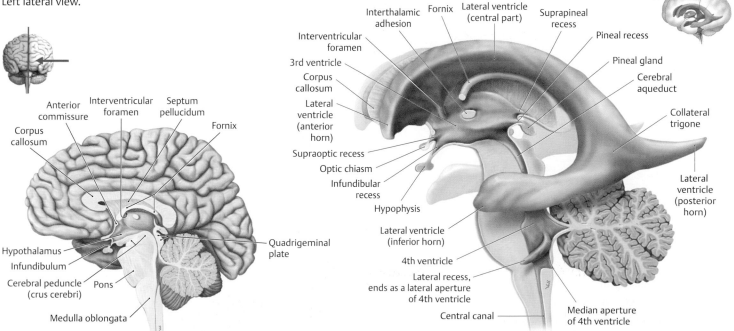

A 3rd and 4th ventricles in midsagittal section.

B Ventricular system with neighboring structures.

48 Blood Vessels of the Brain
Veins & Venous Sinuses of the Brain

Additional information on the venous sinus system and dural folds of the cranial cavity can be found on **pp. 590–593**.

Fig. 48.1 **Superficial cerebral veins**

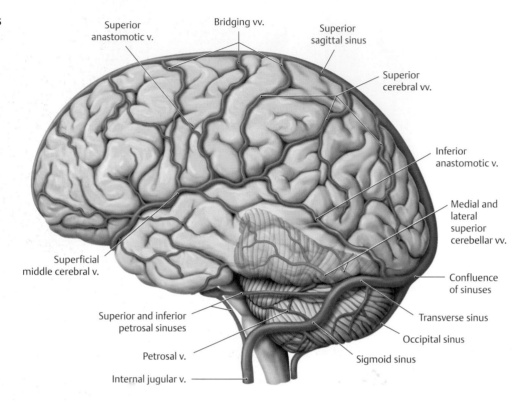

Superior anastomotic v.

Bridging vv.

Superior sagittal sinus

Superior cerebral vv.

Inferior anastomotic v.

Medial and lateral superior cerebellar vv.

Confluence of sinuses

Transverse sinus

Occipital sinus

Sigmoid sinus

Superficial middle cerebral v.

Superior and inferior petrosal sinuses

Petrosal v.

Internal jugular v.

A Left hemisphere, lateral view.

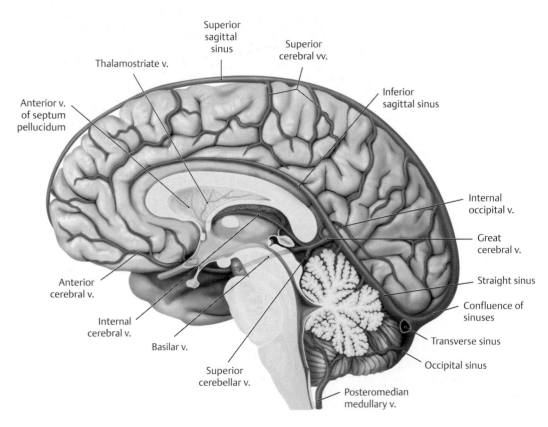

Superior sagittal sinus

Superior cerebral vv.

Thalamostriate v.

Inferior sagittal sinus

Anterior v. of septum pellucidum

Internal occipital v.

Great cerebral v.

Straight sinus

Confluence of sinuses

Transverse sinus

Occipital sinus

Anterior cerebral v.

Internal cerebral v.

Basilar v.

Superior cerebellar v.

Posteromedian medullary v.

B Right hemisphere, medial view.

Fig. 48.2 Basal cerebral venous system
Basal (inferior) view.

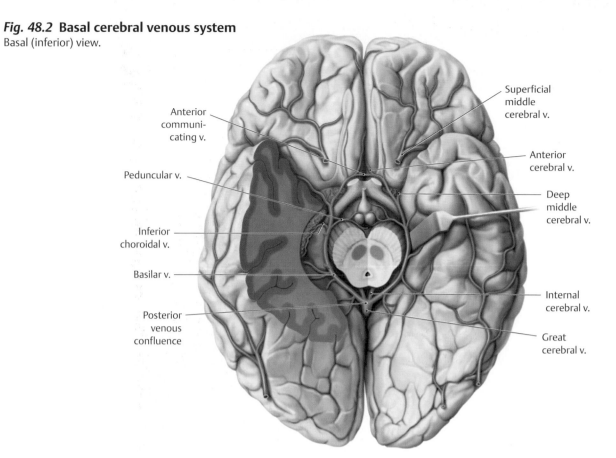

Anterior communicating v.

Superficial middle cerebral v.

Peduncular v.

Anterior cerebral v.

Inferior choroidal v.

Deep middle cerebral v.

Basilar v.

Internal cerebral v.

Posterior venous confluence

Great cerebral v.

Fig. 48.3 Veins of the brainstem
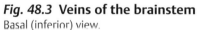

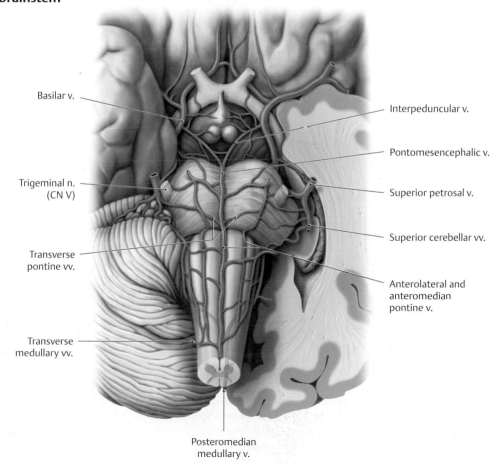

Basilar v.

Interpeduncular v.

Trigeminal n. (CN V)

Pontomesencephalic v.

Superior petrosal v.

Transverse pontine vv.

Superior cerebellar vv.

Anterolateral and anteromedian pontine v.

Transverse medullary vv.

Posteromedian medullary v.

Arteries of the Brain

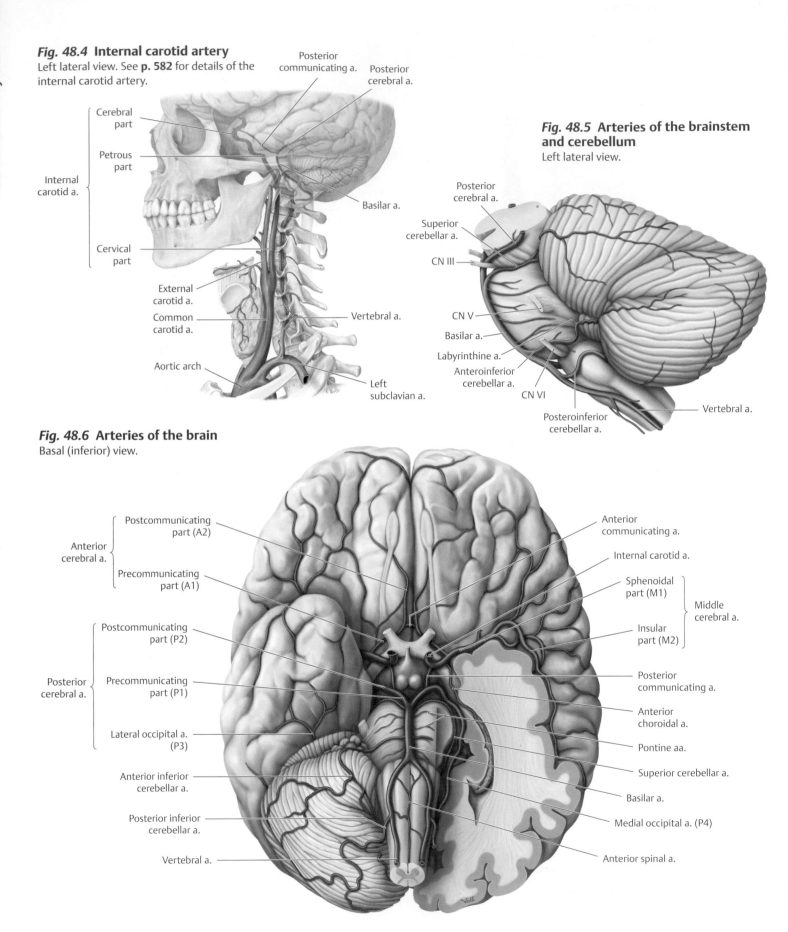

Fig. 48.4 Internal carotid artery
Left lateral view. See **p. 582** for details of the internal carotid artery.

Posterior communicating a.

Posterior cerebral a.

Cerebral part

Petrous part

Internal carotid a.

Cervical part

Basilar a.

External carotid a.

Common carotid a.

Vertebral a.

Aortic arch

Left subclavian a.

Fig. 48.5 Arteries of the brainstem and cerebellum
Left lateral view.

Posterior cerebral a.

Superior cerebellar a.

CN III

CN V

Basilar a.

Labyrinthine a.

Anteroinferior cerebellar a.

CN VI

Posteroinferior cerebellar a.

Vertebral a.

Fig. 48.6 Arteries of the brain
Basal (inferior) view.

Anterior cerebral a.

Postcommunicating part (A2)

Precommunicating part (A1)

Posterior cerebral a.

Postcommunicating part (P2)

Precommunicating part (P1)

Lateral occipital a. (P3)

Anterior inferior cerebellar a.

Posterior inferior cerebellar a.

Vertebral a.

Anterior communicating a.

Internal carotid a.

Sphenoidal part (M1)

Insular part (M2)

Middle cerebral a.

Posterior communicating a.

Anterior choroidal a.

Pontine aa.

Superior cerebellar a.

Basilar a.

Medial occipital a. (P4)

Anterior spinal a.

Fig. 48.7 Cerebral arteries

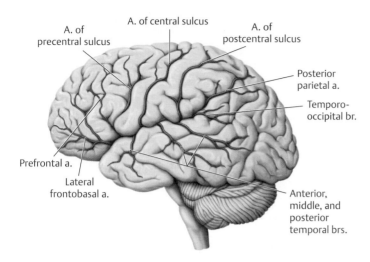

A Middle cerebral artery. Left hemisphere, lateral view.

A. of precentral sulcus
A. of central sulcus
A. of postcentral sulcus
Posterior parietal a.
Temporo-occipital br.
Prefrontal a.
Lateral frontobasal a.
Anterior, middle, and posterior temporal brs.

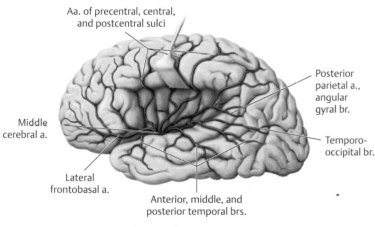

B Middle cerebral artery. Left lateral view with the lateral sulcus retracted.

Aa. of precentral, central, and postcentral sulci
Posterior parietal a., angular gyral br.
Middle cerebral a.
Temporo-occipital br.
Lateral frontobasal a.
Anterior, middle, and posterior temporal brs.

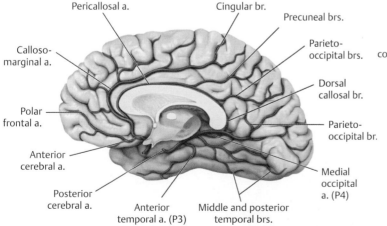

C Anterior and posterior cerebral arteries. Right hemisphere, medial view.

Pericallosal a.
Cingular br.
Precuneal brs.
Calloso-marginal a.
Parieto-occipital brs.
Polar frontal a.
Dorsal callosal br.
Anterior cerebral a.
Parieto-occipital br.
Posterior cerebral a.
Anterior temporal a. (P3)
Middle and posterior temporal brs.
Medial occipital a. (P4)

Fig. 48.8 Cerebral arteries: Distribution areas

The central gray and white matter have a complex blood supply (yellow) that includes the anterior choroidal artery.

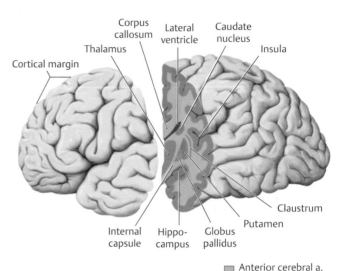

A Left hemisphere, lateral view.

Corpus callosum
Thalamus
Lateral ventricle
Caudate nucleus
Insula
Cortical margin
Claustrum
Putamen
Internal capsule
Hippo-campus
Globus pallidus

☐ Anterior cerebral a.
☐ Middle cerebral a.
☐ Posterior cerebral a.

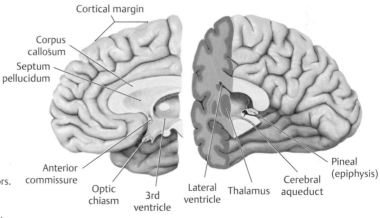

B Right hemisphere, medial view.

Cortical margin
Corpus callosum
Septum pellucidum
Anterior commissure
Optic chiasm
3rd ventricle
Lateral ventricle
Thalamus
Cerebral aqueduct
Pineal (epiphysis)

49 Functional Systems
Anatomy & Organization of the Spinal Cord

Fig. 49.1 Anatomy of a spinal cord segment

Three dimensional representation, oblique anterior view from upper left. The gray matter of the spinal cord is found internally, surrounding the central canal in an H-shaped, or butterfly-like, configuration. This is the reverse of what was seen in the brain where the gray matter was on the external aspect in a cortical configuration. The primary function of the spinal cord is to conduct impulses to and from the brain. To facilitate this, both gray and white matter are organized into longitudinal groupings.

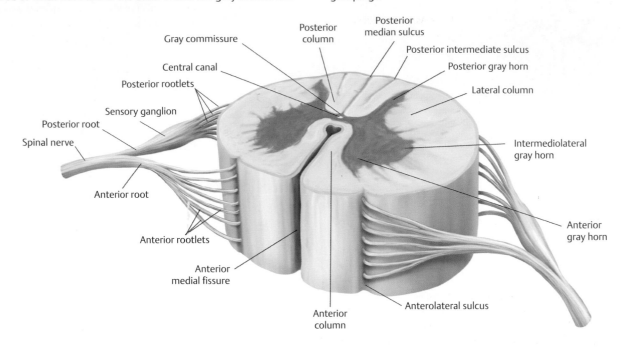

Fig. 49.2 Organization of the gray matter

Left oblique anterosuperior view. The gray matter of the spinal cord is divided into three columns (horns).

- Anterior column (horn): contains motor neurons
- Lateral column (horn): contains sympathetic or parasympathetic (visceromotor) neurons in selected regions
- Posterior column (horn): contains sensory neurons

Sensory (blue) and motor (red) neurons within these columns are clustered in nuclei according to function.

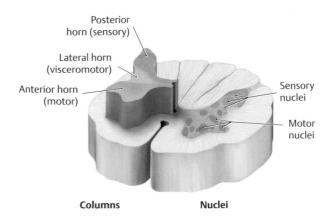

Fig. 49.3 Innervation of muscles

Motor neurons that innervate specific muscles are arranged into vertical columns in the anterior horn of gray matter, the columns themselves can be called nuclei, in a fashion similar to that seen in brainstem motor nuclei. Most muscles (intersegmental muscles) receive innervation from numerous motor nuclei spanning several spinal cord segments. Monosegmental (or indicator) muscles have their motor neurons located entirely within a single spinal cord segment.

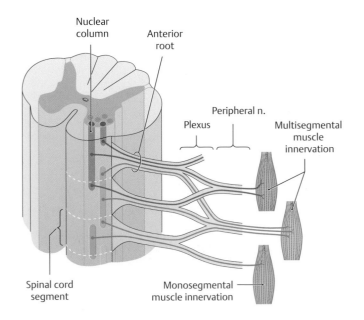

Fig. 49.4 **Organization of the white matter**

Left oblique anterosuperior view. The gray matter columns partition the white matter analogously into anterior, lateral, and posterior columns or funiculi. The white matter of the spinal cord contains ascending and descending tracts which are the CNS equivalent of peripheral nerves.

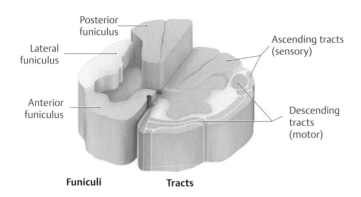

Posterior funiculus

Lateral funiculus

Anterior funiculus

Ascending tracts (sensory)

Descending tracts (motor)

Funiculi   **Tracts**

Fig. 49.5 **Overview of sensorimotor integration**

Schematic illustrates the pathway of incoming primary sensory neuron impulses, the axon of which ascends to synapse with the secondary and tertiary sensory neurons in the brainstem and cerebrum ending in a synapse on a neuron in the sensory cortex. An interneuron links this with an upper motor neuron in the motor cortex which then descends through the white matter funiculi of the spinal cord to a motor neuron, which then synapses with a lower motor neuron, the axon of which passes out the spinal nerve to the effector organ.

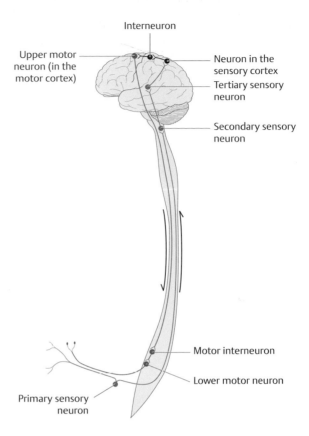

Interneuron

Upper motor neuron (in the motor cortex)

Neuron in the sensory cortex

Tertiary sensory neuron

Secondary sensory neuron

Motor interneuron

Lower motor neuron

Primary sensory neuron

Fig. 49.6 **Principle intrinsic fascicles of the spinal cord (shaded yellow)**

Left oblique anterosuperior view. The majority of muscles have a multi-segmental mode of innervaton that necessitates axons to ascend/descend multiple spinal cord segments to coordinate spinal reflexes. The neurons of these axons originate from interneurons in the gray matter forming intrinsic reflex pathways of the spinal cord. These axons are collected into intrinsic fascicles which are arranged chiefly around the gray matter. These bundles make up the intrinsic circuits of the spinal cord.

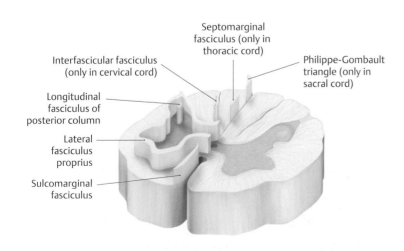

Septomarginal fasciculus (only in thoracic cord)

Interfascicular fasciculus (only in cervical cord)

Philippe-Gombault triangle (only in sacral cord)

Longitudinal fasciculus of posterior column

Lateral fasciculus proprius

Sulcomarginal fasciculus

Fig. 49.7 **Intrinsic circuits of the spinal cord**

Sensory neurons are shown in blue, motor neurons in red. The neurons of the spinal reflex circuits are in black. These chains of interneurons, which are entirely contained within the spinal cord, comprise the intrinsic circuits of the cord. The axons of these intrinsic circuits pass to adjacent segments in intrinsic fascicles located along the edge of the gray matter.

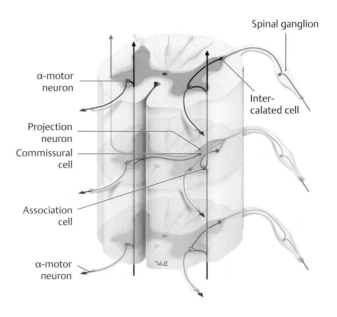

Spinal ganglion

α-motor neuron

Projection neuron

Commissural cell

Association cell

α-motor neuron

Inter-calated cell

691

Sensory & Motor Pathways

Fig. 49.8 **Sensory pathways (ascending tracts)**

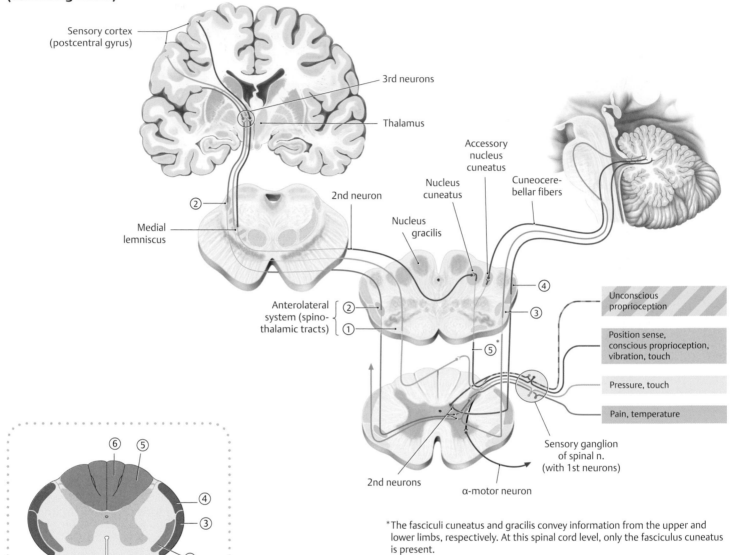

Sensory cortex (postcentral gyrus)

3rd neurons

Thalamus

Accessory nucleus cuneatus

Nucleus cuneatus

Cuneocerebellar fibers

2nd neuron

Medial lemniscus

Nucleus gracilis

Anterolateral system (spinothalamic tracts)

Unconscious proprioception

Position sense, conscious proprioception, vibration, touch

Pressure, touch

Pain, temperature

Sensory ganglion of spinal n. (with 1st neurons)

2nd neurons

α-motor neuron

*The fasciculi cuneatus and gracilis convey information from the upper and lower limbs, respectively. At this spinal cord level, only the fasciculus cuneatus is present.

	Tract	Location	Function		Neurons
①	Anterior spinothalamic tract	Anterior funiculus	Pathway for crude touch and pressure sensation		1st afferent neurons located in spinal ganglia; contain 2nd neurons and cross in the anterior commissure
②	Lateral spinothalamic tract	Anterior and lateral funiculi	Pathway for pain, temperature, tickle, itch, and sexual sensation		
③	Anterior spinocerebellar tract	Lateral funiculus	Pathway for unconscious coordination of motor activities (unconscious proprioception, automatic processes, e.g., jogging, riding a bike) to the cerebellum		Projection (2nd) neurons receive proprioceptive signals from 1st afferent fibers originating at the 1st neurons of spinal ganglia
④	Posterior spinocerebellar tract				
⑤	Fasciculus cuneatus	Posterior funiculus	Pathway for position sense (conscious proprioception) and fine cutaneous sensation (touch, vibration, fine pressure sense, two-point discrimination)	Conveys information from *upper* limb (not present below T3)	Cell bodies of 1st neuron located in spinal ganglion; pass uncrossed to the dorsal column nuclei
⑥	Fasciculus gracilis			Conveys information from *lower* limb	

Table 49.1   Sensory pathways (ascending tracts) of the spinal cord

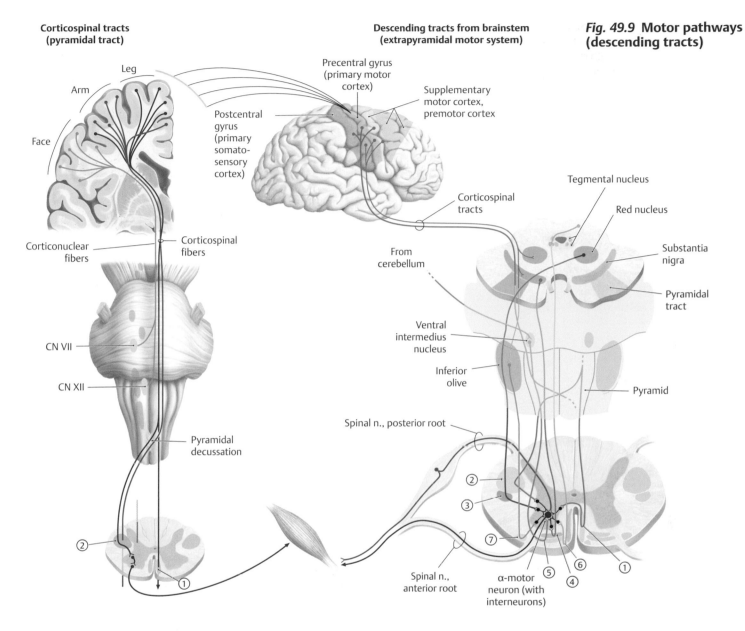

Corticospinal tracts (pyramidal tract)

Leg
Arm
Face

Postcentral gyrus (primary somato-sensory cortex)

Corticonuclear fibers — Corticospinal fibers

CN VII

CN XII

Pyramidal decussation

②

①

Descending tracts from brainstem (extrapyramidal motor system)

Precentral gyrus (primary motor cortex)

Supplementary motor cortex, premotor cortex

Corticospinal tracts

From cerebellum

Ventral intermedius nucleus

Inferior olive

Spinal n., posterior root

②
③
⑦

Spinal n., anterior root

α-motor neuron (with interneurons)

⑤
④
⑥
①

Tegmental nucleus

Red nucleus

Substantia nigra

Pyramidal tract

Pyramid

Fig. 49.9 **Motor pathways (descending tracts)**

Table 49.2	Descending tracts of the spinal cord		
Tract			**Function**
Corticospinal tract (pyramidal tract)	①	Anterior corticospinal tract	Most important pathway for voluntary motor function
	②	Lateral corticospinal tract	Originates in the motor cortex. *Corticonuclear* fibers to motor nuclei of cranial nerves. *Corticospinal* fibers to motor cells in anterior horn of the spinal cord. *Corticoreticular* fibers to nuclei of the reticular formation
Descending tracts from the brainstem (Extrapyramidal motor system)	③	Rubrospinal tract	Pathway for automatic and learned motor processes (e.g., walking, running, cycling)
	④	Reticulospinal tract	
	⑤	Vestibulospinal tract	
	⑥	Tectospinal tract	
	⑦	Olivospinal tract	

693

50 Autonomic Nervous System

Autonomic Nervous System (I): Overview

Fig. 50.1 Autonomic nervous system

The autonomic nervous system is the part of the peripheral nervous system that innervates smooth muscle, cardiac muscle, and glands. It is subdivided into the sympathetic (red) and the parasympathetic (blue) nervous systems, which often act in antagonistic fashion to regulate blood flow, secretions, and organ function. Both the sympathetic and parasympathetic nervous systems have a two-neuron pathway, which is under central nervous system control via an upper motor neuron with its cell body in the hypothalamus. In the sympathetic system, the preganglionic neuron synapses within the ganglia of the sympathetic trunk (paired, one on each side of vertebral column) or on one of the unpaired prevertebral ganglia located at the base of the artery for which the ganglion was named (celiac, superior and inferior mesenteric). Sympathetic postganglionic neurons then either reenter spinal nerves via gray rami communicans and are distributed to their target structure or they reach their target structure by travelling with arteries.

Except in the head, parasympathetic preganglionic neurons synapse in ganglia in the wall of the target organ. Short postganglioinc parasympathetic neurons then innervate the organ. In the head there are four parasympathetic ganglia: ciliary, pterygopalatine, submandibular, and otic, which are associated with cranial nerves III, VII, and IX, respectively. These four ganglia are responsible for distributing fibers to smooth muscle within the eye and to the salivary glands and glands of the nasal cavity, paranasal sinuses, hard and soft palate, and pharynx. Both sympathetic and parasympathetic preganglionic neurons secrete acetylcholine, which acts upon nicotinic receptors in the ganglia. Sympathetic postganglionic neurons secrete norepinephrine, which acts upon adrenoceptors (α or β) in target tissues. Parasympathetic postganglionic neurons secrete acetylcholine, which acts upon muscarinic receptors in target tissues.

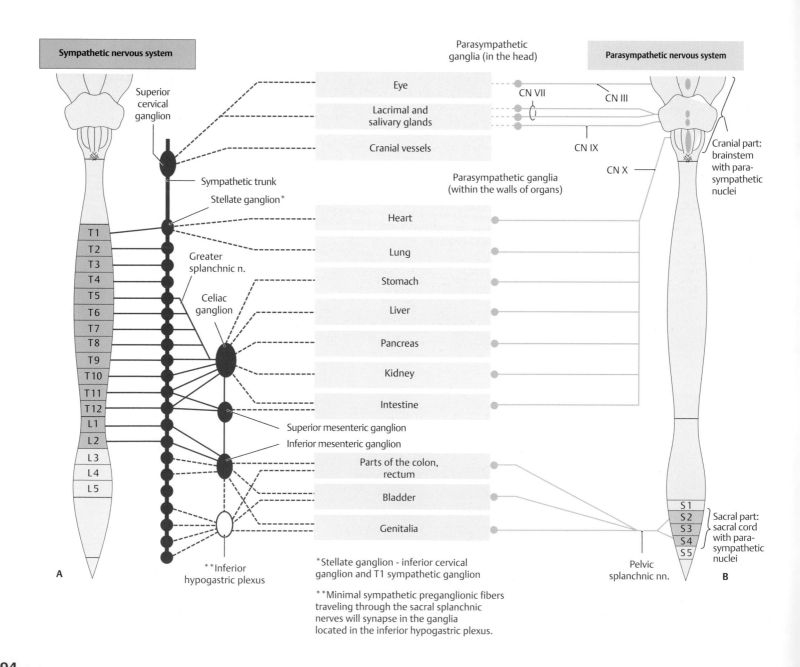

*Stellate ganglion - inferior cervical ganglion and T1 sympathetic ganglion

**Minimal sympathetic preganglionic fibers traveling through the sacral splanchnic nerves will synapse in the ganglia located in the inferior hypogastric plexus.

Table 50.1 Parasympathetic pathways

Neuron	Location of cell body	
Upper motor neuron	**Hypothalamus:** The cell bodies of parasympathetic upper motor neurons are located in the hypothalamus. Their axons descend via white matter tracts to synapse with the lower motor neuron in the brainstem and sacral spinal cord (S2–S4).	
Preganglionic neuron (lower motor neuron)	The parasympathetic nervous system is divided into two parts (cranial and sacral), based on the location of the preganglionic parasympathetic neurons.	
	Brainstem cranial nerve nuclei: The axons of these secondary neurons leave the CNS as the motor root of cranial nn. III, VII, IX, and X.	**Spinal cord (S2–S4):** The axons of the sacral parasympathetics originate from the S2–S4 spinal segments in a region of the spinal cord gray matter similar to that of the lateral horns where the sympathetic division arises from. These axons initially travel through the S2–S4 anterior roots before con-tinuing within the S2–S4 anterior rami. The axons then pass through pelvic splanchnic nerves that arise from the S2–S4 anterior rami before reaching the inferior hypogastric plexus, which then distributes the axons to the pelvic and hindgut structures.
Postganglionic neuron	**Cranial nerve parasympathetic ganglia:** The parasympathetic cranial nn. of the head each have at least one ganglion: • CN III: Ciliary ganglion • CN VII: Pterygopalatine ganglion and submandibular ganglion • CN IX: Otic ganglion • CN X: Small unnamed (intramural) ganglia close to target structures	
Distribution of postganglionic fibers	Parasympathetic fibers course with other fiber types to their targets. In the head, the postganglionic fibers from the pterygopalatine ganglion (CN VII) and otic ganglion (CN IX) are distributed via branches of the trigeminal n. (CN V). Postganglionic fibers from the ciliary ganglion (CN III) course with sympathetic and sensory fibers in the short ciliary nn. (preganglionic fibers travel with the somatomotor fibers of CN III). In the thorax, abdomen, and pelvis, preganglionic parasympathetic fibers from CN X and the pelvic splanchnic nn. combine with postganglionic sympathetic fibers to form plexuses (e.g., cardiac, pulmonary, esophageal).	

Table 50.2 Sympathetic pathways

Neuron	Location of cell body	
Upper motor neuron	**Hypothalamus:** The cell bodies of sympathetic upper motor neurons are located in the hypothalamus. Their axons descend via white matter tracts to synapse with the lower motor neuron in the lateral horn of the spinal cord (T1–L2).	
Preganglionic neuron (lower motor neuron)	**Intermediolateral gray horn of spinal cord (T1–L2):** The lateral horn is the middle portion of the gray matter of the spinal cord, situated between the anterior and posterior horns. It contains exclusively autonomic (sympathetic) neurons. The axons of these neurons leave the CNS as the motor root of the spinal nn. and enter the paravertebral ganglia via the white rami communicans (myelinated).	
Preganglionic neurons in paravertebral ganglia	All preganglionic sympathetic neurons enter the sympathetic chain. There they may synapse in a chain ganglion or ascend or descend to synapse. Preganglionic sympathetic neurons synapse in one of two places, yielding two types of sympathetic ganglia.	
	Synapse in the paravertebral ganglia	Pass without synapsing through the sympathetic ganglia. These fibers travel in the thoracic, lumbar, and sacral splanchnic nn. to synapse in the prevertebral ganglia.
Postganglionic neuron	**Paravertebral ganglia:** These ganglia form the sympathetic nerve trunks that flank the spinal cord. Postganglionic axons leave the sympathetic trunk via the gray rami communicans (unmyelinated).	**Prevertebral ganglia:** Associated with peripheral plexuses, which spread along the abdominal aorta. There are three primary prevertebral ganglia: • Celiac ganglion • Superior mesenteric ganglion • Inferior mesenteric ganglion
Distribution of postganglionic fibers	Postganglionic fibers are distributed in two ways: 1. Spinal nerves: Postganglionic neurons may re-enter the spinal nn. via the gray rami communicans. These sympathetic neurons induce constriction of blood vessels of the skin and dilate the blood vessels of skeletal muscles, sweat glands, and arrector pili (muscle fibers attached to hair follicles, "goose bumps"). 2. Arteries and ducts: Nerve plexuses may form along existing structures. Postganglionic sympathetic fibers may travel with arteries to target structures. Viscera are innervated by this method (e.g., sympathetic innervation concerning vasoconstriction, bronchial dilatation, glandular secretions, pupillary dilatation, smooth muscle contraction).	

Autonomic Nervous System (II)

Fig. 50.2 Typical spinal nerve

All spinal nerves arising from the spinal cord contain somatic sensory (or afferent, from body wall) and somatic motor (or efferent, to body wall) fibers. Sensory fibers come from the posterior (back) region via the posterior ramus and anterolateral regions of the body wall via the anterior ramus of the spinal nerve. The somatic sensory fibers approach the spinal cord via the posterior root. The cell bodies for these fibers lie in the sensory (spinal/dorsal root) ganglion. They synapse with sensory neurons in the posterior horn of gray matter within the spinal cord sending the majority to the brain for interpretation. Somatic motor fibers have their neurons in the anterior horn of gray matter and send their fibers to the spinal n. via the anterior root. This pattern of somatic innervation occurs in all spinal nerves from C1 through S5, whether they are involved in a plexus or not.

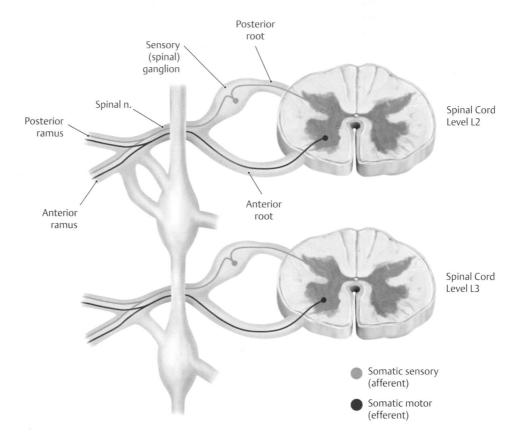

Fig. 50.3 ANS Circuitry

Body wall dermatomes also require sympathetic fibers to contract smooth muscle and cause glands in the dermatome to secrete. Preganglionic sympathetic fibers (purple) arise from cell bodies in the intermediolateral gray horn of the spinal cord. They exit the spinal cord via the outgoing/efferent (anterior) root—along with the somatic motor (efferent) fibers—and enter the spinal nerve. The smooth muscle of the body wall requires innervation by postganglionic sympathetic fibers so the preganglionic fiber looks for the closest synapse site—the paravertebral sympathetic ganglia—found in a chain-like arrangement on either side of the vertebral column. Each ganglion is connected to the spinal n. by communicating branches—the rami communicans. The white ramus communicans is found most lateral and conveys the preganglionic (myelinated = white) sympathetic fiber to the ganglion. Once in the paravertebral ganglion one of two things can happen:

a) The preganglionic sympathetic fiber can synapse in the ganglion and the postganglionic sympathetic fiber (orange) passes along the gray ramus communicans (unmyelinated) back to the spinal n. Now postganglionic sympathetic fibers can be distributed to structures in the dermatome via the anterior and posterior rami—along with somatic motor and sensory fibers.

b) The preganglionic fiber can run up or down the sympathetic trunk to synapse in an upper or lower paravertebral ganglion. This is especially important as the source of sympathetic innervation is limited to spinal cord levels T1 to L2. This figure depicts sympathetic innervation from the last spinal cord segment to contain it (L2) descending along the sympathetic trunk to the paravertebral ganglion at L3. It synapses here and the postganglionic sympathetic fiber exits into the spinal nerve of L3. Note that there is only a gray ramus communicans at this level as white rami communicans are input fibers (T1–L2), while the gray are output fibers above and below T1 and L2. Therefore, there are more gray rami than white rami. Both anterior and posterior rami now contain postganglionic sympathetic fibers distributed to the dermatome of L3 along with the typical somatic sensory and motor fibers of each vertebral level.

Now that the body wall has been supplied with postganglionic sympathetic innervation, we'll turn our attention to the viscera. In the third option for preganglionic sympathetic fibers entering a prevertebral ganglion, the fibers pass through the paravertebral ganglion at that level without synapsing and pass into a splanchnic n. to synapse in one of 3 primary prevertebral (or collateral) ganglia found in the abdomen along the anterior surface of the aorta at the base of one of the three main visceral branches (celiac a., superior mesenteric a., and inferior mesenteric a.). The postganglionic sympathetic fibers (orange) are distributed by following arterial branches to the viscera where they decrease the activity of the glands and peristalsis, constrict sphincters, and vasoconstrict the blood vessels.

The body wall does not receive any parasympathetic innervation. Dilation of the blood vessel walls occurs as the postganglionic sympathetics stop firing to cause vasoconstriction. However, the intricate control of movement of the wall of the intestine, or secretion of the glands within its wall, does require the antagonistic input of the parasympathetic division. Parasympathetic innervation to the viscera of the thorax and much of the abdomen (to the mid transverse colon) is supplied by the vagus n. (dark blue). The vagus n. sends branches to the various sympathetic prevertebral ganglia of the abdomen but they do not synapse there. They pass through, following the branches of the blood vessel to the wall of the organs supplied. There they synapse in

tiny parasympathetic (intramural) ganglion within the wall of the organ. The postganglionic parasympathetic fibers (light blue) are therefore extremely short. The remainder of the abdominal and pelvic viscera receive their parasympathetic supply in a similar fashion but from preganglionic parasympathetic fibers from spinal cord levels S2-4. Viscera also exhibit pain, relayed back to the CNS as visceral afferents (dark green). Note that the visceral afferent fibers follow the pathway of the sympathetic pre- and postganglionic fibers back from the viscera. They pass through the prevertebral ganglion (without synapsing), and then back along the splanchnic n. and through the paravertebral ganglion (again, without synapsing). From there they travel along the white ramus communicans (as visceral afferent fibers, they are also myelinated) and follow the posterior root back to the sensory ganglion where the cell body is found interspersed amongst those for the body wall. They finally synapse in the posterior horn of gray matter in the spinal cord amongst the somatic afferents also synapsing there. This is the basis for referred pain as the brain finds it difficult to distinguish visceral pain from somatic pain as the latter outnumber the former very significantly. Therefore, pain from internal organs is often referred to sites on the body wall.

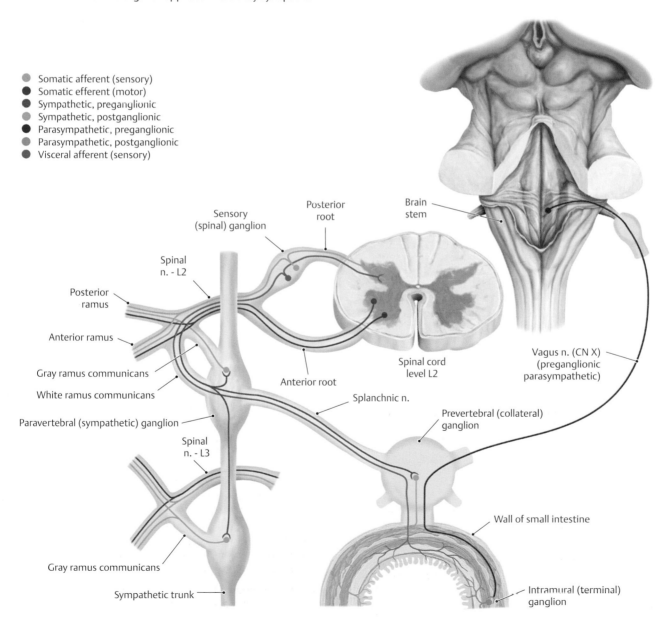

- ● Somatic afferent (sensory)
- ● Somatic efferent (motor)
- ● Sympathetic, preganglionic
- ● Sympathetic, postganglionic
- ● Parasympathetic, preganglionic
- ● Parasympathetic, postganglionic
- ● Visceral afferent (sensory)

Sensory (spinal) ganglion

Posterior root

Brain stem

Spinal n. - L2

Posterior ramus

Anterior ramus

Gray ramus communicans

White ramus communicans

Paravertebral (sympathetic) ganglion

Spinal n. - L3

Anterior root

Spinal cord level L2

Splanchnic n.

Vagus n. (CN X) (preganglionic parasympathetic)

Prevertebral (collateral) ganglion

Wall of small intestine

Gray ramus communicans

Sympathetic trunk

Intramural (terminal) ganglion

51 Sectional & Radiographic Anatomy

Sectional Anatomy of the Nervous System

Fig. 51.1 Sagittal section through the midline of the brain

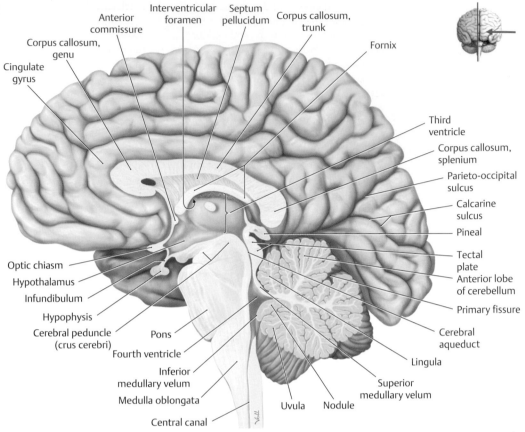

Labels (clockwise):
Corpus callosum, genu
Cingulate gyrus
Anterior commissure
Interventricular foramen
Septum pellucidum
Corpus callosum, trunk
Fornix
Third ventricle
Corpus callosum, splenium
Parieto-occipital sulcus
Calcarine sulcus
Pineal
Tectal plate
Anterior lobe of cerebellum
Primary fissure
Cerebral aqueduct
Lingula
Superior medullary velum
Nodule
Uvula
Central canal
Medulla oblongata
Inferior medullary velum
Fourth ventricle
Pons
Cerebral peduncle (crus cerebri)
Hypophysis
Infundibulum
Hypothalamus
Optic chiasm

Fig. 51.2 Frontal section through the brain I

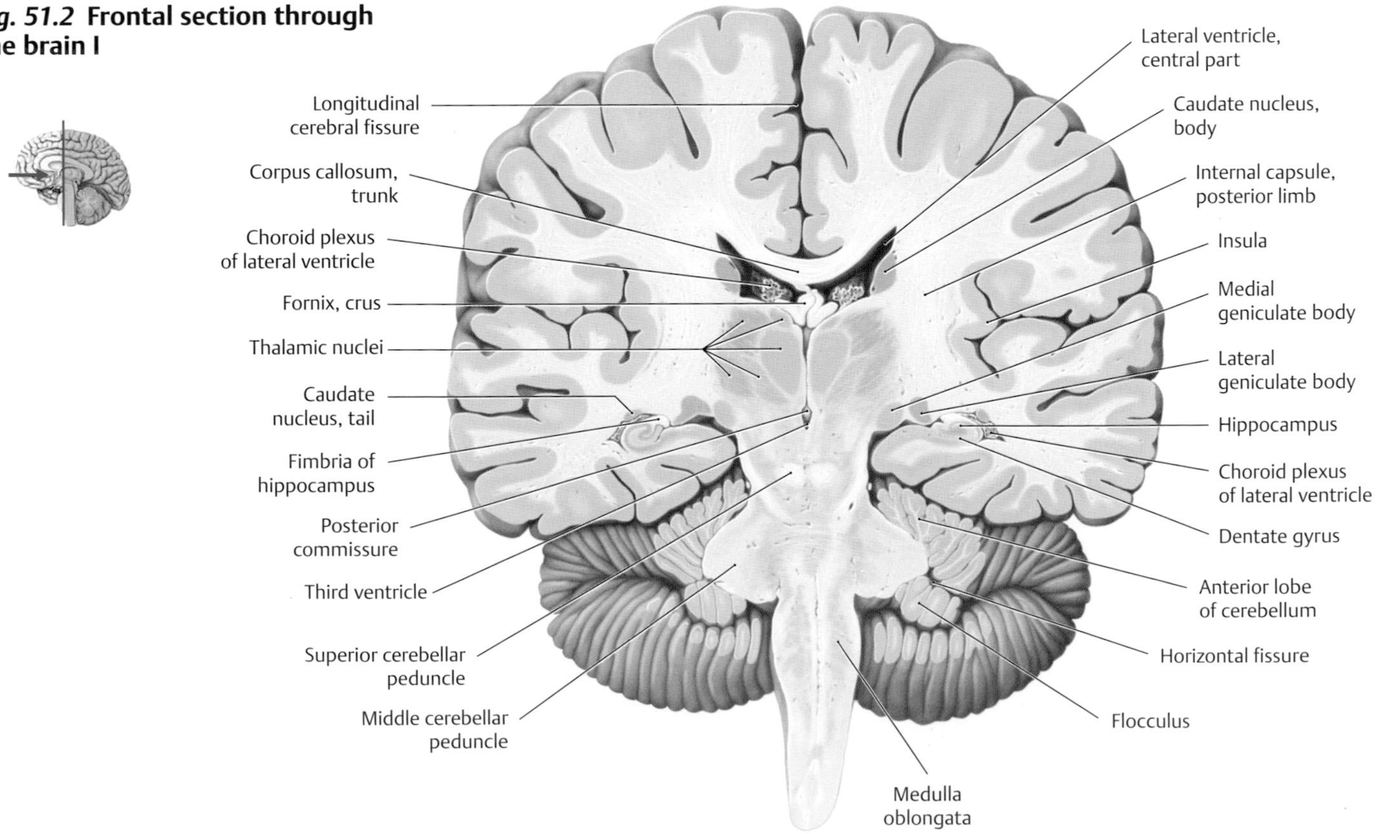

Labels:
Longitudinal cerebral fissure
Corpus callosum, trunk
Choroid plexus of lateral ventricle
Fornix, crus
Thalamic nuclei
Caudate nucleus, tail
Fimbria of hippocampus
Posterior commissure
Third ventricle
Superior cerebellar peduncle
Middle cerebellar peduncle
Medulla oblongata
Lateral ventricle, central part
Caudate nucleus, body
Internal capsule, posterior limb
Insula
Medial geniculate body
Lateral geniculate body
Hippocampus
Choroid plexus of lateral ventricle
Dentate gyrus
Anterior lobe of cerebellum
Horizontal fissure
Flocculus

Fig. 51.3 Frontal section through the brain II

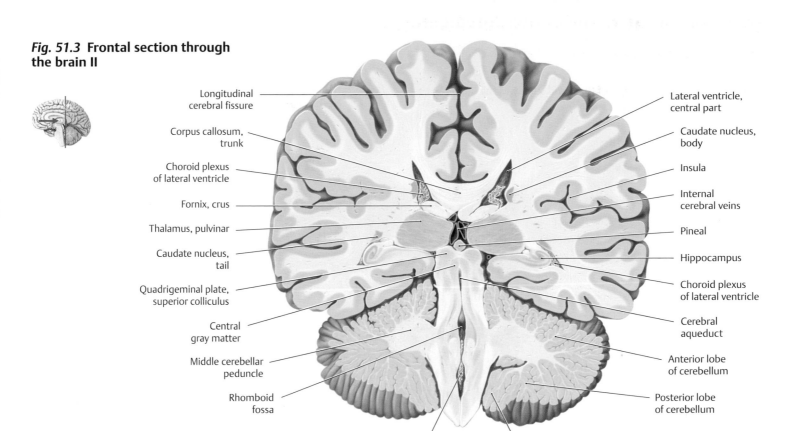

Longitudinal cerebral fissure

Corpus callosum, trunk

Choroid plexus of lateral ventricle

Fornix, crus

Thalamus, pulvinar

Caudate nucleus, tail

Quadrigeminal plate, superior colliculus

Central gray matter

Middle cerebellar peduncle

Rhomboid fossa

Choroid plexus of fourth ventricle

Cerebellar tonsil

Lateral ventricle, central part

Caudate nucleus, body

Insula

Internal cerebral veins

Pineal

Hippocampus

Choroid plexus of lateral ventricle

Cerebral aqueduct

Anterior lobe of cerebellum

Posterior lobe of cerebellum

Fig. 51.4 Transverse section of the brain through the upper region of the brainstem

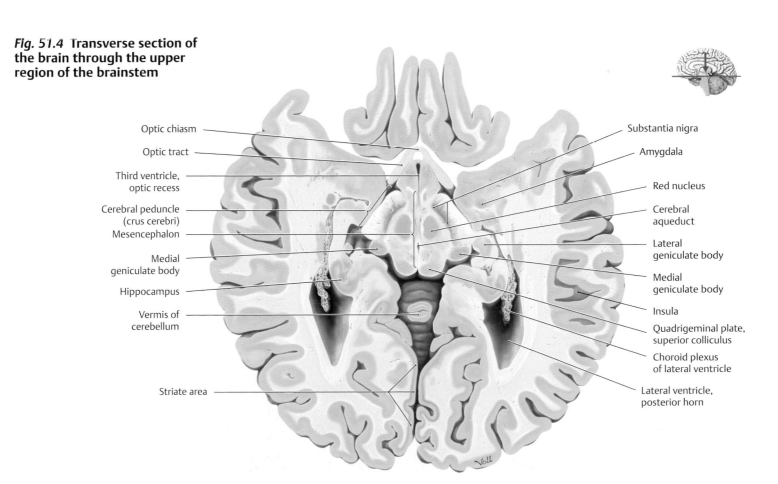

Optic chiasm

Optic tract

Third ventricle, optic recess

Cerebral peduncle (crus cerebri)

Mesencephalon

Medial geniculate body

Hippocampus

Vermis of cerebellum

Striate area

Substantia nigra

Amygdala

Red nucleus

Cerebral aqueduct

Lateral geniculate body

Medial geniculate body

Insula

Quadrigeminal plate, superior colliculus

Choroid plexus of lateral ventricle

Lateral ventricle, posterior horn

Radiographic Anatomy of the Nervous System

Additional radiological images of the blood supply to the brain can be
found on **p. 671.**

Fig. 51.5 **MRI of the brain**
Midsagittal section, left lateral view.
(Reproduced from Moeller TB, Reif E.
Pocket Atlas of Sectional Anatomy,
Vol 1, 4th ed. New York, NY: Thieme;
2014.)

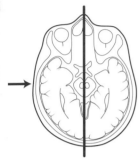

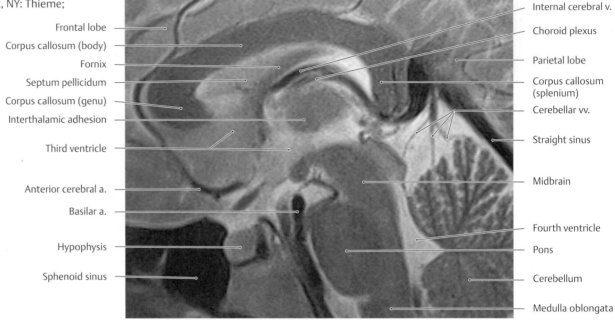

Frontal lobe

Corpus callosum (body)

Fornix

Septum pellicidum

Corpus callosum (genu)

Interthalamic adhesion

Third ventricle

Anterior cerebral a.

Basilar a.

Hypophysis

Sphenoid sinus

Internal cerebral v.

Choroid plexus

Parietal lobe

Corpus callosum
(splenium)

Cerebellar vv.

Straight sinus

Midbrain

Fourth ventricle

Pons

Cerebellum

Medulla oblongata

Fig. 51.6 **MRI of the brain**
Transverse (axial) section through the
cerebral hemispheres, inferior view.
(Reproduced from Moeller TB, Reif E.
Pocket Atlas of Sectional Anatomy,
Vol 1, 4th ed. New York, NY:
Thieme; 2014.)

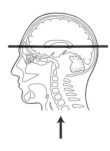

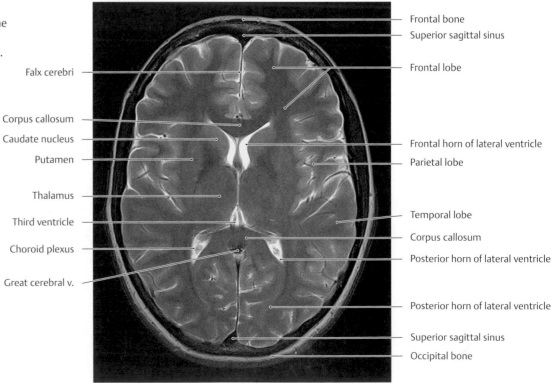

Falx cerebri

Corpus callosum

Caudate nucleus

Putamen

Thalamus

Third ventricle

Choroid plexus

Great cerebral v.

Frontal bone

Superior sagittal sinus

Frontal lobe

Frontal horn of lateral ventricle

Parietal lobe

Temporal lobe

Corpus callosum

Posterior horn of lateral ventricle

Posterior horn of lateral ventricle

Superior sagittal sinus

Occipital bone

Fig. 51.7 MRI of the brain

Coronal section through the ventricular system. (Reproduced from Moeller TB, Reif E. Pocket Atlas of Sectional Anatomy, Vol 1, 4th ed. New York, NY: Thieme; 2014.)

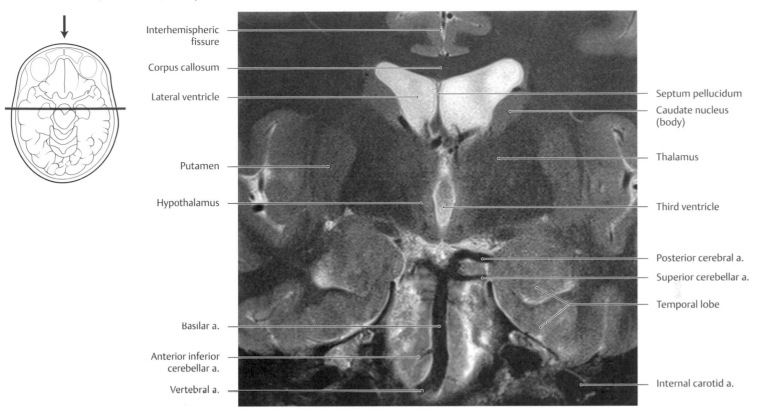

Interhemispheric fissure

Corpus callosum

Lateral ventricle

Putamen

Hypothalamus

Basilar a.

Anterior inferior cerebellar a.

Vertebral a.

Septum pellucidum

Caudate nucleus (body)

Thalamus

Third ventricle

Posterior cerebral a.

Superior cerebellar a.

Temporal lobe

Internal carotid a.

Fig. 51.8 MRI of the neck

Coronal section through the cervical spinal cord, anterior view. (Reproduced from Moeller TB, Reif E. Pocket Atlas of Sectional Anatomy, Vol 1, 4th ed. New York, NY: Thieme; 2014.)

Atlas (C1)

Parotid gland

Internal jugular v.

Spinal n. roots C4, C5, C6

Middle scalene

Spinal n. root C8

Temporal lobe

Medulla oblongata

Dens of C2

Vertebral a.

Intervertebral foramen

Sternocleidomastoid

Spinal cord

Index

cancer of, 77
lymph nodes and lymphatics of, 76, 76t
mammography of, 77
nerves of, 74
structures of, 75
Breast cancer, lymph nodes in, 367
Bronchiole, 121, 126
terminal, 121
Bronchus/bronchi. *See also* Tree, bronchial
foreign body in, *120*
lobar
bronchogram of, *133*
computed tomography (CT) of, 136
inferior, 89, 90, 106, 116, 117, 120, 126,
127, 136
left, 120
right, 120
middle, 90, 117, 120, 127
superior, 90, 117, 120, 127
main, 111
bronchogram of, 133
left, 80, 81, 91, 92, 108, 109, 111, 113,
120, 124, 126, 127, 129, 131, 132
computed tomography (CT) of, 79, 136
MRI of, 133
origin of, 88
right, 79, 80, 89, 108, 111, 113, 120, 124,
125, 129, 133
computed tomography (CT) of, 79, 136
MRI of, 133
segmental subsegmental, 118, 118t
Bulb
carotid, calcified plaque in, *583*
duodenal, 168
olfactory, 549, 562, 620, 621, 659, 677
penile, 245, 255, 264
MRI of, 290
veins of, 269
vestibular, 246, 254, 262, 263, 275, 285
artery of, 261, 275, 285
venous plexus of, 275
Bulbourethral glands, 266, 267, 284
Bulla, ethmoid, 550, 617, 618, 621
Bundle
accessory muscle, 653
anteromedial, 475
atrioventricular (of His), 98, 102
interatrial, 102
intermodal, 102
anterior, 102
middle, 102
posterior, 102
neurovascular
intercostal, 71
of the rectum, 259
posterolateral, 475
Bundle branches, 102

Bursa(e)
acromial, subcutaneous, 307
of calcaneal tendon, 457
gastrocnemius-semimembranous (Baker's
cyst), *437*
iliopectineal, 413, 489
infrapatellar, 442, 443
olecranon, 327
omental, 156, 157, 158, 159, 160, 166, 180,
181, 220
boundaries and walls of, 162–163, 163t
location of, 163
recess of
inferior, 163
splenic, 163, 174
superior, 163
vestibule of, 162, 163, 173
periarticular, 437
prepatellar, 435, 443
semimembranosus, 437, 495
subacromial, 306–307
MRI of, 401
subcoracoid, 304
subcutaneous, 495
subdeltoid, 306, 307, 383
subtendinous
of gastrocnemius, 495
lateral, 437
medial, 437
of subscapularis, 304, 306, 307, 383
trochanteric, 413, 415, 491, 493
Buttocks, regions of, 3

C

Caesarean section, *232*
Calcaneus, 410, 445, 446, 448, 450, 452, 454,
455, 456, 458, 459, 460, 461, 462, 468, 471
MRI of, 509
Calvaria, 545, *587*
diploë, 545
inner table of, 545
muscles of, 556t
outer table of, 545
structure of, 545
Calyx
major, 184, 189
computed tomography (CT) of, 224
minor, 184, 189
Canaliculus
lacrimal
inferior, 611
superior, 611
tympanic, 573, 629
Canal(s)
adductor, 472, 473, 474, 492
anal, 248–249, 287
MRI of, 290

muscularis mucosae of, 274
regions of, 249t
auditory
external, 5, 411, 626, 627, 629
curvature of, *626*
parts of, 626
carotid, 546, 548, 624
opening of, 643
central, 685, 698
cervical, 257
cervical axis in, 256
MRI of, 288, 289
cochlear, 634
condylar, 546, 548
Dorello's, 593
facial, 547, 568, 571, 629
for greater petrosal nerve, 568
hypoglossal, 21, 546, 547, 548, 577
incisive, 548, 616
infraorbital, 602, 602t, 603
MRI of, 669
inguinal, 150, 151, 151t, 255, 489t
gender differences in, *150*
opening of, 151
structures of, 151, 151t
malleolar, 485
mandibular, 567, 598, 644, 656, 657
radiograph of, 668
nasolacrimal, 602t
obturator, 237, 238, 258, 268t
optic, 547, 548, 551, 563, 602, 603, 604, 608,
636, 662
osseofibrous, 25
palatine, 622, 636
palatovaginal (pharyngeal), 546, 622
pelvic, female
narrowest diameter of, 235
true conjugate of, 235
pterygoid, 551, 569, 579, 622
artery of, 601
fossa of, 546
nerve of, 579, 621, 623
pudendal (Alcock's), 268t, 491
pyloric, 166, 167
sacral, 7, 7t, 12, 13, 45, 232, 233, 237
MRI of, 51
of Schlemm, 612, 613, 614
semicircular, 570, 634
anterior, 571, 625, 626, 628, 629, 633, 634
lateral, 571, *625*, 626, 628, 629, 634
prominence of, 629
posterior, 571, *625*, 626, 628, 629, 634
of spinal cord, central, 684
supraorbital, 602, 602t
vertebral, 5, 14, 22, 23, 40
cauda equina in, 41
computed tomography (CT) of, 223

Index